D1637448

Benders' dictionary of nutrition and food technology

Related titles:

Food dehydration: A dictionary and guide
(ISBN-13: 978-1-85573-360-2; ISBN-10: 1-85573-360-9)
This authoritative guide examines the background and principles of food dehydration as well as providing a complete dictionary of food dehydration terms, with detailed definitions and a directory of dehydrated foods. It is an ideal reference work for students of food science as well as a quick and easy source of information for food science professionals.

Food, diet and obesity
(ISBN-13: 978-1-85573-958-1; ISBN-10: 1-85573-958-5)
Obesity is a global epidemic, with large numbers of adults and children overweight or obese in many developed and developing countries. As a result, there is an unprecedented level of interest and research in the complex interactions between our genetic susceptibility, diet and lifestyle in determining individual risk of obesity. With its distinguished editor and international team of contributors, this collection sums up the key themes in weight control research, focusing on their implications and applications for food product development and consumers.

Improving the fat content of foods
(ISBN-13: 978-1-85573-965-9; ISBN-10: 1-85573-965-8)
Dietary fats have long been recognised as having a major impact on health, negative in the case of consumers' excessive intake of saturated fatty acids, positive in the case of increasing consumers' intake of long chain n-3 polyunsaturated fatty acids (PUFAs). However, progress in ensuring that consumers achieve a nutritionally optimal fat intake has been slow. This important collection reviews the range of steps needed to improve the fat content of foods whilst maintaining sensory quality.

Details of these books and a complete list of Woodhead's titles can be obtained by:

- visiting our web site at www.woodheadpublishing.com
- contacting Customer Services (e-mail: sales@woodhead-publishing.com; fax: +44 (0) 1223 893694; tel.: +44 (0) 1223 891358 ext. 30; address: Woodhead Publishing Ltd, Abington Hall, Abington, Cambridge CB1 6AH, England)

Benders' dictionary of nutrition and food technology

Eighth edition

David A. Bender
BSc, PhD, RNutr

Senior Lecturer in Biochemistry,
University College London

CRC Press
Boca Raton Boston New York Washington, DC

WOODHEAD PUBLISHING LIMITED

Cambridge, England

Published by Woodhead Publishing Limited, Abington Hall, Abington
Cambridge CB1 6AH, England
www.woodheadpublishing.com

Published in North America by CRC Press LLC, 6000 Broken Sound Parkway, NW
Suite 300, Boca Raton, FL 33487, USA

First published 1960
Second edition 1965
Third edition 1968
Fourth edition Newnes-Butterworth 1975
Fifth edition Butterworth Scientific 1982
Reprinted 1984
Sixth edition 1990
Reprinted 1998 Woodhead Publishing Limited
Seventh edition 1999, Woodhead Publishing Limited and CRC Press LLC
Eighth edition 2006, Woodhead Publishing Limited and CRC Press LLC

British Library Cataloguing in Publication Data
A catalogue record for this book is available from the British Library.

Library of Congress Cataloging in Publication Data
A catalog record for this book is available from the Library of Congress.

Woodhead Publishing ISBN-13: 978-1-84569-051-9 (book)
Woodhead Publishing ISBN-10: 1-84569-051-6 (book)
Woodhead Publishing ISBN-13: 978-1-84569-165-3 (e-book)
Woodhead Publishing ISBN-10: 1-84569-165-2 (e-book)
CRC Press ISBN-10: 0-8493-7601-7
CRC Press order number: WP7601

The publishers' policy is to use permanent paper from mills that operate a
sustainable forestry policy, and which has been manufactured from pulp which is
processed using acid-free and elementary chlorine-free practices. Furthermore,
the publishers ensure that the text paper and cover board used have met
acceptable environmental accreditation standards.

Typeset by SNP Best-set Typesetter Ltd., Hong Kong.
Printed by TJ International Ltd, Padstow, Cornwall, England.

Contents

Preface

The study of food and nutrition covers a wide range of disciplines, from agriculture and horticulture, through the chemistry, physics and technology of food processing and manufacture (including domestic food preparation), the physiology and biochemistry of nutrition and metabolism, molecular biology, genetics and biotechnology, via social sciences and the law, anthropology and epidemiology to clinical medicine, disease prevention and health promotion. This means that anyone interested in food and nutrition will be reading articles written from a variety of disciplines and hearing lectures by specialists in a variety of fields. We will all come across unfamiliar terms, or terms that are familiar but used in a new context as the jargon of a different discipline.

At the same time, new terms are introduced as our knowledge increases, and as new techniques are introduced, old terms become obsolete, dropping out of current textbooks, so that the reader of earlier literature may be at a loss.

All of this provides the *raison d'être* of this Dictionary, the first edition of which was published in 1960, with definitions of 2000 terms. Over the years it has grown so that in this edition it includes more than 6100 entries.

At the front of the first and following editions, there was the following note:

> *Should this book become sufficiently familiar through usage to earn the title 'Bender's Dictionary', it would probably be more correct to call it 'Benders' Dictionary', in view of the valuable assistance of D., D.A. and B.G., guided, if not driven, by A.E.*

The publisher suggested that the seventh edition should indeed be called 'Bender's Dictionary of Nutrition and Food Technology'. I was proud that my father invited me to join him as a full co-author, so that it could be called Benders' Dictionary. Sadly he died in February 1999, before the typescript of that edition was completed. I hope that in this eighth edition I have done justice to his memory and to the book that was the first of many that he wrote. For the first edition my main task was to read widely, and make a note of terms I did not know. This is still my role, but now I have to find the definitions as well.

David A. Bender

A note on food composition

This book contains nutrient composition data for 340 foods, from the US Department of Agriculture National Nutrient Database for Standard Reference, Release 17, which is freely available from the USDA Nutrient Data Laboratory website: http://www.nal.usda.gov/fnic/foodcomp/.

In addition to the nutrient content per 100 g, we have calculated nutrient yields per serving, and shown the information as a note that a specified serving is a source, good source or rich source of various nutrients. A rich source means that the serving provides more than 30%, a good source 20–30%, and a source 10–20% of the recommended daily amount of that nutrient (based on the EU nutrition labelling figures shown in Table 2 of the Appendix).

Any specified food will differ in composition from one variety to another, and from sample to sample of the same variety, depending on the conditions under which the animal was raised or the plant grown, so that the values quoted here should not be considered to be accurate to better than about ±10%, at best; the variation in micronutrient content may be even greater.

List of figures

A

abalone A SHELLFISH (mollusc), *Haliotus splendens, H. rufescens, H. cracherodii*, also sometimes called ormer, or sea ear. Found especially in waters around Australia, and also California and Japan, the Channel Islands and France.

Composition/100 g: water 75 g, 440 kJ (105 kcal), protein 17 g, fat 0.8 g, cholesterol 85 mg, carbohydrate 6 g, ash 1.6 g, Ca 31 mg, Fe 3.2 mg, Mg 48 mg, P 190 mg, K 250 mg, Na 301 mg, Zn 0.8 mg, Cu 0.2 mg, Se 45 µg, vitamin A 2 µg retinol, E 4 mg, K 23 mg, B_1 0.19 mg, B_2 0.1 mg, niacin 1.5 mg, B_6 0.15 mg, folate 5 µg, B_{12} 0.7 µg, pantothenate 3 mg, C 2 mg. An 85 g serving is a source of Cu, Fe, Mg, vitamin B_1, a good source of P, a rich source of Se, vitamin E, B_{12}, pantothenate.

abscisic acid Plant hormone with growth inhibitory action; the dormancy-inducing hormone, responsible for shedding of leaves by deciduous trees. In herbaceous plants can lead to dwarf or compact plants with normal or enhanced fruit production. Used horticulturally to inhibit growth, and as a defoliant.

absinthe A herb LIQUEUR flavoured with wormwood (*Artemisia absinthium*); it is toxic and banned in many countries. Originally imported from Switzerland (where it was a patent medicine) to France in 1797 by Henri Louis Pernod; sale outlawed in USA in 1912, and in France and other countries in 1915 because of the toxicity of α-thujone. Now available in the EU with an upper limit of 10 ppm thujone.

absolute alcohol Pure ethyl ALCOHOL.

absorption spectrometry Analytical technique based on absorbance of light of a specific wavelength by a solute.

acarbose The name of a group of complex CARBOHYDRATES (oligosaccharides) which inhibit the enzymes of STARCH and DIS-ACCHARIDE digestion; used experimentally to reduce the digestion of starch and so slow the rate of absorption of carbohydrates. Has been marketed for use in association with weight-reducing diet regimes as a 'starch blocker', but there is no evidence of efficacy.

acaricides Pesticides used to kill mites and ticks (Acaridae) which cause animal diseases and the spoilage of flour and other foods in storage.

accelase   A mixture of enzymes that HYDROLYSE PROTEINS, including an EXOPEPTIDASE from the bacterium *Streptococcus lactis*, which is one of the starter organisms in dairy processing. The mixed enzymes are used to shorten the maturation time of cheeses and intensify the flavour of processed cheese.

accelerated freeze drying   *See* FREEZE DRYING.

Acceptable Daily Intake (ADI)   The amount of a food additive that could be taken daily for an entire lifespan without appreciable risk. Determined by measuring the highest dose of the substance that has no effect on experimental animals, then dividing by a safety factor of 100. Substances that are not given an ADI are regarded as having no adverse effect at any level of intake.

See also NO EFFECT LEVEL.

accoub   Edible thistle (*Goundelia tournefortii*) growing in Mediterranean countries and Middle East. The flower buds when cooked have a flavour resembling that of ASPARAGUS or globe ARTICHOKE; the shoots can be eaten in the same way as ASPARAGUS and the roots as SALSIFY.

accuracy   Of an assay; the closeness of the result to the 'true' result.

See also PRECISION.

ACE   Angiotensin converting enzyme (EC 3.4.15.1), a peptidase in the blood vessels of the lungs which converts angiotensin I to active angiotensin II. Many of the drugs for treatment of HYPERTENSION are ACE inhibitors.

acerola   *See* CHERRY, WEST INDIAN.

acesulphame (acesulfame)   Methyl-oxathiazinone dioxide, a nonnutritive or intense (artificial) SWEETENER. The potassium salt, acesulphame-K, is some 200 times as sweet as SUCROSE. It is not metabolised, and is excreted unchanged.

acetanisole   A synthetic flavouring agent (*p*-methoxyacetophenone) with a hawthorn-like odour.

acetic acid (ethanoic acid)   One of the simplest organic acids, CH_3COOH. It is the acid of VINEGAR and is formed, together with LACTIC ACID, in pickled (fermented) foods. It is added to foods and sauces as a preservative.

Acetobacter   Genus of bacteria (family Bacteriaceae) that oxidise ethyl alcohol to ACETIC ACID (secondary fermentation). *Acetobacter pasteurianus* (also known as *Mycoderma aceti*, *Bacterium aceti* or *B. pasteuranum*) is used in the manufacture of VINEGAR.

acetoglycerides   One or two of the long-chain fatty acids esterified to glycerol in a TRIACYLGLYCEROL is replaced by ACETIC ACID. There are three types: diacetomonoglycerides (e.g. diacetomonostearin); monoacetodiglycerides (e.g. monoacetodistearin); monoacetomonoglycerides (e.g. monoacetomono-stearin) in which one hydroxyl group of the glycerol is free. Also known as partial glyceride esters.

They are non-greasy and have lower melting points than the corresponding triacylglycerol. They are used in shortenings and spreads, as films for coating foods and as plasticisers for hard fats.

acetohexamide   Oral HYPOGLYCAEMIC AGENT used to treat non-insulin-dependent DIABETES mellitus.

acetoin   Acetyl methyl carbinol, a precursor of DIACETYL, which is one of the constituents of the flavour of butter. Acetoin and DIACETYL are produced by bacteria during the ripening of BUTTER.

acetomenaphthone   Synthetic compound with VITAMIN K activity; vitamin K_3, also known as menaquinone-0.

acetone   One of the KETONE BODIES formed in the body in FASTING. Also used as a solvent, e.g. in varnishes and lacquer. Chemically dimethyl ketone or propan-2-one $((CH_3)_2C{=}O)$.

acetylated monoglyceride   An EMULSIFIER manufactured by INTER-ESTERIFICATION of fats with glyceryl triacetate (triacetin) or acetylation of monoglycerides with acetic anhydride. Characterised by sharp melting points and stability to oxidative rancidity.

acetylcholine   The acetyl ester of CHOLINE, produced as a neuro-transmitter at cholinergic nerve endings in the brain and at neuromuscular junctions.

achalasia   Difficulty in swallowing owing to disturbance of the normal muscle activity of the OESOPHAGUS, sometimes causing regurgitation and severe chest pain. Also known as cardiospasm.

achene   Botanical term for small, dry one-seeded fruit which does not open to liberate the seed, e.g. nuts.

ACH index   Arm, chest, hip index. A method of assessing a person's nutritional status by measuring the arm circumference, chest diameter and hip width.

   See also ANTHROPOMETRY.

achlorhydria   Failure of secretion of gastric acid and INTRINSIC FACTOR, which are secreted by the gastric parietal (oxyntic) cells. Commonly associated with atrophy of the gastric mucosa with advancing age.

   See also ANAEMIA, PERNICIOUS; GASTRIC SECRETION.

acholia   Absence or deficiency of BILE secretion.

achote   *See* ANNATTO.

achrodextrin   DEXTRINS formed during enzymic hydrolysis of STARCH which give no colour (achromos) when tested with iodine.

achromotricia   Loss of the pigment of hair. One of the signs of PANTOTHENIC ACID deficiency in animals, but there is no evidence that pantothenic acid affects loss of hair colour in human beings.

achylia   Absence of a secretion; e.g. achylia gastrica is absence of gastric secretion.

acid–base balance   Body fluids are maintained just on the alkaline side of neutrality, pH 7.35–7.45, by buffers in the blood and tissues. Buffers include proteins, phosphates and carbon dioxide/bicarbonate, and are termed the alkaline reserve.

Acidic products of metabolism are excreted in the urine combined with bases such as sodium and potassium which are thus lost to the body. The acid–base balance is maintained by replacing them from the diet.

acid dip   Immersion of some fruits in an acid dip (commonly ascorbic and malic acids) prior to drying to improve the colour of the dried product by retarding enzymic browning.

acid drops   Boiled sweets with sharp flavour from tartaric acid (originally acidulated drops); known as sourballs in USA.

acid foods, basic foods   These terms refer to the residue of the METABOLISM of foods. The minerals SODIUM, POTASSIUM, MAGNESIUM and CALCIUM are base-forming, while PHOSPHORUS, SULPHUR and CHLORINE are acid-forming. Which of these predominates in foods determines whether the residue is acidic or basic (alkaline); meat, cheese, eggs and cereals leave an acidic residue, while milk, vegetables and some fruits leave a basic residue. Fats and sugars have no mineral content and so leave a neutral residue. Although fruits have an acid taste caused by organic acids and their salts, the acids are completely oxidised and the sodium and potassium salts yield an alkaline residue.

acidity regulators   *See* BUFFERS.

acid number, acid value   Of a fat, a measure of RANCIDITY due to hydrolysis (*see* HYDROLYSE), releasing free FATTY ACIDS from the TRIACYLGLYCEROL of the fat; serves as an index of the efficiency of refining since the fatty acids are removed during refining and increase with deterioration during storage. Defined as milligrams of potassium hydroxide required to neutralise the free fatty acids in 1 g of fat.

acidosis   An increase in the acidity of BLOOD PLASMA to below the normal range of pH 7.35–7.45, resulting from a loss of the buffering capacity of the plasma, alteration in the excretion of carbon dioxide, excessive loss of base from the body or metabolic overproduction of acids.

See also ACID–BASE BALANCE.

acids, fruit   Organic acids such as citric, malic, and tartaric, which give the sharp or sour flavour to fruits; often added to processed foods for taste.

acidulants   Various organic acids used in food manufacture as flavouring agents, preservatives, chelating agents, buffers, gelling and coagulating agents. CITRIC, FUMARIC, MALIC and TARTARIC ACIDS are general purpose acidulants, other acids have more specialist uses.

ackee (akee) Fruit of Caribbean tree *Blighia sapida*. Toxic when unripe because of the presence of hypoglycin (α-amino-β-methylene-cyclopropanyl-propionic acid), which can reduce blood sugar levels and cause 'vomiting sickness', coma and death.

Aclame^{TM} *See* ALITAME.

acorn Fruit of oak trees (*Quercus* spp.) used to make flour, as animal feed and historically a COFFEE substitute.

Composition/100 g: (edible portion 62%) water 28 g, 1620 kJ (387 kcal), protein 6.2 g, fat 23.9 g (of which 14% saturated, 66% mono-unsaturated, 20% polyunsaturated), carbohydrate 41 g, ash 1.4 g, Ca 41 mg, Fe 0.8 mg, Mg 62 mg, P 79 mg, K 539 mg, Zn 0.5 mg, Cu 0.6 mg, Mn 1.3 mg, vitamin A 2 µg RE, B$_1$ 0.11 mg, B$_2$ 0.12 mg, niacin 1.8 mg, B$_6$ 0.53 mg, folate 87 µg, pantothenate 0.7 mg.

acorn sugar Quercitol, pentahydroxycyclohexane, extracted from ACORNS.

ACP Acid calcium phosphate, *see* PHOSPHATE.

acraldehyde *See* ACROLEIN.

acrodermatitis enteropathica Severe functional ZINC deficiency, leading to dermatitis, due to failure to secrete an endogenous zinc binding ligand in pancreatic juice, and hence failure to absorb zinc. The zinc binding ligand has not been unequivocally identified, but may be the TRYPTOPHAN metabolite picolinic acid.

acrodynia Dermatitis seen in VITAMIN B$_6$ deficient animals; no evidence for a similar dermatitis in human deficiency.

acrolein (acraldehyde) An ALDEHYDE formed when GLYCEROL is heated to a high temperature. It is responsible for the acrid odour and lachrymatory (tear-causing) vapour produced when fats are overheated. Chemically $CH_2{=}CH{-}CHO$.

Acronize^{TM} The ANTIBIOTIC CHLORTETRACYCLINE; 'acronized' is used to describe products that have been treated with chlortetracycline, as, for example, 'acronized ice'.

ACTH *See* ADRENOCORTICOTROPHIC HORMONE.

Actilight^{TM} Short-chain fructose oligosaccharide used as a PREBIOTIC food additive.

Actimel^{TM} YOGURT fortified with PROBIOTICS to boost immunity.

actin One of the contractile PROTEINS of MUSCLE.

active oxygen method A method of measuring the stability of fats and oils to oxidative damage by bubbling air through the heated material and following the formation of peroxides. Also known as the Swift stability test.

actomyosin *See* MUSCLE.

acute phase proteins A variety of serum proteins synthesised in increased (or sometimes decreased) amounts in response to trauma and infection, so confounding their use as indices of nutritional status.

ADA American Dietetic Association, founded Cleveland, Ohio, 1917; web site http://webdietitians.org/Public/index.cfm/.

adai Indian; pancakes made from ground rice and legumes, the dough is left to undergo lactic acid bacterial fermentation before frying.

Adam's fig *See* PLANTAIN.

adaptogens Name coined for the active ingredients of GINSENG and other herbs that are reputed to be anti-stress compounds.

Addisonian pernicious anaemia *See* ANAEMIA, PERNICIOUS.

Addison's disease Degeneration or destruction of the cortex of the adrenal glands, leading to loss of GLUCOCORTICOID and MINERALOCORTICOID adrenal hormones, and resulting in low blood pressure, anaemia, muscular weakness, sodium loss and a low METABOLIC RATE. Treatment is by administration of synthetic adrenocortical hormones.

adenine A NUCLEOTIDE, one of the PURINE bases of the NUCLEIC ACIDS (DNA and RNA). The compound formed between adenine and RIBOSE is the nucleoside adenosine, which can form four phosphorylated derivatives important in metabolism: adenosine monophosphate (AMP, also known as adenylic acid); adenosine diphosphate (ADP); adenosine triphosphate (ATP) and cyclic adenosine monophosphate (cAMP).
See also ATP; ENERGY; METABOLISM.

adenosine *See* ADENINE.

adermin Obsolete name for VITAMIN B_6.

ADH Antidiuretic hormone, *see* VASOPRESSIN.

ADI *See* ACCEPTABLE DAILY INTAKE.

adiabatic A process that involves change in temperature without transfer of heat, as for example cooling by expanding the volume of a gas, or heating by compressing it; also known as constant entropy processes. No heat is added or removed from a system.
See also ISOBARIC; ISOTHERMAL.

adipectomy Surgical removal of subcutaneous fat.

adipocytes Cells of ADIPOSE TISSUE.

adipocytokines, adipokines CYTOKINES secreted by ADIPOSE TISSUE.

adiponectin HORMONE secreted by ADIPOCYTES that seems to be involved in energy homeostasis; it enhances INSULIN sensitivity and GLUCOSE tolerance, as well as oxidation of fatty acids in muscle. Its blood concentration is reduced in obese people and those with type II DIABETES mellitus.

adipose tissue   Body fat, the cells that synthesise and store FAT, releasing it for METABOLISM in FASTING. Also known as white adipose tissue, to distinguish it from the metabolically more active brown adipose tissue. Much of the body's fat reserve is subcutaneous; in addition there is adipose tissue around the organs, which serves to protect them from physical damage.

In lean people, between 20 and 25% of body weight is adipose tissue, increasing with age; the proportion is greater in people who are OVERWEIGHT or OBESE. Adipose tissue contains 82–88% fat, 2–2.6% protein and 10–14% water. The energy yield of adipose tissue is 34–38 MJ (8000–9000 kcal)/kg or 15.1–16.8 MJ (3600–4000 kcal)/lb.

adipose tissue, brown   Metabolically highly active adipose tissue, unlike white adipose tissue, which has a storage function; is involved in heat production to maintain body temperature as a result of partial uncoupling of electron transport (*see* ELECTRON TRANSPORT CHAIN) and OXIDATIVE PHOSPHORYLATION. Colour comes from its high content of MITOCHONDRIA.

See also UNCOUPLING PROTEINS.

adiposis   Presence of an abnormally large accumulation of fat in the body, also known as liposis. Adiposis dolorosa is painful fatty swellings associated with nervous system defects.

See also OBESITY.

adipsia   Absence of thirst.

adirondack bread   American baked product made from ground MAIZE, butter, wheat flour, eggs and sugar.

adlay   The seeds of a wild grass (Job's tears, *Coix lachryma-jobi*) botanically related to MAIZE, growing wild in parts of Africa and Asia and eaten especially in the SE Pacific region.

ADP   Adenosine diphosphate, *see* ADENINE; ATP.

adrenal glands   Also called the suprarenal glands, small ENDOCRINE GLANDS situated just above the kidneys. The inner medulla secretes the HORMONES ADRENALINE and NORADRENALINE, while the outer cortex secretes STEROID hormones known as corticosteroids, including CORTISOL and ALDOSTERONE.

adrenaline (epinephrine)   A hormone secreted by the medulla of the ADRENAL GLAND, especially in times of stress or in response to fright or shock. Its main actions are to increase blood pressure and to mobilise tissue reserves of GLUCOSE (leading to an increase in the blood glucose concentration) and fat, in preparation for flight or fighting.

adrenocorticotrophic hormone (ACTH)   A HORMONE secreted by the anterior part of the pituitary gland which stimulates the ADRENAL GLAND to secrete CORTICOSTEROIDS.

aduki beans   *See* BEAN, ADZUKI.

adulteration   The addition of substances to foods, etc., in order to increase the bulk and reduce the cost, with the intent to defraud the purchaser. Common adulterants were starch in spices, water in milk and beer, etc. The British Food and Drugs Act (1860) was the first legislation to prevent such practices.

adverse reactions to foods   (1) Food aversion, unpleasant reactions caused by emotional responses to certain foods rather than to the foods themselves, which are unlikely to occur in blind testing when the foods are disguised.

(2) Food ALLERGY, physiological reactions to specific foods or ingredients due to an immunological response. ANTIBODIES to the ALLERGEN are formed as a result of previous exposure or sensitisation, and cause a variety of symptoms when the food is eaten, including gastrointestinal disturbances, skin rashes, asthma and, in severe cases, anaphylactic shock, which may be fatal.

(3) Food intolerance, physiological reactions to specific foods or ingredients which are not due to immunological responses, but may result from the irritant action of spices, pharmacological actions of naturally occurring compounds or an inability to metabolise a component of the food as a result of an enzyme defect.

See also AMINO ACID DISORDERS; DISACCHARIDE INTOLERANCE; GENETIC DISEASES.

adzuki bean   *See* BEAN, ADZUKI.

aerobic   (1) Aerobic micro-organisms (aerobes) are those that require oxygen for growth; obligate aerobes cannot survive in the absence of oxygen. The opposite are anaerobic organisms, which do not require oxygen for growth; obligate anaerobes cannot survive in the presence of oxygen.

(2) Aerobic exercise is a sustained level of exercise without excessive breathlessness; the main metabolic pathways are aerobic GLYCOLYSIS and citric acid cycle, and β-oxidation of fatty acids, as opposed to maximum exertion, when muscle can metabolise anaerobically, producing LACTIC ACID, which is metabolised later, creating a need for increased respiration after the exercise has ceased (so-called oxygen debt).

See also ANAEROBIC THRESHOLD.

***Aeromonas* spp.**   Food poisoning micro-organisms that produce ENDOTOXINS after adhering to epithelial cells in the gut. Infective dose 10^6–10^8 organisms, onset 6–48 h, duration 24–48 h; TX 3.1.1.1.

aerophagy   Swallowing of air.

aerosol cream   Cream sterilised and packaged in aerosol canisters with a propellant gas to expel it from the container, giving conveniently available whipped CREAM. Gelling agents and STABILIS-ERS may also be added.

aerosporin *See* POLYMYXINS.

aesculin (esculin) A glucoside of dihydroxycoumarin found in the leaves and bark of the horse chestnut tree (*Aesculus hippocastanum*) which has an effect on CAPILLARY FRAGILITY.

AFD Accelerated freeze drying, *see* FREEZE DRYING.

aflata West African; part of a fermented dough that is boiled, then mixed with the remaining dough to make AKPITI or KENKEY.

aflatoxins Group of carcinogenic MYCOTOXINS formed by *Aspergillus flavus*, *A. parasiticus* and *A. nominus* growing on nuts, cereals, dried fruit and cheese, especially when stored under damp warm conditions. Fungal spoilage of foods with *A. flavus* is a common problem in many tropical areas, and aflatoxin is believed to be a cause of liver cancer in parts of Africa. Aflatoxins can be secreted in milk, so there is strict control of the level in cattle feed.

AFM Atomic force microscopy, *see* MICROSCOPE, ATOMIC FORCE.

agalactia Failure of the mother to secrete enough milk to feed a suckling infant.

agar Dried extracts from various seaweeds, including *Gelidium* and *Gracilaria* spp. It is a partially soluble NON-STARCH POLYSAC-CHARIDE, composed of GALACTOSE units, which swells with water to form a GEL, and is used in soups, jellies, ice cream and meat products. Also used as the basis of bacteriological culture media, as an adhesive, for sizing silk and as a stabiliser for emulsions. Also called agar-agar, macassar gum, vegetable gelatine. Blood agar is a microbiological culture medium containing 5–10% horse blood.

agave nectar A bulk sweetener from the blue agave (*Agave tequilana*). Mainly fructose, 30% sweeter than sucrose.

ageing (1) As wines age, they develop bouquet and a smooth mellow flavour, associated with slow oxidation and the formation of ESTERS.

(2) The ageing of meat by hanging in a cool place for several days results in softening of the muscle tissue, which stiffens after death (rigor mortis), due to anaerobic metabolism leading to the formation of lactic acid.

(3) Ageing of wheat flour for bread making is due to oxidation, either by storage for some weeks after milling or by chemical action. Freshly milled flour produces a weaker and less resilient dough, and hence a less 'bold' loaf, than flour that has been aged. Chemicals used to age (improve) flour include ammonium persulphate, ascorbic acid, chlorine, SULPHUR DIOXIDE, potassium bromate and CYSTEINE. In addition, nitrogen peroxide

or benzoyl peroxide may be used to bleach flour, and chlorine dioxide both to bleach and age.

agene Nitrogen trichloride, first introduced in 1919 as a bleaching and improving agent for wheat flour in bread making. It reacts with the AMINO ACID METHIONINE in proteins to form the toxic compound methionine sulphoximine, and is no longer used.

ageusia Loss or impairment of the sense of TASTE.

agglomeration The process of producing a free-flowing, dust-free powder from substances such as dried milk powder and wheat flour, by moistening the powder with droplets of water and then redrying in a stream of air. The resulting agglomerates can readily be wetted.

agglutinins *See* LECTINS.

agidi West African; thick gruel prepared by soaking maize, then grinding and leaving to undergo lactic acid bacterial fermentation before the paste (koko) is cooked.

aginomoto *See* MONOSODIUM GLUTAMATE.

agouti mouse A genetically obese mouse; the agouti gene is normally expressed only in hair follicles, and only during hair growth, when it antagonises MELANOCORTIN receptors. In the obese yellow mutant the gene is expressed in all tissues, and at all times, when it antagonises the melanocortin receptors in the hypothalamus that normally inhibit feeding. Expression of the agouti gene is variable, depending on maternal nutrition; this is an EPIGENETIC event, linked to failure of methylation of CPG ISLANDS in DNA.

Agrobacterium tumefaciens A bacterium that transforms plant cells into tumorous crown gall cells by introducing bacterial DNA into the host cell. Widely exploited as a means of creating TRANSGENIC plants.

AI Adequate Intake, level of intake of a micronutrient that is more than adequate to meet requirements; based on observed levels of intake, used when there is inadequate information to derive REFERENCE INTAKES.

air broom A device used for cooling and dislodging powder deposits from the inner wall of a spray-drying chamber. A perforated pipe rotates inside the chamber, close to the inner wall, and directs cool air onto it. This disturbs any powder that has accumulated on the wall and cools it, making it easier to handle and transport.

air classification A way of separating the particles of powdered materials in a current of air, on the basis of their weight and size or density. Particularly applied to the fractionation of the ENDOSPERM of milled wheat flour; smaller particles are richer in protein. Various fractions range from 3 to 25% protein.

air cycle   *See* HEAT PUMP.

airfuge   Air-driven bench-top ultra-CENTRIFUGE using frictionless magnetic suspension of the rotor; can achieve $160\,000\,g$ in $30\,\text{s}$.

air/powder separator   A device for separating powder from an air or other gas stream, used to recover fine dried powder from the exhaust air leaving a spray-drying chamber.

ajinomoto   *See* MONOSODIUM GLUTAMATE

ajowan   Thyme-flavoured seed of *Carum ajowan*, used in Indian and Middle Eastern cuisine.

akee   *See* ACKEE.

akpiti   West African; fried doughnuts made from maize (and sometimes plantain flour); the dough is left to undergo a lactic acid bacterial fermentation. Part of the fermented dough is boiled (aflata), mixed with the remainder and fried. Awule bolo is similar, but made with rice flour, banku from sorghum, millet or barley.

ala   *See* BULGUR.

alactasia   Partial or complete deficiency of the enzyme LACTASE in the small intestine, resulting in an inability to digest the sugar LACTOSE in milk, and hence intolerance of milk and milk products.

   See also DISACCHARIDE INTOLERANCE.

alanine   A non-essential AMINO ACID; abbr Ala (A), M_r 89.1, pK_a 2.35, 9.87, CODONS GCNu.

β-alanine   An ISOMER of alanine in which the amino group is attached to carbon-3 rather than carbon-2 as in alanine; it is important as part of PANTOTHENIC ACID, CARNOSINE and ANSERINE, M_r 89.1, pK_a 3.55, 10.24.

alant starch   *See* INULIN.

albacore   A long-finned species of tunny fish, *Thunnus alalunga*, usually canned as TUNA fish.

albedo   The white pith (mesocarp) of the inner peel of citrus fruits, accounting for some 20–60% of the whole fruit. It consists of sugars, CELLULOSE and PECTINS, and is used as a commercial source of pectin.

albumin (albumen)   A specific class of relatively small PROTEINS that are soluble in water and readily coagulated by heat. Ovalbumin is the main protein of egg white, lactalbumin occurs in milk, and plasma or serum albumin is one of the major blood proteins. Serum albumin concentration is sometimes measured as an index of PROTEIN–ENERGY MALNUTRITION. Often used as a non-specific term for proteins (e.g. albuminuria is the excretion of proteins in the urine).

albumin index   A measure of the quality or freshness of an egg – the ratio of the height: width of the albumin when the egg is broken onto a flat surface. As the egg deteriorates, so the albumin spreads further, i.e. the albumin index decreases.

albumin milk   *See* MILK, PROTEIN.

albuminoids   Fibrous proteins that have a structural or protective rather than enzymic role in the body. Also known as scleroproteins. The main proteins of the CONNECTIVE TISSUES of the body. There are three main types:

(1) COLLAGEN in skin, tendons and bones is resistant to enzymic digestion with TRYPSIN and PEPSIN, and can be converted to soluble GELATINE by boiling with water;

(2) ELASTIN in tendons and arteries, which is not converted to gelatine on boiling;

(3) KERATIN, the proteins of hair, feathers, scales, horns and hooves, which are insoluble in dilute acid or alkali, and resistant to digestive enzymes.

albumin water   Beverage made from lightly whisked egg white and cold water, seasoned with lemon juice and salt.

alcaptonuria (alkaptonuria)   A GENETIC DISEASE of PHENYLALANINE and TYROSINE metabolism, owing to lack of the enzyme homogentisic acid oxidase (EC 1.13.11.5). As a result, homogentisic acid accumulates and is excreted in the urine; it oxidises in air and turns the urine black. The defect does not appear to be harmful.

alcohol   Chemically alcohols are compounds with the general formula $C_nH_{(2n+1)}OH$. The alcohol in ALCOHOLIC BEVERAGES is ethanol (ethyl alcohol, C_2H_5OH); pure ethyl alcohol is also known as absolute alcohol. The ENERGY yield of alcohol is 29 kJ (7 kcal)/g.

The strength of alcoholic beverages is most often shown as the percentage of alcohol by volume (sometimes shown as % v/v or ABV). This is not the same as the percentage of alcohol by weight (% w/v) since alcohol is less dense than water (density 0.79): 5% v/v alcohol = 3.96% by weight (w/v); 10% v/v = 7.93% w/v and 40% v/v = 31.7% w/v.

See also PROOF SPIRIT.

alcohol, denatured   Drinkable alcohol is subject to tax in most countries and for industrial use it is denatured to render it unfit for consumption by the addition of 5% methanol CH_3OH, which is poisonous. This is industrial rectified spirit. For domestic use a purple dye and pyridine (which has an unpleasant odour) are also added; this is methylated spirit.

alcoholic beverages   Made by fermenting sugars in fruit juices with YEAST to form ALCOHOL. These include BEER, CIDER and PERRY, 4–6% alcohol by volume; WINES, 9–13% alcohol; SPIRITS (e.g. BRANDY, GIN, RUM, VODKA, WHISKY) made by distilling fermented liquor, 37–45% alcohol; LIQUEURS made from distilled spirits, sweetened and flavoured, 20–40% alcohol; and fortified wines (*see* MADEIRA; PORT; SHERRY; WINE, APÉRITIF) made by adding spirit to wine, 18–25% alcohol.

See also ALCOHOL; PROOF SPIRIT.

alcoholism Physiological addiction to ALCOHOL, associated with persistent heavy consumption of ALCOHOLIC BEVERAGES. In addition to the addiction, there may be damage to the liver (cirrhosis), stomach (gastritis) and pancreas (pancreatitis), as well as behavioural changes and peripheral nerve damage.

See also WERNICKE–KORSAKOFF SYNDROME.

alcohol units For convenience in calculating intakes of alcohol, a unit of alcohol is defined as 8 g (10 mL) of absolute alcohol; this is the approximate amount in $\frac{1}{2}$ pint (300 mL) beer, a single measure of spirit (25 mL) or a single glass of wine (100 mL). The upper limit of prudent consumption of alcohol is 21 units (168 g alcohol) per week or 4 units per day, for men and 14 units (112 g alcohol) per week or 3 units per day, for women.

aldehydes Compounds containing a carbonyl (C$=$O) group, in which one remaining valency of the carbon is occupied by hydrogen and the other by an aliphatic or aromatic group. Formed by oxidation of ALCOHOLS; further oxidation yields carboxylic acids.

alderman's walk The name given in London to the longest and finest cut from the haunch of venison or lamb.

aldosterone A MINERALOCORTICOID STEROID HORMONE secreted by the zona glomerulosa of the adrenal cortex (*see* ADRENAL GLAND); acts to regulate sodium and potassium transport by stimulating the renal tubule resorption of sodium. Synthesis and secretion stimulated by ANGIOTENSIN. Aldosteronism is overproduction of aldosterone leading to HYPERTENSION.

ale *See* BEER.

alecost An aromatic herbaceous plant, *Tanacetum (Chrysanthemum) balsamita*, related to TANSY, used in salads and formerly used to flavour ale.

aleurone layer The single layer of large cells under the bran coat and outside the endosperm of CEREAL grains. It forms about 3% of the weight of the grain, and is rich in protein, as well as containing about 20% of the VITAMIN B_1, 30% of the VITAMIN B_2 and 50% of the NIACIN of the grain. Botanically the aleurone layer is part of the endosperm, but in milling it remains attached to the inner layer of the BRAN.

alewives River herrings, *Pomolobus (Alosa) pseudoharengus*, commonly used for canning after salting.

alexanders   A herb, black lovage (*Smyrnium olisatrum*) with a celery-like flavour.

alfacalcidiol   1α-Hydroxycholecalciferol; synthetic VITAMIN D analogue used in treatment of conditions associated with failure of the renal 1-hydroxylation of calcidiol to active CALCITRIOL. Undergoes 25-hydroxylation to CALCITRIOL in the liver.

alfalfa   Or lucerne, *Medicago sativa*, commonly grown for animal feed or silage, and widely consumed as BEAN SPROUTS.

Sprouted beans, composition/100 g: water 91 g, 121 kJ (29 kcal), protein 4 g, fat 0.7 g, carbohydrate 3.8 g (0.2 g sugars), fibre 2.5 g, ash 0.4 g, Ca 32 mg, Fe 1 mg, Mg 27 mg, P 70 mg, K 79 mg, Na 6 mg, Zn 0.9 mg, Cu 0.2 mg, Mn 0.2 mg, Se 0.6 µg, vitamin A 8 µg RE (99 µg carotenoids), K 30.5 mg, B_1 0.08 mg, B_2 0.13 mg, niacin 0.5 mg, B_6 0.03 mg, folate 36 µg, pantothenate 0.6 mg, C 8 mg.

algae   Simple plants that do not show differentiation into roots, stems and leaves. They are mostly aquatic, either seaweeds or pond and river-weeds. Some seaweeds, such as DULSE and IRISH MOSS, have long been eaten, and a number of unicellular algae, including *Chlorella*, *Scenedesmus* and *SPIRULINA* spp. have been grown experimentally as novel sources of food (50–60% of the dry weight is protein), but are used only as dietary supplements.

algin   Gum derived from alginic acid (*see* ALGINATES).

alginates   Salts of alginic acid found in many seaweeds as calcium salts or the free acid. Chemically, alginic acid is a NON-STARCH POLYSACCHARIDE of mannuronic acid. Iron, magnesium and ammonium salts of alginic acid form viscous solutions and hold large amounts of water.

Used as thickeners, stabilisers and gelling, binding and emulsifying agents in food manufacture, especially ICE CREAM and synthetic CREAM. Trade name Manucol.

Used in combination with magnesium and aluminium hydroxides in ANTACIDS; alginate-containing antacids form a 'raft' floating on the gastric contents, so reducing oesophageal reflux.

alimentary canal   *See* GASTROINTESTINAL TRACT.

alimentary pastes   *See* PASTA.

aliphatic   ORGANIC compounds with (branched or straight) open chain structure, as distinct from cyclic compounds which contain rings of carbon atoms. Cyclic organic compounds that are not aromatic are called alicyclic.

alitame   Synthetic intense SWEETENER, an amide of aspartyl D-alanine (L-aspartyl-*N*-(2,2,4,4-tetramethyl-3-thietanyl)-D-alaninamide).

See also ASPARTAME.

alkali formers   *See* ACID FOODS.

alkaline dip Immersion of some fruits, which are to be dried whole, in an alkaline solution to increase the rate of drying, as a result of forming fine cracks in the skin of the fruit.

alkaline phosphatase Enzyme (EC 3.1.3.1) that hydrolyses a variety of phosphate esters; has alkaline pH optimum. Serum enzyme comes from a variety of tissues, but especially bone, and elevated serum levels indicate metabolic bone disease or VITAMIN D deficiency, hence a sensitive index of preclinical RICKETS or OSTEOMALACIA. The enzyme in raw milk has a similar D-value to heat-resistant pathogens, and measurement is used to test the effectiveness of pasteurisation.

alkaline tide Small increase in pH of blood after a meal as a result of the secretion of gastric acid.

alkali reserve *See* BUFFERS.

alkaloids Term proposed by Meissner (1819) for naturally occurring nitrogen-containing organic bases that have pharmacological actions in humans and other animals, usually basic, normally contain nitrogen in a heterocyclic ring; most are derivatives of AMINO ACIDS. Many are found in plant foods, including potatoes and tomatoes (the *Solanum* alkaloids), or as the products of fungal action (e.g. ERGOT), although they also occur in animal foods (e.g. tetrodotoxin in PUFFER FISH, tetramine in SHELLFISH). Alkylamines, CHOLINE, PURINES and PYRIMIDINES are not usually considered as alkaloids.

See also PROTOALKALOIDS; PSEUDOALKALOIDS.

alkalosis Increase in blood pH above pH 7.45; may be caused by excessive loss of carbon dioxide (e.g. in hyperventilation), excessive intake of bases, as in antacid drugs, loss of gastric juice by vomiting, high intake of sodium and potassium salts of weak organic acids.

See also ACID–BASE BALANCE; ACIDOSIS.

alkannet (alkanet, alkannin, alkanna) A colouring obtained from the root of *Anchusa (Alkanna) tinctoria* which is insoluble in water but soluble in alcohol and oils. Blue in alkali (or in the presence of lead), crimson with tin, and violet with iron. Used for colouring fats, cheese, essences, etc. Also known as orcanella.

allantoin Oxidation product of URIC ACID; excretory end-product of PURINE metabolism in most animals other than humans and other primates, which lack the enzyme uric acid oxidase (EC 1.7.3.3) and therefore excrete uric acid. Some allantoin is formed non-enzymically by reaction of uric acid with oxygen RADICALS, and uric acid may be considered to be part of the body's antioxidant defence.

allergen   A compound, commonly a protein, which causes the production of antibodies, and hence an allergic reaction.
See also ADVERSE REACTIONS TO FOODS; ALLERGY.

allergy   Often used indiscriminately to cover a number of ADVERSE REACTIONS TO FOOD, true allergy is an immune response to a food leading to the formation of immunoglobulin E (IgE) which results in the release of histamine and leucotrienes, among other substances, into the tissues. They are released from mast cells in eyes, skin, respiratory system and intestinal system. Allergy requires an initial sensitisation; reactions may range from relatively short-lived discomfort to anaphylactic shock, which can be fatal.

Over 170 foods have been shown to cause allergic reactions. The main serious food allergens include milk and eggs (and their products), wheat, soya, nuts, shellfish and fruits, and also, to a lesser extent, sunflower and cottonseeds, molluscs and certain beans. Allergens are usually active in extremely small amounts so that contamination from offending foodstuffs can result from traces left on processing machinery and utensils.

allicin   A sulphur-containing compound (diallyl thiosulphinate; thio-2-propene-L-sulfinic acid-5-allyl ester), partially responsible for the flavour of GARLIC. Formed by the action of allinase on alliin (*S*-(2-propenyl)-L-cysteine sulphoxide) when the cells are disrupted, releasing the enzyme to act on the substrate. Has antibacterial properties.

alligator pear   *See* AVOCADO.

alliin, alliinase   *See* ALLICIN.

Allinson bread   A wholewheat BREAD named after Allinson, who advocated its consumption in England at the end of the 19th century, as did Graham in the USA (hence GRAHAM bread). Now trade name for a wholemeal loaf.

Allkream™   FAT REPLACER made from protein.

alloisoleucine   Isomer of ISOLEUCINE.

allolactose   Isomer of LACTOSE, β1,6-galactosyl-glucose.

allotriophagy   An unnatural desire for abnormal foods; also known as cissa, cittosis and pica.

alloxan   Pyrimidine derivative used experimentally to induce insulin-dependent DIABETES mellitus; specifically cytotoxic to β-cells of the pancreatic islets of Langerhans, which secrete INSULIN. Now largely superseded by STREPTOZOTOCIN.

alloxazine   The tricyclic structure that is the central part of the molecule of riboflavin (VITAMIN B_2).

allspice   Dried fruits of the evergreen plant *Pimenta officinalis*, also known as pimento (as distinct from PIMIENTO) or Jamaican pepper. The name allspice derives from the aromatic oil, which has an aroma similar to a mixture of CLOVES, CINNAMON and NUTMEG.

allysine Semi-aldehyde of amino-adipic acid in connective tissue proteins; forms cross-links with lysine in COLLAGEN, and complex links between three or four peptide chains in elastin (DESMOSINES and ISODESMOSINES). It is formed by oxidative deamination of peptide-bound lysine by the enzyme lysyl oxidase (EC 1.4.3.13), which is copper-dependent, and its activity is impaired in dietary COPPER deficiency and by β-aminopropionitrile, one of the toxins in *Lathyrus* spp. (*see* ODORATISM).

almond A nut, the seed of *Prunus amygdalus* var. *dulcis*. All varieties contain the GLYCOSIDE AMYGDALIN, which forms hydrogen cyanide when the nuts are crushed. The bitter almond, used for ALMOND OIL (*P. amygdalus* var. *amara*), may yield dangerous amounts of cyanide.

Composition/100 g: (edible portion 40%) water 5.3 g, 2420 kJ (578 kcal), protein 21.3 g, fat 50.6 g (of which 8% saturated, 67% mono-unsaturated, 25% polyunsaturated), carbohydrate 19.7 g (4.8 g sugars), fibre 11.8 g, ash 3.1 g, Ca 248 mg, Fe 4.3 mg, Mg 275 mg, P 474 mg, K 728 mg, Na 1 mg, Zn 3.4 mg, Cu 1.1 mg, Mn 2.5 mg, Se 2.8 µg, vitamin E 26 mg, B_1 0.24 mg, B_2 0.81 mg, niacin 3.9 mg, B_6 0.13 mg, folate 29 µg, pantothenate 0.3 mg. A 20 g serving (20 nuts) is a source of Cu, Mg, P, a good source of Mn, a rich source of vitamin E.

almond oil Essential oil from the seeds of either the almond tree (*Prunus amygdalis*) or more commonly the apricot tree (*P. armeniaca*), containing benzaldehyde, hydrogen cyanide and benzaldehyde cyanohydrin. After removal of the hydrogen cyanide, used as a flavour and in perfumes and cosmetics. Composition 9% saturated, 73% mono-unsaturated, 18% polyunsaturated, vitamin E 39 mg, K 7 mg/100 g.

almond paste Ground almonds mixed with powdered sugar, bound with egg, used to decorate cakes and make petits fours. Also known as marzipan.

aloe vera *See* LAXATIVES.

Alpha–Laval™ **(Alfa–Laval) centrifuge** A continuous bowl centrifuge for separating liquids of different densities and for clarification. Widely used for cream separation.

alum ALUMINUM sulphate and aluminium potassium sulphate, used in pickles and to prevent discoloration of potatoes.

aluminium (aluminum) The third most abundant element in the earth's crust (after oxygen and silicon) but with no known biological function. Present in small amounts in many foods but only a small proportion (0.01%) is absorbed. Aluminium is used in cooking vessels and as foil for wrapping food, as well as in cans and tubes.

The 'silver' beads used to decorate confectionery are coated with either silver foil or an alloy of aluminium and COPPER. BAKING POWDERS containing sodium aluminium sulphate as the acid agent were used at one time (alum baking powders), and aluminium hydroxide and silicates are commonly used in ANTACID medications.

Aluminium salts are found in the abnormal nerve tangles in the brain in Alzheimer's disease, and it has been suggested that aluminium poisoning may be a factor in the development of the disease, although there is little evidence.

ALV Available lysine value, *see* AVAILABLE LYSINE.

alveograph A device for measuring the stretching quality of dough as an index of its protein quality for baking. A standard disc of dough is blown into a bubble and the pressure curve and bursting pressure are measured to give the stability, extensibility and strength of the dough.

alverine citrate Bulking agent and antispasmodic used to treat IRRITABLE BOWEL SYNDROME and other colon disorders.

AMA American Medical Association; web site http://www. ama-assn.org/.

amaranth (1) A Burgundy red colour (E-123), stable to light; trisodium salt of 1-(4-sulpho-1-naphthylazo)-2-naphthol-3,6-disulphonic acid.

amaranth (2) Some *Amaranthus* spp. (*A. paniculatus*) are cultivated for their leaves (a good source of carotene) and seeds and others only for their leaves (*A. polygamus* and *A. gracilis*). Paste made from the seeds from *A. hypochondrachus* were widely eaten in central America, and used in religious ceremonies by the Aztecs.

Composition/100 g: (edible portion 94%) water 91.7 g, 96 kJ (23 kcal), protein 2.5 g, fat 0.3 g, carbohydrate 4 g, ash 1.5 g, Ca 215 mg, Fe 2.3 mg, Mg 55 mg, P 50 mg, K 611 mg, Na 20 mg, Zn 0.9 mg, Cu 0.2 mg, Mn 0.9 mg, Se 0.9 µg, K 1140 mg, B_1 0.03 mg, B_2 0.16 mg, niacin 0.7 mg, B_6 0.19 mg, folate 85 µg, pantothenate 0.1 mg, C 43 mg.

amarwa *See* ORUBISI.

ambali Indian; sour millet and rice cake; the dough is left to undergo a lactic acid bacterial fermentation before cooking.

ambergris A waxy concretion obtained from the intestine of the sperm whale, containing CHOLESTEROL, ambrein and BENZOIC ACID. Used in drugs and perfumery.

Amberlite^{TM} Group of polystyrene ION-EXCHANGE RESINS. Sulphonic acid derivatives are used for cation exchange, basic types for anion exchange.

ambient-stable foods   Foods that have been cooked in a can or plastic microwaveable container, so that only reheating is required prior to consumption.

See also RETORT POUCHES.

amblyopia   Poor sight not due to any detectable disease of the eye. May occur in VITAMIN B_2 deficiency.

amenorrhoea   Cessation of menstruation, normally occurring between the ages of 45 and 55 (the menopause), but sometimes at an early age, especially as a result of severe undernutrition (as in ANOREXIA NERVOSA) when body weight falls below about 45 kg.

Amer Picon^{TM} Pungent BITTERS invented in 1830 by Gaston Picon; contains quinine, gentian and orange.

Ames test   An *in vitro* test for the ability of chemicals, including potential food ADDITIVES, to cause mutation in bacteria (the mutagenic potential). Commonly used as a preliminary screening method to detect substances likely to be carcinogenic. The test is based on treating bacteria that are already mutant at an easily detectable locus for reversal of the mutation (e.g. a strain of bacteria that cannot grow in the absence of histidine to a form that can do so).

amines   Formed by the decarboxylation of AMINO ACIDS. Physiologically active amines with vasoconstrictor (pressor) activity present in foods or formed by intestinal bacteria include tyramine, tryptamine, phenylethylamine and histamine.

   Have been proposed as triggers for diet-induced migraine, and in patients taking MONOAMINE OXIDASE inhibitors as antidepressant medication; intake of foods such as cheese, chocolate and fermented foods that are rich in these amines may provoke a potentially lethal hypertensive crisis.

amino acid disorders   A number of extremely rare GENETIC DISEASES, occurring between 1 and 80 per million live births, which affect the metabolism of individual AMINO ACIDS; if untreated many result in mental retardation. Screening for those conditions that can be treated is carried out shortly after birth in most countries. Treatment is generally by feeding specially formulated diets providing minimal amounts of the amino acid involved.

   See also ARGININAEMIA; ARGININOSUCCINIC ACIDURIA; CITRULLINAEMIA; CYSTATHIONINURIA; CYSTINURIA; HARTNUP DISEASE; HOMOCYSTINURIA; HYPERAMMONAEMIA; MAPLE SYRUP URINE DISEASE; PHENYLKETONURIA.

amino acid, limiting   The essential AMINO ACID present in a protein in the lowest amount relative to the requirement for that amino acid. The ratio between the amount of the limiting amino acid in a protein and the requirement for that amino acid provides a chemical estimate of the nutritional value (PROTEIN QUALITY) of that protein (CHEMICAL SCORE). Most cereal proteins are limited by LYSINE, and most animal and other vegetable proteins by the sum of METHIONINE + CYSTEINE (the sulphur amino acids). In complete diets it is usually the sulphur amino acids that are limiting.

amino acid profile Amino acid composition of a protein.

amino acids The basic units from which PROTEINS are made. Chemically compounds with an amino group (—NH₂) and a carboxyl group (—COOH) attached to the same carbon atom (*see* p. 22).

Thirteen of the amino acids involved in proteins can be synthesised in the body, and so are called non-essential or dispensable amino acids, since they do not have to be provided in the diet. They are alanine, arginine, aspartic acid, asparagine, cysteine, cystine, glutamic acid, glutamine, glycine, hydroxyproline, proline, serine and tyrosine.

Nine amino acids cannot be synthesised in the body at all and so must be provided in the diet; they are called the essential or indispensable amino acids: histidine, isoleucine, leucine, lysine, methionine, phenylalanine, threonine, tryptophan and valine. Arginine may be essential for infants, since their requirement is greater than their ability to synthesise it.

Two of the non-essential amino acids are made in the body from essential amino acids: cysteine (and cystine) from methionine, and tyrosine from phenylalanine.

A number of other amino acids also occur in proteins, including hydroxyproline, hydroxylysine, γ-carboxyglutamate and methylhistidine, but are nutritionally unimportant since they cannot be reutilised for protein synthesis. Other amino acids occur as intermediates in metabolic pathways, but are not required for protein synthesis and are nutritionally unimportant, although they may occur in foods. These include HOMOCYSTEINE, citrulline and ornithine. Some of the non-protein amino acids that occur in plants are toxic.

The amino acids are sometimes classified by the chemical nature of the side chain. Two are acidic: glutamic acid (glutamate) and aspartic acid (aspartate) with a carboxylic acid (—COOH) group in the side chain. Three, lysine, arginine and histidine, have basic groups in the side chain. Three, phenylalanine, tyrosine and tryptophan, have an aromatic group in the side chain. Three, leucine, isoleucine and valine, have a branched chain structure. Two, methionine and cysteine, contain sulphur in the side chain; although cysteine is not an essential amino acid, it can be synthesised only from methionine, and it is conventional to consider the sum of methionine plus cysteine (the sulphur amino acids) in consideration of PROTEIN QUALITY.

An alternative classification of the amino acids is by their metabolic fate; whether they can be utilised for glucose synthesis or not. Those that can give rise to glucose are termed glucogenic (or sometimes antiketogenic); those that give rise to KETONES or acetyl CoA when they are metabolised are termed ketogenic. Only leucine and lysine are purely ketogenic. Isoleucine, phenylalanine, tyrosine and tryptophan give rise to both ketogenic and glucogenic fragments; the remainder are purely glucogenic.

amino acids, acidic Two of the amino acids, GLUTAMIC ACID and ASPARTIC ACID, which have a carboxylic acid (—COOH) group in the side chain.

amino acids, antiketogenic *See* AMINO ACIDS, GLUCOGENIC.

amino acids, aromatic Three of the amino acids, PHENYLALANINE, TYROSINE and TRYPTOPHAN, which have an aromatic group in the side chain. HISTIDINE is technically also aromatic, but is not generally grouped with the aromatic amino acids.

amino acids, basic Three of the amino acids, LYSINE, ARGININE and HISTIDINE, which have basic groups in the side chain.

amino acids, branched chain Three of the amino acids, LEUCINE, ISOLEUCINE and VALINE, which have a branched aliphatic side chain.

See also MAPLE SYRUP URINE DISEASE.

amino acids, glucogenic Those amino acids that can give rise to glucose when they are metabolised. Sometimes known as antiketogenic, since the glucose formed in their metabolism reduce the rate of production of KETONE bodies. All except LYSINE and LEUCINE can be used for glucose synthesis in the body, although some are also KETOGENIC.

amino acids, ketogenic Those amino acids that give rise to KETONE BODIES or acetyl CoA when they are metabolised. LEUCINE is purely ketogenic, and ISOLEUCINE, PHENYLALANINE, TYROSINE and TRYPTOPHAN give rise to both ketogenic and glucogenic fragments.

amino acids, non-protein A number of amino acids occur as metabolic intermediates, but are not involved in protein synthesis and are nutritionally unimportant, although they may occur in foods. These include ORNITHINE and CITRULLINE. Some in higher plants are toxic to animals and potentially so to humans, e.g. mimosine (in ALFALFA), djenkolic acid (djenkola bean), hypoglycin (unripe ACKEE fruit), oxalylaminoalanine (*Lathyrus* spp.).

amino acids, sulphur Three amino acids, METHIONINE, CYSTEINE and CYSTINE, contain sulphur in the side chain; although cysteine

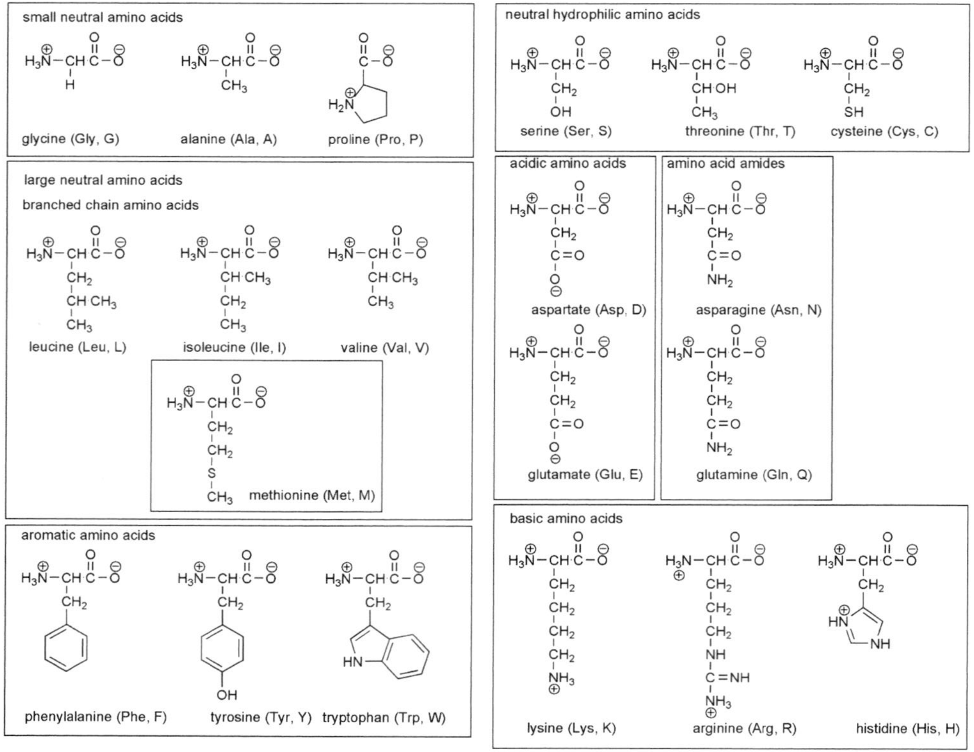

22

THE PROTEIN AMINO ACIDS

small neutral amino acids

glycine (Gly, G) alanine (Ala, A) proline (Pro, P)

large neutral amino acids

branched chain amino acids

leucine (Leu, L) isoleucine (Ile, I) valine (Val, V)

methionine (Met, M)

aromatic amino acids

phenylalanine (Phe, F) tyrosine (Tyr, Y) tryptophan (Trp, W)

neutral hydrophilic amino acids

serine (Ser, S) threonine (Thr, T) cysteine (Cys, C)

acidic amino acids

aspartate (Asp, D) glutamate (Glu, E)

amino acid amides

asparagine (Asn, N) glutamine (Gln, Q)

basic amino acids

lysine (Lys, K) arginine (Arg, R) histidine (His, H)

is not an essential amino acid, it can only be synthesised from methionine, and it is conventional to consider the sum of methionine + cysteine in determinations of PROTEIN QUALITY.

aminoaciduria Excretion of abnormally large amounts of an amino acid or a group of metabolically related amino acids. Overflow aminoaciduria occurs when the plasma concentration exceeds the renal threshold, as a result of impaired metabolism; renal aminoaciduria occurs with normal or lower than normal plasma concentrations, as a result of impaired renal resorption of a group of amino acids that share a common transport system. In either case aminoaciduria may be due to a genetic defect or acquired (i.e. secondary to toxicity or disease).

aminoacylase Enzyme (EC 3.5.1.14) which catalyses esterification specifically of D-amino acids; used in resolution of RACEMIC mixtures of amino acids resulting from chemical synthesis.

aminogram A diagrammatic representation of the amino acids in a protein or peptide. A plasma aminogram represents the amounts of free amino acids in blood plasma.

amino group The —NH$_2$ group of AMINO ACIDS and AMINES.

aminopeptidase Enzyme (EC 3.4.11.1) secreted in the intestinal juice which removes amino acids sequentially from the free amino terminal of a peptide or protein, i.e. an EXOPEPTIDASE.

aminopterin Aminopteroylglutamic acid; metabolic antagonist (antivitamin) of FOLIC ACID.

aminosalicylates 5-Aminosalicylate and its derivatives (balsalazide, mesalazine, olsalazine, sulphasalazine) used in treatment of ulcerative COLITIS.

aminotransferase *See* TRANSAMINASE.

amla Indian gooseberry, *Emblica officinalis* Gaertn., important in Ayurvedic medicine and reported to reduce HYPERCHOLESTEROLAEMIA. An extremely rich source of vitamin C (600 mg/100 g).

amoebiasis (amoebic dysentery) Infection of the intestinal tract with pathogenic amoeba (commonly *Entamoeba histolytica*) from contaminated food or water, causing profuse diarrhoea, intestinal bleeding, pain, jaundice, anorexia and weight loss.

amomum A group of tropical plants including CARDAMOM and MELEGUETA PEPPER, which have pungent and aromatic seeds.

AMP Adenosine monophosphate, *see* ADENINE.

amphetamine A chemical at one time used as an appetite suppressant, addictive and a common drug of abuse ('speed'), its use is strictly controlled by law. Also known as benzedrine.

amphoteric *See* ISOELECTRIC POINT.

amulum Roman; starch used to thicken sauces, made by soaking wheat grains in water, then straining the liquid and pouring onto a tiled floor to thicken in the sun.

amydon A traditional starchy material made by steeping wheat flour in water, then drying the starch sediment in the sun, used for thickening broths, etc.

amygdalin (1) A GLYCOSIDE in ALMONDS and apricot and cherry stones which is hydrolysed by the enzyme EMULSIN to yield glucose, cyanide and benzaldehyde. It is therefore highly poisonous, although it has been promoted, with no evidence, as a nutrient, laetrile or so-called vitamin B_{17}. Unfounded claims have been made for its value in treating cancer.

(2) French name for cakes and sweets made with almonds.

amylases Enzymes that hydrolyse STARCH. α-Amylase (dextrinogenic amylase or diastase, EC 3.2.1.1) acts randomly on α-1,4-glucoside bonds in the molecule, and produces small DEXTRIN fragments. β-Amylase (maltogenic or glucoamylase, EC 3.2.1.2) acts at the non-reducing end of the molecule to liberate maltose plus some free glucose, and isomaltose from the branch points in AMYLOPECTIN. Salivary amylase (sometimes called by its obsolete name of ptyalin) and pancreatic amylase are both α-amylases.

Major sources of α-amylase in the baking and brewing industries are *Aspergillus oryzae* (fungal amylase) and *Bacillus subtilis*, in addition to malted (sprouted) cereals added to increase the hydrolysis of starch to fermentable sugars.

See also DEBRANCHING ENZYMES; DIASTATIC ACTIVITY; Z-ENZYME.

amyli Dried TAMARIND.

amylin A peptide that is secreted together with INSULIN from the pancreatic β-islet cells during and after food intake; it has a potent anorectic (appetite suppressant) action.

amylo-amylose Obsolete name for AMYLOSE.

amylodyspepsia An inability to digest starch.

amyloglucosidase *See* DEBRANCHING ENZYMES.

amylograph A device to measure the viscosity of flour paste as it is heated from 25 °C to 90 °C (as occurs in baking), which serves as a measure of the DIASTATIC ACTIVITY of the flour.

amyloins Carbohydrates that are complexes of dextrins with varying proportions of maltose.

amylopectin The branched chain form of STARCH, about 75% of the total, the remainder being straight chain AMYLOSE. Consists of chains of glucose units linked α-1,4, with 5% of the glucose linked α-1,6 at branch points; gives purplish colour with iodine.

amylopeptic A general term for enzymes that are able to hydrolyse STARCH to soluble products.

amyloplasts Organelles in the ENDOSPERM of cereal grains in which starch granules are synthesised.

amylopsin Alternative name for pancreatic AMYLASE.

amylose The straight chain form of STARCH, ~25% of the total, consisting of glucose units linked α-1,4; gives blue colour with iodine.

See also AMYLOPECTIN.

anabiosis Suspended animation with stoppage of respiration and heart beat caused by freeze drying, e.g. of insects during cold spells.

anabolic agents Those HORMONES (and hormone-like drugs) that stimulate growth and the development of muscle tissue.

anabolism The process of building up or synthesising, *see* METABOLISM.

anaemia Shortage of HAEMOGLOBIN in blood (less than 85% of the reference range; <130 g/L in adult men, or <120 g/L in women) leading to chronic pallor and shortness of breath on exertion. Most commonly due to dietary deficiency of iron or chronic blood loss resulting in a reduced number of smaller red blood cells (microcytic) which also include less haemoglobin (hypochromic anaemia).

Other dietary deficiencies can lead to anaemia: VITAMIN B$_6$ deficiency impairs haemoglobin synthesis; VITAMIN C deficiency impairs iron absorption; FOLIC ACID and VITAMIN B$_{12}$ deficiencies result in megaloblastic anaemia, the release of immature precursors of red blood cells into the circulation.

anaemia, haemolytic ANAEMIA caused by premature and excessive destruction of red blood cells, commonly in response to a toxic stress (*see* FAVISM). Rarely due to nutritional deficiency, but may be a result of vitamin E deficiency in premature infants. Measurement of haemolysis *in vitro*, induced by dialuronic acid or hydrogen peroxide, provides an index of VITAMIN E status.

anaemia, megaloblastic Release into the circulation of immature precursors of red BLOOD CELLS, due to deficiency of either FOLIC ACID or VITAMIN B$_{12}$.

See also ANAEMIA, PERNICIOUS; FIGLU TEST; dUMP SUPPRESSION TEST; SCHILLING TEST.

anaemia, pernicious ANAEMIA due to deficiency of VITAMIN B$_{12}$, most commonly as a result of failure to absorb the vitamin from the diet. There is release into the circulation of immature precursors of red BLOOD CELLS, the same type of megaloblastic anaemia as is seen in FOLIC ACID deficiency. There is also progressive irreversible damage to the spinal cord (sub-acute combined degeneration). The underlying cause of the condition may be the production of ANTIBODIES against either the INTRINSIC FACTOR that is required for absorption of the vitamin, or the cells of the gastric mucosa that secrete intrinsic factor. Atrophy of the gastric mucosa with ageing also impairs vitamin B$_{12}$ absorption, and causes pernicious anaemia. Dietary deficiency of vitamin B_{12} may occur in strict VEGETARIANS (vegans).

See also dUMP SUPPRESSION TEST; INTRINSIC FACTOR; SCHILLING TEST.

anaerobes *See* AEROBIC.

anaerobic threshold The level of exercise at which the rate of oxygen uptake into muscle becomes limiting and there is an increasing proportion of anaerobic GLYCOLYSIS to yield lactate.

See also AEROBIC (2).

analysis, gastric *See* FRACTIONAL TEST MEAL.

analysis, proximate *See* PROXIMATE ANALYSIS.

analyte A compound that is analysed or assayed.

ananas *See* PINEAPPLE.

anaphylactic (anaphylaxic) shock Abnormally severe allergic reaction to an antigen in which HISTAMINE is released from mast cells, causing widespread symptoms.

anatto *See* ANNATTO.

anchovy Small oily FISH, *Engraulis* spp., usually semipreserved with 10–12% salt and sometimes BENZOIC ACID.

Composition (fresh)/100 g: water 73 g, 548 kJ (131 kcal), protein 20 g, fat 4.8 g (of which 31% saturated, 29% mono-unsaturated, 49% polyunsaturated), cholesterol 60 mg, ash 1.4 g, Ca 147 mg, Fe 3.3 mg, Mg 41 mg, P 174 mg, K 383 mg, Na 104 mg, Zn 1.7 mg, Cu 0.2 mg, Se 36.5 µg, vitamin A 15 µg retinol, E 0.6 mg, K 0.1 mg, B_1 0.06 mg, B_2 0.26 mg, niacin 14 mg, B_6 0.14 mg, folate 9 µg, B_{12} 0.6 µg, pantothenate 0.6 mg.

Anchovy butter is prepared from pounded fillets of anchovy mixed with butter as a savoury spread; anchovy paste from pounded fillets of anchovy mixed with vinegar and spices.

ancyclostomiasis Infestation with HOOKWORM.

androgens Male sex hormones (STEROIDS), testosterone, dihydrotestosterone and androsterone. Sometimes used as ANABOLIC AGENTS.

aneurine Obsolete name for VITAMIN B_1.

aneurysm Local dilatation (swelling and weakening) of the wall of a blood vessel, usually the result of ATHEROSCLEROSIS and HYPERTENSION; especially serious in the aorta, where rupture may prove fatal.

angelica Crystallised young stalks of the umbelliferous herb *Angelica archangelica*, which grows in southern Europe. They are bright green in colour, and are used to decorate and flavour confectionery goods. The roots are used together with JUNIPER berries to flavour GIN, and the seeds are used in VERMOUTH and CHARTREUSE. ESSENTIAL OILS are distilled from the root, stem and leaves.

angels on horseback   Shelled oysters wrapped in bacon, skewered on a toothpick and then grilled.

See also DEVILS ON HORSEBACK.

angina (angina pectoris)   Paroxysmal thoracic pain and choking sensation, especially during exercise or stress, due to partial blockage of the coronary artery (the blood vessel supplying the heart), as a result of ATHEROSCLEROSIS.

angiotensin   Peptide hormone formed in the circulation by the action of RENIN (EC 3.4.23.15) on α-globulin; converted to the active vasoconstrictor angiotensin II by angiotensin converting enzyme (ACE, EC 3.4.15.1) in the lungs. Angiotensin II also stimulates secretion of ALDOSTERONE and VASOPRESSIN, so increasing blood pressure.

angiotensinogenase   *See* RENIN.

Angostura   The best known of the BITTERS, widely used in cocktails; a secret blend of herbs and spices, including the bitter aromatic bark of either of two trees of the orange family (*Galipea officinalis, Cusparia felorifuga*). Invented in 1818 by Dr Siegert in the town of Angostura in Venezuela (now called Ciudad Bolivar), originally as a medicine, and now made in Trinidad. A few drops of Angostura in GIN makes a 'pink gin'.

angstrom   A unit of length equal to 10^{-8} cm (10^{-10} m) and hence = 10 nm; not an official SI unit, but commonly used in structural chemistry and crystallography.

angular stomatitis   A characteristic cracking and fissuring of the skin at the angles of the mouth, a symptom of VITAMIN B_2 deficiency, but also seen in other conditions.

anhydrovitamin A   Isomer of retinol in which the —OH group has been removed by treatment with hydrochloric acid, with corresponding shift in the double bonds. Once incorrectly called cyclised or spurious VITAMIN A, it has very slight biological activity.

animal charcoal   *See* BONE CHARCOAL.

animal protein factor   A name given to a growth factor or factors which were found to be present in animal but not vegetable proteins, one of which was identified as VITAMIN B_{12}.

anion   A negatively charged ION.

aniseed (anise)   The dried fruit of *Pimpinella anisum*, a member of the parsley family, which is used to flavour baked goods, meat dishes and drinks, including anise, anisette and ouzo. Chief component of the volatile oil is anethole (methoxypropenyl benzene).

See also ANISE, STAR.

anise pepper   A pungent spice from the Sichuan region of China (the fruit of *Zanthoxylum piperitum*); the flavour develops gradually after biting into the pepper.

28

anise, star A spice, the seeds of *Illicium verum*, widely used in Chinese cooking. Distinct from ANISEED.

annatto (anatto) Also known as bixin, butter colour or rocou; a yellow colouring (E-160b) extracted from the pericarp of the fruit of the tropical shrub *Bixa orellana*. The main component is the CAROTENOID BIXIN, which is fat-soluble. It is used to colour cheese, dairy produce and baked goods. The seeds are used for flavouring in Caribbean foods.

annealing Heating to control the ductility of a material.

anomers A pair of stereo-ISOMERS related in the same way as α- and β-glucose are related to one another.

anona *See* CUSTARD APPLE.

anorectic drugs (anorexigenic drugs) Drugs that depress the appetite, used as an aid to weight reduction. Diethylpropion, FEN-FLURAMINE (and dexfenfluramine), phenmetrazine hydrochloride and mazindol have been used, but are no longer recommended. AMPHETAMINES were used at one time, but are addictive and subject to special control.

anorexia Lack of appetite.

anorexia nervosa A psychological disturbance resulting in a refusal to eat, possibly with restriction to a very limited range of foods, and often accompanied by a rigid programme of vigorous physical exercise, to the point of exhaustion. Anorectic subjects generally do not feel sensations of hunger. The result is a very considerable loss of weight, with tissue atrophy and a fall in BASAL METABOLIC RATE. It is especially prevalent among adolescent girls; when body weight falls below about 45 kg there is a cessation of menstruation as a result of low secretion of LEPTIN from the low reserves of ADIPOSE TISSUE.

See also BULIMIA NERVOSA.

anosmia Lack or impairment of the sense of smell.

anserine A DIPEPTIDE of β-ALANINE and 3-METHYLHISTIDINE found in MUSCLE, of unknown function.

Antabuse™ The drug disulfiram (tetraethyl thiuramdisulphide), used in the treatment of ALCOHOLISM. It inhibits the further metabolism of acetaldehyde arising from the metabolism of alcohol, and so causes headache, nausea, vomiting and palpitations if alcohol is consumed.

antacids Alkalis or BUFFERS that neutralise acids, used generally to counteract excessive gastric acidity and treat INDIGESTION. Antacid preparations generally contain such compounds as SODIUM BICARBONATE, aluminium hydroxide, magnesium carbonate or magnesium hydroxide.

anthelmintic Drugs used to treat infestation with parasitic worms (helminths).

See also FLUKES; HOOKWORM; TAPEWORM.

anthocyanidins The aglycones of ANTHOCYANINS.

anthocyanins Violet, red and blue water-soluble pigments in many flowers, fruits and leaves, used in food colours (E-163). Relatively stable to heat, light and oxygen. They can react with iron or tin, giving rise to discoloration in canned foods.

anthoxanthins Alternative name for FLAVONOIDS.

anthrone method *See* CLEGG ANTHRONE METHOD.

anthropometry Measurement of the physical dimensions and gross composition of the body as an index of development and nutritional status; a non-invasive way of assessing body composition.

Weight-for-age provides information about the overall nutritional status of children; weight-for-height is used to detect acute malnutrition (wasting); height-for-age to detect chronic malnutrition (stunting). Mid-upper arm circumference provides an index of muscle wastage in undernutrition.

SKINFOLD THICKNESS is related to the amount of subcutaneous fat as an index of over- or undernutrition.

Head circumference for age provides an index of chronic undernutrition during intrauterine development or the first two years of life.

See also BODY COMPOSITION; BODY MASS INDEX; CRISTAL HEIGHT; KNEE HEIGHT; STUNTING; TUXFORD'S INDEX; WETZEL GRID.

antibiotics Substances produced by living organisms that inhibit the growth of other organisms. The first antibiotic to be discovered was PENICILLIN, which is produced by the MOULD *Penicillium notatum* and inhibits the growth of sensitive bacteria. Many antibiotics are used to treat bacterial infections in human beings and animals; different compounds affect different bacteria.

Small amounts of antibiotics may be added to animal feed (a few grams per tonne), resulting in improved growth, possibly by controlling mild infections or changing the population of intestinal bacteria and so altering the digestion and absorption of food. To prevent the development of antibiotic-resistant strains of disease-causing bacteria, only those antibiotics that are not used clinically are permitted in animal feed (e.g. NISIN, which is also used as a food preservative (E-234)).

See also TETRACYCLINES.

antibodies A class of proteins formed in the body in response to the presence of ANTIGENS (foreign proteins and other compounds), which bind to the antigen, so inactivating it. Immunity to infection is due to the production of antibodies against specific proteins of bacteria, viruses or other disease-causing organisms, and immunisation is the process of giving these marker proteins, generally in an inactivated form, to stimulate the production of antibodies. ADVERSE REACTIONS TO FOODS (food allergies) may be due to the production of antibodies against specific food proteins. Chemically the antibodies form a class of proteins known as the γ-globulins or immunoglobulins; there are five types, classified as IgA, IgD, IgE, IgG and IgM.

A monoclonal antibody consists of a single protein species. They are produced by fusing sensitised B-lymphocytes from the spleen of an animal immunised with the ANTIGEN with myeloma cells, *in vitro*. The hybrid cells are selected by use of appropriate culture media, diluted so that individual colonies can be raised from a single cell, and therefore produce a single antibody. Theoretically permits very much more specific IMMUNOASSAY than mixed antisera raised *in vivo*, which are polyclonal antibodies.

anticaking agents Substances added in small amounts to powdered foodstuffs such as salt, icing sugar and baking powder to prevent CAKING, e.g. polyphosphates (E-544, 545), aluminium calcium silicate (E-556), calcium silicate (E-552), magnesium carbonate (E-504), calcium carbonate (E-170).

anticoagulants Compounds that prevent or slow the process of blood clotting or coagulation, either in samples of blood taken for analysis or in the body. One of the most commonly used is HEPARIN, which is formed in the lungs and liver. People at risk of thrombosis are often treated with WARFARIN and similar compounds as an anticoagulant, to reduce the risk of intravenous blood clotting. These act as antagonists of VITAMIN K in the synthesis of blood clotting proteins. Oxalate and citrate function as anticoagulants *in vitro* because they remove calcium from the blood clotting system; hirudin (from leeches) inactivates prothrombin.

See also BLOOD CLOTTING.

antidiarrhoeal agents Two groups of compounds are used to treat diarrhoea: adsorbants such as attapulgite (hydrated aluminium magnesium silicate) and kaolin (hydrated aluminium silicate), and compounds that decrease intestinal motility, such as codeine, diphenoxylate and loperamide.

See also ANTIMOTILITY AGENTS.

antidiuretic Drug used to reduce the excretion of urine and so conserve fluid in the body.

See also WATER BALANCE.

antidiuretic hormone (ADH) *See* VASOPRESSIN.

antiemetics A variety of compounds used to treat persistent vomiting, including dopamine, serotonin and muscarinic cholinergic antagonists, antihistamines, cannabinoids, corticosteroids and some of the neuroleptic agents.

antienzymes Substances that specifically inhibit the action of enzymes. Many specifically inhibit digestive enzymes and are present in raw legumes (antitrypsin and antiamylase), anti-cholinesterase (solanine), anti-invertase. Most are proteins and are therefore inactivated by heat. Many intestinal parasites are protected by antienzymes.

antifoaming agents Octanol, sulphonated oils, silicones, etc. used to reduce foaming caused by the presence of dissolved protein.

antigalactic Drug that reduces or prevents the secretion of milk in women after parturition.

antigen Any compound that is foreign to the body (e.g. bacterial, food or pollen protein, or some complex carbohydrates) which, when introduced into the circulation, stimulates the formation of an ANTIBODY.

See also ADVERSE REACTIONS TO FOODS.

anti-grey hair factor Deficiency of the VITAMIN PANTOTHENIC ACID causes loss of hair colour in black and brown rats, and at one time the vitamin was known as the anti-grey hair factor. It is not related to the loss of hair pigment in human beings.

antihaemorrhagic vitamin *See* VITAMIN K.

antihistamine Drug that antagonises the actions of HISTAMINE; those that block histamine H_1 receptors are used to treat allergic reactions; those that block H_2 receptors are used to treat peptic ULCERS.

antihypertensive Drug, diet or other treatment used to treat HYPERTENSION by lowering blood pressure.

antilipidaemic Drug, diet or other treatment used to treat HYPER-LIPIDAEMIA by lowering blood lipids.

antimetabolite Compound that inhibits a normal metabolic process, acting as an analogue of a normal metabolite. Some are useful in chemotherapy of cancer, others are naturally occurring toxins in foods, frequently causing vitamin deficiency diseases by inhibiting the normal metabolism of the vitamin.

See also ANTIVITAMINS.

antimicrobial agents Compounds used to preserve food by preventing growth of micro-organisms (bacteria and fungi).

antimony Toxic metal of no known metabolic function, so not a dietary essential. Antimony compounds are used in treatment of some parasitic diseases.

antimotility agents Drugs used to reduce gastrointestinal motility, and hence reduce the discomfort associated with DIARRHOEA: codeine phosphate, co-phenotrope (diphenoxylate plus ATROPINE SULPHATE), loperamide, morphine.

antimutagen Compound acting on cells and tissues to decrease initiation of mutation by a MUTAGEN.

antimycotics (antimould agents) Substances that inhibit the growth of MOULDS and FUNGI. Sorbates (E-200–203), benzoates

(E-210–213), propionates (E-280–283), hydroxybenzoates (E-214–219) are used in foods.

antineuritic vitamin   Obsolete name for VITAMIN B₁.

antioxidant   (1) A substance that retards the oxidative RANCIDITY of fats in stored foods. Many fats, and especially vegetable oils, contain naturally occurring antioxidants, including VITAMIN E (E-306–309), which protect them against rancidity for some time. Synthetic antioxidants include propyl, octyl and dodecyl gallates (E-310–312), butylated hydroxyanisole (BHA, E-320) and butylated hydroxytoluene (BHT, E-321).

See also INDUCTION PERIOD.

(2) Highly reactive oxygen RADICALS are formed both during normal oxidative METABOLISM and in response to infection, radiation and some chemicals. They cause damage to FATTY ACIDS in cell membranes, and the products of this damage can then cause damage to proteins and DNA. The most widely accepted theory of the biochemical basis of much CANCER, and also of ATHEROSCLEROSIS and possibly KWASHIORKOR, is that the key factor in precipitating the condition is tissue damage by radicals.

A number of different mechanisms are involved in protection against, or repair after, oxygen radical damage, involving a number of nutrients, especially VITAMIN E, CAROTENE, VITAMIN C and SELENIUM. Collectively these are known as antioxidant nutrients.

antiracchitic   Preventing or curing RICKETS.

antiscorbutic   Preventing or curing SCURVY. VITAMIN C was originally known as the antiscorbutic vitamin.

antisialagogues   Substances that reduce the flow of SALIVA.

antispasmodic   Drugs that relieve spasm of smooth muscle (e.g. intestinal muscle).

antispattering agents   Compounds such as lecithin (E-322), sucrose esters of fatty acids (E-473) and esters of mono- and diglycerides (E-472) which are added to frying oils and fats to prevent potentially dangerous spattering. They function by preventing the coalescence of water droplets.

antistaling agents   Substances that soften the crumb and retard STALING of baked products; e.g. sucrose stearate (E-473), polyoxyethylene monostearate (E-430, 431), glyceryl monostearate (E-472), stearoyl tartrate (E-483).

antivitamins   Substances that interfere with the normal metabolism or function of VITAMINS, or destroy them. Dicoumarol in spoiled sweet clover inhibits the metabolism of VITAMIN K, thiaminase in raw fish hydrolyses VITAMIN B₁, the drug methotrexate antagonises folic acid action (this is part of its mechanism of action in treating cancer), the drug isoniazid forms an inactive adduct with VITAMIN B$_6$.

antixerophthalmic vitamin *See* VITAMIN A.

antral chalone Peptide hormone secreted by the stomach; decreases gastric secretion.

antralectomy Surgical removal of the ANTRUM of the stomach, for treatment of peptic ULCERS that are resistant to other therapy.

antrum The region of the stomach adjacent to the pylorus; it secretes most of the gastric acid, PEPSIN and GASTRIN. *See* GASTROINTESTINAL TRACT.

AOAC International Originally the Association of Official Agricultural Chemists, formed in 1884 to adopt uniform methods of analysis of fertilisers; name changed in 1965 to the Association of Official Analytical Chemists. Its main purpose is to promote validation and quality assurance in analytical science, and to develop new methods. Web site http://www.aoac.org/.

AOM *See* ACTIVE OXYGEN METHOD.

aortic aneurysm *See* ANEURYSM.

apastia Refusal to take food, as an expression of a psychiatric disturbance.

> *See also* ANOREXIA NERVOSA.

aperient Any mild LAXATIVE.

APF *See* ANIMAL PROTEIN FACTOR.

APHA American Public Health Association; web site http://www.apha.org/.

aphagia Inability to swallow. Difficulty in swallowing is dysphagia.

aphagosis Inability to eat.

aphtha Small ulcers occurring singly or in groups in the mouth as small red or white spots. Cause unknown.

apiculture Bee keeping for HONEY production; derives from the Latin name of the honey bee, *Apis mellifera*.

apio Root vegetable from the legume *Apios tuberosa*, eaten like potatoes.

apo-carotenals *See* CAROTENALS.

apoenzyme The protein part of an enzyme which requires a COENZYME for activity, and is therefore inactive if the COENZYME is absent.

> *See also* ENZYME ACTIVATION ASSAYS; PROSTHETIC GROUP.

apoferritin The protein part of FERRITIN. *See* IRON STORAGE.

apolipoprotein The protein part of LIPOPROTEINS, without the associated lipid. *See* LIPOPROTEINS, PLASMA.

Apollinaris water An alkaline, highly aerated, mineral water (*see* WATER, MINERAL) containing sodium chloride and calcium, sodium and magnesium carbonates, from a spring in the valley of Ahr (in Germany).

apoptosis The process of programmed or organised cell death, as opposed to NECROSIS.

aporrhegma Any of the toxic substances formed from AMINO ACIDS during the bacterial decomposition of a protein.

aposia Absence of sensation of thirst.

apositia Aversion to food.

appendix (vermiform appendix) A residual part of the intestinal tract, a small sac-like process extending from the caecum, some 4–8 cm long. Acute inflammation, caused by an obstruction (appendicitis) can lead to perforation and peritonitis if surgery is not performed in time.

    See also GASTROINTESTINAL TRACT.

appenzeller Swiss hard cheese, washed with white wine and herbs while maturing.

appertisation French term for the process of destroying all the micro-organisms of significance in food, i.e. 'commercial sterility'; a few organisms remain alive but quiescent. Named after Nicholas Appert (1752–1841), a Paris confectioner who invented the process of CANNING, and opened the first vacuum bottling factory in 1804.

appestat *See* APPETITE CONTROL.

appetite control Hunger centres found in the lateral hypothalamus initiate feeding; satiety centres found in the ventromedial hypothalamus signal satiety. Centres found in the temporal lobe (amygdala) control learnt food behaviour.

    See also LEPTIN.

apple Fruit of the tree *Malus sylvestris* and its many cultivars and hybrids; there are more than 2000 varieties in the British National Fruit Collection. Crab apples are grown mainly for decoration and for pollination of fruit-bearing trees, although the sour fruit can be used for making jelly. Cooking apples are generally sourer varieties than dessert apples and normally have flesh which crumbles on cooking; cider apples are sour varieties especially suited to the making of CIDER.

    Composition/100 g: (edible portion 92%) water 86 g, 218 kJ (52 kcal), protein 0.3 g, fat 0.2 g, carbohydrate 13.8 g (10.4 g sugars), fibre 2.4 g, ash 0.2 g, Ca 6 mg, Fe 0.1 mg, Mg 5 mg, P 11 mg, K 107 mg, Na 1 mg, vitamin A 3 µg RE (67 µg carotenoids), E 0.2 mg, K 2.2 mg, B_1 0.02 mg, B_2 0.03 mg, niacin 0.1 mg, B_6 0.04 mg, folate 3 µg, pantothenate 0.1 mg, C 5 mg.

apple brandy SPIRIT made by distillation of CIDER, known in France as calvados.

    See also APPLE JACK.

apple butter   Apple that has been boiled in an open pan to a thick consistency; similar to apple sauce, but darker in colour owing to the prolonged boiling.

apple jack   American name for APPLE BRANDY, normally distilled, but traditionally prepared by leaving cider outside in winter, when the water froze out as ice crystals, leaving the alcoholic spirit.

apple nuggets   Crisp granules of apple of low moisture content, used commercially for manufacture of apple sauce.

apple-pear   Not a cross between apple and pear but a distinctive type of pear-shaped fruit with apple texture. Also called Japanese pear, pear-apple, and shalea or chalea.

apricot   Fruit of the tree *Prunus armeniaca*.

Composition/100 g: (edible portion 93%) water 86.3 g, 201 kJ (48 kcal), protein 1.4 g, fat 0.4 g, carbohydrate 11.1 g (9.2 g sugars), fibre 2 g, ash 0.8 g, Ca 13 mg, Fe 0.4 mg, Mg 10 mg, P 23 mg, K 259 mg, Na 1 mg, Zn 0.2 mg, Cu 0.1 mg, Mn 0.1 mg, Se 0.1 μg, vitamin A 96 μg RE (1306 μg carotenoids), E 0.9 mg, K 3.3 mg, B_1 0.03 mg, B_2 0.04 mg, niacin 0.6 mg, B_6 0.05 mg, folate 9 μg, pantothenate 0.2 mg, C 10 mg.

Apricot kernels are used to prepare ALMOND OIL; apricot kernel oil is 7% saturated, 63% mono-unsaturated, 31% polyunsaturated, vitamin E 4 mg/100 g.

AQL   Acceptable quality limit.

aquaculture   The farming of aquatic organisms, including fish, molluscs, crustaceans, echinoderms (sea urchins), cephalopods (octopus, squid, cuttlefish), reptiles (alligators, sea turtles, freshwater turtles), amphibians (frogs) and aquatic plants. Includes fresh, salt and brackish water cultivation.

aquamiel   *See* PULQUE.

aquavit (akvavit or akavit)   Scandinavian; spirit flavoured with herbs (commonly caraway, cumin, dill or fennel). Also known as snaps, and in Germany as schnapps.

aquocobalamin   *See* VITAMIN B_{12}.

arabinogalactan   Gum extracted from sap of larch trees (*Larix* spp.), also known as larch gum.

araboascorbic acid   *See* ERYTHORBIC ACID.

arachidonic acid   Polyunsaturated FATTY ACID (C20:4 ω6). Not strictly essential, since it can be formed from LINOLEIC ACID, but three times more potent than linoleic acid in curing the signs of essential fatty acid deficiency.

arachin   One of the GLOBULIN proteins from the PEANUT.

arachis oil   *See* PEANUT oil.

aragula   *See* ROCKET.

Arbroath smokie   Smoked haddock; unlike FINNAN HADDOCK not split but smoked whole to a dull copper colour.

arbute   Fruit of the South European strawberry tree (*Arbutus unedo*); resembles strawberries in appearance but with little taste and a grainy texture.

archaea   Formerly classified as bacteria, then archaebacteria, now recognised as a separate type of prokaryotic organism, genetically distinct from bacteria; they are chemo-autrophic EXTREMOPHILES, surviving at very high or very low temperatures.

areca nut   *See* BETEL.

arginase   Enzyme (EC 3.5.3.1) that hydrolyses arginine to urea and ornithine, the last stage of UREA synthesis.

argininaemia   A GENETIC DISEASE due to lack of ARGINASE affecting the formation of urea and elimination of nitrogenous waste. Depending on the severity of the condition, affected infants may become comatose and die after a moderately high intake of protein. Treatment is by severe restriction of protein intake.

  Sodium benzoate (*see* BENZOIC ACID) may be given to increase the excretion of nitrogenous waste as hippuric acid.

arginine   A basic amino acid; abbr Arg (R), M_r 174.2, pK_a 1.83, 8.99, 12.48 (guanido), CODONS CGNu, AGPu. Not a dietary essential for adult human beings, but infants may not be able to synthesise enough to meet the high demands of growth so some may be required in infant diets.

argininosuccinic aciduria   A GENETIC DISEASE due to lack of argininosuccinase (EC 4.32.2.1) affecting the formation of urea and elimination of nitrogenous waste. Depending on the severity of the condition, affected infants may become comatose and die after a moderately high intake of protein. Treatment is by restriction of protein intake and feeding supplements of the amino acid arginine, which permits elimination of nitrogenous waste as argininosuccinic acid.

  Sodium benzoate (*see* BENZOIC ACID) may be given to increase the excretion of nitrogenous waste as hippuric acid.

argol   Crust of crude CREAM OF TARTAR (potassium acid tartrate) which forms on the sides of wine vats, also called wine stone. It consists of 50–85% potassium hydrogen tartrate and 6–12% calcium tartrate, and will be coloured by the grapes, so white argol comes from white grapes and red argol from red grapes. Used in VINEGAR fermentation, in the manufacture of TARTARIC ACID and as a mordant in dyeing.

ariboflavinosis   Deficiency of riboflavin (VITAMIN B$_2$) characterised by swollen, cracked, bright red lips (cheilosis), an enlarged, tender magenta-red tongue (glossitis), cracking at the corners of the mouth (angular stomatitis), congestion of the blood vessels of the conjunctiva and a characteristic dermatitis with filiform (wire-like) excrescences.

arkshell *See* COCKLES.

armagnac BRANDY made from white wine from one of three defined areas of France: Bas-Armagnac, Haut-Armagnac or Ténarèze.

See also COGNAC.

Armenian bole Ferric oxide (iron oxide), either occurring naturally as haematite or prepared by heating ferrous sulphate and other iron salts. Used in metallurgy, polishing compounds, paint pigment and as a food colour (E-172).

Arogel^{TM} Potato starch preparation that is stable to heating and is used as a thickener in gravies, sauces and canned foods.

Aros *See* P. 4000.

arracacha Also know as Peruvian carrot, Andean (Colombian) root vegetable from the legume *Arracacia xanthoriza*, eaten like potatoes or to make a flour.

arrowhead Aquatic plants (*Sagittaria sagittifolia* and *S. chinensis*); both leaves and starchy root used in Chinese cooking. Also known as tule potato or wappato.

Composition/100 g: (edible portion 75%) water 72.5 g, 414 kJ (99 kcal), protein 5.3 g, fat 0.3 g, carbohydrate 20.2 g, ash 1.7 g, Ca 10 mg, Fe 2.6 mg, Mg 51 mg, P 174 mg, K 922 mg, Na 22 mg, Zn 0.3 mg, Cu 0.2 mg, Mn 0.4 mg, Se 0.7 µg, B_1 0.17 mg, B_2 0.07 mg, niacin 1.6 mg, B_6 0.26 mg, folate 14 µg, pantothenate 0.6 mg, C 1 mg.

arrowroot Tuber of the Caribbean plant *Maranta arundinacea*, mainly used to prepare arrowroot starch, a pure starch, used to thicken sauces and in bland, low-salt and protein-restricted diets.

Composition/100 g: (edible portion 85%) water 80.8 g, 272 kJ (65 kcal), protein 4.2 g, fat 0.2 g, carbohydrate 13.4 g, fibre 1.3 g, ash 1.4 g, Ca 6 mg, Fe 2.2 mg, Mg 25 mg, P 98 mg, K 454 mg, Na 26 mg, Zn 0.6 mg, Cu 0.1 mg, Mn 0.2 mg, Se 0.7 µg, vitamin A 1 µg RE (11 µg carotenoids), B_1 0.14 mg, B_2 0.06 mg, niacin 1.7 mg, B_6 0.27 mg, folate 338 µg, pantothenate 0.3 mg, C 2 mg.

Arrowroot flour, composition/100 g: water 11.4 g, 1494 kJ (357 kcal), protein 0.3 g, fat 0.1 g, carbohydrate 88.2 g, fibre 3.4 g, ash 0.1 g, Ca 40 mg, Fe 0.3 mg, Mg 3 mg, P 5 mg, K 11 mg, Na 2 mg, Zn 0.1 mg, Mn 0.5 mg, folate 7 µg, pantothenate 0.1 mg.

arroz fermentado (arroz amarillo) *See* RICE, FERMENTED.

arsenic A toxic metal, with no known metabolic function. Organic arsenic derivatives (arsenicals) have been used as pesticides and in treatment of diseases such as syphilis, leprosy and yaws. Arsenic can accumulate in crops treated with arsenical pesticides, and in fish and shellfish living in arsenic-polluted water.

arteriolsclerosis Thickening of the walls of the arterioles due to ageing or HYPERTENSION.

arteriosclerosis   Thickening and calcification of the arterial walls, leading to loss of elasticity, occurring with ageing and especially in HYPERTENSION.

See also ATHEROMA; ATHEROSCLEROSIS.

artichoke, Chinese   Tubers of *Stachys affinis*, similar to Jerusalem ARTICHOKE but smaller.

artichoke, globe   Young flower heads of *Cynara scolymus*; the edible part is the fleshy bracts and the base; the choke is the inedible filaments.

Composition/100 g: (edible portion 40%) water 84.9 g, 197 kJ (47 kcal), protein 3.3 g, fat 0.2 g, carbohydrate 10.5 g, fibre 5.4 g, ash 1.1 g, Ca 44 mg, Fe 1.3 mg, Mg 60 mg, P 90 mg, K 370 mg, Na 94 mg, Zn 0.5 mg, Cu 0.2 mg, Mn 0.3 mg, Se 0.2 µg, K 14 mg, B_1 0.07 mg, B_2 0.07 mg, niacin 1 mg, B_6 0.12 mg, folate 68 µg, pantothenate 0.3 mg, C 12 mg. A 100 g serving (1 artichoke) is a source of Cu, Mn, P, a good source of Mg, vitamin C, a rich source of folate.

artichoke, Japanese   Tubers of the perennial plant *Stachys sieboldi*, similar to Jerusalem ARTICHOKE.

artichoke, Jerusalem   Tubers of *Helianthus tuberosus*. The origin of the name Jerusalem is from the Italian *girasole* (sunflower). Introduced to Europe from Canada by Samuel de Champlain in 1616, and originally called Canadian artichoke. Much of the carbohydrate is the NON-STARCH POLYSACCHARIDE INULIN.

Composition/100 g: (edible portion 69%) water 78 g, 318 kJ (76 kcal), protein 2 g, fat 0 g, carbohydrate 17.4 g (9.6 g sugars), fibre 1.6 g, ash 2.5 g, Ca 14 mg, Fe 3.4 mg, Mg 17 mg, P 78 mg, K 429 mg, Na 4 mg, Zn 0.1 mg, Cu 0.1 mg, Mn 0.1 mg, Se 0.7 µg, vitamin A 1 µg RE (12 µg carotenoids), E 0.2 mg, K 0.1 mg, B_1 0.2 mg, B_2 0.06 mg, niacin 1.3 mg, B_6 0.08 mg, folate 13 µg, pantothenate 0.4 mg, C 4 mg. A 120 g serving is a source of P, vitamin B_1, a good source of Fe.

artificial sweeteners   *See* SWEETENERS, INTENSE.

asafoetida   A resin extracted from the oriental umbelliferous plant *Narthex asafoetida*, with a bitter flavour and strong garlic-like odour, used widely in oriental and Middle Eastern cooking, and in small amounts in sauces and pickles. (The strength of its aroma is suggested by its French and German names: *merde du diable* Fr, *Teufelsdreck* Ger.)

ascariasis   Intestinal infestation with the parasitic nematode worm *Ascaris lumbricoides*.

ascites   Abnormal accumulation of fluid in the peritoneal cavity, occurring as a complication of cirrhosis of the liver, congestive heart failure, cancer and infectious diseases. Depending on the underlying cause, treatment may sometimes consist of a high-energy, high-protein, low-sodium diet, together with diuretic drugs and fluid restriction.

ascorbic acid VITAMIN C, chemically L-xyloascorbic acid, to distinguish it from the ISOMER D-araboascorbic acid (isoascorbic acid or erythorbic acid), which has only slight vitamin C activity. Both ascorbic acid and erythorbic acid have strong chemical reducing properties, and are used as ANTIOXIDANTS in foods and to preserve the red colour of fresh and preserved meats, and in the curing of hams.

ascorbate   monodehydroascorbate   dehydroascorbate
(semidehydroascorbate)

ASCORBIC ACID AND DEHYDROASCORBATE

ascorbic acid, monodehydro Or semidehydro, a free RADICAL which is the intermediate stage in the oxidation of ASCORBIC ACID to dehydroascorbic acid; it has a relatively long half-life compared with other radicals, and can undergo enzymic or non-enzymic reaction to yield ascorbic acid and dehydroascorbic acid.

ascorbic acid oxidase An enzyme (EC 1.10.3.3) in plant tissues that oxidises ASCORBIC ACID to dehydroascorbic acid. In the intact fresh plant the enzyme is separated from the ascorbic acid, and is only released when the plant wilts or is cut; in addition to the loss of vitamin C, this is important in BROWNING REACTIONS.

ascorbyl palmitate An ester of ASCORBIC ACID and PALMITIC ACID used as an ANTISTALING compound in bakery goods (E-304).

ascorbyl stearate An ester of ASCORBIC ACID and STEARIC ACID; a fat-soluble form of the vitamin used as an ANTIOXIDANT.

aseptic processing Heat sterilisation of foods before filling into pre-sterilised (aseptic) containers.

See also CANNING.

ash The residue left behind after all organic matter has been burnt off, a measure of the total content of mineral salts in a food.

ASN American Society for Nutrition; web site http://www. asnutrition.org/.

ASO Association for the Study of Obesity; web site http://www.aso.org.uk/.

asparagine A non-essential AMINO ACID, chemically the β-amide of ASPARTIC ACID; abbr Asn (N), M_r 132.1, pK_a 2.1, 8.84, CODONS AAPy.

asparagus The young shoots of the plant *Asparagus officinalis*, originally known in England as sparrow grass (17th century).

Composition/100 g: (edible portion 53%) water 93.2 g, 84 kJ (20 kcal), protein 2.2 g, fat 0.1 g, carbohydrate 3.9 g (1.9 g sugars), fibre 2.1 g, ash 0.6 g, Ca 24 mg, Fe 2.1 mg, Mg 14 mg, P 52 mg, K 202 mg, Na 2 mg, Zn 0.5 mg, Cu 0.2 mg, Mn 0.2 mg, Se 2.3 μg, vitamin A 38 μg RE (1168 μg carotenoids), E 1.1 mg, K 41.6 mg, B$_1$ 0.14 mg, B$_2$ 0.14 mg, niacin 1 mg, B$_6$ 0.09 mg, folate 52 μg, pantothenate 0.3 mg, C 6 mg. A 60 g serving (5 spears) is a source of folate.

aspartame An artificial SWEETENER, β-aspartyl-phenylalanine methyl ester, some 200 times as sweet as sucrose. Stable for a few months in solution, then gradually breaks down. Used in soft drinks, dessert mixes and as a 'table top sweetener'. Trade names Canderel, Equal, Nutrasweet, Sanecta.

Because aspartame contains PHENYLALANINE, it is specifically recommended that children with PHENYLKETONURIA avoid consuming it, although the amounts that would be consumed are extremely small.

See also ALITAME.

aspartic acid (aspartate) A non-essential AMINO ACID; abbr Asp (D), M_r 133.1, pK_a 1.99, 3.90, 9.90, CODONS GAPy.

aspartyl-phenylalanine methyl ester *See* ASPARTAME.

ASPEN American Society for Parenteral and Enteral Nutrition; web site http://www.clinnutr.org/.

Aspergillus A family of moulds, important in the spoiling of stored nuts and grains because *A. flavus* produces AFLATOXINS. *A. oryzae* is grown commercially as a source of TAKADIASTASE (fungal AMYLASE).

aspic jelly A clear jelly made from fish, chicken or meat stock, sometimes with added GELATINE, flavoured with lemon, tarragon, vinegar, sherry, peppercorns and vegetables, used to glaze foods such as meat, fish and game. The name may be derived from the herb espic or spikenard.

assize of bread English; courts to prosecute bakers selling under-weight or over-priced bread (established 1266, repealed 1815).

astaxanthin A CAROTENOID, the pink colour of salmon and trout muscle; not VITAMIN A active.

astringency The action of unripe fruits and cider apples, among other foods, to cause a contraction of the epithelial tissues of the tongue (literally astringency means 'a drawing together'). It is believed to result from a destruction of the lubricant properties of SALIVA because of precipitation by TANNINS.

Ateromixol™ *See* POLICOSANOLS.

atheroma The fatty deposit composed of lipids, complex carbohydrates and fibrous tissue which forms on the inner wall of blood vessels in ATHEROSCLEROSIS.

atherosclerosis Degenerative disease of the arteries in which there is accumulation on the inner wall of lipids together with complex carbohydrates and fibrous tissue, called ATHEROMA. This leads to narrowing of the lumen of the arteries. When it occurs in the coronary artery it can lead to failure of the blood supply to the heart muscle (ISCHAEMIA).

See also ARTERIOSCLEROSIS.

athletae Roman; unleavened bread mixed with curd cheese.

atholl brose Scottish beverage made from malt whisky, honey, cream and oatmeal.

Atkins diet A KETOGENIC DIET originally proposed in 1972, in which carbohydrate intake is strictly limited but fat and protein are permitted in unlimited amounts. It is effective for weight loss, since ketonaemia reduces appetite; fat and protein may be more satiating than carbohydrates, and the energy cost of GLUCONEO-GENESIS from amino acids to maintain blood glucose increases metabolic rate, but it runs counter to all modern advice on a prudent diet.

atomic absorption spectrometry Technique for measurement of a variety of metals in a flame or heated gas, in the atomic state, by absorption of light at a wavelength specific for each element.

atomisation The process of converting a liquid or slurry into a fine spray suitable for spray drying.

atomiser Apparatus for ATOMISATION of liquids or slurries.

ATP Adenosine triphosphate, the coenzyme that acts as an intermediate between energy-yielding (catabolic) METABOLISM (the oxidation of metabolic fuels) and ENERGY EXPENDITURE as physical work and in synthetic (anabolic) reactions. ADP (adenosine diphosphate) is phosphorylated to ATP linked to oxidations; in energy expenditure ATP is hydrolysed to ADP and phosphate ions.

See also ADENINE; PURINES.

atrophy Wasting of normally-developed tissue or muscle as a result of disuse, ageing or undernutrition.

atropine One of the belladonna ALKALOIDS; anticholinergic compound acting on muscarinic receptors. Acts as a smooth muscle relaxant, used as the sulphate in treatment of DYSPEPSIA, IRRITABLE BOWEL SYNDROME and DIVERTICULAR DISEASE. Synthetic compounds with similar action and uses, but fewer central nervous system actions, include dicyclomine, dicycloverine, propantheline and hyoscine.

See also ANTIMOTILITY AGENTS.

attapulgite   *See* ANTIDIARRHOEAL AGENTS.

Atwater factors   *See* ENERGY CONVERSION FACTORS.

aubergine   The fruit of *Solanum melongena*, a native of SE Asia, widely cultivated and eaten as a vegetable, also known as eggplant and (in W Africa) field egg.

Composition/100 g: (edible portion 81%) water 92.4 g, 100 kJ (24 kcal), protein 1 g, fat 0.2 g, carbohydrate 5.7 g (2.3 g sugars), fibre 3.4 g, ash 0.7 g, Ca 9 mg, Fe 0.2 mg, Mg 14 mg, P 25 mg, K 230 mg, Na 2 mg, Zn 0.2 mg, Cu 0.1 mg, Mn 0.3 mg, Se 0.3 µg, vitamin A 1 µg RE (16 µg carotenoids), E 0.3 mg, K 3.5 mg, B_1 0.04 mg, B_2 0.04 mg, niacin 0.6 mg, B_6 0.08 mg, folate 22 µg, pantothenate 0.3 mg, C 2 mg. A 230 g serving (half fruit) is a source of Cu, pantothenate, a good source of folate, a rich source of Mn.

audit ale   Strong BEER originally brewed at Oxford and Cambridge Universities to be drunk on 'audit days'.

aurantiamarin   A GLUCOSIDE present in the ALBEDO of the bitter orange which is partly responsible for its flavour.

aureomycin   Oxytetracycline, one of the TETRACYCLINE ANTIBIOTICS.

autoclave   A vessel in which high temperatures can be achieved by using high pressure; the domestic pressure cooker is an example.

At atmospheric pressure water boils at 100 °C; at 5 lb (35 kPa) above atmospheric pressure the boiling point is 109 °C; at 10 lb (70 kPa), 115 °C; at 15 lb (105 kPa), 121 °C and at 20 lb (140 kPa), 126 °C.

Autoclaves have two major uses. In cooking, the higher temperature reduces the time needed. At these higher temperatures and under moist conditions, bacteria are destroyed more rapidly, so permitting sterilisation of foods, surgical dressings and instruments, etc.

autocrine   Production by a cell of hormones or growth factors that influence the growth of the cell producing them.

See also ENDOCRINE GLANDS; PARACRINE.

autoimmune disease   Condition in which ANTIBODIES are produced against normal body tissues (autoantibodies). May be a cause of pernicious ANAEMIA, some forms of HYPOTHYROIDISM and perhaps insulin-dependent DIABETES mellitus.

autolysis   Process of self-digestion catalysed by the hydrolytic enzymes normally contained in lysosomes. Responsible for the softening of meat when hung, as a result of hydrolysis of CON-NECTIVE TISSUE proteins. YEAST EXTRACT is produced by autolysis of yeast.

automat Automatic restaurant in which customers place a coin in the slot to permit them to open glass doors and obtain food, originally developed in Germany; the first in USA was opened by Horn and Hardart in Philadelphia in 1902; the last, in New York, closed in 1991.

autopyron Roman; coarse unleavened bread made from bran and only a little flour, mainly fed to slaves.

Autotrak™   *See* DEFT.

autotrophes Organisms that can synthesise all the compounds required for growth from simple inorganic salts, as distinct from heterotrophes, which must be supplied with complex organic compounds. Plants are autotrophes, whereas animals are heterotrophes. Bacteria may be of either type; heterotrophic bacteria are responsible for food spoilage and disease.

autoxidation Radical chain reaction leading to oxidation of unsaturated fatty acids in fats and oils, forming hydroperoxides that decompose to form off-flavour compounds (secondary oxidation products).

auxin A plant hormone produced by shoot tips, responsible for controlling cell growth and differentiation, and frequently used as a rooting hormone for cuttings. Chemically indoleacetic acid and related compounds.

auxotrophe Mutant strain of micro-organism that requires one or more nutrients for growth that are not required by the parent organism. Commonly used for microbiological assay of vitamins, amino acids, etc.

availability Also known as bioavailability or biological availability. In some foodstuffs, nutrients that can be demonstrated to be present chemically may not be available, or only partially so, when they are eaten. This is because the nutrients are chemically bound in a form that is not susceptible to enzymic digestion, although it is susceptible to the strong acid or alkali HYDROLYSIS used in chemical analysis. For example, the NIACIN in cereal grains, CALCIUM bound to PHYTIC ACID, and LYSINE combined with sugars in the Maillard complex (*see* MAILLARD REACTION), are all biologically unavailable.

See also AVAILABLE LYSINE.

available carbon dioxide *See* BAKING POWDER; FLOUR, SELF-RAISING.

available lysine Not all of the LYSINE in proteins is biologically available, since some is linked through the ε-amino group, either to sugars in the Maillard complex (*see* MAILLARD REACTION), or to

other AMINO ACIDS. These linkages are not HYDROLYSED by digestive enzymes, and so the lysine cannot be absorbed.

Available lysine is that proportion of the protein-bound lysine
in which the ε-amino group is free, so that it can be absorbed
after digestion of the protein.

avenalin, avenin   PROTEINS present in oats. Avenalin is a globulin,
avenin a PROLAMIN, and the major storage protein in the cereal.

avern jelly   Scottish; jelly made from wild strawberries.

aversion to foods   *See* ADVERSE REACTIONS TO FOODS.

Avicel^{TM} FAT REPLACER made from NON-STARCH POLYSACCHARIDE.

avidin   Protein in white of eggs that binds BIOTIN with very high
affinity.

avitaminosis   The absence of a VITAMIN; may be used specifically,
as, for example, avitaminosis A, or generally, to mean any vitamin
deficiency disease.

avocado   Fruit of the tree *Persica americana*, also known as the
avocado pear or alligator pear, because of its rough skin and pear
shape, although it is not related to the PEAR. It is unusual among
fruits for its high fat content, of which 12% is LINOLEIC ACID, and
also for the fact that it does not ripen until after it has been
removed from the tree.

Composition/100 g: (edible portion 74%) water 73.2 g, 670 kJ
(160 kcal), protein 2 g, fat 14.7 g (of which 15% saturated, 72%
mono-unsaturated, 13% polyunsaturated), carbohydrate 8.5 g
(0.7 g sugars), fibre 6.7 g, ash 1.6 g, Ca 12 mg, Fe 0.6 mg, Mg 29 mg,
P 52 mg, K 485 mg, Na 7 mg, Zn 0.6 mg, Cu 0.2 mg, Mn 0.1 mg, Se
0.4 µg, I 2 µg, vitamin A 7 µg RE (385 µg carotenoids), E 2.1 mg,
K 21 mg, B_1 0.07 mg, B_2 0.13 mg, niacin 1.7 mg, B_6 0.26 mg, folate
81 µg, pantothenate 1.4 mg, C 10 mg. A 75 g serving (half fruit)
is a source of Cu, vitamin E, pantothenate, C, a rich source of
folate.

avron   *See* CLOUDBERRY.

awule bolo   *See* AKPITI.

axerol, axerophthol   Early names for VITAMIN A.

azeotrope   A mixture of two liquids that boils at a constant composition, so that the composition of the vapour is the same as
that of the liquid.

azlon   Textile fibres produced from proteins such as CASEIN and
ZEIN.

azodicarbonamide   A dough conditioner used in ageing and
bleaching FLOUR.

azo dyes   Synthetic chemicals used as dyestuffs and food colours,
made by reacting a diazonium salt with a phenol or aromatic
AMINE. Also known as diazo or diazonium compounds.

azorubin(e)   A red colour, carmoisine (E-122).

Azotobacter   Genus of free-living soil bacteria of family Bacteri-aceae which can reduce nitrogen gas to ammonia, and hence fix nitrogen for incorporation into amino acids, etc.
See also NITROGENASE.

B

baba   A French cake supposedly invented by King Stanislas I of Poland and named after Ali Baba. 'Rum baba' is flavoured with rum; a French modification using a 'secret' syrup was called brillat-savarin or savarin.

babaco   The seedless fruit of the tree *Carica pentagona*, related to the PAWPAW, discovered in Ecuador in the 1920s, introduced into New Zealand in 1973, and more recently into the Channel Islands.

babassu oil   Edible oil from the wild Brazilian palm nut (*Orbignya matiana* or *O. oleiferae*), similar in fatty acid composition to COCONUT oil, and used for food and in soaps and cosmetics. 86% saturated, 12% mono-unsaturated, 2% polyunsaturated, vitamin E 19 mg/100 g.

Babcock test   For fat in milk; the sample is mixed with sulphuric acid in a long-necked Babcock bottle, centrifuged, diluted and recentrifuged. The amount of fat is read off the neck of the bottle.

bacalao   *See* KLIPFISH.

Bacillus cereus   SPORE-forming bacterium in cereals (especially rice), cause of food poisoning by production of ENTEROTOXINS in the food (emetic type TX 1.3.6.1) or in the gut (diarrhoeal type TX 2.1.1.1–2). Infective dose 10^5–10^7 organisms, emetic type onset 1–6 h, duration 6–24 h; diarrhoeal type onset 6–12 h, duration 12–24 h.

bacon   Cured (and sometimes smoked) meat from the back, sides and belly of a pig; variety of cuts with differing fat contents. Gammon is bacon made from the top of the hind legs; green bacon has been cured but not smoked.

Composition/100 g: water 40 g, 1917 kJ (458 kcal), protein 11.6 g, fat 45 g (of which 38% saturated, 50% mono-unsaturated, 12% polyunsaturated), carbohydrate 0.7 g, ash 2.5 g, Ca 6 mg, Fe 0.5 mg, Mg 12 mg, P 188 mg, K 208 mg, Na 833 mg, Zn 1.2 mg, Cu 0.1 mg, Se 20.2 μg, vitamin A 11 μg RE (11 μg retinol), E 0.3 mg, B_1 0.28 mg, B_2 0.11 mg, niacin 3.8 mg, B_6 0.21 mg, folate 2 μg, B_{12} 0.7 μg, pantothenate 0.5 mg. An 80 g serving (2 rashers) is a source of P, vitamin B_1, niacin, a good source of Se, a rich source of vitamin B_{12}.

bacteria   Unicellular micro-organisms, ranging between 0.5 and 5 μm in size. They may be classified on the basis of their shape: spherical (coccus); rodlike (bacilli); spiral (spirillum); comma-shaped (vibrio); corkscrew-shaped (spirochaetes) or filamentous.

Other classifications are based on whether or not they are stained by Gram stain, AEROBIC or anaerobic, and autotrophic (*see* AUTOTROPHES) or heterotrophic.

Some bacteria form spores, which are relatively resistant to heat and sterilising agents. Bacteria are responsible for much food spoilage, and for disease (pathogenic bacteria that produce toxins), but they are also made use of, for example in the PICK-LING process and FERMENTATION of milk, as well as in the manufacture of VITAMINS and AMINO ACIDS and a variety of enzymes and HORMONES.

Between 45 and 85% of the dry matter of bacteria is protein, and some can be grown on petroleum residues, methane or methanol, for use in animal feed.

bacterial count *See* PLATE COUNT.

bacterial filter A filter 0.5–5 µm in diameter (fine enough to prevent the passage of BACTERIA); permits removal of bacteria and hence sterilisation of solutions. Viruses are considerably smaller, and will pass through a bacterial filter.

bactericidal Conditions or compounds that are capable of killing bacteria.

See also BACTERIOSTATIC.

bacteriocins Antibiotic peptides produced by lactic acid bacteria and some other micro-organisms to inhibit the growth of others.

See also PROBIOTICS.

bacteriophage Viruses that attack bacteria, commonly known as phages. They pass through BACTERIAL FILTERS, and can be a cause of considerable trouble in bacterial cultures (e.g. milk starter cultures). Each phage acts specifically against a particular species of bacterium; this can be exploited in phage typing as a means of identifying bacteria.

bacteriostatic Conditions or compounds that are capable of inhibiting growth of bacteria, but are not BACTERICIDAL.

Bacterium aceti *See* ACETOBACTER.

Bactofoss™ *See* BIOLUMINESCENCE.

bactofugation Belgian process for removing bacteria from milk using a high-speed CENTRIFUGE.

bactometer A device for the rapid estimation of bacterial contamination (within a few hours) based on measuring the early stages of breakdown of nutrients by the bacteria through changes in the electrical impedance of the medium.

Bactoscan™ *See* DEFT.

badderlocks   Edible seaweed (*Alaria esculenta*) found on northern British coasts and around Faroe Islands. Known as honeyware in Scotland.

bagasse   The residue from sugar-cane milling, consisting of the crushed stalks from which the juice has been expressed; it consists of 50% CELLULOSE, 25% HEMICELLULOSES and 25% LIGNIN. It is used as a fuel, for cattle feed and in the manufacture of paper and fibre board. The name is sometimes also applied to the residues of other plants, such as sugar beet, which is sometimes incorporated into foods as a source of dietary fibre.

bagel   A circular BREAD roll with a hole in the middle, made from fermented wheat flour dough with egg, which is boiled before being baked. Traditionally a Jewish specialty.

bagoong   Philippines; salted paste made from shrimps and small fish.

baguette   A French BREAD, a long thin loaf about 60 cm long, weighing 250 g, with a crisp crust.

bain marie   A double saucepan named after the medieval alchemist Maria de Cleofa.

bajoa   *See* MILLET.

baked apple berry   *See* CLOUDBERRY.

baker's cheese   *See* COTTAGE CHEESE.

baker's yeast glycan   Dried cell walls of yeast, *Saccharomyces cerevisiae*, used as an emulsifier and thickener.

baking additives   Materials added to flour products for a variety of purposes, including bleaching the flour, AGEING, slowing the rate of staling and improving the texture of the finished product.

baking blind   A pastry case for a tart or flan, baked empty and then filled.

baking powder   A mixture that liberates carbon dioxide when moistened and heated. The source of carbon dioxide is sodium bicarbonate, and an acid is required. This may be CREAM OF TARTAR (in fast-acting baking powders which liberate carbon dioxide in the dough before heating) or calcium acid phosphate, sodium pyrophosphate or sodium aluminium sulphate (in slow-acting powders, which liberate most of the carbon dioxide during heating).

Legally, baking powder must contain not less than 8% available, and not more than 1.5% residual, carbon dioxide.

Golden raising powder is similar, but is coloured yellow (formerly known as egg substitute), and must contain not less than 6% available, and not more than 1.5% residual, carbon dioxide.

baking soda   *See* SODIUM BICARBONATE.

Balade™ Low-CHOLESTEROL butter, prepared by mixing CYCLODEXTRIN with the melted butter.

balance (1) With reference to diet, positive balance is a net gain to the body and negative balance a net loss from the body. When intake equals excretion the body is in equilibrium or balance with respect to the nutrient in question. Used in reference to nitrogen (protein), mineral salts and energy.

(2) A balanced diet is one containing all nutrients in appropriate amounts.

(3) A weighing device.

balanced coil system For detection of metal in foods. The food is passed between coils that produce a balanced electrical field. When metal is introduced, the balanced state is disturbed, generating a voltage in the coils. Detects magnetic and non-magnetic metals, but not in aluminium cans. *See also* MAGNETIC FIELD SYSTEM.

balantidiasis Infestation of the large intestine with the parasitic protozoan *Balantidum coli*. A rare cause of DYSENTERY.

Balling A table of specific gravity of sugar solutions published by von Balling in 1843, giving the weight of cane sugar in 100 g of a solution for the specific gravity determined at 17.5 °C. It is used to calculate the percentage extract in BEER WORT. The original table was corrected for slight inaccuracies by Plato in 1900, and extracts are referred to as per cent Plato.

ball mill Machine for COMMINUTION of dry foods; a rotating cylinder containing steel balls. With small balls or slow rotation shearing forces predominate; at higher speeds or with larger balls impact forces predominate.

See also ROD MILL.

balm A herb (*Melissa officinalis*) with hairy leaves and a lemon scent, therefore often known as lemon balm. Used for its flavour in fruit salads, sweet or savoury sauces, etc., as well as for preparation of herb teas. Claimed to have calming medicinal properties, and promoted at one time as an elixir of life and a cure for impotence; it is rich in tannins.

balsalazide *See* AMINOSALICYLATES.

balsam peru oil A flavouring agent with a sweet balsamic odour, extracted from Peruvian balsam (*Myroxylon pereirae*).

bambarra groundnut Also known as the Madagascar peanut or earth pea, *Voandseia subterranea*. It resembles the true GROUND-NUT, but the seeds are low in oil. They are hard and require soaking or pounding before cooking.

bamboo shoots Thick pointed young shoots of *Bambusa vulgaris* and *Phyllostachys pubescens* eaten as a vegetable.

Composition/100 g: (edible portion 29%) water 91 g, 113 kJ (27 kcal), protein 2.6 g, fat 0.3 g, carbohydrate 5.2 g (3 g sugars), fibre 2.2 g, ash 0.9 g, Ca 13 mg, Fe 0.5 mg, Mg 3 mg, P 59 mg, K 533 mg, Na 4 mg, Zn 1.1 mg, Cu 0.2 mg, Mn 0.3 mg, Se 0.8 µg, vitamin A 1 µg RE (12 µg carotenoids), E 1 mg, B_1 0.15 mg, B_2 0.07 mg, niacin 0.6 mg, B_6 0.24 mg, folate 7 µg, pantothenate 0.2 mg, C 4 mg.

bamboo tea Chinese; bitter black tea, so-called because it is encased in bamboo leaves.

bamies, bamya *See* OKRA.

banana Fruit of the genus *Musa*; cultivated kinds are sterile hybrids, and so cannot be given species names. Dessert bananas have a high sugar content (17–19%) and are eaten raw; PLANTAINS (sometimes known as green bananas) have a higher starch and lower sugar content and are picked when too hard to be eaten raw.

Composition/100 g: (edible portion 64%) water 74.9 g, 373 kJ (89 kcal), protein 1.1 g, fat 0.3 g, carbohydrate 22.8 g (12.2 g sugars), fibre 2.6 g, ash 0.8 g, Ca 5 mg, Fe 0.3 mg, Mg 27 mg, P 22 mg, K 358 mg, Na 1 mg, Zn 0.2 mg, Cu 0.1 mg, Mn 0.3 mg, Se 1 µg, I 8 µg, vitamin A 3 µg RE (73 µg carotenoids), E 0.1 mg, K 0.5 mg, B_1 0.03 mg, B_2 0.07 mg, niacin 0.7 mg, B_6 0.37 mg, folate 20 µg, pantothenate 0.3 mg, C 9 mg. A 100 g serving (one banana) is a source of Mn, vitamin B_6, C.

banana, baking American name for PLANTAIN.

banana, false The fruit of *Ensete ventricosum*, related to the banana. The fruits are small and, unlike bananas, contain seeds. The rhizome and inner tissue of the stem are eaten after cooking; a major part of the diet in southern Ethiopia.

banana figs Bananas that have been split longitudinally and sundried without treating with SULPHUR DIOXIDE. The product is dark in colour and sticky.

banian days Days on which no meat was served; named after Banian (Hindu) merchants who abstained from eating meat. An obsolete term for 'days of short commons'.

banku *See* AKPITI.

bannock A flat round cake made from oat, rye or barley meal and baked on a hearth or griddle. Pitcaithly bannock is a type of almond shortbread containing CARAWAY seeds and chopped peel.

Bantu beer *See* BEER.

bap Traditionally a soft, white, flat, flour-coated Scottish breakfast roll. Now also used for any relatively large soft-crusted roll, made from white, brown or wholemeal flour.

BAPEN British Association for Parenteral and Enteral Nutrition; web site http://www.bapen.org.uk/.

bara brith *See* BARM BRACK.

bara lawr *See* LAVER.

Barbados cherry *See* CHERRY, WEST INDIAN.

Barbados sugar *See* SUGAR.

barbecue   Originally native American name for a wooden frame used to smoke and dry meat over a slow smoky fire; the whole animal was placed on a spit over burning coals. Now outdoor cooking of meat, sausages, etc., on a charcoal or gas fire; also the fire on which they are cooked.

barberry   Fruits of *Berberis* spp.

barberry fig   *See* PRICKLY PEAR.

Barcelona nut   Spanish variety of HAZEL NUT (*Corylus avellana*).

barium   A metal of no known metabolic function, so not a dietary essential. Barium sulphate is opaque to X-rays and a suspension is used (a barium meal) to allow examination of the shape and movements of the stomach for diagnostic purposes, and as a barium enema for X-ray investigation of the lower intestinal tract.

barley   Grain of *Hordeum vulgare*, one of the hardiest of the CEREALS; mainly used as animal feed and for malting and brewing. The whole grain with only the outer husk removed (pot, Scotch or hulled barley) requires several hours cooking; the commercial product is usually pearl barley, where most of the husk and germ is removed. Barley flour is ground pearl barley; barley flakes are the flattened grain.

Composition/100 g: water 9.4 g, 1482 kJ (354 kcal), protein 12.5 g, fat 2.3 g (of which 26% saturated, 16% mono-unsaturated, 58% polyunsaturated), carbohydrate 73.5 g (0.8 g sugars), fibre 17.3 g, ash 2.3 g, Ca 33 mg, Fe 3.6 mg, Mg 133 mg, P 264 mg, K 452 mg, Na 12 mg, Zn 2.8 mg, Cu 0.5 mg, Mn 1.9 mg, Se 37.7 μg, vitamin A 1 μg RE (173 μg carotenoids), E 0.6 mg, K 2.2 mg, B_1 0.65 mg, B_2 0.28 mg, niacin 4.6 mg, B_6 0.32 mg, folate 19 μg, pantothenate 0.3 mg. A 100 g serving is a source of Zn, vitamin B_2, B_6, a good source of Fe, niacin, a rich source of Cu, Mg, Mn, P, Se, vitamin B_1.

barleycorn   An obsolete measure of length; the size of a single grain of barley, 0.85 cm.

barley, malted   *See* MALT.

barley sugar   SUGAR confectionery made by melting and cooling sugar, originally made by boiling with a decoction of barley.

barley water   A drink made by boiling pearl barley with water, commonly flavoured with orange or lemon.

barley wine   Fermented malted barley, stronger than BEER (8–10% ALCOHOL by volume), bottled under pressure, so sparkling.

Barlow's disease   Infantile SCURVY, also known as Moeller's disease or Cheadle's disease.

barm   An alternative name for YEAST or leaven, or the froth on fermenting malt liquor. Spon (short for spontaneous) or virgin barm is made by allowing wild yeast to fall into sugar medium and multiply.

barm brack Irish; yeast cake made with butter, egg, buttermilk and dried fruit, flavoured with caraway seed. Similar Welsh cake is bara brith.

Barmene™ YEAST EXTRACT, prepared from autolysed brewer's yeast, plus vegetable juices, used for flavouring.

baron of beef The pair of sirloins of BEEF, left uncut at the bone.

baroresistance Resistance to high pressure.

barosensitivity Sensitivity to high pressure.

barquette Small boat-shaped pastry cases, used for savoury or sweet mixtures.

barrel A standard barrel contains 36 gallons. (36 Imperial gallons (UK) = 163.6 L; 36 US gallons = 136.3 L.)

basal metabolic rate (BMR) The ENERGY cost of maintaining the metabolic integrity of the body, nerve and muscle tone, respiration and circulation. For children the BMR also includes the energy cost of growth.

It depends on the amount of metabolically active body tissue, and hence can be calculated from body weight, height and age:

$$MJ/day = 0.0418 \times weight\ (kg) + 0.026 \times height\ (cm) - 0.0209 \times age\ (y) - 0.674\ (for\ males)\ or - 0.0291\ (for\ females)$$

$$kcal/day = 9.99 \times weight\ (kg) + 6.25 \times height\ (cm) - 5 \times age\ (y) - 161\ (males)\ or - 5\ (females)$$

Experimentally, BMR is measured as the heat output from the body, or the rate of oxygen consumption, under strictly standardised conditions, 12–14 h after the last meal, completely at rest (but not asleep) and at an environmental temperature of 26–30 °C, to ensure thermal neutrality. Measurement of metabolic rate under less rigorously controlled conditions gives the resting metabolic rate (RMR).

For people with a sedentary lifestyle and relatively low physical activity, BMR accounts for about 70% of total energy expenditure. The energy costs of different activities are generally expressed as the physical activity ratio, the ratio of energy expenditure in the activity to BMR.

Basedow's disease *See* THYROTOXICOSIS.

basella Leaves of *Basella rubra*, also known as Ceylon, Indian, Malabar, or red vine, or vine spinach.

Composition/100 g: water 93 g, 80 kJ (19 kcal), protein 1.8 g, fat 0.3 g, carbohydrate 3.4 g, ash 1.4 g, Ca 109 mg, Fe 1.2 mg, Mg 65 mg, P 52 mg, K 510 mg, Na 24 mg, Zn 0.4 mg, Cu 0.1 mg, Mn 0.7 mg, Se 0.8 µg, vitamin A 400 µg RE, B_1 0.05 mg, B_2 0.16 mg, niacin 0.5 mg, B_6 0.24 mg, folate 140 µg, pantothenate 0.1 mg, C 102 mg.

basic foods *See* ACID FOODS.

basic foods plan A grouping of foods used for public health education with a recommendation to eat some food from each group every day; foods may be divided into four, five or seven groups. For the seven group plan, the groups are: (1) green and yellow vegetables; (2) oranges, grapefruit, tomatoes and raw salads; (3) potatoes and other vegetables and fruits; (4) milk and cheese; (5) meat, poultry, fish and eggs; (6) bread, pasta, flour and other cereal products; (7) butter, margarine, oils and fats.

   See also FOOD PYRAMID.

basil An aromatic herb *Ocimum basilicum* and *O. minimum*; other members of the genus *Ocimum* are also used as seasoning.

basmati Long-grain Indian variety of rice, much prized for its delicate flavour (the name means 'fragrant' in Hindi).

bass A white FISH, *Dicentrarchus labrax*. Composition/100 g: water 76 g, 477 kJ (114 kcal), protein 18.9 g, fat 3.7 g (of which 24% saturated, 42% mono-unsaturated, 33% polyunsaturated), cholesterol 68 mg, carbohydrate 0 g, ash 1.5 g, Ca 80 mg, Fe 1.5 mg, Mg 30 mg, P 200 mg, K 356 mg, Na 70 mg, Zn 0.6 mg, Cu 0.1 mg, Mn 0.9 mg, Se 12.6 µg, vitamin A 30 µg retinol, B_1 0.08 mg, B_2 0.07 mg, niacin 1.3 mg, B_6 0.12 mg, folate 15 µg, B_{12} 2 µg, pantothenate 0.8 mg, C 2 mg. An 80 g serving is a source of Se, a good source of P, a rich source of Mn, vitamin B_{12}.

baste To ladle hot fat (or other liquid) over meat, poultry, etc., at intervals while it is baking or roasting, in order to improve the texture, flavour and appearance.

batata *See* POTATO, SWEET.

Bath bun A small English cake made from milk-based yeast dough, with dried fruit and a topping of sugar crystals, attributed to Dr W. Oliver of Bath (18th century).

Bath chap The cheek and jawbones of the pig, salted and smoked. Originated in Bath.

Bath cheese A small English CHEESE, made from cow's milk with the subsequent addition of cream.

Bath Oliver A biscuit made with yeast, attributed to Dr W. Oliver of Bath (18th century).

Baudouin test A colour test for the presence of sesame oil. In some countries sesame oil is added to all food oils except olive oil, hence permitting detection of the adulteration of olive oil with cheaper vegetable oils.

bauernspeck Austrian; pork cured in brine with juniper berries and smoked.

Baumé A scale used to measure the density of liquids. For all liquids heavier than water, the density at 15.5 °C corresponds to degrees Baumé.

bavarois(e) (1) A hot drink made from eggs, milk and tea, sweetened and flavoured with a liqueur; 17th-century Bavarian.

(2) French; (*crème bavarois*) a cold dessert made from egg custard with gelatine and cream.

(3) Hollandaise sauce with CRAYFISH garnish.

bay (bay leaf) A herb, the leaf of the Mediterranean sweet bay tree (*Lauris nobilis*) with a strong characteristic flavour. Rarely used alone, but an important component of BOUQUET GARNI, and used with other herbs in MARINADES, pickles, stews and stuffing.

bayberry Root bark of the tree *Myricia cerifera*, containing FLAVONOIDS, TANNINS and TERPENES, stated to possess antipyretic, circulatory stimulant, emetic, and mild diaphoretic properties.

Baycovin™ *See* DIETHYL PYROCARBONATE.

bay lobster Or Moreton Bay bug; a variety of sand lobster found in Australia.

BDA British Dietetic Association; web site http://www.bda.uk.com/.

bdelygmia An extreme loathing for food.

bean, adzuki Also known as aduki or feijoa bean, the seed of the Asian adzuki plant *Phaseolus* (*Vigna*) *angularis*. Sweet tasting, the basis of Cantonese red bean paste used to fill DIM-SUM. Also ground to a flour and used in bread, pastry and sweets or eaten after sprouting as BEAN SPROUTS.

Composition/100 g: water 13.4 g, 1377 kJ (329 kcal), protein 19.9 g, fat 0.5 g, carbohydrate 62.9 g, fibre 12.7 g, ash 3.3 g, Ca 66 mg, Fe 5 mg, Mg 127 mg, P 381 mg, K 1254 mg, Na 5 mg, Zn 5 mg, Cu 1.1 mg, Mn 1.7 mg, Se 3.1 μg, vitamin A 1 μg RE, B_1 0.46 mg, B_2 0.22 mg, niacin 2.6 mg, B_6 0.35 mg, folate 622 μg, pantothenate 1.5 mg. An 85 g serving is a source of vitamin B_2, niacin, B_6, a good source of Zn, vitamin B_1, pantothenate, a rich source of Cu, Fe, Mg, Mn, P, folate.

bean, black eyed Also known as black eyed pea or cow pea, *Vigna sinensis*; creamy white bean with a black mark on one edge.

Composition/100 g: water 11 g, 1427 kJ (341 kcal), protein 21.6 g, fat 1.4 g (of which 36% saturated, 9% mono-unsaturated, 55% polyunsaturated), carbohydrate 62.4 g (2.3 g sugars), fibre 15.2 g, ash 3.6 g, Ca 123 mg, Fe 5 mg, Mg 171 mg, P 352 mg, K 1483 mg, Na 5 mg, Zn 3.7 mg, Cu 0.8 mg, Mn 1.1 mg, Se 3.2 μg, vitamin E 0.2 mg, K 6 mg, B_1 0.9 mg, B_2 0.19 mg, niacin 2 mg, B_6 0.29 mg, folate 444 μg, pantothenate 0.9 mg. An 85 g serving is a source of Ca, vitamin B_6, pantothenate, a good source of Zn, a rich source of Cu, Fe, Mg, Mn, P, vitamin B_1, folate.

bean, borlotti Italian variety of *Phaseolus vulgaris*. *See* BEAN, HARICOT.

bean, broad Also known as fava or horse bean, *Vicia faba*.

Composition/100 g: water 11 g, 1427 kJ (341 kcal), protein 26.1 g, fat 1.5 g (of which 25% saturated, 25% mono-unsaturated, 50% polyunsaturated), carbohydrate 58.3 g (5.7 g sugars), fibre 25 g, ash 3.1 g, Ca 103 mg, Fe 6.7 mg, Mg 192 mg, P 421 mg, K 1062 mg, Na 13 mg, Zn 3.1 mg, Cu 0.8 mg, Mn 1.6 mg, Se 8.2 μg, vitamin A 3 μg RE (32 μg carotenoids), E 0.1 mg, K 9 mg, B_1 0.56 mg, B_2 0.33 mg, niacin 2.8 mg, B_6 0.37 mg, folate 423 μg, pantothenate 1 mg, C 1 mg. An 85 g serving is a source of Zn, vitamin B_2, niacin, B_6, pantothenate, a rich source of Cu, Fe, Mg, Mn, P, vitamin B_1, folate.

bean, butter Several large varieties of *Phaseolus vulgaris*, also known as Lima, curry, Madagascar and sugar bean.

Composition/100 g: water 10.2 g, 1415 kJ (338 kcal), protein 21.5 g, fat 0.7 g, carbohydrate 63.4 g (8.5 g sugars), fibre 19 g, ash 4.3 g, Ca 81 mg, Fe 7.5 mg, Mg 224 mg, P 385 mg, K 1724 mg, Na 18 mg, Zn 2.8 mg, Cu 0.7 mg, Mn 1.7 mg, Se 7.2 μg, vitamin E 0.7 mg, K 6 mg, B_1 0.51 mg, B_2 0.2 mg, niacin 1.5 mg, B_6 0.51 mg, folate 395 μg, pantothenate 1.4 mg. An 85 g serving is a source of Zn, pantothenate, a good source of vitamin B_6, a rich source of Cu, Fe, Mg, Mn, P, vitamin B_1, folate.

bean curd *See* TOFU.

bean, French Unripe seeds and pods of *Phaseolus vulgaris*; ripe seeds are HARICOT BEANS.

Composition/100 g: (edible portion 88%) water 90.3 g, 130 kJ (31 kcal), protein 1.8 g, fat 0.1 g, carbohydrate 7.1 g (1.4 g sugars), fibre 3.4 g, ash 0.7 g, Ca 37 mg, Fe 1 mg, Mg 25 mg, P 38 mg, K 209 mg, Na 6 mg, Zn 0.2 mg, Cu 0.1 mg, Mn 0.2 mg, Se 0.6 μg, vitamin A 35 μg RE (1088 μg carotenoids), E 0.4 mg, K 14.4 mg, B_1 0.08 mg, B_2 0.1 mg, niacin 0.8 mg, B_6 0.07 mg, folate 37 μg, pantothenate 0.1 mg, C 16 mg. A 60 g serving is a source of folate, vitamin C.

bean, haricot Ripe seed of small variety of *Phaseolus vulgaris* (the unripe seed is the FRENCH BEAN). Also known as navy, string, pinto or snap bean.

Composition/100 g: water 12.1 g, 1411 kJ (337 kcal), protein 22.3 g, fat 1.5 g (of which 8% saturated, 17% mono-unsaturated, 75% polyunsaturated), carbohydrate 60.8 g (3.9 g sugars), fibre 24.4 g, ash 3.3 g, Ca 147 mg, Fe 5.5 mg, Mg 175 mg, P 407 mg, K 1185 mg, Na 5 mg, Zn 3.7 mg, Cu 0.8 mg, Mn 1.4 mg, Se 11 μg, K 2.5 mg, B_1 0.77 mg, B_2 0.16 mg, niacin 2.2 mg, B_6 0.43 mg, folate 364 μg, pantothenate 0.7 mg. An 85 g serving is a source of Ca, Se, vitamin B_6, a good source of Zn, a rich source of Cu, Fe, Mg, Mn, P, vitamin B_1, folate.

bean, Lima *See* BEAN, BUTTER.

bean, mung Whole or split seed of *Vigna radiata* (*Phaseolus aureus, P. radiatus*), green gram.

Composition/100 g: water 9.1 g, 1453 kJ (347 kcal), protein 23.9 g, fat 1.1 g (of which 33% saturated, 22% mono-unsaturated, 44% polyunsaturated), carbohydrate 62.6 g (6.6 g sugars), fibre 16.3 g, ash 3.3 g, Ca 132 mg, Fe 6.7 mg, Mg 189 mg, P 367 mg, K 1246 mg, Na 15 mg, Zn 2.7 mg, Cu 0.9 mg, Mn 1 mg, Se 8.2 μg, vitamin A 6 μg RE (68 μg carotenoids), E 0.5 mg, K 9 mg, B_1 0.62 mg, B_2 0.23 mg, niacin 2.3 mg, B_6 0.38 mg, folate 625 μg, pantothenate 1.9 mg, C 5 mg. An 85 g serving is a source of Ca, Zn, vitamin B_2, B_6, a good source of pantothenate, a rich source of Cu, Fe, Mg, Mn, P, vitamin B_1, folate.

bean, red kidney Ripe seed of large variety of *Phaseolus vulgaris*.

Composition/100 g: water 11.8 g, 1394 kJ (333 kcal), protein 23.6 g, fat 0.8 g, carbohydrate 60 g (2.2 g sugars), fibre 24.9 g, ash 3.8 g, Ca 143 mg, Fe 8.2 mg, Mg 140 mg, P 407 mg, K 1406 mg, Na 24 mg, Zn 2.8 mg, Cu 1 mg, Mn 1 mg, Se 3.2 μg, vitamin E 0.2 mg, K 19 mg, B_1 0.53 mg, B_2 0.22 mg, niacin 2.1 mg, B_6 0.4 mg, folate 394 μg, pantothenate 0.8 mg, C 5 mg. An 85 g serving is a source of Ca, Zn, vitamin B_2, B_6, pantothenate, a rich source of Cu, Fe, Mg, Mn, P, vitamin B_1, folate.

bean, runner *Phaseolus multiflorus*.

Composition/100 g: (edible portion 88%) water 90.3 g, 130 kJ (31 kcal), protein 1.8 g, fat 0.1 g, carbohydrate 7.1 g (1.4 g sugars), fibre 3.4 g, ash 0.7 g, Ca 37 mg, Fe 1 mg, Mg 25 mg, P 38 mg, K 209 mg, Na 6 mg, Zn 0.2 mg, Cu 0.1 mg, Mn 0.2 mg, Se 0.6 μg, vitamin A 35 μg RE (1088 μg carotenoids), E 0.4 mg, K 14.4 mg, B_1 0.08 mg, B_2 0.1 mg, niacin 0.8 mg, B_6 0.07 mg, folate 37 μg, pantothenate 0.1 mg, C 16 mg. A 60 g serving is a source of folate, vitamin C.

beans, baked Usually mature haricot beans, cooked in sauce; often canned with tomato sauce and starch with added sugar (or sweetener) and salt.

bean, soya *See* SOYA.

bean sprouts A number of peas, beans and seeds can be germinated and the sprouts eaten raw or cooked. The sprouting causes the synthesis of vitamin C. One of the commonest sprouts is that of the MUNG BEAN, but ALFALFA and ADZUKI BEANS are also used.

bean, string Either RUNNER BEANS or FRENCH BEANS which have a climbing habit rather than growing as small bushes. The name derives from the method of growing them up strings.

béarnaise sauce A thick French sauce made with egg yolk, butter, wine vinegar or white wine and chopped SHALLOTS, named after Béarn in SW France.

béchamel sauce Also known as white sauce. One of the basic French sauces, made with milk, butter and flour. Louis de Béchamel, of the court of Louis XIV of France, invested heavily in Newfoundland fisheries, and invented the sauce in 1654 to mask the flavour of dried cod he shipped across the Atlantic.

bêche-de-mer The sea slug, *Stichopus japonicus*, an occasional food in many parts of the world; also called trepang.

beechwood sugar *See* XYLOSE.

beef Flesh of the ox (*Bos taurus*); flesh from young calves is VEAL. Composition/100g (varying with joint of meat): water 57.3g, 1218kJ (291kcal), protein 17.3g, fat 24g (of which 46% saturated, 50% mono-unsaturated, 4% polyunsaturated), cholesterol 74mg, carbohydrate 0g, ash 0.8g, Ca 8mg, Fe 1.8mg, Mg 17mg, P 154mg, K 267mg, Na 59mg, Zn 3.6mg, Cu 0.1mg, Se 18.1µg, I 10µg, vitamin B_1 0.08mg, B_2 0.16mg, niacin 3.5mg, B_6 0.33mg, folate 7µg, B_{12} 2.7µg, pantothenate 0.3mg. A 100g serving is a source of Fe, P, niacin, vitamin B_6, a good source of Se, Zn, a rich source of vitamin B_{12}.

beefalo A cross between the domestic cow (*Bos taurus*) and the buffalo (*Bubalus* spp.) which can be fattened on range grass, rather than requiring cereal and protein supplements.

Composition/100g: water 70.9g, 599kJ (143kcal), protein 23.3 g, fat 4.8g (of which 48% saturated, 48% mono-unsaturated, 5% polyunsaturated), cholesterol 44mg, carbohydrate 0g, ash 0.9g, Ca 18mg, Fe 2.3mg, P 224mg, K 436mg, Na 78mg, Zn 4.9mg, Se 9.8µg, vitamin B_1 0.04mg, B_2 0.09mg, niacin 4.6mg, folate 15µg, B_{12} 2.4µg, pantothenate 0.6mg. A 100g serving is a source of Fe, Se, a good source of P, niacin, a rich source of Zn, vitamin B_{12}.

beefburger *See* HAMBURGER.

beef, corned *See* CORNED BEEF.

beef, pressed (Salt beef); boned brisket beef that has been salted, cooked and pressed. Known as corned beef in USA.

beefsteak fungus Large edible fungus (*Fistulina hepatica*) with a stringy, meat-like texture and deep red juice. *See* MUSHROOMS.

beer ALCOHOLIC BEVERAGE made by the fermentation of CEREALS; traditionally barley, but also maize, rice or sorghum. The first step is the malting of barley; it is allowed to sprout, when the enzyme AMYLASE hydrolyses some of the starch to dextrins and maltose. The sprouted (malted) barley is dried, then extracted with hot water (the process of mashing) to produce wort. After the addition of HOPS for flavour, the wort is allowed to ferment. Two types of YEAST are used in brewing: top fermenting yeasts which float on the surface of the wort and bottom or deep fermenters.

Most traditional British beers (ale, bitter, stout and porter) are brewed with top fermenting yeasts. UK beers, brown ale and stout, around 3–4% alcohol by volume; strong ale is 6.6% alcohol. Ale is a light-coloured beer, relatively high in alcohol content, and relatively heavily hopped. Bitter beers are darker and contain even more hops. Lager is the traditional mainland European type of beer, sometimes called Pilsner lager or Pils, since the original lager was brewed in Pilsen in Bohemia. It is brewed by deep fermentation.

Porter (first brewed in London in 1722, as a low cost beer for market porters) and stout are almost black in colour; they are made from wort containing some partly charred malt; milk stout is made from wort containing added LACTOSE.

Lite beer is beer that has been allowed to ferment until virtually all of the carbohydrate has been converted to alcohol and so is lower in carbohydrate and higher in alcohol.

Low-alcohol beer may be made either by fermentation of a low carbohydrate wort, or by removal of much of the alcohol after fermentation (de-alcoholised beer).

Sorghum beer (African, made also from millet, maize or plantain) is a thick sour beverage consumed while still fermenting. Also known by numerous local names, kaffir beer, bouza, pombé, Bantu beer. 3–8% alcohol, 3–10% carbohydrate.

bees' royal jelly *See* ROYAL JELLY.

beestings The first milk given by the cow after calving, the COLOSTRUM, rich in immunoglobulins.

beeswax Wax from the honeycomb of the bee, used to glaze confectionery, in chewing gum, and as a flavouring agent.

beet, leaf, or silver spinach *See* SWISS CHARD.

beetroot The root of *Beta vulgaris*, eaten cooked or pickled. Known simply as beet in N America. The violet-red pigment, betanin, is used as a food colour (E-162).

Composition/100g: (edible portion 67%) water 88g, 180kJ (43kcal), protein 1.6g, fat 0.2g, carbohydrate 9.6g (6.8g sugars), fibre 2.8g, ash 1.1g, Ca 16mg, Fe 0.8mg, Mg 23mg, P 40mg, K 325mg, Na 78mg, Zn 0.3mg, Cu 0.1mg, Mn 0.3mg, Se 0.7µg, vitamin A 2µg RE (20µg carotenoids), K 0.2mg, B_1 0.03mg, B_2 0.04mg, niacin 0.3mg, B_6 0.07mg, folate 109µg, pantothenate 0.2mg, C 5mg. An 80g serving is a rich source of folate.

Composition/100g beet greens: (edible portion 56%) water 91g, 92kJ (22kcal), protein 2.2g, fat 0.1g, carbohydrate 4.3g (0.5g sugars), fibre 3.7g, ash 2.3g, Ca 117mg, Fe 2.6mg, Mg 70mg, P 41mg, K 762mg, Na 226mg, Zn 0.4mg, Cu 0.2mg, Mn 0.4mg, Se 0.9µg, vitamin A 316µg RE (5300µg carotenoids), E 1.5mg, K 400mg, B_1 0.1mg, B_2 0.22mg, niacin 0.4mg, B_6 0.11mg, folate 15µg, pantothenate 0.3mg, C 30mg. A 32g serving (1 leaf) is a source of vitamin A, C.

58

beet sugar *See* SUGAR; SUGAR BEET.

beeturia Excretion of red-coloured urine after eating BEETROOT, due to excretion of the pigment betanin. It occurs, not consistently, in about one person in eight.

bee wine Wine produced by fermentation of sugar, using a clump of yeast and lactic bacteria which rises and falls with the bubbles of carbon dioxide formed during fermentation, hence the name 'bee'.

behenic acid Long-chain saturated FATTY ACID (C22:0).

beikost Any additional food used in infant feeding other than human milk and infant milk formula; weaning foods.

belching *See* ERUCTATION.

bell pepper *See* PEPPER, SWEET.

beluga Russian name for the white sturgeon (*Acipenser huro*), whose ROE forms the most prized CAVIAR.

Benecol™ Spreads and yogurt containing STANOLS that inhibit the absorption of cholesterol from the intestinal tract.

Bénédictine French LIQUEUR invented about 1510 by the monks of the Benedictine Abbey of Fécamp in France. The Abbey was closed, and the recipe lost after the French revolution, then rediscovered about 1863. It is based on double-distilled BRANDY, flavoured with some 75 herbs and spices; 40% alcohol by volume and 30% sugar; 1.3 MJ (300 kcal)/100 mL.

Benedict–Roth spirometer *See* SPIROMETER.

Benedict's reagent Alkaline copper reagent (sodium citrate, sodium carbonate and copper sulphate) used for detection and semi-quantitative determination of GLUCOSE and other reducing sugars. Benedict's quantitative reagent also includes potassium thiocyanate and potassium ferrocyanide. The colour of the precipitate on boiling gives an indication of the concentration of glucose between 0.05 and 2%.

See also FEHLING'S REAGENT; SOMOGYI–NELSON REAGENT.

benniseed *See* SESAME.

Benn's index Ratio of weight divided by height^p, where p is derived from weight/height ratio and the regression coefficient of log(weight) on log(height) for the population group. Values of p range between 1.60 and 1.83.

bentonite *See* FULLER'S EARTH.

bentoo no tomo Japanese seasoning consisting of dried fish, salt, soy sauce and MONOSODIUM GLUTAMATE.

benzedrine *See* AMPHETAMINE.

benzidine test Very sensitive test for blood; a green colour is developed when the sample is treated with a saturated solution of benzidine in glacial acetic acid, followed by hydrogen peroxide.

benzoic acid A preservative normally used as the sodium, potassium or calcium salts and their derivatives (E-210–219), especially in acid foods such as pickles and sauces.

Occurs naturally in a number of fruits, including CRANBERRIES, prunes, GREENGAGES, CLOUDBERRIES and CINNAMON. Cloudberries contain so much benzoic acid that they can be stored for long periods of time without any precautions being taken against bacterial or fungal spoilage.

Benzoic acid and its derivatives are excreted conjugated with the AMINO ACIDS glycine (forming hippuric acid) and alanine. Because of this, benzoic acid is sometimes used in the treatment of ARGININAEMIA, ARGININOSUCCINIC ACIDURIA and CITRULLINAEMIA, permitting excretion of nitrogenous waste as these conjugates.

benzoyl peroxide   Used as a bleaching agent for flour, see AGEING.

bergamot   (1) A pear-shaped orange, *Citrus bergamia*, grown mainly in Calabria, Italy, for its peel oil.

(2) An ornamental herb, *Monarda didyma*, the dried leaves of which were used to make Oswego tea.

(3) A type of PEAR, *Pyrus persica*.

beriberi   The result of severe and prolonged deficiency of VITAMIN B₁, still a problem in parts of SE Asia where the diet is high in carbohydrate (polished RICE) and poor in vitamin B₁. In developed countries vitamin B₁ deficiency is associated with alcohol abuse; while it may result in beriberi, more commonly the result is central nervous system damage, the WERNICKE–KORSAKOFF SYNDROME.

In beriberi there is degeneration of peripheral nerves, starting in the hands and feet and ascending the arms and legs, with a loss of sensation and deep muscle pain. There is also enlargement of the heart, which may lead to OEDEMA (wet beriberi), and death results from heart failure. Fatal heart failure may develop without the nerve damage being apparent (Shoshin or sudden beriberi).

The name is derived from the Bahasa-Malay word for sheep, to describe the curious sheep-like gait adopted by sufferers.

berry   Botanical term for fleshy juicy fruits with one or more seeds not having a stone, e.g. grape, gooseberry, tomato, banana, black-currant, cranberry.

best before   *See* DATE MARKING.

beta-carotene (β-carotene)   *See* CAROTENE.

betacyanins   *See* BETALAINS.

betaine   *N*-Trimethyl glycine, a source of methyl groups in various reactions, especially the methylation of HOMOCYSTEINE to METHIONINE in tissues other than the brain; an intermediate in the metabolism of CHOLINE. Occurs in beetroot and cottonseed. (Obsolete names lycine, oxyneurine.)

betalains   Red and yellow N-containing pigments (chromoalkaloids) in plants. Betacyanins (e.g. BETANIN and isobetanin in

BEETROOT) are red, betaxanthins yellow. Unlike ANTHOCYANINS the colour is little affected by pH.

betanin   Red-purple betacyanin pigment in beetroot; permitted food colour E-162.

Betatene™   Mixed CAROTENOIDS from the alga *Dunaliella salina*.

betaxanthins   *See* BETALAINS.

betel   Leaves of the creeper *Piper betel*, chewed in some parts of the world for their stimulating effect, due to the presence of the ALKALOIDS arecoline and guvacoline. The leaves are chewed with the nuts of the areca palm, *Arecha catechu*, which is therefore often called the betel palm, and the nut is called betel nut.

The Indian delicacy pan is based on betel leaf and areca nut, together with aromatic spices and herbs.

beurre manié   Butter with an equal amount of flour blended in, used for thickening sauces.

bezafibrate   *See* FIBRIC ACID.

bezoar   A hard ball of undigested food, sometimes together with hair, which forms in the stomach or intestine and can cause obstruction. Foods with a high content of PECTIN can form bezoars if swallowed without chewing. The name is derived from the Arabic meaning *protection against poison*, since bezoars were formerly believed to have protective properties.

See also GASTROLITH; TRICHOBEZOAR.

BHA   *See* BUTYLATED HYDROXYANISOLE.

bhaji   (1) Chinese spinach (*Amaranthus gangeticus*) also known as callaloo.

(2) Also bhajia, Indian vegetable fritters, normally made with gram (lentil) flour.

bhatura   Indian; deep fried flat bread; the dough is leavened with yogurt (dahi PURI) or curds (khamiri puri) and fermented overnight before cooking.

bhindi   *See* OKRA.

BHT   *See* BUTYLATED HYDROXYTOLUENE.

BIE   *See* BIOELECTRICAL IMPEDANCE.

biffins   Apples that have been peeled, partly baked, then pressed and dried.

bifidobacteria   *See* PROBIOTICS.

bifidogenic   Promoting the growth of (beneficial) bifidobacteria in the intestinal tract; *see* BIFIDUS FACTOR; PREBIOTICS; PROBIOTICS.

bifidus factor   A carbohydrate in human milk that contains nitrogen and stimulates the growth of *Lactobacillus bifidus* in the intestine. In turn, this organism lowers the pH of the intestinal contents and suppresses the growth of *E. COLI* and other pathogenic bacteria.

See also LACTULOSE; PREBIOTICS.

bigarade (bigaradier) *See* ORANGE, BITTER.

biguanides *See* HYPOGLYCAEMIC AGENTS.

bijon South-east Asian; noodles made from fermented maize kernels and cornflour.

bilberry The berry of wild shrubs of the genus *Vaccinium*, not generally cultivated. Variously known as whortleberry, blaeberry, whinberry, huckleberry.

bile Fluid produced by the liver and stored in the gall bladder before secretion into the small intestine (duodenum) via the bile duct. It contains the BILE SALTS, bile pigments (BILIRUBIN and biliverdin) and CHOLESTEROL. It is alkaline, and neutralises the acid from the stomach as the food reaches the small intestine.

Relatively large amounts of VITAMIN B_{12} and FOLIC ACID are secreted in the bile and then reabsorbed from the small intestine (enterohepatic circulation). Most of the cholesterol and bile salts are also reabsorbed from the small intestine.

See also GASTROINTESTINAL TRACT.

bile salts (bile acids) Salts of cholic and chenodeoxycholic acids, secreted in the bile as glycine and taurine conjugates; act as emulsifying agents in the absorption of fats. Also important as the cofactor of CAROTENE dioxygenase (EC 1.13.11.21).

Bacterial metabolism in the colon leads to hydrolysis of the conjugates and formation of the secondary bile salts, lithocholic and deoxycholic acids, which are absorbed and then resecreted in the bile, again as glycine and taurine conjugates. Total secretion of bile salts is about 30 g/day; faecal output 1–2 g/day.

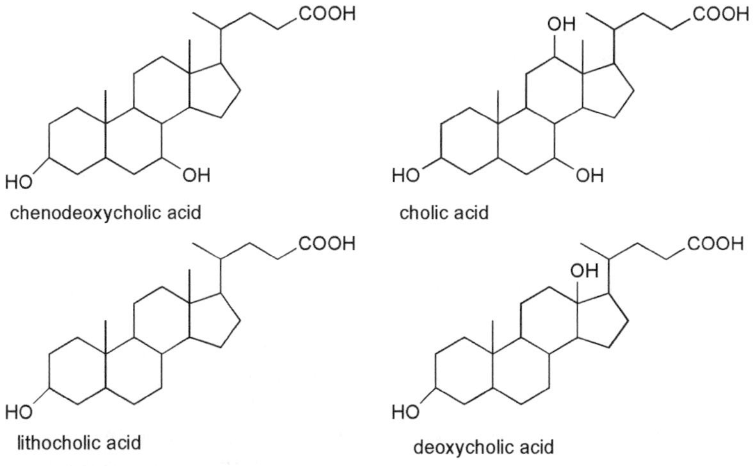

chenodeoxycholic acid

cholic acid

lithocholic acid

deoxycholic acid

BILE SALTS

bilirubin, biliverdin   The BILE pigments, formed by catabolism of HAEMOGLOBIN. Blood bilirubin is normally <17 μmol/L; when it rises above 20–30 μmol/L there is visible jaundice.

biltong   South African; strips of dried meat, salted, spiced and dried in air for 10–14 days.

binge–purge syndrome   A feature of the eating disorder BULIMIA NERVOSA, characterised by the ingestion of excessive amounts of food and the excessive use of LAXATIVES.

Bingham fluid   *See* PLASTIC FLUIDS.

bio   Commonly used to indicate probiotic yogurt containing live bacterial culture. *See* PROBIOTICS.

bioactive polymers   In food packaging, polymers that have enzymes or other active compounds (e.g. antimicrobial peptides) covalently bound to the surface or embedded in the polymer film, so that the active material does not migrate into the food.

bioassay   Biological assay; measurement of biologically active compounds (e.g. vitamins and essential amino acids) by their ability to support growth of micro-organisms or animals.

biocytin   BIOTIN bound to the ε-amino group of lysine, the form in which biotin is present in enzymes. Normally hydrolysed to release free biotin by the enzyme biotinidase (EC 3.5.1.12).

bioelectrical impedance (BIE)   A method of measuring the proportion of fat in the body by the difference in the resistance to passage of an electric current between fat and lean tissue.

   Correctly measures the impedance, since a 50 MHz alternating current (800 μA) is passed between electrodes attached to the hand and foot, and the fall in voltage is measured.

   See also TOTAL BODY ELECTRICAL CONDUCTIVITY.

bioflavonoids   *See* FLAVONOIDS.

biofortification   The process of breeding varieties of food crops that are naturally rich in micronutrients.

Biofoss^{TM} *See* DEFT.

biolistics   Acceleration of heavy microparticles coated with DNA to introduce foreign DNA into plant cells as a means of creating TRANSGENIC plants.

biological oxygen demand (BOD)   A way of assessing bacterial contamination of water, milk, etc. by micro-organisms which take up oxygen for their metabolism.

biological value (BV)   A measure of PROTEIN QUALITY.

bioluminescence   Emission of light by reaction of the enzyme LUCIFERASE with ATP. Exploited as a rapid and sensitive way of detecting bacteria (and other cells) in milk and other foods, since all living cells contain ATP. Trade names for bioluminescence instruments include Biotrace, Bactofoss, Bio-Orbit and Hy-Lite.

biomarkers Metabolic, chemical or functional changes that can be measured in response to nutritional, drug or other interventions. Sometimes regarded as surrogate end-points, since they respond more rapidly and more sensitively than clinical disease or overt signs of toxicity.

Bio-Orbit^{TM} *See* BIOLUMINESCENCE.

biopterin Pterin coenzyme required by PHENYLALANINE (EC 1.14.16.1), TYROSINE (EC 1.14.16.2) and TRYPTOPHAN (EC 1.14.16.4) hydroxylases. Not a dietary requirement, but synthesised from cGMP. Rare patients with a variant form of PHENYLKETONURIA cannot synthesise biopterin, and have to receive supplements.

bios A name given to a factor in cell-free extract of yeast which is essential for the growth of yeast, by Wildiers in 1901. Three components were subsequently identified: INOSITOL, β-ALANINE and BIOTIN. Of these, only biotin is a VITAMIN and essential for human beings.

biosensor An enzyme or antibody (or intact cells), coupled to a physical or chemical reporting system to measure a specific component of a food or other product. Among other applications, used in intelligent PACKAGING.

biotin A VITAMIN, sometimes known as vitamin H, required as coenzyme for carboxylation reactions in synthesis of fatty acids and glucose, and in the control of cell division. Widely distributed in foods; dietary deficiency is unknown. There is no evidence on which to base REFERENCE INTAKES other than to state that current average intakes (between 15 and 70 µg/day) are obviously more than adequate to prevent deficiency.

The protein, avidin, in raw egg white, binds biotin strongly, preventing its absorption, and individuals who consume abnormally large amounts of uncooked egg (several dozen eggs per week) have been reported to show biotin deficiency. Avidin is denatured (*see* DENATURATION) on cooking, and does not combine with biotin; indeed cooked egg is a rich source of available biotin.

See also BIOCYTIN.

BIOTIN

biotinidase   *See* BIOCYTIN.

Biotrace™   *See* BIOLUMINESCENCE.

biphenyl   *See* DIPHENYL.

birch beer   A non-alcoholic carbonated beverage flavoured with oil of wintergreen or oils of sweet birch and SASSAFRAS.

bisacodyl   A stimulant LAXATIVE.

biscuit   A baked flour confectionery dried down to low moisture content. The name is derived from the Latin *bis coctus*, meaning cooked twice. Known as cookie in the USA, where 'biscuit' means a small cake-like bun.

biscuit check   The development of splitting and cracking in BISCUITS immediately after baking.

Biskoids™   *See* SACCHARIN.

Bismarck herring   Pickled and spiced whole HERRING.

bismuth   Mineral of no known metabolic function. A variety of bismuth salts are used as ANTACIDS and astringents in treating gastrointestinal disorders; the carbonate is used in treatment of peptic ULCER, especially when *HELICOBACTER PYLORI* is the causative agent.

bisque   Thick rich soup, generally made from FISH or SHELLFISH stock.

Bitot's spots   Irregular shaped foam-like plaques on the conjunctiva of the eye, characteristically seen in VITAMIN A deficiency, but not considered to be a diagnostic sign without other evidence of deficiency.

bitterroot   Roots of *Lewisia rediviva* (purslane family), N American vegetable.

bitters   Extracts of herbs, spices, roots and bark, steeped in, or distilled with, SPIRITS. Originally prepared for medicinal use (tinctures or alcoholic extracts of the natural products); now used mainly to flavour spirits and cocktails, or as apéritifs.

See also ANGOSTURA; WINE, APÉRITIF.

biuret reaction   Method for colorimetric determination of protein using an alkaline copper sulphate plus tartrate reagent which forms a coordination complex with four —NH groups in peptide bonds; sensitivity 1 mg/mL, maximum absorbance 540–560 nm.

bixin   A CAROTENOID pigment found in the seeds of the tropical plant *Bixa orellana*; the crude extract is the colouring agent ANNATTO (E-160).

blaanda bread   Shetland; unleavened bread made from barley and oat meal, with milk and butter, baked slowly on a griddle.

blackberry   Berry of the bramble, *Rubus fruticosus*.

Composition/100 g: (edible portion 96%) water 88 g, 180 kJ (43 kcal), protein 1.4 g, fat 0.5 g, carbohydrate 9.6 g (4.9 g sugars), fibre 5.3 g, ash 0.4 g, Ca 29 mg, Fe 0.6 mg, Mg 20 mg, P 22 mg, K 162 mg, Na 1 mg, Zn 0.5 mg, Cu 0.2 mg, Mn 0.6 mg, Se 0.4 µg, vitamin A 11 µg RE (246 µg carotenoids), E 1.2 mg, K 19.8 mg, B_1 0.02 mg, B_2 0.03 mg, niacin 0.6 mg, B_6 0.03 mg, folate 25 µg, pantothenate 0.3 mg, C 21 mg. A 110 g serving is a source of Cu, vitamin E, folate, a good source of Mn, a rich source of vitamin C.

blackcock   *See* GROUSE.

blackcurrants   Fruit of the bush *Ribes nigra*, of special interest because of their high vitamin C content. The British National Fruit Collection has 120 varieties.

Composition/100 g: (edible portion 98%) water 82 g, 264 kJ (63 kcal), protein 1.4 g, fat 0.4 g, carbohydrate 15.4 g, ash 0.9 g, Ca 55 mg, Fe 1.5 mg, Mg 24 mg, P 59 mg, K 322 mg, Na 2 mg, Zn 0.3 mg, Cu 0.1 mg, Mn 0.3 mg, vitamin A 12 µg RE , E 1 mg, B_1 0.05 mg, B_2 0.05 mg, niacin 0.3 mg, B_6 0.07 mg, pantothenate 0.4 mg, C 181 mg. A 110 g serving is a source of Fe, Mn, vitamin E, a rich source of vitamin C.

black forest mushroom   Or shiitake, *Lentinula (Lentinus) edodes*, *see* MUSHROOMS.

black fungus   Or woodears, edible wild fungus, *Auriculia polytricha*, *see* MUSHROOMS.

black jack   *See* CARAMEL.

black PN   A black food colour (E-151), also known as brilliant black BN.

black pudding   Also known as blood pudding. Traditional European dish made with sheep or pig blood and suet, originally together with oatmeal, liver and herbs, stuffed into membrane casings shaped like a horseshoe. Although it is already cooked, it is usually sliced and fried. German *Blutwurst* and French *boudin noir* are made without cereal.

blackthorn   *See* SLOE.

black tongue disease   A sign of NIACIN deficiency in dogs, the canine equivalent of PELLAGRA, historically important in isolation of the VITAMIN.

blaeberry   *See* BILBERRY.

blanching   Partial precooking by treating food with hot gas, hot water, steam, super-heated steam, microwave, for a short time. Also known as scalding, a preferred term, since the original reason for blanching was to whiten food, but the process is also used to preserve colour.

Fruits and vegetables are blanched before dehydrating or freezing, to soften the texture, shrink the food or remove air, destroy enzymes that may cause spoilage when frozen, and remove undesirable flavours. Blanching is also performed to remove excess salt from preserved meat, and to aid the removal of skin, e.g. from almonds and tomatoes.

There can be a loss of 10–20% of the sugars, salts and protein, as well as some of the vitamins B_1, B_2 and niacin, and up to one-third of the vitamin C.

blancmange powder   Usually a cornflour base with added flavour and colour, mixed with hot milk to make a dessert.

bland diet   A diet that is non-irritating, does not overstimulate the digestive tract and is soothing to the intestines, generally avoiding alcohol, strong tea or coffee, pickles, spices and high intake of dietary FIBRE.

blawn fish   Scottish (Orkney); fresh fish, rubbed with salt and hung in a windy passage for a day, then grilled.

bleach figure (for flour)   A measure of the extent of bleaching of the flour from the relative paleness of the extracted (yellow) pigments.

bleaching   The removal or destruction of colour. In the context of food it usually refers to the bleaching of flour. It also refers to the bleaching of oils, a stage in the purification by which dispersed impurities and natural colouring materials are removed by activated CHARCOAL or FULLER'S EARTH.

See also AGEING (3).

bleeding bread   A bacterial infection with *Bacillus prodigiosus* or *Serratia marcescens*, which stains the bread bright red. Under warm and damp conditions the infection can appear overnight, and contamination of the shewbread in churches has led to accusations and riots against religious minorities over the centuries.

blewits   Edible wild fungus, *Tricholoma (Lepista) saevum*, also known as bluetail; also wood blewits, *T. nudum*, *see* MUSHROOMS.

blinding   Blocking of a sieve by small particles.

blind loop syndrome   Or stagnant loop syndrome; stasis of the small intestine, permitting bacterial overgrowth and causing malabsorption and STEATORRHOEA. Usually the result of chronic obstruction or surgical by-pass operations producing a stagnant length of bowel.

blind staggers   Acute VITAMIN B_1 deficiency in horses and other animals, caused by eating bracken, which contains THIAMINASE.

bloaters   Salted, cold-smoked HERRINGS.

blood   Various BLOOD CELLS suspended in plasma; carries nutrients and oxygen to tissues, and removes waste metabolic products from the tissues. Oxygenated blood travels from the lungs in arteries, while deoxygenated blood returns to the lungs in veins; in the tissues the blood from the arteries enters smaller vessels, the arterioles, then capillaries, which then drain into venules, then the veins.

Average blood volume is 5.3 L (78 mL/kg body weight) in males and 3.8 L (56 mL/kg body weight) in females.

blood cells   Three main types of cell are present in blood: erythrocytes or red cells, LEUCOCYTES or white cells and platelets. Red blood cells contain HAEMOGLOBIN, which is responsible for the transport of oxygen from the lungs to tissues, and of carbon dioxide from tissues. White blood cells are generally concerned with protection against invading micro-organisms, and platelets with the process of BLOOD CLOTTING.

blood charcoal (or blood char)   Charcoal prepared by treating whole blood or blood meal with activating agents and heating in airtight containers at 650–750 °C for 6–8 h. Contains 80% carbon, used for absorption of gases, as an industrial decolourising agent, and as an antidote for chemical poisoning.

blood clotting   The process by which the soluble protein fibrinogen in BLOOD PLASMA is converted to insoluble fibrin, thus preventing blood loss through cuts, etc. VITAMIN K is required and deficiency is characterised by excessive bleeding.

See also ANTICOAGULANTS; THROMBOSIS.

blood plasma   The liquid component of blood, accounting for about half the total volume of the blood. Plasma is a solution of nutrients and proteins, mainly albumin and globulins, including the immunoglobulins which are responsible for defence against infection, as well as some ADVERSE REACTIONS TO FOODS. When blood has clotted (*see* BLOOD CLOTTING), the resultant fluid is known as serum.

See also LIPOPROTEINS, PLASMA.

blood pressure   Blood pressure (bp) is measured as millimetres of mercury (Hg) at systole (when the heart contracts) and diastole (when the heart relaxes), and increases with age due to loss of elasticity of the arteries.

Normal systolic bp is 120 mmHg at the age of 12 rising to 160 (men) or 175 (women) at 70. Normal diastolic bp is 70 mmHg at age 12, rising to 85 (men) or 95 (women) at age 70.

Diastolic bp above 105 is moderate, and above 115 severe, HYPERTENSION.

blood sausage   *See* BLACK PUDDING.

blood serum   *See* BLOOD PLASMA.

blood sugar   GLUCOSE; normal concentration is about 3.5–5 mmol (60–90 mg)/L, and is maintained in the fasting state by mobilisation of tissue reserves of GLYCOGEN and gluconeogenesis (synthesis from AMINO ACIDS). Only in prolonged starvation does it fall below about 3.5 mmol (60 mg)/L. If it falls to 2 mmol (35 mg)/L there is loss of consciousness (hypoglycaemic coma, *see* HYPOGLYCAEMIA).

After a meal the concentration of glucose rises, but this rise is limited by the hormone INSULIN, which is secreted by the pancreas to stimulate the uptake of glucose into tissues. DIABETES mellitus is the result of failure of the insulin mechanism.

See also GLUCOSE TOLERANCE test.

bloom Fat bloom is the whitish appearance on the surface of chocolate which sometimes occurs on storage. It is due either to a change in the form of the fat at the surface or to fat diffusing outwards and being deposited as crystals on the surface. Sugar bloom is due to the deposition of sugar crystals on the surface, but is less common than fat bloom.

See also TEMPERING.

Bloom gelometer An instrument for measuring the strength of jellies, and also for any test of firmness, e.g. the staleness of bread.

blotting A series of techniques involving the transfer of DNA, RNA or protein after gel ELECTROPHORESIS onto an inert nitrocellulose membrane, under denaturing conditions, so that it remains bound to the membrane. Southern blotting uses fragments of DNA produced using RESTRICTION ENZYMES, and they are identified by annealing with radioactive cDNA. Northern blotting is essentially similar, for identification of RNA fragments. Western blotting is for proteins, which are identified using labelled antibodies.

blueberry Fruit of *Vaccinium corymbosum* (the high-bush blueberry) or *V. augustifolium* (low-bush blueberry) grown mainly in N America.

Composition/100 g: (edible portion 98%) water 84.2 g, 239 kJ (57 kcal), protein 0.7 g, fat 0.3 g, carbohydrate 14.5 g (10 g sugars), fibre 2.4 g, ash 0.2 g, Ca 6 mg, Fe 0.3 mg, Mg 6 mg, P 12 mg, K 77 mg, Na 1 mg, Zn 0.2 mg, Cu 0.1 mg, Mn 0.3 mg, Se 0.1 µg, vitamin A 3 µg RE (112 µg carotenoids), E 0.6 mg, K 19.3 mg, B_1 0.04 mg, B_2 0.04 mg, niacin 0.4 mg, B_6 0.05 mg, folate 6 µg, pantothenate 0.1 mg, C 10 mg. A 110 g serving is a source of Mn, vitamin C.

BMI *See* BODY MASS INDEX.

BMNES British Meat Nutrition Education Service; web site http://www.meatandhealth.co.uk/.

BMR *See* BASAL METABOLIC RATE.

BNF British Nutrition Foundation; web site http://www.nutrition. org.uk/.

boar, wild Meat of *Sus scrofa*. Hunted in parts of Europe, farmed on small scale in UK and elsewhere.

Composition/100 g: water 72 g, 511 kJ (122 kcal), protein 21.5 g, fat 3.3 g (of which 36% saturated, 46% mono-unsaturated, 18% polyunsaturated), carbohydrate 0 g, ash 1 g, Ca 12 mg, P 120 mg, Se 9.8 µg, vitamin B_1 0.39 mg, B_2 0.11 mg, niacin 4 mg. A 100 g serving is a source of P, Se, a good source of vitamin B$_1$, niacin.

bockwurst   German; white sausage made from pork and veal with chives, parsley, eggs and milk.

BOD   *See* BIOLOGICAL OXYGEN DEMAND.

body composition   Various methods are used to assess gross body composition, including ANTHROPOMETRY, BIOELECTRICAL IMPEDANCE, TOTAL BODY ELECTRICAL CONDUCTIVITY, SKINFOLD THICKNESS and BODY DENSITY.

body density   Body fat has a density of 0.90, while fat-free body mass is 1.10. Direct determination of density by weighing in air and in water, or by determination of body volume by PLETHYSMOGRAPHY, therefore permits calculation of the proportions of fat and lean body tissue.

body mass index (BMI)   An index of fatness and obesity. The weight (in kg) divided by the square of height (in m). The acceptable (desirable) range is 20–25. Above 25 is overweight, and above 30 is OBESITY. BMI below the lower end of the acceptable range indicates undernutrition and wasting.

Also called Quetelet's index.

body surface area   Heat loss from the body is related to surface area; BASAL METABOLIC RATE and energy expenditure are sometimes expressed per unit body surface area. It is commonly calculated according to the formulae of Du Bois or Meeh:

$$\text{Du Bois: area (cm}^2\text{)} = 71.84 \times \text{weight}^{0.425} \text{ (kg)} \times \text{height}^{0.725} \text{ (cm)}$$

$$\text{Meeh: area (cm}^2\text{)} = 11.9 \times \text{weight}^{2/3} \text{ (kg)}$$

The surface area of adults is about $18\,000\,\text{cm}^2$ (men) or $16\,000\,\text{cm}^2$ (women).

bog butter   Norsemen, Finns, Scots and Irish used to bury firkins of butter in bogs to ripen and develop a strong flavour.

bog myrtle   A wild plant (*Myrica gale*) with a strong resinous flavour. The leaves and seeds are used to flavour soups and stews.

boiler water additives   Compounds used in a steam or boiler water as anticorrosion agents, to prevent scale.

bole   *See* ARMENIAN BOLE.

boletus   Edible wild MUSHROOM, *Boletus edulis* or *B. granulatus*, also known as the yellow mushroom or cep (cèpe).

bologna   Italian smoked pork and veal SAUSAGE, also known as polony.

bolus   Soft mass of chewed food that is ready to be swallowed.

Bombay duck   Bombil, a fish found in Indian waters, *Harpodon nehereus* or *Saurus ophiodon*, eaten either fresh or after salting and curing.

Bombay mix *See* CHEVDA.

bomb calorimeter *See* CALORIMETER.

bombil *See* BOMBAY DUCK.

Bond's law Equation to calculate the energy cost of reducing particle size, based on the diameter of a sieve that allows 80% of the feedstock to pass and that of a sieve that allows 80% of the ground material to pass.

See also COMMINUTION; KICK'S LAW; RITTINGER'S LAW.

bone Bones consist of an organic matrix composed of COLLAGEN and other proteins and crystalline mineral, mainly HYDROXYAPATITE (calcium phosphate and hydroxide), together with magnesium phosphate, fluorides and sulphates.

Cortical (compact) bone forms the outer shell of bones; it is a solid mass of bony tissue.

Spongy (cancellous) bone beneath the cortical bone consists of a meshwork of trabeculae with interconnecting spaces containing bone MARROW.

Bone density can be assessed as an index of calcium and VITAMIN D status by X-ray, photon absorptiometry or NEUTRON ACTIVATION ANALYSIS.

See also CALCIUM; MARROW (1); OSTEOMALACIA; OSTEOPOROSIS; RICKETS.

bone broth Prepared by prolonged boiling of bones to break down the COLLAGEN and extract it as GELATINE. Of little nutritive value, consisting of 2–4% gelatine, with little calcium.

bone charcoal Animal charcoal, produced by heating pieces of bone sufficiently to burn off the organic matter, leaving the carbon deposited on a framework of calcium carbonate. It is used to purify solutions because it will absorb colouring matter and other impurities.

bone meal Prepared from degreased bones and used as a supplement in both animal and human foods as a source of calcium and phosphate. Also used as a plant fertiliser; a slowly released source of phosphate.

bongkrek Indonesian; fermented coconut PRESS CAKE. *Rhizopus oligosporus* and *Neurospora sitophila* are the fermenting fungi. If the pH is above 6, it can be infected with *Pseudomonas cocovenenans*, which produces the toxins bongkrekic acid and toxoflavin.

bonito Any of the various species of TUNA.

Bontrae™ TEXTURED VEGETABLE PROTEIN prepared by spinning or extrusion.

boracic acid *See* BORIC ACID.

borage A herb, *Borago officinalis*. The flowers and leaves have a cucumber-like flavour and are used to flavour drinks, salads and cheese. Contains potentially toxic alkaloids. The seed oil is a rich source of γ-LINOLENIC ACID.

Composition/100g: (edible portion 80%) water 93g, 88kJ (21kcal), protein 1.8g, fat 0.7g, carbohydrate 3.1g, ash 1.4g, Ca 93mg, Fe 3.3mg, Mg 52mg, P 53mg, K 470mg, Na 80mg, Zn 0.2mg, Cu 0.1mg, Mn 0.3mg, Se 0.9μg, vitamin A 210μg RE (as carotenoids), B_1 0.06mg, B_2 0.15mg, niacin 0.9mg, B_6 0.08mg, folate 13μg, C 35mg. A 50g serving is a source of Fe, vitamin A, a good source of vitamin C.

borborygmos (plural **borborygmi**)   Audible abdominal sound produced by excessive intestinal motility.

borderline substances   Foods that may have characteristics of medication in certain circumstances, and which may then be prescribed under the National Health Service in the UK, e.g. nutritional supplements for treatment of short bowel disease, lactose-free milk for children with LACTOSE intolerance, GALACTOSAEMIA and galactokinase deficiency, GLUTEN-FREE FOODS for patients with COELIAC DISEASE, specially formulated foods for treatment of a variety of GENETIC DISEASES.

borecole   *See* KALE.

boric acid H_3BO_4; has been used in the past as a preservative in bacon and margarine, but BORON accumulates in the body. Formerly used as an anti-infective agent and eye-wash (boracic acid) but there was a high incidence of toxic reactions.

Borneo tallow (green butter)   *See* COCOA BUTTER EQUIVALENTS.

boron   An element, known to be essential for plant growth, but not known to have any physiological function in animals. Suggested to modify the actions and metabolism of OESTROGENS, and sometimes used in preparations to alleviate premenstrual syndrome, although there is little evidence of efficacy; toxic in excess. Occurs mainly as salts of BORIC ACID.

Boston brown bread   An American spiced pudding, steamed in the can.

bottle   The traditional wine bottle holds 700, 720 or 750mL of wine, depending on the variety. A 2-bottle size is a magnum, 4 a Jeroboam or double magnum, 6 a Methuselah, 12 a Salmanazar and 20 a Nebuchadnezzar.

bottled sweat   *See* SPORTS DRINKS.

bottlers' sugar   *See* SUGAR.

botulinum cook   The degree of heat required to ensure destruction of (virtually) all spores of *Clostridium botulinum*, the causative organism of BOTULISM, the most resistant of bacterial spores.

botulism   A rare form of food poisoning caused by the extremely potent neurotoxins (TX1.2.5.1–7) produced by *Clostridium bot-*

ulinum. At least seven different toxins have been identified; they can be inactivated by heating. Although rare, it is often fatal unless the antitoxin is given.

The name is derived from *botulus*, for sausage, since the disease was originally associated with sausages in Germany (1735). A wide range of foods has been involved, including meat, fish, milk, fruits and vegetables which have been incorrectly preserved or treated, so that competing micro-organisms have been destroyed; spores of *C. botulinum* are extremely resistant to heat, and dangerous amounts of toxins can accumulate in contaminated foods without apparent spoilage.

boucanning A Caribbean process by which meat was preserved by sun-drying and smoking while resting on a wooden grid known as a boucan.

bouillabaisse French; fish stew or soup flavoured with saffron, spices and herbs; specialty of the Mediterranean region.

boundary film (or surface film) Film of fluid adjacent to the surface it flows over, that causes a resistance to heat transfer.

bound moisture Water physically or chemically bound to a solid food matrix which exerts a lower vapour pressure than free water at the same temperature.

bouquet garni A small bundle of parsley, thyme, marjoram and bay leaves, tied together with cotton and added to the dish being cooked. Now also the same mixture of herbs in a porous paper sack. Also known as a FAGGOT.

bourbon American WHISKEY made by distilling fermented MAIZE mash. Sour mash bourbon is made from mash that has yeast left in it from a previous fermentation.

bourbonal Ethyl vanillin. *See* VANILLA.

Bournvita^{TM} A preparation of malt, milk, sugar, cocoa, eggs and flavouring, to make a beverage when mixed with milk.

bovine somatotrophin (BST) *See* SOMATOTROPHIN, BOVINE.

bovine spongiform encephalopathy *See* BSE.

Bovril^{TM} A preparation of MEAT EXTRACT, hydrolysed beef, beef powder and YEAST EXTRACT, used as a beverage, flavouring agent and for spreading on bread.

boysenberry A fruit, a hybrid of BLACKBERRY, RASPBERRY and LOGANBERRY developed by Rudolph Boysen (1920).

brachyose *See* ISOMALTOSE.

bracken Young unopened leaves (fronds) of bracken (*Pteridium* spp.), eaten as a vegetable and regarded as a delicacy in the Far East. Known as fiddleheads in Canada and USA.

Composition/100 g: water 88.7 g, 142 kJ (34 kcal), protein 4.6 g, fat 0.4 g, carbohydrate 5.5 g, ash 0.8 g, Ca 32 mg, Fe 1.3 mg, Mg 34 mg, P 101 mg, K 370 mg, Na 1 mg, Zn 0.8 mg, Cu 0.3 mg, Mn

0.5 mg, vitamin A 181 µg RE (2301 µg carotenoids), B_1 0.02 mg, B_2 0.21 mg, niacin 5 mg, C 27 mg.

Contains THIAMINASE, which cleaves VITAMIN B_1; cattle and horses eating large amounts suffer from BLIND STAGGERS due to acute vitamin B_1 deficiency; also contains a number of known or suspected CARCINOGENS.

Bradford method *See* COOMASSIE BRILLIANT BLUE.

bradycardia An unusually slow heart beat, less than 60 beats/min; may be normal in trained athletes.

bradyphagia Eating very slowly.

brain sugar Obsolete name for GALACTOSE.

bramble Wild BLACKBERRY.

bran The outer layers of cereal grain, which are largely removed when the grain is milled (i.e. in the preparation of white flour or white rice). The germ is discarded at the same time, and there is a considerable loss of iron and other minerals, and particularly of the B vitamins, as well as of dietary FIBRE.

See also FLOUR, EXTRACTION RATE; WHEATFEED.

branched-chain amino acids *See* AMINO ACIDS.

brander Scottish name for gridiron or grill.

brandy A SPIRIT distilled from wine, and containing 37–45% (most usually 40%) alcohol by volume. The name is derived from the German *brandtwein*, meaning burnt wine, corrupted to brandy wine. First produced in 1300 at the Montpellier medical school by Arnaud de Villeneuve. Most wine-producing countries also make brandy.

The age of brandy is generally designated as three-star (3–5 years old before bottling); VSOP (very special old pale, aged 4–10 or more years, the name indicating that it has not been heavily coloured with caramel); Napoleon (premium blend aged 6–20 years); XO, extraordinary old (extra or grand reserve, possibly 50 years old).

COGNAC and ARMAGNAC are brandies made in defined regions of France. Fruit brandies are either distilled from fruit wines (e.g. plum and apple brandies) or are prepared by soaking fruit in brandy (e.g. cherry and apricot brandies).

See also MARC.

Brannan plan USA; plan to increase food production without reducing profitability by paying farmers directly the difference between the market price and the price needed to yield a fair profit. Proposed in 1950 by Secretary of Agriculture Charles F. Brannan.

Brassica Genus of vegetables that includes broccoli, Brussels sprouts, cabbage, cauliflower, kale, kohlrabi, mustard, swede.

brat, bratwurst *See* SAUSAGES, EMULSION.

brawn Made from pig meat, particularly the head, boiled with peppercorns and herbs, minced and pressed into a mould. Mock brawn (head cheese) differs in that other meat by-products are used.

Brazil nuts Fruit of the tree *Bertholletia excelsa*.

Composition/100 g (edible portion 50%): water 305 g, 2750 kJ (656 kcal), protein 14 g, fat 66 g (of which 31% saturated, 29% mono-unsaturated, 49% polyunsaturated), carbohydrate 12 g (2.3 g sugars), fibre 7.5 g, ash 3.5 g, Ca 160 mg, Fe 2.4 mg, Mg 376 mg, P 725 mg, K 659 mg, Na 3 mg, Zn 4.1 mg, Cu 1.7 mg, Mn 1.2 mg, Se 1917 µg, vitamin E 5.7 mg, B_1 0.62 mg, B_2 0.04 mg, niacin 0.3 mg, B_6 0.1 mg, folate 22 µg, pantothenate 0.2 mg, C 0.7 g.

bread Baked dough made from cereal flour, usually wheat, although rye, barley and other cereals are also used. Normally leavened by fermentation of the dough with yeast, or addition of SODIUM BICARBONATE. Soda bread is an Irish specialty, made with whey or buttermilk, and leavened with SODIUM BICARBONATE and acid in place of yeast, although yeast may also be used.

Unleavened bread is flat bread made by baking dough that has not been leavened with yeast or baking powder. MATZO is baked to a crisp texture, while PITTA and CHAPATTIS have a softer texture.

Aerated bread is made from dough that is prepared with water saturated with carbon dioxide under pressure, rather than being leavened with yeast. The aim was to produce an aerated loaf without the loss of carbohydrate involved in a yeast fermentation (7% of the total ingredients). The resultant loaf was insipid in flavour and the method went out of use.

Wholemeal bread is baked with 100% extraction flour, i.e. containing the whole of the cereal grain. White bread is made from 72% extraction flour. Brown bread is made with flour of extraction rate intermediate between that of white bread and wholemeal. A loaf may not legally be described as brown unless it contains at least 0.6% FIBRE on a dry weight basis. Black bread is a coarse wholemeal wheat or rye bread leavened with sourdough (*sauerteig*).

Rye bread is baked wholly or partly with RYE flour, of varying extraction rate, so that it can vary from very light to grey or black. It is commonly a sourdough bread and may contain CARAWAY seeds.

Sourdough bread is commonly wholemeal wheat or rye bread, but may also be white bread, that has been leavened with sourdough (*sauerteig*), dough that has been left to ferment overnight, and contains a mixture of fermenting micro-organisms, including peptonising bacteria that turn the dough to a more plastic state, yeast and lactic or acetic bacteria that produce the sour flavour.

There is a wide variety of different types of bread, with loaves baked in different shapes, or with various additions to the dough. For batch bread, the moulded pieces of dough touch each other in the oven, so that when baked and separated only the top and bottom of the loaf have crusts. Traditional French bread is made with soft-wheat flour, and has a more open texture and crisp crust. Focaccia is Italian white bread made with olive oil (9%) and herbs; ciabatta (also Italian) is a flat white bread with large holes, made with olive oil (5%), literally *old slipper*. Bank Holiday bread is made with extra fat to soften the crumb so that it will last over a long (Bank Holiday) weekend. Cornell bread was originally developed at Cornell University, with increased nutritional value from the addition of 6% soya flour and 8% skim milk solids. Lactein bread has added milk, usually about 6% milk solids (3–4% milk solids are often added to the ordinary loaf in the USA).

See also CHORLEYWOOD PROCESS; FLOUR, EXTRACTION RATE; HOVIS; QUICK BREADS.

breadfruit Large, spherical, starchy fruit of the tree *Artocarpus communis* or *A. incisa* (fig family). Seasonal staple food in the Caribbean, eaten roasted whole when ripe, or boiled in pieces when green. Discovered in 1688 in the Pacific island of Guam by William Dampier.

Composition/100 g: (edible portion 78%) water 70.7 g, 431 kJ (103 kcal), protein 1.1 g, fat 0.2 g, carbohydrate 27.1 g (11 g sugars), fibre 4.9 g, ash 0.9 g, Ca 17 mg, Fe 0.5 mg, Mg 25 mg, P 30 mg, K 490 mg, Na 2 mg, Zn 0.1 mg, Cu 0.1 mg, Mn 0.1 mg, Se 0.6 µg, 22 µg carotenoids, vitamin E 0.1 mg, K 0.5 mg, B_1 0.11 mg, B_2 0.03 mg, niacin 0.9 mg, B_6 0.1 mg, folate 14 µg, pantothenate 0.5 mg, C 29 mg. A 100 g serving is a rich source of vitamin C.

bread, prebaked (or part-baked) Bread that has been partially baked, then allowed to cool, or frozen, for final baking later, to produce a freshly baked loaf.

breadspreads General term for fats used to spread on bread, including BUTTER, MARGARINE and low-fat SPREADS that may not legally be called margarine.

bread, starch-reduced Bread is normally 9–10% protein and about 50% starch; if the starch is reduced, either by washing some of it out of the dough or by adding extra protein, the bread is referred to as starch-reduced, and is often claimed to be of value in slimming and diabetic diets (*see* DIABETIC FOODS). Legally, the name 'starch-reduced bread' may be applied only to bread containing less than 50% carbohydrate, and any claims for its value as a slimming aid are strictly controlled.

breadstick *See* GRISSINI.

breakfast cereal (breakfast food)   Legally defined as any food obtained by the swelling, roasting, grinding, rolling or flaking of any cereal.

break middlings   *See* DUNST.

break rolls   *See* MILLING.

bream   White FISH, *Abramis brama* (N American bluegill bream is *Leponis macrochinus*).

Bredsoy™   An unheated (i.e. enzyme active) full-fat SOYA FLOUR.

brem   Indonesian; sweet or sweet-sour starchy rice paste produced by fermenting cooked rice with moulds (*Mucor* and *Rhizopus* spp.) and yeasts (*Candida* and *Saccharomyces* spp.) for several days, then boiled down and sun dried.

brenza   Eastern European soft buttery cheese made from goat and sheep milk.

bretzels   *See* PRETZELS.

brewers' grains   Cereal residue from brewing, containing about 25% protein; used as animal feed.

brewnzyme   Mixture of bacterial PROTEASES and AMYLASES with barley β-amylase, used to mash unmalted starch for BEER making.

brie   French soft CHEESE.

Composition/100 g: water 48.4 g, 1398 kJ (334 kcal), protein 20.8 g, fat 27.7 g (of which 66% saturated, 31% mono-unsaturated, 3% polyunsaturated), cholesterol 100 mg, carbohydrate 0.4 g (0.4 g sugars), ash 2.7 g, Ca 184 mg, Fe 0.5 mg, Mg 20 mg, P 188 mg, K 152 mg, Na 629 mg, Zn 2.4 mg, Se 14.5 μg, I 16 μg, vitamin A 174 μg RE (173 μg retinol, 9 μg carotenoids), E 0.2 mg, K 2.3 mg, B_1 0.07 mg, B_2 0.52 mg, niacin 0.4 mg, B_6 0.23 mg, folate 65 μg, B_{12} 1.6 μg, pantothenate 0.7 mg. A 40 g serving is a source of vitamin B_2, folate, a rich source of vitamin B_{12}.

Brillat-Savarin   A French gourmet (1755–1826) whose name is given to a consommé (clear soup), BABA and several other dishes.

brilliant acid green BS   *See* GREEN S.

brine   Salt solutions of varying concentrations used in PICKLING. 'Fresh' brine may have added NITRITE; 'live' brine contains micro-organisms that convert nitrate to nitrite (pickling salts).

brining   The process of soaking vegetables in BRINE before pickling in vinegar, in order to remove some of the water, and retain a crisp texture. Dry brining is when the vegetables are covered with dry salt, rather than immersed in a salt solution.

brisling   Young SPRAT, *Clupea sprattus*.

British Farm Standard   Voluntary labelling of foods with a red tractor logo meaning that the requirements of specific farm quality assurance schemes have been met. Under EU legislation the mark is not restricted to British produce, but may be used for produce of other EU countries providing it meets the required standards.

Brix A table of specific gravity based on the BALLING tables, calculated in grams of cane sugar in 100g of solution at 20°C; degree Brix = percentage sugar. It is used to refer to the concentration of sugar syrups used in canned fruits.

broasting A cooking method in which the food is deep fried under pressure, which is quicker than without pressure, and the food absorbs less fat.

broccoli, Chinese (Chinese kale) *Brassica oleracea* var. *alboglabra*; similar to CALABRESE and sprouting BROCCOLI.

broccoli, sprouting Member of the cabbage family, *Brassica oleracea italica* group with purple and white clusters of flower buds (which turn green when boiled) with smaller heads than CALABRESE (broccoli = *little shoots*, It). Originally known in France as Italian asparagus (17th century).

Composition/100g: (edible portion 61%) water 89.3g, 142kJ (34kcal), protein 2.8g, fat 0.4g, carbohydrate 6.6g (1.7g sugars), fibre 2.6g, ash 0.9g, Ca 47mg, Fe 0.7mg, Mg 21mg, P 66mg, K 316mg, Na 33mg, Zn 0.4mg, Mn 0.2mg, Se 2.5µg, vitamin A 33µg RE (2100µg carotenoids), E 0.8mg, K 102mg, B_1 0.07mg, B_2 0.12mg, niacin 0.6mg, B_6 0.17mg, folate 63µg, pantothenate 0.6mg, C 89mg. An 85g serving is a good source of folate, a rich source of vitamin C.

broiling Cooking by direct heat over a flame, as in a barbecue; American term for grilling. Pan broiling is cooking through hot dry metal over direct heat.

bromatology The science of foods; from the Greek *broma*, food.

bromelains Enzymes (EC 3.4.22.32 and 33) in the PINEAPPLE and related bromelids, which hydrolyse proteins. They are available as by-products from commercial pineapple production, usually from the stems, and are used to tenderise meat, treat sausage casings and CHILLPROOF beer.

See also TENDERISERS.

brominated oils Oils from a variety of sources, including peach and apricot kernels, olive and soya oils which have been reacted with bromine to add across the carbon–carbon double bonds. They are used to help stabilise emulsions of flavouring substances in soft drinks. Also known as weighting oils.

bronze diabetes *See* HAEMOCHROMATOSIS.

brose A Scottish dish made by pouring boiling water on to oatmeal or barley meal; fish, meat and vegetables may be added.

brown colours Three brown colours are used in foods: brown FK (E-154), synthetic, which is used to colour KIPPERS; chocolate brown HT (E-155), synthetic; and CARAMEL (E-150).

brown fat *See* ADIPOSE TISSUE, BROWN.

brownie American cake made with chocolate.

browning reactions Chemical reactions in foods that result in the formation of a brown colour. *See* MAILLARD REACTION; PHENOL OXIDASES; STRECKER DEGRADATION.

brugnon Hybrid fruit, a cross between plum and peach. Resembles nectarine, and name sometimes used in France for nectarines.

brûlé Literally burnt; food grilled or otherwise heated sufficiently to give it a brown colour.

brunch Combination meal of breakfast and lunch, a hearty late breakfast. Term first used in the magazine *Punch* in 1896.

Brunner's glands MUCUS-secreting glands embedded in the submucosa of the duodenum and upper jejunum.

brush border *See* MICROVILLI.

Brussels sprouts Leaf buds of *Brassica oleracea gemmifera*.
Composition/100 g: (edible portion 90%) water 86 g, 180 kJ (43 kcal), protein 3.4 g, fat 0.3 g, carbohydrate 8.9 g (2.2 g sugars), fibre 3.8 g, ash 1.4 g, Ca 42 mg, Fe 1.4 mg, Mg 23 mg, P 69 mg, K 389 mg, Na 25 mg, Zn 0.4 mg, Cu 0.1 mg, Mn 0.3 mg, Se 1.6 µg, vitamin A 38 µg RE (2046 µg carotenoids), E 0.9 mg, K 177 mg, B_1 0.14 mg, B_2 0.09 mg, niacin 0.7 mg, B_6 0.22 mg, folate 61 µg, pantothenate 0.3 mg, C 85 mg. A 90 g serving is a source of Mn, a good source of folate, a rich source of vitamin C.

BS 5750 British Standard of excellence in quality management; originally an engineering standard but applicable to food companies, hospitals, etc.; incorporates the EU equivalent IS0 9002.

BSE Bovine spongiform encephalopathy; a degenerative brain disease, transmitted between animals by feeding slaughter-house waste from infected animals. Commonly known as 'mad cow disease'. The infective agent is believed to be a PRION, and can be transmitted to human beings, causing a form of Creutzfeldt–Jakob disease.

BST *See* SOMATOTROPHIN, BOVINE.

BTU British thermal unit, the amount of heat required to raise the temperature of one pound of water through one degree Fahrenheit.

bubble and squeak English; originally cold boiled beef fried with cooked potatoes and cabbage (the name comes from the sound made as it cooks). More commonly now, a fried mixture of left-over cabbage and potatoes. Colcannon is a similar Irish dish.

buccal glands Small glands in the mucous membrane of the mouth that secrete material that mixes with saliva.

buchu oil Essential oil from South African shrub (*Barosma* spp.) used in artificial fruit flavours.

buckling A hot-smoked HERRING (the KIPPER is cold-smoked).

buck rarebit *See* WELSH RAREBIT.

buck's fizz Sparkling wine mixed with orange juice; known in USA as a mimosa.

buckwheat A cereal, the grains of *Fagopyrum esculentum* and other spp., also known as Saracen corn, and, when cooked, as kasha (Russian). It is unsuitable for breadmaking, and is eaten as the cooked grain, a porridge or baked into pancakes.

Composition/100 g: water 9.8 g, 1436 kJ (343 kcal), protein 13.3 g, fat 3.4 g (of which 26% saturated, 37% mono-unsaturated, 37% polyunsaturated), carbohydrate 71.5 g, fibre 10 g, ash 2.1 g, Ca 18 mg, Fe 2.2 mg, Mg 231 mg, P 347 mg, K 460 mg, Na 1 mg, Zn 2.4 mg, Cu 1.1 mg, Mn 1.3 mg, Se 8.3 µg, B_1 0.1 mg, B_2 0.43 mg, niacin 7 mg, B_6 0.21 mg, folate 30 µg, pantothenate 1.2 mg. A 30 g serving is a source of Mn, P, niacin, a good source of Cu, Mg.

buffalo berry N American yellow berry, fruit of *Shepherdia argentea*.

buffalo currant Two varieties of N American currant: *Ribes odoratum*, which has a distinctive smell, and *R. aureum*, the golden or Missouri currant.

buffer Substance that prevents a change in the pH when acid or alkali is added. Salts of weak acids and bases are buffers and are commonly used to control the acidity of foods. Amino acids and proteins also act as buffers.

The pH of blood (*see* ACID–BASE BALANCE) is maintained by physiological buffers including phosphates, bicarbonate and proteins.

bulbogastrone Peptide hormone secreted by the duodenum; decreases gastric secretion.

bulgur The oldest processed food known, originally from the Middle East. Wheat is soaked, cooked and dried, then lightly milled to remove the outer bran and cracked. It is eaten in soups and cooked with meat (when it is known as kibbe). Also called ala, burghul, cracked wheat and American rice.

Composition/100 g: water 9 g, 1432 kJ (342 kcal), protein 12.3 g, fat 1.3 g (of which 22% saturated, 22% mono-unsaturated, 56% polyunsaturated), carbohydrate 75.9 g (0.4 g sugars), fibre 18.3 g, ash 1.5 g, Ca 35 mg, Fe 2.5 mg, Mg 164 mg, P 300 mg, K 410 mg, Na 17 mg, Zn 1.9 mg, Cu 0.3 mg, Mn 3 mg, Se 2.3 µg, 225 µg carotenoids, vitamin E 0.1 mg, K 1.9 mg, B_1 0.23 mg, B_2 0.12 mg, niacin 5.1 mg, B_6 0.34 mg, folate 27 µg, pantothenate 1 mg. A 30 g serving is a source of Mg, P, a rich source of Mn.

bulimia nervosa An eating disorder, especially of women aged between 15 and 30, characterised by powerful and intractable urges to overeat, followed by self-induced vomiting and the excessive use of purgatives.

See also ANOREXIA NERVOSA.

bulking agents Non-nutritive substances (commonly NON-STARCH POLYSACCHARIDES) added to foods to increase the bulk and hence sense of SATIETY, especially in foods designed for weight reduction.

bulk sweeteners *See* SUGAR ALCOHOLS.

bullace Fruit of the wild DAMSON, *Prunus insititia*; similar to SLOE, very acidic.

bullnose pepper *See* PEPPER, SWEET.

bullock's heart *See* CUSTARD APPLE.

bully beef The name given by troops during the First World War to CORNED BEEF (canned salted beef).

bulrush A wild plant common in ponds and marshes (correctly the false bulrush or common reedmace, *Typha latifolia*). The young sprouts and shoots can be eaten in salads, the pollen is used as a flavouring, and the roots and unripe flower heads may be boiled as a vegetable.

bunderfleisch Swiss; beef, brined, rubbed with spices and air-dried.

buni Coffee beans left in the field to dry; generally hard and of poor quality.

bunt *See* SMUT.

burbot Freshwater FISH, *Lota lota*, also known as ling, eelpout, loche, freshwater cod.

Composition/100 g: water 79.3 g, 377 kJ (90 kcal), protein 19.3 g, fat 0.8 g, cholesterol 60 mg, carbohydrate 0 g, ash 1.2 g, Ca 50 mg, Fe 0.9 mg, Mg 32 mg, P 200 mg, K 404 mg, Na 97 mg, Zn 0.8 mg, Cu 0.2 mg, Mn 0.7 mg, Se 12.6 μg, vitamin A 5 μg retinol, B_1 0.37 mg, B_2 0.14 mg, niacin 1.6 mg, B_6 0.3 mg, folate 1 μg, B_{12} 0.8 μg, pantothenate 0.2 mg. A 100 g serving is a source of Cu, Se, vitamin B_6, a good source of P, vitamin B_1, a rich source of Mn, vitamin B_{12}.

burdock Wild thistle-like plant (*Arctium lappa*); leaves used in salads, and to flavour traditional carbonated beverage (dandelion and burdock); called gobo in Japan.

burger *See* HAMBURGER.

burghul *See* BULGUR.

burnet Salad burnet, a wild plant (*Poterium sanguisorba*) growing in grassland on chalky soil. The leaves have the flavour of cucumber, and can be used to flavour fruit wines, vinegar and butter, and are used in salads. Also called pimpernel.

burning foot syndrome Nutritional melalgia (neuralgic pain); severe aching, throbbing and burning pain in the feet, associated with nerve damage, observed in severely undernourished prisoners of war in the Far East. It results from long periods on a diet poor in protein and B VITAMINS, and may (doubtfully) be due specifically to a deficiency of PANTOTHENIC ACID.

burstin Orkneys, historical; barley grains toasted by placing in a pot beside the fire, then ground and used to make a porridge.

busa *See* MILK, FERMENTED.

bushel A traditional dry measure of volume, equivalent to the volume of 80 lb of distilled water at 17 °C with a barometer reading of 30 inches, i.e. 8 Imperial gallons (36.4 L); used as a measure of corn, potatoes, etc. The American (Winchester) bushel is 3% larger.

The weight of a bushel varies with the product: wheat 27 kg, maize and rye 25 kg, barley 22 kg, paddy rice 20 kg, oats 14.5 kg.

butt A cask for beer or wine, containing 108 Imperial gallons (491 L).

butter Made from separated CREAM by churning (sweet cream butter); legally not less than 80% fat (and not more than 16% water). Lactic butter is made by first ripening the cream with a bacterial culture to produce lactic acid and increase the flavour (due to diacetyl). This is normally unsalted or up to 0.5% salt added. Sweet cream butter may be salted up to 2%.

Composition/100 g: water 15.9 g, 3001 kJ (717 kcal), protein 0.9 g, fat 81.1 g (of which 68% saturated, 28% mono-unsaturated, 4% polyunsaturated), cholesterol 215 mg, carbohydrate 0.1 g (0.1 g sugars) ash 2.1 g, Ca 24 mg, Mg 2 mg, P 24 mg, K 24 mg, Na 576 mg, Zn 0.1 mg, Se 1 μg, I 38 μg, vitamin A 684 μg RE (671 μg retinol, 158 μg carotenoids), E 2.3 mg, K 7 mg, B_2 0.03 mg, folate 3 μg, B_{12} 0.2 μg, pantothenate 0.1 mg. A 15 g serving is a source of vitamin A.

Clarified butter is butter fat, prepared by heating butter and separating the fat from the water. It does not become RANCID as rapidly as butter. Also known as GHEE or ghrt (India) and samna (Egypt).

Process or renovated butter has been melted and rechurned with the addition of milk, cream or water.

Drawn butter is melted butter used as a dressing for cooked vegetables. Devilled butter is mixed with lemon juice, cayenne and black pepper and curry powder. Ravigote butter is creamed with chopped fresh aromatic herbs (tarragon, parsley, chives, chervil), usually served with grilled meat. Green butter is mixed with chopped herbs and other seasonings to produce a savoury spread. Black butter is browned by heating, then vinegar, salt, pepper or other seasonings are added.

See also VEGETABLE BUTTERS.

butterbur   *See* FUKI.

butterine   US term for MARGARINE.

buttermilk   The residue left after churning butter, 0.1–2% fat, with the other constituents of milk increased proportionally. Slightly acidic, with a distinctive flavour due to the presence of DIACETYL and other substances. Usually made by adding lactic bacteria to skim milk; 90–92% water, 4% lactose with acidic flavour from lactic acid.

butternut   Fruit of the N American tree *Juglans cinerea*, also known as white walnut, lemon walnut, oilnut.

Composition/100 g: (edible portion 27%) water 3.3 g, 2562 kJ (612 kcal), protein 24.9 g, fat 57 g (of which 2% saturated, 19% mono-unsaturated, 78% polyunsaturated), carbohydrate 12.1 g, fibre 4.7 g, ash 2.7 g, Ca 53 mg, Fe 4 mg, Mg 237 mg, P 446 mg, K 421 mg, Na 1 mg, Zn 3.1 mg, Cu 0.4 mg, Mn 6.6 mg, Se 17.2 µg, vitamin A 6 µg RE, B_1 0.38 mg, B_2 0.15 mg, niacin 1 mg, B_6 0.56 mg, folate 66 µg, pantothenate 0.6 mg, C 3 mg. A 20 g serving is a source of Mg, P, a rich source of Mn.

butterscotch   *See* TOFFEE.

butter, whey (serum butter)   Butter made from the small amount of fat left in WHEY; it has a slightly different FATTY ACID composition from ordinary butter.

butylated hydroxyanisole (BHA)   An ANTIOXIDANT (E-320) used in fats and fatty foods; stable to heating, and so is useful in baked products.

butylated hydroxytoluene (BHT)   An ANTIOXIDANT (E-321) used in fats and fatty foods.

butyric acid   Short-chain saturated FATTY ACID (C4:0). It occurs as 5–6% of butter fat, and in small amounts in other fats and oils.

BV   Biological value, a measure of PROTEIN QUALITY.

C

CA   Controlled   atmosphere.   *See*   PACKAGING,   MODIFIED ATMOSPHERE.

cabbage   Leaves of *Brassica oleracea capitata*.

Composition/100 g: (edible portion 80%) water 92.5 g, 100 kJ (24 kcal), protein 1.2 g, fat 0.2 g, carbohydrate 5.4 g, fibre 2.3 g, ash 0.7 g, Ca 47 mg, Fe 0.6 mg, Mg 15 mg, P 23 mg, K 246 mg, Na 18 mg, Zn 0.2 mg, Mn 0.2 mg, Se 0.9 µg, vitamin A 6 µg RE, B_1 0.05 mg, B_2 0.03 mg, niacin 0.3 mg, B_6 0.09 mg, folate 57 µg, pantothenate 0.1 mg, C 51 mg. An 85 g serving is a good source of folate, a rich source of vitamin C.

cabbage, Chinese   Name given to two oriental vegetables: *Brassica pekinensis* (pe-tsai, Pekin cabbage, snow cabbage); pale green compact head resembling lettuce, and *B. chinensis* (pak choi, Chinese greens, Chinese chard); loose bunch of dark green leaves and thick stalks.

Pe tsai, composition/100g: (edible portion 93%) water 94.4g, 67kJ (16kcal), protein 1.2g, fat 0.2g, carbohydrate 3.2g (1.4g sugars), fibre 1.2g, ash 1g, Ca 77mg, Fe 0.3mg, Mg 13mg, P 29mg, K 238mg, Na 9mg, Zn 0.2mg, Mn 0.2mg, Se 0.6µg, vitamin A 16µg RE (239µg carotenoids), E 0.1mg, K 42.9mg, B_1 0.04mg, B_2 0.05mg, niacin 0.4mg, B_6 0.23mg, folate 79µg, pantothenate 0.1mg, C 27mg. A 40g serving is a source of folate, vitamin C.

Pak choi, composition/100g: (edible portion 88%) water 95.3g, 54kJ (13kcal), protein 1.5g, fat 0.2g, carbohydrate 2.2g (1.2g sugars), fibre 1g, ash 0.8g, Ca 105mg, Fe 0.8mg, Mg 19mg, P 37mg, K 252mg, Na 65mg, Zn 0.2mg, Mn 0.2mg, Se 0.5µg, vitamin A 223µg RE (2722µg carotenoids), E 0.1mg, K 35.8mg, B_1 0.04mg, B_2 0.07mg, niacin 0.5mg, B_6 0.19mg, folate 66µg, pantothenate 0.1mg, C 45mg. A 40g serving is a source of vitamin A, folate, a rich source of vitamin C.

cabbage palm Several types of palm tree that have edible inner leaves, terminal buds or inner part of the stem (HEART OF PALM).

cabbie-claw Scottish (Shetland); fresh codling, salted and hung in open air for 1–2 days, then simmered with horseradish. The name derives from the Shetland dialect name for COD, kabbilow.

caboc Scottish; double cream cheese (60% fat), rolled in oatmeal.

cabrales Spanish goat or sheep milk hard cheese.

cacao butter *See* COCOA BUTTER.

cacen-gri Welsh; soda scones made with currants and BUTTERMILK.

cachectin (cachexin) *See* CACHEXIA; TUMOUR NECROSIS FACTOR.

cachexia The condition of extreme emaciation and wasting seen in patients with advanced diseases such as cancer and AIDS, owing to both an inadequate intake of food and the effects of the disease in increasing METABOLIC RATE (hypermetabolism) and the breakdown of tissue protein.

See also NITROGEN BALANCE; PROTEIN–ENERGY MALNUTRITION; TUMOUR NECROSIS FACTOR.

cachou Small scented tablets for sweetening the breath.

cactus pear *See* PRICKLY PEAR.

cadmium A mineral of no known function in the body and therefore not a dietary essential. It accumulates in the body throughout life, reaching a total body content of 20–30mg (200–300µmol). It is toxic and cadmium poisoning is a recognised industrial disease.

In Japan, cadmium poisoning has been implicated in itai-itai disease, a severe and sometimes fatal loss of calcium from the bones; the disease occurred in an area where rice was grown on land irrigated with contaminated waste water.

Accidental contamination of drinking water with cadmium salts also leads to kidney damage, and enough cadmium can leach out from cooking vessels with cadmium glaze to pose a hazard.

caecum   The first part of the large intestine, separated from the small intestine by the ileocolic sphincter. It is small in carnivorous animals and very large in herbivores, since it is involved in the digestion of cellulose. In omnivorous animals, including humans, it is of intermediate size.

See also GASTROINTESTINAL TRACT.

Caerphilly   Welsh hard cheese with sour flavour and crumbly texture.

cafestol   Diterpene in COFFEE oil, associated with reversible HYPER-CHOLESTEROLAEMIA and hypertriglyceridaemia and also possibly an anticarcinogenic effect by enhancement of PHASE II METABO-LISM of foreign compounds. Only released into the beverage when coffee is boiled for a prolonged period of time.

See also KAHWEOL.

caffeine   A PURINE, trimethylxanthine, an ALKALOID found in coffee and tea, also known as theine. It raises blood pressure, acts as a DIURETIC and temporarily averts fatigue, so has a stimulant action.

It acts to potentiate the action of hormones and neurotransmitters that act via cAMP, since it inhibits phosphodiesterase (EC 3.1.4.17). It can also be a cause of insomnia in some people, and decaffeinated coffee and tea are commonly available.

COFFEE beans contain about 1% caffeine, and the beverage contains about 70 mg/100 mL. Tea contains 1.5–2.5% caffeine, about 50–60 mg/100 mL of the beverage. COLA DRINKS contain 12–18 mg/100 mL.

See also THEOBROMINE; XANTHINE.

caffeol   A volatile oil in coffee beans, giving the characteristic flavour and aroma.

caking   Undesirable AGGLOMERATION of powders as a result of exposure to humidity. *See also* ANTICAKING AGENTS.

calabasa   West Indian or green pumpkin, with yellow flesh.

calabash   *See* GOURD.

calabrese   An annual plant (*Brassica oleracea italica*), a variety of BROCCOLI that yields a crop in the same year as it is sown. Also called American, Italian or green sprouting broccoli.

calamondin   A CITRUS fruit resembling a small tangerine, with a delicate pulp and a lime-like flavour.

calandria A heat exchanger consisting of a closed cylindrical vessel containing a vertical bundle of tubes used for falling film evaporation of milk, which is passed as a thin film down the inside of the tubes, which are surrounded by a steam jacket.

calbindin An intracellular calcium binding protein induced by VITAMIN D; it is involved in CALCIUM transport.

calcidiol 25-Hydroxycholecalciferol, 25-hydroxy derivative of VITAMIN D, the main storage and circulating form of the vitamin in the body.
    See also CALCITRIOL.

calciferol Used at one time as a name for ercalciol (ergocalciferol or vitamin D_2) made by ultraviolet irradiation of ergosterol. Also used as a general term to include both VITAMERS of VITAMIN D (vitamins D_2 and D_3).

calcinosis Abnormal deposition of CALCIUM salts in tissues. May be due to excessive intake of VITAMIN D.

calciol Official name for cholecalciferol, the naturally occurring form of VITAMIN D (vitamin D_3).

calcipotriol VITAMIN D analogue used as ointment for treatment of psoriasis.

calcitonin Peptide hormone secreted by the C cells of the thyroid gland; lowers blood CALCIUM by suppressing the activity of osteoclasts, so inhibiting the release of calcium from bone.

calcitonin-gene-related peptide Peptide hormone secreted throughout gut; decreases gastric acid secretion.

calcitriol 1,25-Dihydroxycholecalciferol, the active metabolite of VITAMIN D in the body.

calcium The major inorganic component of bones and teeth; the total body content of an adult is about 1–1.5 kg (15–38 mol). The small amounts in blood plasma (2.1–2.6 mmol/L, 85–105 mg/L) and in tissues play a vital role in the excitability of nerve tissue, the control of muscle contraction and the integration and regulation of metabolic processes. An unacceptably high plasma concentration of calcium is HYPERCALCAEMIA.
    The absorption of calcium from the intestinal tract requires VITAMIN D, and together with parathyroid hormone, vitamin D also controls the body's calcium balance, mobilising it from the bones to maintain the plasma concentration within a very narrow range.
    Although a net loss of calcium from bones occurs as a normal part of the ageing process, and may lead to OSTEOPOROSIS, there is little evidence that higher intakes of calcium in later life will affect the process.

calcium acid phosphate Also known as monocalcium phosphate and acid calcium phosphate or ACP, $Ca(H_2PO_4)_2$. Used as the acid ingredient of BAKING POWDER and self-raising FLOUR, since it reacts with bicarbonate to liberate carbon dioxide. Calcium phosphates are permitted food additives (E-341).

calculi (calculus) Stones formed in tissues such as the gall bladder (biliary calculus or GALLSTONE), kidney (renal calculus) or ureters. Renal calculi may consist of URIC ACID and its salts (especially in GOUT) or of OXALIC ACID salts. Oxalate calculi may be of metabolic or dietary origin and people at metabolic risk of forming oxalate renal calculi are advised to avoid dietary sources of oxalic acid and its precursors. Rarely, renal calculi may consist of the amino acid CYSTINE.

See also TARTAR.

calf's foot jelly GELATINE, stock made by boiling calves' feet in water; it sets to a stiff jelly on cooling.

calmodulin Small intracellular calcium-binding protein that acts to regulate adenylate cyclase (EC 4.6.1.1) and protein kinases in response to changes in intracellular calcium concentrations.

calorie A unit of ENERGY used to express the energy yield of foods and energy expenditure by the body. One calorie (cal) is the amount of heat required to raise the temperature of 1 g of water through 1 °C (from 14.5 to 15.5 °C).

Nutritionally the kilocalorie (1000 calories) is used, the amount of heat required to raise the temperature of 1 kg of water through 1 °C, and is abbreviated as either kcal or Cal.

The calorie is not an SI unit, and correctly the JOULE is used as the unit of energy, although kcal are widely used. 1 kcal = 4.18 kJ; 1 kJ = 0.24 kcal.

See also ENERGY; ENERGY CONVERSION FACTORS.

calorimeter (bomb calorimeter) An instrument for measuring the amount of oxidisable energy in a substance, by burning it in oxygen and measuring the heat produced.

The energy yield of a foodstuff in the body is equal to that obtained in a bomb calorimeter only when the metabolic end-products are the same as those obtained by combustion. Thus, proteins liberate 23.64 kJ (5.65 kcal)/g in a calorimeter, when the nitrogen is oxidised to the dioxide, but only 18.4 kJ (4.4 kcal)/g in the body, when the nitrogen is excreted as urea (which has a heat of combustion equal to the 'missing' 5.23 kJ (1.25 kcal)).

See also ENERGY CONVERSION FACTORS.

calorimetry The measurement of energy expenditure by the body.

Direct calorimetry is the measurement of heat output from the body as an index of energy expenditure, and hence energy requirement. The subject is placed inside a small thermally insulated room, and the heat produced is measured. Few such difficult studies have been performed, and only a limited range of activities can be studied under these confined conditions.

Indirect calorimetry is a means of estimating energy expenditure indirectly, rather than by direct measurement of heat production. Two methods are in use:

(1) Measurement of the rate of oxygen consumption, using a SPIROMETER; permits calculation of energy expenditure. Most studies of the energy cost of activities have been performed by this method.

(2) Estimation of the total production of carbon dioxide over a period of 7–10 days, after consumption of dual isotopically labelled water (i.e. water labelled with both ^{2}H and ^{18}O, see DOUBLE-LABELLED WATER).

caltrops *See* WATER CHESTNUT.

Camembert French soft CHEESE made from cows' milk, originating from Auge in Normandy. Covered with a white mould (*Penicillium candidum* or *P. camembertii*) which participates in the ripening process.

Composition/100g: water 51.8g, 1256kJ (300kcal), protein 19.8g, fat 24.3g (of which 67% saturated, 30% mono-unsaturated, 3% polyunsaturated), cholesterol 72mg, carbohydrate 0.5g (0.5g sugars), ash 3.7g, Ca 388mg, Fe 0.3mg, Mg 20mg, P 347mg, K 187mg, Na 842mg, Zn 2.4mg, Se 14.5µg, I 16µg, vitamin A 241µg RE (240µg retinol, 12µg carotenoids), E 0.2mg, K 2mg, B_1 0.03mg, B_2 0.49mg, niacin 0.6mg, B_6 0.23mg, folate 62µg, B_{12} 1.3µg, pantothenate 1.4mg. A 40g serving is a source of Ca, P, vitamin A, B_2, folate, a rich source of vitamin B_{12}.

camomile Either of two herbs, *Anthemis nobilis* or *Matricaria recutica*. The essential oil is used to flavour LIQUEURS; camomile tea is a TISANE prepared by infusion of the dried flower heads and the whole herb can be used to make a herb beer.

Campden process The preservation of food by the addition of sodium bisulphite (E-222), which liberates sulphur dioxide. Also known as cold preservation, since it replaces heat STERILISATION.

Campden tablets Tablets of sodium bisulphite (E-222), used for sterilisation of bottles and other containers and in the preservation of foods.

Campylobacter A genus of pathogenic organisms which are the most commonly reported cause of gastroenteritis in UK, although it is not known what proportion of cases are foodborne. Campylobacteriosis has been associated with the consumption of undercooked meats, milk that has been inadequately pasteurised or contaminated by birds, and contaminated water. *C. jejuni* (*C. coli*, TX 4.1.2.1) invades intestinal epithelial cells. Infective

dose 10^3 organisms, onset 3–8 days, duration weeks. HELICOBAC-
TER PYLORI was formerly classified as a *Campylobacter*.

camu-camu   Fruit of the Peruvian bush *Myrciaria paraensis*;
burgundy red in colour, weighing 6–14 g and about 3 cm in diameter; contains 3000 mg vitamin C/100 g.

cananga oil   A lipid-soluble flavouring agent, obtained by distillation of flowers of *Cananga odorato*.

canavanine   Toxic amino acid (an analogue of ARGININE in which
the final methylene group is replaced by oxygen), originally isolated from the jack bean, *Canavalia ensiformis*, and also found
in a variety of other plants, including especially alfalfa bean
sprouts. It is incorporated into proteins in place of arginine, and
also inhibits nitric oxide synthetase.

canbra oil   Oil extracted from selected strains of RAPESEED containing not more than 2% ERUCIC ACID.

   See also CANOLA.

cancer   A wide variety of diseases characterised by uncontrolled
growth of tissue. Dietary factors may be involved in the initiation of some forms of cancer, and a high-fat diet has been
especially implicated. There is some evidence that ANTIOXI-
DANT nutrients such as CAROTENE, VITAMINS C and E and the
mineral SELENIUM may be protective, as may NON-STARCH
POLYSACCHARIDES.

   See also CARCINOGEN; CACHEXIA.

candelilla wax   A hydrocarbon wax from the candelilla plant
(*Euphorbia cerifera*). Used as a lubricant and surface finishing
agent in chewing gum and hard candy.

Canderel™   The SWEETENER ASPARTAME, in tablets

Candida   Genus of yeasts that inhabit the gut. *C. albicans* can,
under some circumstances, cause candidiasis (thrush) in the
vagina, mouth and skin folds.

candy   (1) Crystallised sugar made by repeated boiling and slow
evaporation.

   (2) USA, general term for SUGAR confectionery.

candy doctor   *See* SUGAR DOCTOR.

cane sugar   SUCROSE extracted from the sugar cane *Saccharum
officinarum*; identical to sucrose prepared from any other source,
such as sugar beet. *See* SUGAR.

canihua   Seeds of *Chenopodium pallidicaule*, grown in the Peruvian Andes; nutritionally similar to cereals.

cannelloni   *See* PASTA.

canner's alkali   A mixture of sodium hydroxide (and sometimes
also sodium carbonate) used to remove the skin from fruit before
canning.

canners' sugar   *See* SUGAR.

canning The process of preserving food by sterilisation and cooking in a sealed metal can, which destroys bacteria and protects from recontamination. If foods are sterilised and cooked in glass jars that are then closed with hermetically sealed lids, the process is known as bottling.

Canned foods are sometimes known as tinned foods, because the cans were originally made using tin-plated steel. Usually now they are made of lacquered steel or aluminium.

In aseptic canning, foods are presterilised at a very high temperature (150–175 °C) for a few seconds and then sealed into cans under sterile (aseptic) conditions. The flavour, colour and retention of vitamins are superior with this short-time high-temperature process compared with conventional canning.

canola Oilseeds of the brassica family that contain less than specified amounts of GLUCOSINOLATES and ERUCIC ACID. Canola oil is 7% saturated, 62% mono-unsaturated, 31% polyunsaturated, vitamin E 17.1 mg, K 122 mg.

See also MUSTARD OIL; RAPESEED.

cantaloupe *See* MELON.

canthaxanthin A red CAROTENOID pigment, not a precursor of VITAMIN A. It is used as a food colour (E-161g), and can be added to the diet of broiler CHICKENS to colour the skin and shanks, and to the diet of farmed TROUT to produce the same bright colour as is seen in wild fish.

CAP Controlled atmosphere packaging.

cape gooseberry Fruit of the Chinese lantern *Physalis peruviana*, *P. pubescens* or *P. edulis*; herbaceous perennial resembling small cherry, surrounded by dry, bladder-like calyx, also known as golden berry, physalis, Chinese lantern, Peruvian cherry and ground tomato.

Composition/100 g: (edible portion 94%) water 85.4 g, 222 kJ (53 kcal), protein 1.9 g, fat 0.7 g, carbohydrate 11.2 g, ash 0.8 g, Ca 9 mg, Fe 1 mg, P 40 mg, vitamin A 36 μg RE, B_1 0.11 mg, B_2 0.04 mg, niacin 2.8 mg, C 11 mg.

caper Unopened flower buds of the subtropical shrub *Capparis spinosa* or *C. inermis* with a peppery flavour; commonly used in pickles and sauces. Unripe seeds of the nasturtium (*Tropaeolum majus*) may be pickled and used as a substitute.

capercaillie (capercailzie) A large GAME bird (*Tetrao urogallus*), also known as wood grouse or cock of the wood.

capillary flow The way in which a liquid will rise inside a capillary tube, above the bulk liquid surface, as a result of surface tension.

capillary fragility A measure of the resistance to rupture of the small blood vessels (capillaries), which would lead to leakage of red blood cells into tissue spaces. Deficiency of VITAMIN C can lead to increased capillary fragility.

See also FLAVONOIDS.

capon A castrated cockerel (male CHICKEN), which has a faster rate of growth, and more tender flesh, than the cockerel. Surgery has generally been replaced by chemical caponisation, the implantation of pellets of OESTROGEN.

caprenin Poorly absorbed fat, two medium-chain fatty acids (CAPRIC and CAPRYLIC ACID) and one very long-chain fatty acid (BEHENIC ACID) esterified to glycerol; used as a FAT REPLACER. Behenic acid is poorly absorbed and caprenin yields only 5 kcal/g, compared with 9 kcal/g for normal fats.

capric acid Medium-chain saturated fatty acid, C10:0.

caprotil An ACE inhibitor.

caprylic acid Medium-chain saturated fatty acid, C8:0.

capsicum *See* PEPPER, CHILLI and PEPPER, SWEET.

carambola Or star fruit, star apple; 8–12 cm long ribbed fruit of *Averrhoa carambola* and *A. bilimbi*.

Composition/100 g: (edible portion 97%) water 91.4 g, 130 kJ (31 kcal), protein 1 g, fat 0.3 g, carbohydrate 6.7 g (4 g sugars), fibre 2.8 g, ash 0.5 g, Ca 3 mg, Fe 0.1 mg, Mg 10 mg, P 12 mg, K 133 mg, Na 2 mg, Zn 0.1 mg, Cu 0.1 mg, Se 0.6 µg, vitamin A 3 µg RE (115 µg carotenoids), E 0.2 mg, B_1 0.01 mg, B_2 0.02 mg, niacin 0.4 mg, B_6 0.02 mg, folate 12 µg, pantothenate 0.4 mg, C 34 mg.

caramel Brown material formed by heating carbohydrates in the presence of acid or alkali; also known as burnt sugar. It can be manufactured from various sugars, starches and starch hydrolysates and is used as a flavour and colour (E-150) in a wide variety of foods.

caramels Sweets similar to TOFFEE but boiled at a lower temperature; may be soft or hard.

caraway Dried ripe fruit of *Carum carvi*, an aromatic spice.

carbachol Parasympathomimetic drug used to restore the function of inactive bowels or bladder after surgery.

carbenoxolone Synthetic derivative of GLYCYRRHIZINIC acid (from LIQUORICE) used in combination with ANTACIDS for treatment of gastric ULCERS and gastro-oesophageal reflux; stimulates secretion of protective mucus.

carbohydrate Sugars and starches, which provide 50–70% of energy intake. Chemically they are composed of carbon, hydrogen and oxygen in the ratio $C_n : H_{2n} : O_n$. The basic carbohydrates are the MONOSACCHARIDE sugars, of which glucose, fructose and galactose are nutritionally the most important.

Disaccharides are composed of two monosaccharides: nutritionally the important disaccharides are SUCROSE, LACTOSE, MALTOSE and TREHALOSE. A number of oligosaccharides occur in foods, consisting of 3–5 monosaccharide units; in general these are not digested, and should be considered among the unavailable carbohydrates.

Larger polymers of carbohydrates are known as polysaccharides or complex carbohydrates. Nutritionally two classes of polysaccharide can be distinguished: (a) starches, polymers of glucose, either as a straight chain (AMYLOSE) or with a branched structure (AMYLOPECTIN); (b) a variety of other polysaccharides which are collectively known as NON-STARCH POLYSACCHARIDES (NSP) and are not digested by human digestive enzymes. The carbohydrate reserve in liver and muscles is glycogen, a glucose polymer with the same branched structure as amylopectin.

The metabolic energy yield of carbohydrates is 17 kJ (4 kcal)/g. More precisely, monosaccharides yield 15.7 kJ (3.74 kcal), disaccharides 16.6 kJ (3.95 kcal) and starch 17.6 kJ (4.18 kcal)/g. GLYCEROL is a three-carbon sugar alcohol, and is classified as a carbohydrate; it yields 18.1 kJ (4.32 kcal)/g.

See also STARCH; SUGAR; SUGAR ALCOHOLS.

CARBOHYDRATES: MONO- AND DISACCHARIDES

carbohydrate by difference   It is relatively difficult to determine the various carbohydrates present in foods, and an approximation is often made by subtracting the measured PROTEIN, FAT, ASH and water from the total weight. It is the sum of nutritionally available carbohydrates (dextrins, starches and sugars); nutritionally unavailable carbohydrate (pentosans, pectins, hemicelluloses and cellulose) and non-carbohydrates such as organic acids and LIGNINS.

carbohydrate loading   Practice of some endurance athletes (e.g. marathon runners) in training for a major event; it consists of exercising to exhaustion, so depleting muscle GLYCOGEN, then eating a large carbohydrate-rich meal so as to replenish glycogen reserves with a higher than normal proportion of straight chain glycogen.

carbohydrate metabolism   *See* GLUCOSE METABOLISM.

carbohydrate, unavailable   A general term for those carbohydrates present in foods that are not digested, and are therefore excluded from calculations of energy intake, although they may be fermented by intestinal bacteria and yield some energy. The term includes both indigestible oligosaccharides and the various NON-STARCH POLYSACCHARIDES.

   See also FATTY ACIDS, VOLATILE; STARCH, RESISTANT.

carbon dioxide, available   *See* BAKING POWDER; FLOUR, SELF-RAISING.

carbon dioxide storage   *See* PACKAGING, MODIFIED ATMOSPHERE.

γ-carboxyglutamate   A derivative of the amino acid glutamate (abbr Gla, M_r 191.1) which is found in PROTHROMBIN and other calcium-binding proteins involved in BLOOD CLOTTING. Its formation requires VITAMIN K. Also occurs in the protein osteocalcin in BONE, where it has a function in ensuring the correct crystallisation of bone mineral.

carboxymethylcellulose   *See* CELLULOSE DERIVATIVES.

carboxypeptidase E   Enzyme (EC 3.4.17.10) that catalyses cleavage of PRO-INSULIN to INSULIN, and post-synthetic modification of PRO-OPIOMELANOCORTIN and other peptide HORMONES.

carboxypeptidases   Enzymes (EC 3.4.17.1 and 2) secreted in the pancreatic juice that remove amino acids sequentially from the free carboxyl end of a peptide or protein, i.e. EXOPEPTIDASES.

carcinogen   Any compound that is capable of inducing cancer.

carcinoid syndrome   Condition in which there are metastases to the liver of a carcinoid tumour of the enterochromaffin cells of the small intestine. The tumour produces a variety of physiologically active AMINES, including HISTAMINE (which causes flushing reactions) and 5-HYDROXYTRYPTAMINE. The depletion of TRYPTO-

PHAN to form 5-hydroxytryptamine can be severe enough to lead to the development of PELLAGRA.

cardamom The dried, nearly ripe, fruit and seeds of *Elettaria cardamomum*, a member of the ginger family. An aromatic spice used as a flavouring in sausages, bakery goods, SUGAR confectionery and whole in mixed pickling spice. It is widely used in Indian cooking (the Hindi name is elaichi), and as one of the ingredients of CURRY POWDER. Arabic coffee (similar to Turkish coffee) is flavoured with ground cardamom seeds.

cardiomyopathy Any chronic disorder affecting the muscle of the heart. May be associated with ALCOHOLISM and VITAMIN B_1 deficiency.

cardiospasm *See* ACHALASIA.

cardoon Leafy vegetable (*Cynara cardunculus*); both the fleshy root and the ribs and stems of the inner (blanched) leaves are eaten. Sometimes called chard, although distinct from true chard or spinach beet.

Composition/100 g: (edible portion 49%) water 94 g, 84 kJ (20 kcal), protein 0.7 g, fat 0.1 g, carbohydrate 4.9 g, fibre 1.6 g, ash 0.3 g, Ca 70 mg, Fe 0.7 mg, Mg 42 mg, P 23 mg, K 400 mg, Na 170 mg, Zn 0.2 mg, Mn 0.1 mg, Se 0.9 µg, vitamin A 6 µg RE, B_1 0.02 mg, B_2 0.03 mg, niacin 0.3 mg, B_6 0.04 mg, folate 28 µg, pantothenate 0.1 mg, C 2 mg.

caries Dental decay caused by attack on the tooth enamel by acids produced by bacteria that are normally present in the mouth. Sugars in the mouth promote bacterial growth and acid production; SUCROSE specifically promotes PLAQUE-forming bacteria, which cause the most damage. A moderately high intake of FLUORIDE increases the resistance of tooth enamel to acid attack.
See also TOOTHFRIENDLY SWEETS.

cariogenic Causing tooth decay (CARIES) by stimulating the growth of acid-forming bacteria on the teeth; the term is applied to sucrose and other fermentable carbohydrates.

carissa Fruit of the evergreen shrub *Carissa macrocarpa* (*C. grandiflora*), also known as natal plum.

Composition/100 g: (edible portion 86%) water 84.2 g, 260 kJ (62 kcal), protein 0.5 g, fat 1.3 g, carbohydrate 13.6 g, ash 0.4 g, Ca 11 mg, Fe 1.3 mg, Mg 16 mg, P 7 mg, K 260 mg, Na 3 mg, Cu 0.2 mg, vitamin A 2 µg RE, B_1 0.04 mg, B_2 0.06 mg, niacin 0.2 mg, C 38 mg. A 20 g serving (1 fruit without skin and seeds) is a source of vitamin C.

carmine Brilliant red colour derived from COCHINEAL (E-120).

carminic acid *See* COCHINEAL.

carmoisine A red colour, also known as azorubine, synthetic azo-dye (E-122).

carnauba wax   A hard wax from the leaf buds and leaves of the Brazilian wax palm *Copernicia cerifera*, used in candy glaze.

carnitine   γ-Amino-β-hydroxybutyric acid trimethylbetaine, required for the transport of fatty acids into MITOCHONDRIA for oxidation. There is no evidence that it is a dietary essential for human beings, since it can readily be formed from lysine, although there is some evidence that increased intake may enhance the work capacity of muscles. A dietary essential for some insects, at one time called vitamin B_T.

carnosine   A dipeptide, β-alanylhistidine, found in the muscle of most animals, function not known.

carob   Seeds and pod of the tree *Ceratonia siliqua*, also known as locust bean and St John's bread. It contains a sweet pulp which is rich in sugar and gums, as well as containing 21% protein and 1.5% fat. It is used as animal feed, and to make confectionery (as a substitute for chocolate).

Carob GUM (locust bean gum) is extracted from the carob and is used as an emulsifier and stabiliser (E-410) as well as in cosmetics and as a size for textiles.

caroenum   Roman; very sweet cooking wine, reduced to one-third its volume by boiling and mixed with honey.

Carophyll^{TM} Apo-8-carotenal, a CAROTENE derivative (*see* CAROTENALS).

carotenals   Also known as apo-carotenals. Aldehydes formed by asymmetric oxidative cleavage of CAROTENE by carotene dioxygenase (EC 1.13.11.21); RETINAL is the carotenal formed by 15-15′ cleavage of carotene. Depending on where the carotene molecule is split, the products are variously 8′-, 10′- and 12′-apocarotenal, which may be oxidised to yield retinaic acid, but cannot form RETINOL.

See also VITAMIN A.

carotene   The red and orange pigments of many plants, obvious in carrots, red palm oil and yellow maize, but masked by CHLOROPHYLL in leaves. Three main carotenes in foods are important as precursors of VITAMIN A: α-, β- and γ-carotene, which are also used as food colours (E-160a). Plant foods contain a considerable number of other carotenes, most of which are not precursors of vitamin A.

Carotene is converted into vitamin A (RETINOL) in the intestinal mucosa, or is absorbed unchanged. 6 μg of β-carotene, and 12 μg of other provitamin A carotenoids, are nutritionally equivalent to 1 μg of preformed vitamin A. About 30% of the vitamin A in western diets, and considerably more in diets in less developed countries, comes from carotene.

In addition to their role as precursors of vitamin A, carotenes are important as ANTIOXIDANT nutrients.

CAROTENES

carotenoids   A general term for the wide variety of red and yellow
compounds chemically related to CAROTENE that are found in
plant foods, some of which are precursors of VITAMIN A, and hence
known as provitamin A carotenoids.

carotenols   Hydroxylated carotenoids, including XANTHOPHYLL.

carotinaemia (carotenaemia)   Presence of excessive amounts of CAROTENE in blood plasma. Also known as xanthaemia.

carp   Freshwater FISH, *Cyprinus carpio.*

Composition/100 g: water 76.3 g, 532 kJ (127 kcal), protein 17.8 g, fat 5.6 g (of which 23% saturated, 48% mono-unsaturated, 29% polyunsaturated), cholesterol 66 mg, carbohydrate 0 g, ash 1.5 g, Ca 41 mg, Fe 1.2 mg, Mg 29 mg, P 415 mg, K 333 mg, Na 49 mg, Zn 1.5 mg, Cu 0.1 mg, Se 12.6 µg, vitamin A 9 µg retinol, E 0.6 mg, K 0.1 mg, B_1 0.12 mg, B_2 0.05 mg, niacin 1.6 mg, B_6 0.19 mg, folate 15 µg, B_{12} 1.5 µg, pantothenate 0.8 mg, C 2 mg. A 100 g serving is a source of Se, pantothenate, a rich source of P, vitamin B_{12}.

carrageen   Edible seaweeds, *Chondrus crispus*, also known as Iberian moss or Irish sea moss, and *Gigartina stellata*; stewed in milk to make a jelly or blancmange. A source of CARRAGEENAN.

carrageenan   A POLYSACCHARIDE extracted from red algae, especially *Chondrus crispus* (Irish moss) and *Gigartina stellata.* One of the plant GUMS, it binds water to form a gel, increases viscosity, and reacts with proteins to form emulsions. It is used as an emulsifier and stabiliser in milk drinks, processed cheese, low-energy foods, etc. (E-407).

carrot   The root of *Daucus carota*, commonly used as a vegetable.

Composition/100 g: water 88.3 g, 172 kJ (41 kcal), protein 0.9 g, fat 0.2 g, carbohydrate 9.6 g (4.5 g sugars), fibre 2.8 g, ash 1 g, Ca 33 mg, Fe 0.3 mg, Mg 12 mg, P 35 mg, K 320 mg, Na 69 mg, Zn 0.2 mg, Mn 0.1 mg, Se 0.1 µg, vitamin A 600 µg RE (8878 µg carotenoids), E 0.7 mg, K 13.2 mg, B_1 0.07 mg, B_2 0.06 mg, niacin 1 mg, B_6 0.14 mg, folate 19 µg, pantothenate 0.3 mg, C 6 mg. A 60 g serving is a rich source of vitamin A.

Carr–Price reaction   Colorimetric assay for VITAMIN A, based on the development of a blue colour after reaction with antimony trichloride in chloroform. The Neeld–Pearson method uses trifluoroacetic acid in place of antimony trichloride.

carthamin   A yellow to red colourant from safflower flowers, *Carthemus tinctorius*, chemically a chalcone.

cartilage   The hard connective tissue of the body, composed mainly of COLLAGEN, together with chondromucoid (a protein combined with chondroitin sulphate) and chondroalbuminoid (a protein similar to ELASTIN). New BONE growth consists of cartilage on which calcium salts are deposited as it develops.

Cartose^TM   A steam hydrolysate of maize starch, used as a carbohydrate modifier in milk preparations for infant feeding. It consists of a mixture of DEXTRIN, MALTOSE and GLUCOSE.

carubin   *See* LOCUST BEAN.

carubinose   *See* MANNOSE.

CAS Controlled atmosphere storage.

casaba American name for winter MELON.

cascara *See* LAXATIVES.

case hardening Formation of a hard impermeable skin on some foods during drying; produces a food with a dry surface and a moist interior.

casein About 75% of the proteins of milk are classified as caseins; a group of 12–15 small hydrophobic proteins, in four main classes (α-, β-, γ- and κ-caseins). They occur in milk as coarse colloidal particles (micelles) some 100 mm in diameter. Often used as a protein supplement, since the casein fraction from milk is more than 90% protein.

Hammarsten's casein is prepared by diluting fat-free milk with water and precipitating the protein with acetic acid. The precipitate is washed three times with water, dissolved in ammonium hydroxide and reprecipitated; this is repeated twice. The final precipitate is washed with alcohol and ether and finally extracted with ether.

caseinogen An obsolete name for the form in which CASEIN is present in solution in milk; when it was precipitated it was then called casein.

cashew nut Fruit of the tropical tree *Anacardium occidentale*, generally eaten roasted and salted. The nut hangs from the true fruit, a large fleshy but sour apple-like fruit, which is very rich in vitamin C.

Composition/100 g: water 1.7 g, 2403 kJ (574 kcal), protein 15.3 g, fat 46.3 g (of which 21% saturated, 62% mono-unsaturated, 18% polyunsaturated), carbohydrate 32.7 g (5 g sugars), fibre 3 g, ash 4 g, Ca 45 mg, Fe 6 mg, Mg 260 mg, P 490 mg, K 565 mg, Na 16 mg, Zn 5.6 mg, Cu 2.2 mg, Mn 0.8 mg, Se 11.7 µg, 23 µg carotenoids, E 0.9 mg, K 34.7 mg, B_1 0.2 mg, B_2 0.2 mg, niacin 1.4 mg, B_6 0.26 mg, folate 69 µg, pantothenate 1.2 mg. A 25 g serving is a source of P, a good source of Mg, vitamin a rich source of Cu.

Casilan™ A CASEIN preparation used as a protein concentrate and nutritional supplement.

cassareep Caribbean; boiled-down juice from grated CASSAVA root, flavoured with cinnamon, cloves and brown sugar; used as a base for sauces. It can also be fermented with MOLASSES.

cassava (manioc) The tuber of the tropical plant *Manihot utilissima*. It is the dietary staple in many tropical countries, although it is an extremely poor source of protein; the plant grows well even in poor soil, and is extremely hardy, withstanding considerable drought. It is one of the most prolific crops, yielding up to 13 million kcal/acre, compared with YAM 9 million, and SORGHUM or MAIZE 1 million. Introduced into Africa by slave ships returning from Brazil in mid-16th century. Fermented cassava meal is gari.

Cassava root contains cyanide, and before it can be eaten it must be grated and left in the open to allow the cyanide to evaporate. The leaves can be eaten as a vegetable, and the tuber is the source of TAPIOCA.

Composition/100 g: water 59.7 g, 670 kJ (160 kcal), protein 1.4 g, fat 0.3 g, carbohydrate 38.1 g (1.7 g sugars), fibre 1.8 g, ash 0.6 g, Ca 16 mg, Fe 0.3 mg, Mg 21 mg, P 27 mg, K 271 mg, Na 14 mg, Zn 0.3 mg, Cu 0.1 mg, Mn 0.4 mg, Se 0.7 µg, vitamin A 1 µg RE (8 µg carotenoids), E 0.2 mg, K 1.9 mg, B_1 0.09 mg, B_2 0.05 mg, niacin 0.9 mg, B_6 0.09 mg, folate 27 µg, pantothenate 0.1 mg, C 21 mg.

cassia The inner bark of a tree grown in the Far East (*Cinnamomium cassia*), used as a flavouring, similar to CINNAMON.

cassina A tea-like beverage made from cured leaves of a holly bush, *Ilex cassine*, containing 1–1.6% CAFFEINE and 8% TANNIN.

Casson fluid *See* PLASTIC FLUIDS.

Casson value A measure of the rheological properties (shear stress and viscosity) of CHOCOLATE.

castor oil Oil from the seeds of the castor oil plant, *Ricinus* spp. The oil itself is not irritating, but in the small intestine it is hydrolysed by LIPASE to release ricinoleic acid, which is an irritant to the intestinal mucosa and therefore acts as a purgative. The seeds also contain the toxic LECTIN ricin.

catabolism Those pathways of METABOLISM concerned with the breakdown and oxidation of fuels and hence provision of metabolic energy. People who are undernourished or suffering from CACHEXIA are sometimes said to be in a catabolic state, in that they are catabolising their body tissues, without replacing them.

catadromous fish Fish that live in fresh water and go to sea to spawn, such as eels.

catalase HAEM-containing enzyme (EC 1.11.1.6) that catalyses the decomposition of HYDROGEN PEROXIDE to water and oxygen. Its main function *in vivo* is removal of hydrogen peroxide formed by a variety of OXYGENASES. Used in food processing to remove hydrogen peroxide used as a sterilant, and together with glucose oxidase (EC 1.1.3.4) to remove traces of oxygen.

catchup *See* KETCHUP.

catecholamines General term for dihydroxyphenylamines, including DOPAMINE, ADRENALINE and NORADRENALINE.

catechol oxidase *See* PHENOL OXIDASES.

catfish Several types of (mainly North American) freshwater fish that have barbells resembling a cat's whiskers, including bullhead and channel catfish.

catharsis Purging or cleansing out of the bowels by giving a LAXATIVE (cathartic) to stimulate intestinal activity.

cathepsins (Also kathepsins); a group of intracellular enzymes in animal tissues that hydrolyse proteins. They are involved in the normal turnover of tissue protein, and the softening of meat when GAME is hung.

CAT scanning Computerised axial tomography, an X-ray technique that permits a three-dimensional X-ray image to be generated. Used nutritionally to determine ADIPOSE TISSUE distribution and BONE mass.

catsup *See* KETCHUP.

caudle Hot spiced wine thickened with eggs. *See also* MULLED WINE.

caul Membrane enclosing the fetus; that from sheep or pig used to cover meat while roasting.

cauliflower The edible flower of *Brassica oleracea botrytis*, normally creamy-white in colour, although some cultivars have green or purple flowers. Horticulturally, varieties that mature in summer and autumn are called cauliflower, and those that mature in winter BROCCOLI, but commonly both are called cauliflower.

Composition/100 g: (edible portion 39%) water 92 g, 105 kJ (25 kcal), protein 2 g, fat 0.1 g, carbohydrate 5.3 g (2.4 g sugars), fibre 2.5 g, ash 0.7 g, Ca 22 mg, Fe 0.4 mg, Mg 15 mg, P 44 mg, K 303 mg, Na 30 mg, Zn 0.3 mg, Mn 0.2 mg, Se 0.6 µg, vitamin A 1 µg RE (41 µg carotenoids), E 0.1 mg, K 16 mg, B_1 0.06 mg, B_2 0.06 mg, niacin 0.5 mg, B_6 0.22 mg, folate 57 µg, pantothenate 0.7 mg, C 46 mg. A 90 g serving is a good source of folate, a rich source of vitamin C.

caviar(e) The salted hard ROE of the sturgeon, *Acipenser* spp.; three main types, sevruga, asetra (ocietre) and BELUGA, the prime variety. Mock caviare (also known as German, Danish or Norwegian caviare) is the salted hard roe of the lumpfish (*Cyclopterus lumpus*).

Composition/100 g: water 47.5 g, 1055 kJ (252 kcal), protein 24.6 g, fat 17.9 g (of which 25% saturated, 29% mono-unsaturated, 46% polyunsaturated), cholesterol 588 mg, carbohydrate 4 g, ash 6.5 g, Ca 275 mg, Fe 11.9 mg, Mg 300 mg, P 356 mg, K 181 mg, Na 1500 mg, Zn 0.9 mg, Cu 0.1 mg, Mn 0.1 mg, Se 65.5 µg, vitamin A 561 µg retinol, E 7 mg, K 0.7 mg, B_1 0.19 mg, B_2 0.62 mg, niacin 0.1 mg, B_6 0.32 mg, folate 50 µg, B_{12} 20 µg, pantothenate 3.5 mg. A 16 g serving (1 tbsp) is a source of Fe, Mg, Se, vitamin A, E, a rich source of vitamin B_{12}.

cavitation Production of bubbles in foods by ULTRASOUND and their rapid expansion/contraction.

cayenne pepper *See* PEPPER, CHILLI.

CBE *See* COCOA BUTTER EQUIVALENTS.

CCK *See* CHOLECYSTOKININ.

CCP *See* CRITICAL CONTROL POINT.

cDNA Copy or complementary DNA; a single-stranded DNA copy of mRNA, synthesised using REVERSE TRANSCRIPTASE, which can then be inserted into a PLASMID or other vector, for the introduction of new DNA into a bacterial or other cell. cDNA libraries represent the information encoded in the mRNA of a particular tissue or organism.

Celacol^{TM} Methyl, hydroxyethyl and other CELLULOSE derivatives.

celeriac A variety of CELERY with a thick root which is eaten grated in salads or cooked as a vegetable, *Apium graveolens* var. *rapaceum*, also known as turnip-rooted or knob celery.

Composition/100 g: (edible portion 86%) water 88 g, 176 kJ (42 kcal), protein 1.5 g, fat 0.3 g, carbohydrate 9.2 g (1.6 g sugars), fibre 1.8 g, ash 1 g, Ca 43 mg, Fe 0.7 mg, Mg 20 mg, P 115 mg, K 300 mg, Na 100 mg, Zn 0.3 mg, Cu 0.1 mg, Mn 0.2 mg, Se 0.7 µg, 1 µg carotenoids, E 0.4 mg, K 41 mg, B_1 0.05 mg, B_2 0.06 mg, niacin 0.7 mg, B_6 0.17 mg, folate 8 µg, pantothenate 0.4 mg, C 8 mg.

celery Edible stems of *Apium graveolens* var. *dulce*.

Composition/100 g: (edible portion 89%) water 95 g, 59 kJ (14 kcal), protein 0.7 g, fat 0.2 g, carbohydrate 3 g (1.8 g sugars), fibre 1.6 g, ash 0.8 g, Ca 40 mg, Fe 0.2 mg, Mg 11 mg, P 24 mg, K 260 mg, Na 80 mg, Zn 0.1 mg, Mn 0.1 mg, Se 0.4 µg, vitamin A 22 µg RE (553 µg carotenoids), E 0.3 mg, K 29.3 mg, B_1 0.02 mg, B_2 0.06 mg, niacin 0.3 mg, B_6 0.07 mg, folate 36 µg, pantothenate 0.2 mg, C 3 mg.

celiac disease *See* COELIAC DISEASE.

cellobiose A disaccharide of glucose linked β-1,4; formed by hydrolysis of CELLULOSE by CELLULASE, and not hydrolysed by mammalian digestive enzymes.

Cellofas^{TM} Derivatives of CELLULOSE: Cellofas A is methylethylcellulose, Cellofas B is sodium carboxymethylcellulose.

Cellophane^{TM} The first transparent, non-porous film, made from wood pulp (CELLULOSE), patented in 1908 by Swiss-French chemist Jacques-Edwin Brandenburger; waterproof cellophane for food wrapping developed by Du Pont in 1926. Still widely used for wrapping foods and other commodities.

celluflour Powdered CELLULOSE, used in experimental diets to provide indigestible bulk.

cellulase Enzymes that hydrolyse CELLULOSE. Present in the digestive juices of some wood-boring insects and various microorganisms, but not mammals.

1:4-β-Glucan cellobiohydrolase (EC 3.2.9.1) is an endohydrolase, yielding soluble cellulose fragments. 1:4-β-Glucan glucanohydrolase (EC 3.2.1.4) is an exohydrolase, yielding CELLOBIOSE. β-Glucosidase (EC 3.7.1.21) catalyses the hydrolysis of cellobiose to glucose.

Cell-free preparations of cellulase from *Trichoderma* spp. (especially the mesophilic fungus *T. resie*) are used to liquefy fruit pulps, and to prepare glucose SYRUPS from waste cellulose from pulp mills, etc.

cellulose   A POLYSACCHARIDE of GLUCOSE units linked β-1,4 which is not hydrolysed by mammalian digestive enzymes. The main component of plant cell walls, but does not occur in animal tissues. It is digested by bacterial CELLULASE, and hence only RUMINANTS and animals that have a large CAECUM have an adequate population of intestinal bacteria to permit them to digest cellulose to any significant extent. There is little digestion of cellulose in the human large intestine; nevertheless, it serves a valuable purpose in providing bulk to the intestinal contents, and is one of the major components of dietary fibre (*see* FIBRE, DIETARY) or NON-STARCH POLYSACCHARIDES.

See also CELLULOSE, MICROCRYSTALLINE.

cellulose derivatives   A number of chemically modified forms of cellulose are used in food processing for their special properties, including:

(1) Carboxymethylcellulose (E-466), which is prepared from the pure cellulose of cotton or wood. It absorbs up to 50 times its own weight of water to form a stable colloidal mass. It is used, together with stabilisers, as a whipping agent, in ice cream, confectionery, jellies, etc., and as an inert filler in 'slimming aids'.

(2) Methylcellulose (E-461), which differs from carboxymethylcellulose (and other GUMS) since its viscosity increases with increasing temperature rather than decreasing. Hence it is soluble in cold water and forms a gel on heating. Used as a thickener and emulsifier, and in foods formulated to be low in GLUTEN.

(3) Other cellulose derivatives used as emulsifiers and stabilisers are hydroxypropylcellulose (E-463), hydroxypropylmethylcellulose (E-464) and ethylmethylcellulose (E-465).

cellulose, microcrystalline   Partially hydrolysed CELLULOSE used as a filler in slimming and other foods (E-460).

celtuce Stem lettuce, *Lactuca sativa*; enlarged stem eaten raw or cooked, with a flavour between celery and lettuce; leaves are not palatable.

Composition/100 g: (edible portion 75%) water 95 g, 75 kJ (18 kcal), protein 0.9 g, fat 0.3 g, carbohydrate 3.7 g, fibre 1.7 g, ash 0.7 g, Ca 39 mg, Fe 0.6 mg, Mg 28 mg, P 39 mg, K 330 mg, Na 11 mg, Zn 0.3 mg, Mn 0.7 mg, Se 0.9 µg, vitamin A 175 µg RE, B_1 0.05 mg, B_2 0.07 mg, niacin 0.6 mg, B_6 0.05 mg, folate 46 µg, pantothenate 0.2 mg, C 20 mg.

centrifuge A machine that exerts a force many thousand times that of gravity, by spinning. Commonly used to clarify liquids by settling the heavier solids or to separate liquids of different density, e.g. cream from milk. High-speed centrifuges run up to 60000g; preparative and analytical ultracentrifuges at 500000–600000g.

cereal Any grain or edible seed of the grass family that may be used as food; e.g. WHEAT, RICE, OATS, BARLEY, RYE, MAIZE and MILLET. Cereals are collectively known as corn in the UK; in the USA corn is specifically maize. Cereals provide the largest single foodstuff in most diets; in some less developed countries up to 90% of the total diet may be cereal; in the UK BREAD and FLOUR provide 25–30% of the total energy and protein of the average diet.

cereals, puffed Whole grains, grain parts, or a shaped dough, expanded by subjecting to heat and pressure to produce a very light and airy product.

See also EXTRUSION; PUFFING GUN.

cerebrose Obsolete name for GALACTOSE.

cerebrosides Glycolipids containing no phosphate, but with a polar head region consisting of neutral oligosaccharides of GALACTOSE. Especially important in nerve membranes and the myelin sheath of nerves. The fatty acids may be esterified to either GLYCEROL or sphingosine (SPHINGOLIPIDS).

See also GANGLIOSIDES.

cerelose A commercial preparation of GLUCOSE containing about 9% water.

ceroid pigment Age spots or liver spots. Patches of brown pigment under the skin, increasing with age, believed to be due to accumulation of the products of oxidation of fatty acids and protein.

ceruloplasmin A copper-containing protein in BLOOD PLASMA, the main circulating form of copper in the body. Has ferrioxidase (EC 1.16.3.1) activity and is important in IRON metabolism. Not useful for assessment of copper status since levels are elevated in pregnancy, lactation, inflammatory diseases and in response to oral contraceptive agents.

cervelat SAUSAGE, originally made with brain, but now minced beef and pork, seasoned and smoked.

cestode *See* TAPEWORM.

CF *See* CITROVORUM FACTOR.

CFC Chlorofluorocarbon, *see* REFRIGERANTS.

CFSAN Centre for Food Safety and Nutrition of the US Food and Drug Administration; web site http://vm.cfsan.fda.gov/.

cfu Colony forming units, a measure of the bacterial content of foods, etc.

chalasia Abnormal relaxation of the cardiac sphincter muscle of the stomach so that gastric contents reflux into the oesophagus, leading to regurgitation.

chamomile Either of two herbs, *Anthemis nobilis* or *Matricaria recutica*. The essential oil is used to flavour LIQUEURS; chamomile tea is a TISANE prepared by infusion of the dried flower heads and the whole herb can be used to make a herb beer.

champagne Sparkling wine from the Champagne region of north-eastern France, made by a second fermentation in the bottle; pioneered by Benedictine cellar master Dom Pierre Pérignon at the Abbey d'Hautvilliers, late 17th century. Sparkling wine from other regions, even when made in the same way, cannot legally be called champagne, but is known as méthode champenoise.

chanterelle Edible wild fungus, *Cantharellus cibarius*, *see* MUSHROOMS.

chapatti (chappati, chuppati) Indian; unleavened whole-grain WHEAT or MILLET bread, baked on an ungreased griddle. Phulka are small chapattis; roti are chapattis prepared with maize flour.

chaptalisation Addition of sugar to grape must during fermentation to increase the alcohol content of the WINE.

charcoal Finely divided carbon, obtained by heating bones (BONE CHARCOAL) or wood in a closed retort to carbonise the organic matter. Used to purify solutions because it will absorb colouring matter and other impurities.

charlotte Dessert made from stewed fruit encased in, or layered alternately with, bread or cake crumbs, e.g. apple charlotte. In charlotte russe there is a centre of a cream mixture surrounded by cake.

charqui (charki) S. American; dried meat, normally prepared from beef, but may also be made from sheep, llama and alpaca. Strips of meat are cut lengthways and pressed after salting, then air-dried. The final form is flat, thin, flaky sheets, so differing from the long strips of BILTONG. Also called jerky or jerked beef.

Chartreuse (1) A LIQUEUR invented in 1605 and still made by the Carthusian monks, named for the great charterhouse (la grande chartreuse), the mother house of the order, near Grenoble in southern France. It is reputed to contain more than 200 ingredients. There are three varieties: green Chartreuse is 55%, yellow 43% and white 30% ALCOHOL.

(2) A dish turned out of a mould; more usually, fruit enclosed in jelly.

Chastek paralysis Acute deficiency of vitamin B_1 in foxes and mink fed on diets high in raw fish, which contains THIAMINASE.

chateaubriand Thick steak cut from BEEF fillet. Originally named in 1822 in honour of the Comte de Chateaubriand.

chaudron (chawdron) Medieval English; sauce served with roast swan, made from the giblets boiled in broth with its blood, vinegar and spices.

chaya Large tropical herb (up to 2 m tall), *Cnidoscolus chayamansa*; the young leaves are eaten like SPINACH.

CHD Coronary heart disease, *see* ISCHAEMIC HEART DISEASE.

cheddar Hard CHEESE dating from 16th century prepared by a particular method (CHEDDARING); originally from the Cheddar area of Somerset, England; matured for several months or even years. Red Cheddar is coloured with ANNATTO.

Composition/100 g: water 36.8 g, 1687 kJ (403 kcal), protein 24.9 g, fat 33.1 g (of which 67% saturated, 30% mono-unsaturated, 3% polyunsaturated), cholesterol 105 mg, carbohydrate 1.3 g (0.5 g sugars), ash 3.9 g, Ca 721 mg, Fe 0.7 mg, Mg 28 mg, P 512 mg, K 98 mg, Na 621 mg, Zn 3.1 mg, Se 13.9 µg, I 30 µg, vitamin A 265 µg RE (258 µg retinol, 85 µg carotenoids), E 0.3 mg, K 2.8 mg, B_1 0.03 mg, B_2 0.38 mg, niacin 0.1 mg, B_6 0.07 mg, folate 18 µg, B_{12} 0.8 µg, pantothenate 0.4 mg. A 40 g serving is a source of vitamin A, a good source of P, a rich source of Ca, vitamin B_{12}.

cheddaring In the manufacture of CHEESE, after coagulation of the milk, heating of the curd and draining, the curds are piled along the floor of the vat, when they consolidate to a rubbery sheet of curd. This is the cheddaring process; for cheeses with a more crumbly texture the curd is not allowed to settle so densely.

cheese Prepared from the curd precipitated from milk by RENNET, purified CHYMOSIN or lactic acid. Cheeses other than cottage and cream cheeses are cured by being left to mature with salt, under various conditions that produce the characteristic flavour of that type of cheese.

Although most cheeses are made from cow's milk, goat's milk and sometimes ewe's milk can be used to make specialty cheeses. These are generally soft cheeses. There is a very wide variety of different types of cheese. There are numerous variants (over 800) including more than 100 from England and Wales alone (eight major regional cheeses: Caerphilly, Derby, Double Gloucester, CHEDDAR, Lancashire, Red Leicester, STILTON and Wensleydale).

Some varieties are regional specialties, and legally may only be made in a defined geographical area; others are defined by the process rather than the region of production. The strength of flavour of cheese increases as it ages; mild or mellow cheeses are younger, and less strongly flavoured, than mature or extra mature cheeses. The flavour that develops on ripening is due to the activity of PROTEINASES and LIPASES, with further metabolism of free fatty acids to a variety of products.

Cheeses differ in their water and fat content and hence their nutrient and energy content, ranging from 50 to 80% water in soft cheeses (mozzarella, Quark, Boursin, cottage) to less than 20% in hard cheese (PARMESAN, Emmental, Gruyère, CHEDDAR) with semi-hard cheeses around 40% water (Caerphilly, Gouda, Edam, Stilton). They contain much of the calcium of the milk and many contain a relatively large amount of sodium from the added salt.

Edam, Gouda composition/100 g: water 41.5 g, 1490 kJ (356 kcal), protein 24.9 g, fat 27.4 g (of which 68% saturated, 30% mono-unsaturated, 3% polyunsaturated), cholesterol 114 mg, carbohydrate 2.2 g (2.2 g sugars) ash 3.9 g, Ca 700 mg, Fe 0.2 mg, Mg 29 mg, P 546 mg, K 121 mg, Na 819 mg, Zn 3.9 mg, Se 14.5 μg, vitamin A 165 μg RE (164 μg retinol, 10 μg carotenoids), E 0.2 mg, K 2.3 mg, B_1 0.03 mg, B_2 0.33 mg, niacin 0.1 mg, B_6 0.08 mg, folate 21 μg, B_{12} 1.5 μg, pantothenate 0.3 mg. A 40 g serving is a good source of P, a rich source of Ca, vitamin B_{12}.

Mozarella composition/100 g: water 50 g, 1256 kJ (300 kcal), protein 22.2 g, fat 22.4 g (of which 64% saturated, 32% mono-unsaturated, 4% polyunsaturated), cholesterol 79 mg, carbohydrate 2.2 g (1 g sugars), ash 3.3 g, Ca 505 mg, Fe 0.4 mg, Mg 20 mg, P 354 mg, K 76 mg, Na 627 mg, Zn 2.9 mg, Se 17 μg, vitamin A 179 μg RE (174 μg retinol, 57 μg carotenoids), E 0.2 mg, K 2.3 mg, B_1 0.03 mg, B_2 0.28 mg, niacin 0.1 mg, B_6 0.04 mg, folate 7 μg, B_{12} 2.3 μg, pantothenate 0.1 mg. A 40 g serving is a source of P, a good source of Ca, a rich source of vitamin B_{12}.

Blue-veined cheeses (Gorgonzola, Stilton, Roquefort, etc.) derive the colour (and flavour) from the growth of the mould *Penicillium roquefortii*, during ripening.

Traditionally, hard cheeses must contain not less than 40% fat on a dry weight basis, and that fat must be milk fat. However, a number of low-fat variants of traditional hard cheeses, and vegetarian cheeses, are now made.

Cottage cheese is soft uncured white cheese made from pasteurised skim milk (or milk powder) by lactic acid starter (with or without added rennet), heated, washed and drained (salt may be added). Contains more than 80% water. Also known as pot cheese, Schmierkäse and, in USA, as Dutch cheese. Baker's or hoop cheese is made in the same way as cottage cheese, but the curd is not washed, and it is drained in bags, giving it a finer grain. It contains more water and acid than cottage cheese.

Composition/100 g: water 79 g, 431 kJ (103 kcal), protein 12.5 g, fat 4.5 g (of which 67% saturated, 30% mono-unsaturated, 2% polyunsaturated), cholesterol 15 mg, carbohydrate 2.7 g (0.3 g sugars) ash 1.4 g, Ca 60 mg, Fe 0.1 mg, Mg 5 mg, P 132 mg, K 84 mg, Na 405 mg, Zn 0.4 mg, Se 9 µg, I 24 µg, vitamin A 44 µg RE (43 µg retinol, 12 µg carotenoids), K 0.4 mg, B_1 0.02 mg, B_2 0.16 mg, niacin 0.1 mg, B_6 0.07 mg, folate 12 µg, B_{12} 0.6 µg, pantothenate 0.2 mg. A 110 g serving (small pot) is a source of I, P, Se, vitamin B_2, a rich source of vitamin B_{12}.

Cream cheese is unripened soft cheese made from cream with varying fat content (20–25% fat or 50–55% fat).

Composition/100 g: water 53.8 g, 1461 kJ (349 kcal), protein 7.6 g, fat 34.9 g (of which 66% saturated, 30% mono-unsaturated, 4% polyunsaturated), cholesterol 110 mg, carbohydrate 2.7 g (0.2 g sugars), ash 1.2 g, Ca 80 mg, Fe 1.2 mg, Mg 6 mg, P 104 mg, K 119 mg, Na 296 mg, Zn 0.5 mg, Se 2.4 µg, vitamin A 366 µg RE (359 µg retinol, 89 µg carotenoids), E 0.3 mg, K 2.9 mg, B_1 0.02 mg, B_2 0.2 mg, niacin 0.1 mg, B_6 0.05 mg, folate 13 µg, B_{12} 0.4 µg, pantothenate 0.3 mg. A 30 g serving is a source of vitamin A, B_{12}.

Processed cheese is made by milling various hard cheeses with emulsifying salts (phosphates and citrates), whey and water, then pasteurising to extend the shelf-life. Typically 40% water, a 30 g portion contains 5 g protein, 8 g fat; provides 100 kcal (410 kJ). Soft version with 50% water is used as a spread.

Feta is Balkan (especially Greek), white, soft, crumbly, salted cheese made from goat's or ewe's milk.

Composition/100 g: water 55.2 g, 1105 kJ (264 kcal), protein 14.2 g, fat 21.3 g (of which 74% saturated, 23% mono-unsaturated, 3% polyunsaturated), cholesterol 89 mg, carbohydrate 4.1 g (4.1 g sugars), ash 5.2 g, Ca 493 mg, Fe 0.6 mg, Mg 19 mg, P 337 mg, K 62 mg, Na 1116 mg, Zn 2.9 mg, Se 15 µg, vitamin A 125 µg RE (125 µg retinol, 3 µg carotenoids), E 0.2 mg, K 1.8 mg, B_1 0.15 mg, B_2 0.84 mg, niacin 1 mg, B_6 0.42 mg, folate 32 µg, B_{12} 1.7 µg, pantothenate 1 mg. A 40 g serving is a source of P, a good source of Ca, vitamin B_2, a rich source of vitamin B_{12}.

Swiss cheese is an American name for any hard cheese that contains relatively large bubbles of air, like the Swiss Emmental and Gruyère. The holes arise during ripening from gases produced by bacteria.

Composition/100 g: water 33.2 g, 1729 kJ (413 kcal), protein 29.8 g, fat 32.3 g (of which 62% saturated, 33% mono-unsaturated,

6% polyunsaturated), cholesterol 110 mg, carbohydrate 0.4 g (0.4 g sugars), ash 4.3 g, Ca 1011 mg, Fe 0.2 mg, Mg 36 mg, P 605 mg, K 81 mg, Na 336 mg, Zn 3.9 mg, Se 14.5 µg, vitamin A 271 µg RE (268 µg retinol, 33 µg carotenoids), E 0.3 mg, K 2.7 mg, B_1 0.06 mg, B_2 0.28 mg, niacin 0.1 mg, B_6 0.08 mg, folate 10 µg, B_{12} 1.6 µg, pantothenate 0.6 mg. A 40 g serving is a source of vitamin A, a rich source of Ca, P, vitamin B_{12}.

Soft goat cheese composition/100 g: water 60.8 g, 1122 kJ (268 kcal), protein 18.5 g, fat 21.1 g (of which 73% saturated, 24% mono-unsaturated, 3% polyunsaturated), cholesterol 46 mg, carbohydrate 0.9 g (0.9 g sugars), ash 1.6 g, Ca 140 mg, Fe 1.9 mg, Mg 16 mg, P 256 mg, K 26 mg, Na 368 mg, Zn 0.9 mg, Cu 0.7 mg, Mn 0.1 mg, Se 2.8 µg, I 51 µg, vitamin A 288 µg RE (283 µg retinol, 54 µg carotenoids), E 0.2 mg, K 1.8 mg, B_1 0.07 mg, B_2 0.38 mg, niacin 0.4 mg, B_6 0.25 mg, folate 12 µg, B_{12} 0.2 µg, pantothenate 0.7 mg. A 40 g serving is a source of I, P, vitamin A, a good source of Cu.

cheese analogues   Cheese-like products made from CASEIN or SOYA and vegetable fat.

cheese, filled   CHEESE made from skimmed milk with the addition of vegetable oil to replace the butterfat of whole milk.

cheese, vegetarian   Cheese in which animal RENNET has not been used to precipitate the curd. Precipitation is achieved using lactic acid alone, or a plant enzyme or biosynthetic CHYMOSIN. Truly vegetarian cheese is made from vegetable protein rather than milk.

cheese, whey   Made from WHEY by heat coagulation of the proteins (lactalbumin and lactoglobulin).

cheilosis   Cracking of the edges of the lips, one of the clinical signs of VITAMIN B_2 (riboflavin) deficiency.

chelating agents   Chemicals that combine with metal ions and remove them from their sphere of action, also called sequestrants. Used in food manufacture to remove traces of metal ions that might otherwise cause foods to deteriorate and clinically to alter absorption of a mineral, or to increase its excretion in cases of metal poisoning, e.g. EDTA, citrates, DESFERRIOXAMINE, tartrates, penicillamine, phosphates.

See also HAEMOCHROMATOSIS; IRON.

chemical caponisation   *See* CAPON.

chemical ice   Ice containing a preservative, e.g. a solution of ANTIBIOTIC or other chemicals; used to preserve fish.

chemical score   A measure of PROTEIN QUALITY based on chemical analysis. *See* AMINO ACIDS.

chenodeoxycholic acid   One of the primary BILE salts synthesised in the liver and secreted in the bile as a GLYCINE or TAURINE conjugate.

chenopods   Seeds of *Chenopodium* spp. eaten in the Peruvian Andes: *C. quinoa* (QUINOA) and *C. pallidicaule* (CANIHUA). Other *Chenopodium* spp. have been considered for poultry feed, including Russian thistle, summer cypress and garden orache.

cherimoya   *See* CUSTARD APPLE.

cherry   Fruits of *Prunus* spp.

Composition/100 g: (edible portion 90%) water 82.3 g, 264 kJ (63 kcal), protein 1.1 g, fat 0.2 g, carbohydrate 16 g (12.8 g sugars), fibre 2.1 g, ash 0.5 g, Ca 13 mg, Fe 0.4 mg, Mg 11 mg, P 21 mg, K 222 mg, Zn 0.1 mg, Cu 0.1 mg, Mn 0.1 mg, vitamin A 3 µg RE (123 µg carotenoids), E 0.1 mg, K 2.1 mg, B_1 0.03 mg, B_2 0.03 mg, niacin 0.2 mg, B_6 0.05 mg, folate 4 µg, pantothenate 0.2 mg, C 7 mg.

Peruvian cherry is CAPE GOOSEBERRY, Surinam cherry is PITANGA.

cherry, ground   Fruit of *Physalis pruinosa*, similar to CAPE GOOSEBERRY; grows wild, eaten raw but more usually boiled or as preserve; also called strawberry tomato, and dwarf Cape gooseberry.

cherry, West Indian   The fruit of a small bush, native to the tropical and subtropical regions of America, *Malpighia punicifolia*. One of the richest known sources of vitamin C. Also known as acerola, Barbados or Antilles cherry.

Composition/100 g: (edible portion 80%) water 91 g, 134 kJ (32 kcal), protein 0.4 g, fat 0.3 g, carbohydrate 7.7 g, fibre 1.1 g, ash 0.2 g, Ca 12 mg, Fe 0.2 mg, Mg 18 mg, P 11 mg, K 146 mg, Na 7 mg, Zn 0.1 mg, Cu 0.1 mg, Se 0.6 µg, vitamin A 38 µg RE, B_1 0.02 mg, B_2 0.06 mg, niacin 0.4 mg, B_6 0.01 mg, folate 14 µg, pantothenate 0.3 mg, C 1678 mg. A 100 g serving (20 cherries) is an exceptionally rich source of vitamin C.

chervil   (1) A herb, *Anthriscus cerefolium*, with parsley-like leaves, used in the fresh green state as a garnish, and fresh or dried to flavour salads and soups.

(2) The turnip-rooted chervil, *Chaerophyllum bulbosum*, a hardy biennial vegetable cultivated for its roots.

(3) Sweet chervil, a wild plant (*Myrrhis odorata*) with a smell of aniseed. The leaves are used to flavour fruit cups, fruit salads and cooked fruit; the main root can be boiled, sliced and used in salads. Also known as sweet cecily.

Cheshire   English hard CHEESE with a crumbly texture.

Cheshire cat   An old English cheese measure.

chestnut   (1) Spanish or sweet chestnut from trees of *Castanea* spp. Unlike other common nuts it contains very little fat, being largely starch and water.

Composition /100 g: water 52 g, 820 kJ (196 kcal), protein 1.6 g, fat 1.3 g (of which 18% saturated, 36% mono-unsaturated, 45% polyunsaturated), carbohydrate 44.2 g, ash 1 g, Ca 19 mg, Fe

0.9 mg, Mg 30 mg, P 38 mg, K 484 mg, Na 2 mg, Zn 0.5 mg, Cu 0.4 mg, Mn 0.3 mg, vitamin A 1 μg RE, B_1 0.14 mg, B_2 0.02 mg, niacin 1.1 mg, B_6 0.35 mg, folate 58 μg, pantothenate 0.5 mg, C 40 mg. A 50 g serving (5 nuts) is a source of Cu, folate, a rich source of vitamin C.

(2) Water chestnut, seeds of *Trapa natans*, also called caltrops or sinharanut; eaten raw or roasted.

Composition /100 g: (edible portion 77%) water 74 g, 406 kJ (97 kcal), protein 1.4 g, fat 0.1 g, carbohydrate 23.9 g (4.8 g sugars), fibre 3 g, ash 1.1 g, Ca 11 mg, Fe 0.1 mg, Mg 22 mg, P 63 mg, K 584 mg, Na 14 mg, Zn 0.5 mg, Cu 0.3 mg, Mn 0.3 mg, Se 0.7 μg, vitamin E 1.2 mg, K 0.3 mg, B_1 0.14 mg, B_2 0.2 mg, niacin 1 mg, B_6 0.33 mg, folate 16 μg, pantothenate 0.5 mg, C 4 mg.

(3) Chinese water chestnut, also called matai or waternut; tuber of the sedge, *Eleocharis tuberosa* or *E. dulcis*; white flesh on a black horned shell. Composition /100 g: (edible portion 84%) water 44 g, 938 kJ (224 kcal), protein 4.2 g, fat 1.1 g (of which 18% saturated, 55% mono-unsaturated, 27% polyunsaturated), carbohydrate 49.1 g, ash 1.7 g, Ca 18 mg, Fe 1.4 mg, Mg 84 mg, P 96 mg, K 447 mg, Na 3 mg, Zn 0.9 mg, Cu 0.4 mg, Mn 1.6 mg, vitamin A 10 μg RE, B_1 0.16 mg, B_2 0.18 mg, niacin 0.8 mg, B_6 0.41 mg, folate 68 μg, pantothenate 0.6 mg, C 36 mg.

chestnut mushroom *See* MUSHROOMS.

chevda (chewda) A dry and highly spiced mixture of deep fried rice, DHAL, CHICKPEAS and small pieces of chickpea batter, with peanuts and raisins, seasoned with sugar and salt, a common N. Indian snack food, also known as Bombay mix.

chewing gum Based on CHICLE and other plant resins, with sugar or other sweetener, balsam of Tolu and various flavours.

chichi South American; effervescent sour alcoholic beverage made from maize, other starch crops or beans; both a lactic acid bacterial and a yeast fermentation.

chicken Domestic fowl, *Gallus domesticus*. There are differences between the white (breast) and dark (leg) meat, the former being lower in fat but also lower in iron and vitamin B_2. Poussin or spring chicken is a young bird, 4–6 weeks old, weighing 250–300 g.

Dark meat composition /100 g: (edible portion 44%) water 76 g, 523 kJ (125 kcal), protein 20.1 g, fat 4.3 g (of which 31% saturated, 37% mono-unsaturated, 31% polyunsaturated), cholesterol 80 mg, carbohydrate 0 g, ash 0.9 g, Ca 12 mg, Fe 1 mg, Mg 23 mg, P 162 mg, K 222 mg, Na 85 mg, Zn 2 mg, Cu 0.1 mg, Se 13.5 μg, I 6 μg, vitamin A 22 μg retinol, E 0.2 mg, K 2.4 mg, B_1 0.08 mg, B_2 0.18 mg, niacin 6.2 mg, B_6 0.33 mg, folate 10 μg, B_{12} 0.4 μg, pantothenate 1.2 mg, C 3 mg. A 100 g serving is a source of

Se, Zn, vitamin B_2, B_6, a good source of P, pantothenate, a rich source of niacin, vitamin B_{12}.

Light meat composition /100 g: (edible portion 55%) water 74.9 g, 477 kJ (114 kcal), protein 23.2 g, fat 1.6 g (of which 33% saturated, 33% mono-unsaturated, 33% polyunsaturated), cholesterol 58 mg, carbohydrate 0 g, ash 1 g, Ca 12 mg, Fe 0.7 mg, Mg 27 mg, P 187 mg, K 239 mg, Na 68 mg, Zn 1 mg, Se 17.8 µg, I 6 µg, vitamin A 8 µg retinol, E 0.2 mg, K 2.4 mg, B_1 0.07 mg, B_2 0.09 mg, niacin 10.6 mg, B_6 0.54 mg, folate 4 µg, B_{12} 0.4 µg, pantothenate 0.8 mg. A 100 g serving is a source of pantothenate, a good source of P, Se, vitamin B_6, a rich source of niacin, vitamin B_{12}.

chicken, broiler   Fast-growing chicken developed by the USDA at Beltsville, Maryland, and first produced commercially in 1930.

chicken, mountain   *See* CRAPAUD.

chickling pea or vetch   *Lathyrus sativus*, *see* LATHYRISM.

chickoo   *See* SAPODILLA.

chickpea   Also known as garbanzo; seeds of *Cicer arietinum*, widely used in Mediterranean and Middle Eastern stews and casseroles. Puréed chickpea is the basis of HUMMUS and deep fried balls of chickpea batter are FELAFEL.

Composition /100 g: water 11.5 g, 1524 kJ (364 kcal), protein 19.3 g, fat 6 g (of which 13% saturated, 30% mono-unsaturated, 57% polyunsaturated), carbohydrate 60.7 g (10.7 g sugars), fibre 17.4 g, ash 2.5 g, Ca 105 mg, Fe 6.2 mg, Mg 115 mg, P 366 mg, K 875 mg, Na 24 mg, Zn 3.4 mg, Cu 0.8 mg, Mn 2.2 mg, Se 8.2 µg, vitamin A 3 µg RE (40 µg carotenoids), E 0.8 mg, K 9 mg, B_1 0.48 mg, B_2 0.21 mg, niacin 1.5 mg, B_6 0.54 mg, folate 557 µg, pantothenate 1.6 mg, C 4 mg. An 85 g serving is a source of Ca, Zn, vitamin B_2, a good source of vitamin B_1, B_6, pantothenate, a rich source of Cu, Fe, Mg, Mn, P, folate.

chickweed   Common garden weed (*Stellaria media*); can be eaten in salads or cooked; a modest source of vitamin C.

chicle   The partially evaporated milky latex of the evergreen sapodilla tree (*Achra sapota*); it contains gutta (which has elastic properties) and resin, together with carbohydrates, waxes and tannins. Used in the manufacture of chewing gum. The same tree also produces the SAPODILLA plum.

chicory   Witloof or Belgian chicory (Belgian endive in USA), *Cichorium intybus*; the root is harvested and grown in the dark to produce bullet-shaped heads of young white leaves (chicons). Also called succory; red variety is radicchio. The leaves are eaten as a salad or braised as a vegetable and the bitter root, dried and partly caramelised, is often added to coffee as a diluent to cheapen the product.

Composition /100 g: (edible portion 89%) water 94.5 g, 71 kJ (17 kcal), protein 0.9 g, fat 0.1 g, carbohydrate 4 g, fibre 3.1 g, ash 0.5 g, Ca 19 mg, Fe 0.2 mg, Mg 10 mg, P 26 mg, K 211 mg, Na 2 mg, Zn 0.2 mg, Cu 0.1 mg, Mn 0.1 mg, Se 0.2 µg, vitamin A 1 µg RE, B_1 0.06 mg, B_2 0.03 mg, niacin 0.2 mg, B_6 0.04 mg, folate 37 µg, pantothenate 0.1 mg, C 3 mg.

chief cells Cells in the stomach that secrete pepsinogen, the precursor of the ENZYME PEPSIN.

chikuwa Japanese; grilled foods prepared from SURIMI. *See also* KAMABOKO.

chilled foods Foods stored at −1 to +1 °C (fresh fish and meats); at 0–5 °C (baked goods, milk, salads); 0–8 °C (cooked meats, butter, margarine, soft fruits). Often combined with controlled gas storage (*see* PACKAGING, MODIFIED ATMOSPHERE).

chill haze *See* HAZE.

chilli (chili) *See* PEPPER, CHILLI.

chilling Reduction of temperature to between −1 and 8 °C.

chilling, cryogenic Use of solid carbon dioxide or liquid nitrogen directly in contact with the food to reduce its temperature; the latent heat of sublimation or vaporization comes from the food being treated.

chilling injury The physiological damage to many plants and plant products as a result of exposure to low temperatures (but not freezing), including surface pitting, poor colour, failure to ripen and loss of structure and texture.

chillproofing A treatment to prevent the development of haziness or cloudiness due to precipitation of proteins when BEER is chilled. Treatments include the addition of TANNINS to precipitate proteins, materials such as bentonite (FULLER'S EARTH) to adsorb them and proteolytic enzymes to hydrolyse them.

chimche Korean; fermented cabbage with garlic, red peppers and pimientos.

chine A joint of meat containing the whole or part of the backbone of the animal. *See also* CHINING.

Chinese cabbage (Chinese leaves) *See* CABBAGE, CHINESE.

Chinese cherry *See* LYCHEE.

Chinese gooseberry *See* KIWI.

Chinese lantern *See* CAPE GOOSEBERRY.

Chinese restaurant syndrome Flushing, palpitations and numbness associated at one time with the consumption of MONOSODIUM GLUTAMATE, and then with HISTAMINE, but the cause of these symptoms after eating various foods is not known.

chining To sever the rib bones from the backbone by sawing through the ribs close to the spine.

See also CHINE.

chips Chipped potatoes; pieces of potato deep fried in fat or oil. Known in French as *pommes frites* or just *frites*; in USA 'chips' are potato crisps and chips are called French fries or fries. Fat content depends on size of chip and the process, commonly about 25% but can be 40% in fine-cut chips and as little as 4–8% in frozen oven-baked chips.

chitin Poly-*N*-acetylglucosamine, the organic matrix of the exoskeleton of insects and crustaceans, and present in small amounts in mushrooms. An insoluble NON-STARCH POLYSACCHA-RIDE. Partial deacetylation results in the formation of chitosans, which are used as protein-flocculating agents. Chitosan also has antibacterial properties, disrupting bacterial cell walls, and is used in active PACKAGING of foods, and as an edible protective coating, e.g. on fish. Also marketed, with no evidence of efficacy, as a slimming aid.

chitosan *See* CHITIN.

chitterlings The (usually fried) small intestine of ox, calf or pig.

chives Small member of the onion family (*Allium schoenoprasum*); the leaves are used as a garnish or dried as a herb; mild onion flavour.

chlonorchiasis Infestation with the liver FLUKE *Chlonorchis sinensis* in the bile ducts. Acquired by eating undercooked fresh-water fish harbouring the larval stage.

chlorella *See* ALGAE.

chlorine An element found in biological tissues as the chloride ION; the body contains about 100 g (3 mol) of chloride and the average diet contains 6–7 g (0.17–0.2 mol), mainly as sodium chloride. Free chlorine is used as a sterilising agent, e.g. for drinking water.

chlorine dioxide A bread improver. *See* AGEING.

chlorophyll The green pigment of leaves, etc; a substituted POR-PHYRIN ring chelating a Mg^{2+} ion. The essential pigment in PHO-TOSYNTHESIS, responsible for the trapping of light energy for the formation of carbohydrates from carbon dioxide and water. Both α- and β-chlorophylls occur in leaves, together with the CAROTENOIDS xanthophyll and carotene.

Chlorophyll has no nutritional value, although it does contain MAGNESIUM as part of its molecule. It is used in breath fresheners and toothpaste but there is no evidence that it has any useful action.

chlorophyllide The dull green pigment found in the water after cooking some vegetables; it is a water-soluble derivative of

CHLOROPHYLL, the product of hydrolysis of the phytol side chain, by either enzymic action (chlorophyllase, EC 3.1.1.14) in the vegetables or alkaline hydrolysis. Also formed enzymically by degradation of chlorophyll as fruit and vegetables ripen or age.

See also PHEOPHORBIDE; PHEOPHYTIN.

chlorothiazide DIURETIC drug used to treat OEDEMA and HYPERTENSION.

chlorpropamide An oral hypoglycaemic agent used in the treatment of DIABETES; it stimulates secretion of INSULIN.

chlortetracycline An ANTIBIOTIC.

chlorthalidone DIURETIC drug used to treat OEDEMA and HYPERTENSION.

chocolate Made from cocoa nibs (husked, fermented and roasted COCOA beans) by refining and the addition of sugar, COCOA BUTTER, flavouring, LECITHIN and, for milk chocolate, milk solids. It may also contain vegetable oils other than cocoa butter. White chocolate contains cocoa butter, but no cocoa powder.

Cocoa beans grow in pods contained in a soft, starchy pulp. This is allowed to ferment to a liquid that drains away, leaving the beans. They are roasted, broken into small pieces and dehusked, leaving 'nibs'; this is finely ground to 'cocoa mass' and some of the fat removed, leaving cocoa powder. The powder is mixed with sugar, cocoa butter (and milk powder for milk chocolate) in a MELANGEUR, then subjected to severe mechanical treatment (CONCHING). The fats can solidify in six polymorphs melting at different temperatures and require cooling and reheating (TEMPERING) before being moulded into a bar.

See also COCOA; COCOA BUTTER EQUIVALENTS; COCOA BUTTER SUBSTITUTES.

chocolate, drinking Partially solubilised COCOA powder for preparation of a chocolate-flavoured milk drink, containing about 75% sucrose.

choke cherry Sour wild N. American CHERRY, fruit of *Prunus virginiana* and *P. edmissa*.

cholagogue A substance that stimulates the secretion of BILE from the GALL BLADDER.

cholangitis Inflammation of the BILE ducts.

cholecalciferol *See* VITAMIN D.

cholecystectomy Surgical removal of the GALL BLADDER.

cholecystitis Inflammation of the GALL BLADDER.

cholecystography X-ray examination of the gall bladder after administration of a radio-opaque compound that is excreted in the BILE. Cholangiography is similar examination of the bile ducts.

cholecystokinin (CCK)   Peptide hormone secreted by the I-cells of the duodenum in response to partially digested food entering from the stomach. Stimulates contraction of the GALL BLADDER, secretion of BILE, secretion of pancreatic enzymes. Also stimulates contraction of the pyloric sphincter, and so controls the rate of gastric emptying. Also known as pancreozymin.

cholelithiasis   *See* GALLSTONES.

choleretic   An agent that stimulates the secretion of BILE.

cholestasis   Failure of normal amounts of BILE to reach the intestine, resulting in obstructive jaundice. May be caused by bile stones or liver disease.

   See also BILIRUBIN, BILIVERDIN.

cholesterol   The principal sterol in animal tissues, an essential component of cell membranes and the precursor for the formation of the STEROID hormones. Not a dietary essential, since it is synthesised in the body.

   Transported in the plasma LIPOPROTEINS. An elevated plasma concentration of cholesterol in low-density lipoprotein is a risk factor for ATHEROSCLEROSIS. The synthesis of cholesterol in the body is increased by a high intake of saturated FATS, but apart from people with a rare genetic defect in the regulation of cholesterol synthesis, a high dietary intake of cholesterol does not affect the plasma concentration, since there is normally strict control over the rate of synthesis.

   See also HMG COA REDUCTASE; HYPERCHOLESTEROLAEMIA; HYPERLIPIDAEMIA; LIPOPROTEINS, PLASMA.

CHOLESTEROL

cholestyramine   Ion-exchange resin used to treat HYPERLIPIDAEMIA by complexing BILE SALTS in the intestinal lumen and increasing their excretion, so increasing the metabolic clearance of CHOLESTEROL.

cholic acid   One of the primary BILE SALTS synthesised in the liver and secreted in the bile as a GLYCINE or TAURINE conjugate.

choline   *N*-Trimethylethanolamine, a derivative of the amino acid SERINE; an important component of cell membranes.

Phosphatidylcholine is also known as LECITHIN, and preparations of mixed phospholipids rich in phosphatidylcholine are generally called lecithin, although they also contain other phospholipids; lecithin from PEANUTS and SOYA beans is widely used as an emulsifying agent (E-322).

Choline released from membrane phospholipids is important for the formation of the neurotransmitter ACETYLCHOLINE, and choline is also important in the metabolism of methyl groups. Synthesised in the body, and a ubiquitous component of cell membranes, it therefore occurs in all foods; dietary deficiency is unknown. Deficiency has been observed in patients on long-term total PARENTERAL NUTRITION, suggesting that the ability to synthesise choline is inadequate to meet requirements without some intake. There is no evidence on which to base estimates of requirements; the average intake is between 0.25–0.5 g/day.

cholla (challa) A loaf of white bread made in a twisted form by plaiting together a large and small piece of dough, the Biblical beehive coil. The dough is made from white flour, enriched with eggs and a pinch of saffron, and the loaf is decorated with poppyseed. It is mentioned in the Bible, translated as 'loaves' and is traditionally used for benediction of the Jewish sabbath and festivals.

chondroitin A polysaccharide, classified as a mucopolysaccharide, a polymer of galactosamine and glucuronic acid. Chondroitin sulphate is a component of cartilage and the organic matrix of bone.

chondrometer An instrument used to determine the specific weight of WHEAT. A wet English wheat may weigh 68 kg, and a dry American wheat 84 kg /hectolitre.

Chondrus crispus A seaweed, the source of CARRAGEENAN.

chopsuey Chinese dishes based on bean sprouts and shredded vegetables, cooked with shredded quick-fried meat, capped with a thin omelette. Not authentically Chinese, but an invention of Chinese restaurateurs in western countries. Unlike true Chinese food, the flavours of a chopsuey are all mixed together; one translation is 'savoury mess', reputedly invented in either New York or San Francisco in 1896, although it may derive from tsap seui from the Guangzhou region of China.

Chorleywood process A method of preparing dough for breadmaking by submitting it to intense mechanical working, so that together with the aid of oxidising agents, the need for bulk fermentation of the dough is eliminated. This is a so-called 'no-time' process and saves $1\frac{1}{2}$–2 h in the process; permits use of an increased proportion of weaker flour, and produces a softer, finer loaf, which stales more slowly. Named after the British Baking Industries Research Association at Chorleywood.

chorote *See* POZOL.

choux (chou) pastry Light airy pastry, invented by the French chef Carême, used in éclairs and profiteroles. The batter is pre-cooked in a saucepan, then baked. The name comes from the French *chou* for cabbage, the characteristic shape of the cream-filled puffs.

chowder Thick soup made from shellfish (especially clams) or other fish, with pork or bacon. Originally French, now mainly New England and Newfoundland. Name derived from the French chaudière, the large cauldron in which it is prepared.

chromatography Technique for separation of solutes by partition between adsorption onto a stationary phase and solution in a mobile phase. The mobile phase may be gas or liquid; the stationary phase may be solid (paper, a thin layer of adsorbent or a column of adsorbent) or liquid.

High-performance liquid chromatography (HPLC) uses a column of extremely uniform particles of stationary phase and a solvent under high pressure; in reverse phase chromatography the stationary phase is more lipophilic than the mobile phase.

In ion-exchange chromatography, the stationary phase is an ion-exchange resin, so achieving separation on the basis of ionic charge.

In gel exclusion chromatography, the stationary phase is a gel that permits molecules up to a given size to penetrate the gel matrix, so achieving separation on the basis of molecular size and shape.

chromium A metallic element that is a dietary essential. It forms an organic complex, the GLUCOSE TOLERANCE FACTOR, and deficiency results in impaired GLUCOSE TOLERANCE. There is little evidence on which to base estimates of requirements; deficiency has been observed at intakes below 6µg (0.12µmol)/day, and a SAFE AND ADEQUATE INTAKE level has been set at 35µg for men and 25µg for women.

High intakes of inorganic chromium salts are associated with kidney and liver damage.

chromoproteins Proteins conjugated with a metal-containing group, such as the haem group of HAEMOGLOBIN, which contains iron.

CHU Centigrade (or Celsius) heat unit, the amount of heat required to raise the temperature of one pound of water through one degree Celsius.

chuck *See* BEEF.

chufa *See* TIGER NUT.

chuño   Traditional dried potato prepared in the highlands of Peru and Bolivia. The tubers are crushed, pressed, frozen during the night then dried in the sunshine during the day.

chutney   Originally Hindi; a strong, sweet relish. It is a type of pickle with a lower acidity and higher sugar content.

chyle   *See* LYMPH.

chylomicrons   Large plasma lipoproteins, assembled in the small intestinal mucosa, and containing mainly triacylglycerol synthesised from the products of intestinal lipid hydrolysis. They are absorbed into the lymphatic system, then enter the bloodstream at the thoracic duct. Tissues take up triacylglycerol by the action of lipoprotein LIPASE, and chylomicron remnants are cleared by the liver.

   See also LIPOPROTEINS, PLASMA.

chymase   Alternative name for CHYMOSIN.

chyme   The partly digested mass of food as it exists in the stomach.

chymosin   Also known as rennin, an enzyme (EC 3.4.23.4), in the abomasum of calves and the stomach of human infants, that clots milk; it hydrolyses the κ-casein surrounding the CASEIN micelles, so permitting coagulation and precipitation. No evidence that is important in digestion in adults. Biosynthetic chymosin is used in cheese-making (vegetable RENNET).

   See also CHEESE; RENNET.

chymotrypsin   An enzyme (EC 3.4.21.1) involved in the DIGESTION of proteins; secreted as the inactive precursor chymotrypsinogen in the pancreatic juice. It is activated by TRYPSIN, and is an ENDOPEPTIDASE, with specificity for esters of aromatic amino acids.

   See also ELASTASE; PEPSIN; TRYPSIN.

chytridiomycetes   Anaerobic fungi with a motile zoospore phase resembling the flagellate protozoa of the RUMEN flora; they make a significant contribution to ruminant digestion of lignocellulose. The vegetative phase colonises lignified regions of the leaves of a variety of tropical grasses.

ciabatta   *See* BREAD.

cibophobia   Dislike of food.

cider, cyder   An ALCOHOLIC BEVERAGE; fermented APPLE juice (in UK may include not more than 25% PEAR juice). In USA the term cider or fresh cider is used for unfermented apple juice; the fermented product is hard or fermented cider.

   Composition: Dry cider, 2.6% sugars, 3.8% alcohol, 460 kJ (110 kcal);. sweet cider, 4.3% sugars, 525 kJ (125 kcal); vintage cider 7.3% sugars, 10.5% alcohol, 1260 kJ (300 kcal)/300 mL (half pint).

cieddu *See* MILK, FERMENTED.

ciguatera Poisoning from eating fish feeding in the region of coral reefs in the Caribbean, Indian and Pacific Oceans. The species of fish are normally edible, and appear to derive the toxins, ciguatoxins, from their diet. Reported in seafarers' tales in the 16th century.

ciguatoxins *See* CIGUATERA.

cimetidine *See* HISTAMINE RECEPTOR ANTAGONISTS.

CIMMYT (Centro Internacional de Mejoramiento de Maíz y Trigo) International Maize and Wheat Improvement Center, Texcoco, Mexico.

cinnamon The aromatic bark of *Cinnamomum* spp.; it is split off the shoots, cured and dried. During drying, the bark shrinks and curls into a cylinder or quill. It is used as a flavour in meat products, bakery goods and confectionery, and may be available either as the whole quill or powdered ready for use. A 2 g serving (1 tsp) is a source of Mn.

Ceylon or true cinnamon (*C. zeylican*) differs from other types and the oil contains mostly cinnamic aldehyde, together with some eugenol. Saigon cinnamon also contains cineol; Chinese cinnamon has no eugenol.

CIP Cleaning-in-place; cleaning food machinery without dismantling pipelines, etc. (as required for manual cleaning), by circulating water and cleaning solutions through the plant.

cis- Chemical description of arrangement about a carbon–carbon double bond when groups are arranged on the same side of the bond; in the *trans*-isomer they are on opposite sides of the double bond. *See* ISOMERS.

cissa An unnatural desire for certain foods; alternative words, cittosis, allotriophagy and pica.

citral An important constituent of many essential oils, especially lemon. Used as the starting material for the synthesis of ionone (the synthetic perfume with an odour of violets), which is an intermediate in the chemical synthesis of retinol (see VITAMIN A).

citrange A hybrid CITRUS fruit.

citric acid A tricarboxylic acid, widely distributed in plant and animal tissues and an important metabolic intermediate, yielding 10.9 kJ (2.47 kcal)/g. Used as a flavouring and acidifying agent (E-330). Citrates are used as acidity regulators (E-331–333). Commercially prepared by the fermentation of sugars by *Aspergillus niger* or extracted from CITRUS fruits: Lemon juice contains 5–8% citric acid.

citrin A mixture of two flavonones found in citrus pith, hesperidin and eriodictin. *See* FLAVONOIDS.

citron   A CITRUS fruit.

citronella   Lemon scented tropical grass *Cymbopogon nardus* used in salads and dressings; the essential oil is also used as an insect repellent.

citronin   A flavonone GLYCOSIDE from the peel of immature ponderosa lemons. *See* FLAVONOIDS.

citrovorum factor   The name given to a growth factor for the micro-organism *Leuconostoc citrovorum*, now known to be formyltetrahydropteroylglutamic acid. *See* FOLIC ACID.

citrullinaemia   A GENETIC DISEASE caused by lack of argininosuccinate synthetase (EC 6.3.4.5) affecting the synthesis of urea, and hence the elimination of nitrogenous waste. The defect may be mild, or so severe that affected infants become comatose and may die after a moderately high intake of protein. Treatment is usually by restriction of protein intake and feeding supplements of the AMINO ACID ARGININE, so as to permit excretion of nitrogenous waste as CITRULLINE.

Sodium benzoate (*see* BENZOIC ACID) may be given to increase the excretion of nitrogenous waste as hippuric acid.

citrulline   An amino acid formed as a metabolic intermediate, but not involved in proteins, and of no nutritional importance.

citrus   Genus of trees with fleshy, juicy fruits; there is considerable confusion over the names because of hybridisation and mutations.

Sweet orange *Citrus sinensis*; various cultivars including Valencia, Washington navel, Shamouti. Sour, bitter, or Seville orange *C. aurantium*; too bitter to eat, used for marmalade.

Lemon *C. limon*. Lime *C. aurantifolia*. Citron *C. medica*, thick, white inner skin; used mainly to make candied peel. Pomelo (shaddock) *C. grandis*, parent of the grapefruit. Grapefruit *C. paradisi* (hybrid of pomelo and sweet orange).

Tangerine or satsuma, mandarin, calamondin, naartje (S. Africa), small citrus fruit with loose skin. Clementine is a hybrid of tangerine and bitter orange, sometimes regarded as variety of tangerine. Mineola is a hybrid of grapefruit and tangerine. Ortanique is a hybrid of orange and tangerine, unique to Jamaica. Citrange is a hybrid of citron and orange. Tangors are hybrids of tangerine and sweet orange. Ugli fruit is a hybrid of grapefruit and tangerine. Tangelo is a hybrid of tangerine and pomelo.

All are a rich source of vitamin C and contain up to 10% sugars.

cittosis   An unnatural desire for foods; alternative words, cissa, allotriophagy, pica.

CLA   Conjugated linoleic acid. *See* LINOLEIC ACID, CONJUGATED.

clabbered milk   Unpasteurised milk that has soured naturally, becoming thick and curdy. Clabber cheese is curd or cottage cheese.

clams   Various marine bivalve molluscs, including SCALLOP, *Tridacna gigas*, quahog, *Mya arenaria* and *Venus mercenaria*.

Composition/100 g: water 82 g, 310 kJ (74 kcal), protein 12.8 g, fat 1 g, cholesterol 34 mg, carbohydrate 2.6 g, ash 1.9 g, Ca 46 mg, Fe 14 mg, Mg 9 mg, P 169 mg, K 314 mg, Na 56 mg, Zn 1.4 mg, Cu 0.3 mg, Mn 0.5 mg, Se 24.3 µg, vitamin A 90 µg retinol, E 0.3 mg, K 0.2 mg, vitamin B_1 0.08 mg, B_2 0.21 mg, niacin 1.8 mg, B_6 0.06 mg, folate 16 µg, B_{12} 49.4 µg, pantothenate 0.4 mg, C 13 mg. A 60 g serving (3 clams) is a source of Cu, Mn, P, Se, vitamin C, a rich source of Fe, vitamin B_{12}.

claret   Name given in UK to red wines from the Bordeaux region of France.

clarification The process of clearing a liquid of suspended particles. It may be carried out by filtration, centrifugation (*see* CENTRIFUGE), the addition of enzymes to hydrolyse and solubilise particulate matter (proteolytic or pectolytic enzymes) or the addition of flocculating agents.

clarifier, centrifugal   CENTRIFUGE used to clarify liquids by removing solids.

clarifixation   A method of homogenising milk in which the cream is separated, homogenised and remixed with the milk in one machine, the clarifixator.

clarifying   Of fats; freeing the fat of water so that it can be used for frying, pastry-making, etc. Clarified fats are less susceptible to RANCIDITY on storage; GHEE is clarified butter fat. Also the process of filtering juices before making jellies, etc.

Clarke degrees   A measure of WATER HARDNESS.

Clegg anthrone method   For determination of total available carbohydrate. The sample is digested with perchloric acid to yield monosaccharides which are determined colorimetrically using anthrone in sulphuric acid (maximum absorbance 630 nm).

clementine   A CITRUS fruit, *Citrus nobilis* var. *deliciosa*; regarded by some as a variety of TANGERINE and by others as a cross between the tangerine and a wild N. African orange.

climacteric   (1) Post-harvesting increase in metabolic rate and production of carbon dioxide and ETHYLENE associated with ripening in some (but not all) fruits, e.g. apple, apricot, avocado, banana, mango, peach, pear, plum and tomato. Stimulated by the low concentrations of ethylene (1 ppm). Non-climacteric fruits include cherry, cucumber, fig, grapefruit, lemon, pineapple, strawberry and vegetables.

(2) Clinically, the menopause in women, or declining sexual drive and fertility in men after middle age.

clinching In food canning, loose attachment of the end of the can before heating to expel air.

clofibrate *See* FIBRIC ACIDS.

clone A colony of micro-organisms, or a plant or animal produced by vegetative (asexual) reproduction from a single cell, so that all cells have identical genetic composition.

cloning vector The DNA of a PLASMID or virus into which a segment of foreign DNA can be inserted in order to introduce a new gene into the cells of another organism.

Clostridium Genus of spore-forming bacteria responsible for food poisoning.

Cl. botulinum causes BOTULISM, a rare but often fatal form of food poisoning where the exotoxins are present in the food. The spores are the most heat-resistant food poisoning organism encountered, and their thermal death time is used as a minimum standard for processing foods with pH above 4.5.

Cl. perfringens produces an ENTEROTOXIN in the gut. Infective dose 10^7–10^8 organisms, onset 8–16 h, duration 16–24 h, TX2.1.1.3.

cloudberry An orange-yellow fruit resembling the raspberry in shape; *Rubus chamaemorus*, known as avron in Scotland, and baked-apple berries in Canada. An extremely rich natural source of BENZOIC ACID and will not ferment; remains fresh for many months without preservation.

clouding agents Compounds added to clear FRUIT JUICES to give them a (desirable) cloudy appearance; including extract of quillaia or various emulsifiers, stabilisers or modified starches.

clove A spice, the dried aromatic flower buds of *Caryophyllus aromaticus*; mother of clove is the ripened fruit, which is inferior in flavour. A 2 g serving (1 tsp) is a good source of Mn.

clupeine *See* PROTAMINES.

cluster analysis Statistical technique to analyse data (e.g. from food consumption records) by classifying into groups or clusters, so that the degree of association is strong between members of the same cluster and weak between members of different clusters. *See also* DIETARY PATTERN ANALYSIS.

CMC Carboxymethylcellulose. *See* CELLULOSE DERIVATIVES.

Co I, Co II Obsolete abbreviations for coenzymes I and II, now known as nicotinamide adenine dinucleotide (NAD) and nicotinamide adenine dinucleotide phosphate (NADP), respectively.

CoA Coenzyme A. *See* COENZYMES; PANTOTHENIC ACID.

coacervation (1) The heat-reversible aggregation of the AMYLOPECTIN form of STARCH, which is believed to be one of the mechanisms involved in the staling of bread.

(2) A technique used to encapsulate flavouring materials. *See* ENCAPSULATION.

coagulase The name given to an enzyme said to be present in milk and to account for the ability of milk to clot a solution of fibrinogen.

coagulation (1) A process involving the denaturation of proteins, loss of their native, soluble, structure, so that they become insoluble; it may be effected by heat, strong acids and alkalis, metals and various other chemical agents. Some proteins are coagulated by specific enzymic action. Denaturation is due to the breaking of hydrogen bonds that maintain the protein in its native structure. As the process continues, there is considerable unfolding of the protein, and interaction between adjacent molecules, forming aggregates which reach such a size that they precipitate.

(2) The final stage in BLOOD CLOTTING is the precipitation of fibrils of insoluble fibrin, formed from the soluble plasma protein fibrinogen, an example of coagulation caused by enzymic action. The enzyme responsible is prothrombin (EC 3.4.21.5), which is normally inactive, and is activated by a cascade of events in response to injury. VITAMIN K is required for the synthesis of prothrombin, and clotting requires calcium ions.

coalfish *See* SAITHE.

cob nut *See* HAZEL NUT.

cobalamin *See* VITAMIN B_{12}.

cobalt A mineral whose main function is in VITAMIN B_{12}, although there are a few cobalt-dependent enzymes. There is no evidence of cobalt deficiency in human beings, and no evidence on which to base estimates of requirements for inorganic cobalt. 'Pining disease' in cattle and sheep is due to cobalt deficiency (their rumen micro-organisms synthesise vitamin B_{12}). Cobalt salts are toxic in excess, causing degeneration of the heart muscle, and habitual intakes in excess of 300 mg/day are considered undesirable.

cobamide Obsolete term for coenzymes derived from VITAMIN B_{12}: adenosyl and methyl cobalamin.

Coca Cola^{TM} A COLA DRINK.
See also COCA LEAVES.

coca leaves From the S American plant *Erythroxylon coca*; they contain the narcotic alkaloid cocaine, and are traditionally chewed by the natives of Peru as a stimulant. Originally the beverage Coca Cola (*see* COLA DRINKS) contained coca leaf extract, although this was removed from the formulation many years ago.

cocarboxylase An obsolete name for thiamin diphosphate, the metabolically active COENZYME derived from VITAMIN B_1.

cocarcinogen A substance that does not itself induce cancer, but potentiates the action of a CARCINOGEN.

  See also PROMOTER.

cochineal A water-soluble red colour obtained from the female conchilla, *Dactilopius coccus* (*Coccus cactus*), an insect found in Mexico, Central America and the Caribbean. Colour is due to anthroquinones such as kermesic and carminic acids. 1 kg of the colour is obtained from about 150 000 insects. Legally permitted in foods in most countries (E-120). Cochineal red A is an alternative name for PONCEAU 4R (E-124), often used to replace cochineal. Carmine is produced from cochineal.

cockles (arkshell) Several types of marine bivalve molluscs of genus *Cardium*, often sold preserved in brine or vinegar.

cock of the wood *See* CAPERCAILLIE.

cocoa Originally known as cacao, introduced into Europe from Mexico by the Spaniards in the early sixteenth century. The powder is prepared from the seed embedded in the fruit of the cocoa plant, *Theobroma cacao*. Also a milk drink prepared with cocoa powder. Used to prepare CHOCOLATE. Contains the ALKALOIDS THEOBROMINE and CAFFEINE.

cocoa butter The fat from the cocoa bean, used in chocolate manufacture and in pharmaceuticals; it has a sharp melting point, between 31 and 35 °C, so melts in the mouth; mostly 2-oleopalmitostearin (62% saturated, 34% mono-unsaturated, 3% polyunsaturated) contains 1.8 mg vitamin E, 24.7 mg vitamin K/100 g).

  See also COCOA BUTTER EQUIVALENTS; COCOA BUTTER SUBSTITUTES.

cocoa butter equivalents Also known as cocoa butter extenders; fats that are physically and chemically similar to COCOA BUTTER and can be mixed with cocoa butter in CHOCOLATE manufacture. Some raise the melting point of the chocolate, making it more suitable for tropical regions. Borneo tallow (green butter) from the Malaysian and Indonesian plant *Shorea stenopiera*; dhupa from the Indian plant *Vateria indica*; illipe butter (mowrah fat) from the Indian plant *Bassia longifolia*; kokum from the Indian tree *Garcinia indica*; sal from the Indian plant *Shorea robusta*; shea butter from the African plant *Butyrospermum parkii*.

cocoa butter extenders *See* COCOA BUTTER EQUIVALENTS.

cocoa butter substitutes Fats that are physically similar to cocoa butter, but chemically different, used with defatted COCOA, to make substitute chocolate or compound coatings for bakery. They cannot be mixed with cocoa butter, but some do not require TEMPERING and can be cooled much more rapidly than cocoa butter.

cocoa, Dutch Cocoa treated with a dilute solution of alkali (carbonate or bicarbonate) to improve its colour, flavour and solubility. The process is known as 'Dutching'.

cocolait A form of coconut 'milk' made by pressing COCONUTS under high pressure and homogenising the oil and water emulsion obtained. Bottled and used (e.g. in Philippines) in place of cow's milk.

coconut Fruit of the tropical palm, *Cocos nucifera*. The dried nut is copra which contains 60–65% oil. The residue after extraction of the oil is used for animal feed. The hollow unripe nut contains a watery liquid known as coconut milk, which is gradually absorbed as the fruit ripens.

Composition/100 g: (edible portion 52%) water 47 g, 1482 kJ (354 kcal), protein 3.3 g, fat 33.5 g (of which 94% saturated, 4% mono-unsaturated, 1% polyunsaturated), carbohydrate 15.2 g (6.2 g sugars), fibre 9 g, ash 1 g, Ca 14 mg, Fe 2.4 mg, Mg 32 mg, P 113 mg, K 356 mg, Na 20 mg, Zn 1.1 mg, Cu 0.4 mg, Mn 1.5 mg, Se 10.1 µg, vitamin E 0.2 mg, K 0.2 mg, B_1 0.07 mg, B_2 0.02 mg, niacin 0.5 mg, B_6 0.05 mg, folate 26 µg, pantothenate 0.3 mg, C 3 mg. A 50 g serving (quarter fruit) is a source of Cu, a rich source of Mn.

Coconut oil is 92% saturated, 6% mono-unsaturated, 2% polyunsaturated, vitamin E 0.1 mg, K 0.5 mg.

cocoyam W. African; new cocoyam is TANNIA, old cocoyam is TARO.

cod A white FISH, *Gadus morrhua*, and other species.

Composition/100 g: water 81 g, 343 kJ (82 kcal), protein 17.8 g, fat 0.7 g, cholesterol 43 mg, carbohydrate 0 g, ash 1.2 g, Ca 16 mg, Fe 0.4 mg, Mg 32 mg, P 203 mg, K 413 mg, Na 54 mg, Zn 0.4 mg, Se 33.1 µg, I 110 µg, vitamin A 12 µg retinol, E 0.6 mg, K 0.1 mg, B_1 0.08 mg, B_2 0.06 mg, niacin 2.1 mg, B_6 0.25 mg, folate 7 µg, B_{12} 0.9 µg, pantothenate 0.2 mg, C 1 mg. A 100 g serving is a source of niacin, vitamin B_6, a good source of P, a rich source of I, Se, vitamin B_{12}.

codeine *See* ANTIDIARRHOEAL AGENTS.

Codes of Practice In the area of food production these refer to standards of procedure that cannot be covered by exact specifications and serve as agreed guidelines. They may originate from government departments, trade organisations, professional institutes or individual companies.

Codex Alimentarius Originally Codex Alimentarius Europaeus; since 1961 part of the United Nations FAO/WHO Commission on Food Standards to simplify and integrate food standards for adoption internationally. Web site: http://www.codexalimentarius.net/.

cod liver oil The oil from codfish liver; the classical source of vitamins A and D, used for its medicinal properties long before the vitamins were discovered. An average sample contains 120–1200 µg vitamin A and 1–10 µg vitamin D per gram. 25% saturated, 51% mono-unsaturated, 25% polyunsaturated, cholesterol 570 mg/100 g.

codon   A sequence of three bases (PURINES or PYRIMIDINES) in DNA or mRNA that codes for an amino acid. Where codons for amino acids are shown in this book, Pu is used to indicate either purine, Py either pyrimidine, and Nu any nucleotide.

coeliac disease (celiac disease)   Intolerance of the proteins of wheat, rye and barley; specifically, the gliadin fraction of the protein GLUTEN. The villi of the small intestine are severely affected and absorption of food is poor. Stools are bulky and fermenting from unabsorbed carbohydrate, and contain a large amount of unabsorbed fat (steatorrhoea). As a result of the malabsorption, affected people are malnourished and children suffer from growth retardation.

Treatment is by exclusion of wheat, rye and barley proteins (the starches are tolerated); rice, oats and maize are generally tolerated. Manufactured foods that are free from gluten, and hence suitable for consumption by people with coeliac disease are usually labelled as 'gluten-free'. Also known as gluten-induced enteropathy, and sometimes as non-tropical sprue.

coenzymes   Organic compounds required for the activity of some enzymes; most are derived from vitamins. A coenzyme that is covalently bound to the enzyme is a PROSTHETIC GROUP.

Other coenzymes act to transfer groups from one enzyme to another, e.g. Coenzyme A transfers acetyl groups between enzymes, NAD transfers hydrogen between enzymes in oxidation and reduction reactions.

An enzyme that requires a tightly bound coenzyme is inactive in the absence of its coenzyme; this can be exploited to assess VITAMIN B_1, B_2 and B_6 NUTRITIONAL STATUS, by measuring the activity of enzymes that require coenzymes derived from these vitamins (*see* ENZYME ACTIVATION ASSAYS).

Coenzyme A (CoA) is derived from the VITAMIN PANTOTHENIC ACID; it is required for the transfer and metabolism of acetyl groups (and other fatty acyl groups). Coenzyme I and coenzyme II are obsolete names for nicotinamide adenine dinucleotide (NAD) and nicotinamide adenine dinucleotide phosphate (NADP). Coenzyme Q is UBIQUINONE; Coenzyme R is obsolete name for BIOTIN.

coextrusion   For manufacture of food packaging materials, a multilayer film in which the distinct layers are formed by a simultaneous extrusion process through a single die rather than by separate stages of coating and lamination.

coffee   A beverage produced from the roasted beans from the berries of two principal types of shrub: *Coffea arabica* (arabica coffee) and *C. canephora* (robusta coffee). A third species (*C. liberica*) is of little commercial importance, but is valuable for development of disease-resistant hybrids. NIACIN is formed from trigonelline during the roasting process, and the coffee can contain 10–40 mg niacin/100 g, making a significant contribution to average intakes.

Instant coffee is dried coffee extract which can be used to make a beverage by adding hot water or milk. It may be manufactured by spray drying (*see* SPRAY DRYER) or FREEZE DRYING. Coffee essence is an aqueous extract of roasted coffee; usually about 400 g of coffee/L.

Coffee contains CAFFEINE; decaffeinated coffee is coffee beans (or instant coffee) from which the caffeine has been extracted with solvent (e.g. methylene or ethylene chloride), carbon dioxide under pressure (supercritical CO_2) or water. Coffee decaffeinated by water extraction is sometimes labelled as 'naturally' decaffeinated.

Coffee-Mate^{TM} Non-dairy creamer (*see* CREAMER, NON-DAIRY) introduced by Carnation Co., 1961.

coffee whitener   *See* CREAMER, NON-DAIRY.

cognac   BRANDY made in the Charentes region of NW France, around the town of Cognac, from special varieties of grape grown on shallow soil and claimed to be distilled only in pot, not continuous, stills; first distilled by Jean Martell in 1715. Sometimes used (incorrectly) as a general name for brandy.

See also ARMAGNAC.

cohort study   Systematic follow-up of a group of people for a defined period of time or until a specified event, also known as longitudinal or prospective study.

cola drinks   Carbonated drinks containing extract of cola bean, the seed of the tree *Cola acuminata*, and a variety of other flavouring ingredients. Cola seed contains CAFFEINE, and the drink contains 10–15 mg caffeine/100 mL, unless decaffeinated.

colcannon   (1) Irish; potato mashed with kale or cabbage, often fried. *See also* BUBBLE AND SQUEAK.

(2) Scottish; cabbage, carrots, potatoes and turnips mashed together.

colchicine   An ALKALOID isolated from the meadow saffron, or autumn crocus (*Colchicum* spp.). An old remedy for GOUT, it inhibits cell division, and is used in experimental horticulture to produce plants with an abnormal number of chromosomes.

cold preservation   *See* CAMPDEN PROCESS.

cold-shortening (of meat)   When the temperature of muscle is reduced below 10 °C while the pH remains above 6–6.2 (early in the post-mortem conversion of glycogen to lactic acid) the muscle contracts in reaction to cold and, when cooked, the meat is tough.

cold sterilisation   *See* IRRADIATION; STERILISATION, COLD.

cold store bacteria   *See* PSYCHROPHILES.

cole, coleseed   *See* RAPESEED.

colectomy   Surgical removal of all or part of the colon, to treat cancer or severe ulcerative COLITIS.

colestipol   Drug used to treat hypercholesterolaemia; it binds BILE SALTS in the gut, preventing their reabsorption and reutilisation, so forcing *de novo* synthesis from cholesterol.

coley   *See* SAITHE.

colic   Severe abdominal pain, of fluctuating severity, with waves of pain a few minutes apart.

coliform bacteria   A group of aerobic, lactose-fermenting bacteria; *Escherichia coli* is the most important member. Many coliforms are not harmful, but since they arise from faeces, they are useful as a test of faecal contamination particularly as a test for water pollution. Some strains of E. COLI produce toxins, or are otherwise pathogenic, and are associated with FOOD POISONING.

colipase   Small protein secreted in pancreatic juice; obligatory activator of pancreatic LIPASE (EC 3.1.1.3).

colitis   Inflammation of the large intestine, with pain, diarrhoea and weight loss; there may be ulceration of the large intestine (ulcerative colitis).

  See also CROHN'S DISEASE; GASTROINTESTINAL TRACT; IRRITABLE BOWEL SYNDROME.

collagen   Insoluble protein in CONNECTIVE TISSUE, bones, tendons and skin of animals and fish; converted into soluble GELATINE by moist heat. The quantity and quality of collagen in meat affects its texture, and hence toughness.

  See also MUSCLE.

collagen sugar   Old name for GLYCINE.

collapse temperature   In freeze drying, the maximum temperature the food can reach before its structure collapses, preventing movement of water vapour.

collard (collard greens)   American name for varieties of cabbage (*Brassica oleracea*) that do not form a compact head. Generally known in UK as greens or SPRING GREENS.

  Composition/100 g: (edible portion 57%) water 91 g, 126 kJ (30 kcal), protein 2.5 g, fat 0.4 g, carbohydrate 5.7 g (0.5 g sugars), fibre 3.6 g, ash 0.9 g, Ca 145 mg, Fe 0.2 mg, Mg 9 mg, P 10 mg, K

169 mg, Na 20 mg, Zn 0.1 mg, Mn 0.3 mg, Se 1.3 µg, vitamin A 333 µg RE (13 092 µg carotenoids), E 2.3 mg, K 510.8 mg, B$_1$ 0.05 mg, B$_2$ 0.13 mg, niacin 0.7 mg, B$_6$ 0.17 mg, folate 166 µg, pantothenate 0.3 mg, C 35 mg. A 90 g serving is a source of Ca, Mn, a good source of vitamin E, a rich source of vitamin A, folate, C.

colloid (colloidal suspension)   A two phase system consisting of a dispersant medium and a separate dispersed phase. Main types are EMULSION; FOAM; GEL; SOL.

Lyophilic colloids are those in which there is a high affinity between the particles of the dispersed phase and the dispersion medium. They include proteins and higher carbohydrates. Very viscous; electrically charged; require large amounts of electrolyte for precipitation, which is reversible. Also known as emulsions.

Lyophobic colloids are those in which there is no affinity between the particles of the dispersed phase and the dispersion medium. The particles carry an electric charge and are flocculated irreversibly by electrolytes. Also called suspensoids. For example, colloids of metals and inorganic salts.

See also EMULSIFIERS; STABILISERS.

colloid mill   Equipment for preparation of a COLLOID by subjecting the immiscible liquids to shear stress using a fast rotor against a static plate, or two contra-rotating rotors.

colocasia   *See* TARO.

cologel   Alternative name for methylcellulose. *See* CELLULOSE DERIVATIVES.

Colombo Plan   A co-operative effort to develop the resources and living standards of the peoples of S. and S.E. Asia, started at meeting held in Colombo in 1950.

colon   Also known as the large intestine or bowel, consisting of three anatomical regions: the ascending, the transverse and the descending colon. The colon normally has a considerable population of bacteria, while it is rare to find a significant bacterial population in the small intestine. The colon terminates at the rectum, where faeces are compacted and stored before voiding.

See also GASTROINTESTINAL TRACT; IRRITABLE BOWEL SYNDROME.

colostomy   Surgical creation of an artificial conduit in the abdominal wall for voiding of intestinal contents following surgical removal of much of the COLON and/or rectum.

colostrum   The milk produced by mammals during the first few days after parturition; compared with mature human milk, human colostrum contains more protein (2 g/100 mL compared with 1.3); slightly less lactose (6.6 g/100 mL compared with 7.2), considerably less fat (2.6 g/100 mL compared with 4.1) and overall slightly less energy, 235 kJ (56 kcal)/100 mL compared with 290 kJ (69 kcal).

Colostrum is a valuable source of antibodies for the new-born infant. Animal colostrum is sometimes known as beestings.

colours   Widely used in foods to increase their aesthetic appeal; may be natural, NATURE-IDENTICAL or synthetic. Natural colours include CAROTENOIDS (red, yellow and orange colours), some of which are VITAMIN A precursors; CHLOROPHYLL (green pigments in all leaves and stems); ANTHOCYANINS (red, blue and violet pigments in beetroot, raspberries, red cabbage); FLAVONES (yellow pigments in most leaves and flowers).

There are 20 permitted synthetic colours (mainly azo dyes).

CARAMEL is used both for flavour and as a brown colour made by heating sugar.

In addition to all these there are various ingredients such as paprika, saffron, turmeric that also provide colour.

See Table 7 of the Appendix.

Colwick   English soft cheese made in cylindrical shape.

colza   *See* RAPESEED.

COMA   Committee on Medical Aspects of Food Policy; permanent Advisory Committee to the UK Department of Health.

co-magaldrox   Mixture of aluminium and magnesium hydroxides, used as an ANTACID.

combining diet   *See* HAY DIET.

comet assay   Technique for rapid quantification of DNA strand breaks in single cells by electrophoresis.

commensal   Micro-organisms that live in close association with another species without either harming or benefiting it, e.g. many of the intestinal bacteria, which find nutrition and a habitat in the gut, but neither harm nor benefit the host.

See also PATHOGEN; SYMBIOTIC.

comminuted   Finely divided; used with reference to minced meat products and fruit drinks made from crushed whole fruit including the peel.

See also COMMINUTION.

comminution   Reduction in particle size of solid foods by grinding, compression or impact forces.

See also BOND'S LAW; KICK'S LAW; MILLS; RITTINGER'S LAW.

competitive radioassay   *See* RADIOIMMUNOASSAY.

Complan™   A mixture of dried skim milk, arachis oil, casein, maltodextrins, sugar and vitamins, used as a nutritional supplement.

complementation   Used with respect to proteins when a relative deficiency of an amino acid in one is compensated by a relative surplus from another protein consumed at the same time. The PROTEIN QUALITY is higher than the average of the individual values.

conalbumin One of the proteins of egg white, constituting 12% of the total solids. It binds iron in a pink-coloured complex; this accounts for the pinkish colour resulting when eggs are stored in rusty containers.

conching Part of the process of making CHOCOLATE in which the mixture is subjected to severe mechanical treatment with heavy rollers to produce a uniform smooth consistency.

conditioning (of meat) After slaughter, muscle GLYCOGEN is broken down to LACTIC ACID, and this acidity gradually improves the texture and keeping qualities of the meat. When all the changes have occurred, the meat is 'conditioned'.

See also RIGOR MORTIS.

confabulation Invention of circumstantial fictitious detail about events supposed to have occurred. May occur with any form of memory loss, but especially associated with KORSAKOFF'S PSYCHOSIS in VITAMIN B$_1$ deficiency.

confectioner's glucose *See* SYRUP.

congee (1) Chinese soft rice soup or gruel; may be sweet or savoury.

(2) Also congie or conje, water from cooking rice; used as a drink and contains much of the thiamin and niacin from the rice.

Conge machine Used, in the manufacture of CHOCOLATE blend for coating, to obtain smoothness by kneading the material.

congeners Flavour substances in alcoholic SPIRITS that distil over with the alcohol; a mixture of higher alcohols and esters. Said to be responsible for many of the symptoms of HANGOVER after excessive consumption.

See also FUSEL OIL.

conidendrin Substance isolated from a number of coniferous woods whose derivatives, norconidendrin and α- and β-conidendrol, are antioxidants. Chemically similar to NORDIHYDROGUAIARETIC ACID.

conjugase Intestinal enzyme, poly-γ-glutamyl hydrolase (EC 3.4.19.9) that hydrolyses the γ-glutamyl side chain of FOLIC ACID conjugates for absorption.

conjugated linolenic acid An isomer of LINOLENIC ACID in which the double bonds are conjugated, rather than methylene-interrupted.

conjunctival impression cytology Microscopic examination of conjunctival epithelial cells to detect morphological changes due to VITAMIN A deficiency.

connective tissue Consists of the proteins COLLAGEN and ELASTIN; in fish, collagen is found between the muscle segments (myotomes); in meat it is spread through the muscle, uniting the muscle fibres into bundles and supporting the blood vessels, and consists of both collagen and elastin. A high content of connective tissue results in tougher meat; collagen is softened to some extent by stewing, but roasting or frying have little effect. Elastin is unaffected by heating, and remains tough, elastic and insoluble.

constipation Difficulty in passing stools or infrequent passage of hard stools. In the absence of intestinal disease, frequently a result of a diet low in NON-STARCH POLYSACCHARIDE, and treated by increasing the intake of fruits, vegetables and especially whole grain cereal products. Severe cases may be treated by CATHARTICS, LAXATIVES or PURGATIVES.

contaminants Undesirable compounds found in foods, as a result of residues of agricultural chemicals (pesticides, fungicides, herbicides, fertilisers, etc.), through the manufacturing process or as a result of pollution. For many such compounds there are limits to the amount that may legally be present in the food.

See also ACCEPTABLE DAILY INTAKE.

controlled atmosphere storage *See* PACKAGING, MODIFIED ATMOSPHERE.

convicine One of the toxins in broad beans, responsible for the acute haemolytic anaemia of FAVISM.

cook–chill A method of catering involving cooking followed by fast chilling and storage at –1 to +5 °C, giving a storage time of only a few days.

cooker, fireless *See* HAYBOX COOKING.

cook–freeze A method of catering involving cooking followed by rapid freezing and storage below –18 °C, giving a storage time of several months.

cookie *See* BISCUIT.

cooking Required to make food more palatable, more digestible and safer. There is breakdown of the CONNECTIVE TISSUE in meat, softening of the CELLULOSE in plant tissues, and proteins are denatured by heating, so increasing their digestibility.

In general, water-soluble vitamins and minerals are lost in the cooking water, the amount depending on the surface area:volume ratio, i.e. greater losses take place from finely cut or minced foods. Fat-soluble vitamins are little affected except at frying temperatures. Proteins suffer reduction of available lysine when they are heated in the presence of reducing substances, and further loss at high temperature. Dry heat, as in baking, results in some loss of vitamin B_1 and available lysine. The most sensitive nutrients are vitamins C and B_1.

cooler shrink Surface dehydration of meat and poultry kept under refrigeration.

cooling agents   Compounds that reduce the temperature of foods through direct contact.

Coomassie brilliant blue   Dye used for detection and determination of proteins (the Bradford method), especially in electrophoretic gels; sensitivity 20 µg/mL, maximum absorbance 595 nm; the dye binding capacity of proteins depends on their content of basic AMINO ACIDS.

coon   American cheddar-type cheese, but manufacture includes scalding the milk.

co-phenotrope   *See* ANTIMOTILITY AGENTS.

copper   A dietary essential trace metal, which forms the PROSTHETIC GROUP of a number of enzymes. The REFERENCE INTAKES are 0.9–1.2 mg/day. Toxic in excess, and it is recommended that not more than 2–10 mg/day should be consumed habitually.

copra   Dried COCONUT used for production of oil for MARGARINE and soap manufacture.

coproducts   In meat processing, everything except the dressed carcase; edible coproducts are OFFAL (organ meat), blood, TALLOW and GELATINE, inedible coproducts include BLOOD CHARCOAL, BONE MEAL, BONE CHARCOAL and feather meal.

coprolith   Mass of hard faeces in colon or rectum due to chronic CONSTIPATION.

coprophagy   Eating of faeces. Since B vitamins are synthesised by intestinal bacteria, animals that eat their faeces can make use of these vitamins, which are not absorbed from the large intestine, the site of bacterial action.

CoQ   *See* UBIQUINONE.

coquille St Jacques   *See* SCALLOPS.

coracan   *See* MILLET.

coral   The ovaries of female LOBSTERS, used as the basis for sauces; red coloured when cooked.

cordial, fruit   Originally a fruit LIQUEUR, and still used in this sense in USA; in UK a cordial is now used to mean any fruit drink, usually a concentrate to be diluted.

cordon bleu   A term to denote first class cooking. Originally the blue sash worn by senior students at the Institut de Saint-Louis, founded in 1686 for the daughters of impoverished nobility; cookery was one of the subjects taught. The Ecole de Cordon Bleu was founded in Paris in 1880 by Marthe Distel, and Le Petit Cordon Bleu cooking school and restaurant in New York in 1942.

coriander   *Coriandrum sativum* (a member of the parsley family); the leaf is used fresh or dried as a herb, and the dried ripe fruit (also called dhanyia) as a spice.

corked   Of wines, the development of an unpleasant flavour due to fungal contamination of the cork.

corm The thickened, underground base of the stem of plants, often called bulbs, as, for example, TARO and ONION.

corn The seed of a cereal plant, especially that of the chief cereal of the district, thus in England WHEAT, in Scotland OATS, in the USA MAIZE.

corned beef In UK a canned product made from low quality BEEF that has been partially extracted with hot water to make MEAT EXTRACT. In USA and elsewhere, corned beef is pickled beef (in UK this is salt beef).

Cornell bread *See* BREAD.

cornflour Purified starch from MAIZE; in the USA called corn starch. Used in custard, blancmange and baking powders and for thickening sauces and gravies.

corn grits *See* HOMINY.

corn, Guinea, kaffir *See* SORGHUM.

Cornish pastie Traditional Cornish pastry turnover with a variety of fillings, commonly seasoned meat and cooked vegetables. Historically meat baked in a pastry crust without a dish.

corn oil (maize oil) Extracted from MAIZE germ, *Zea mays*; 13% saturated, 27% mono-unsaturated, 60% polyunsaturated fatty acids.

corn pone Small corn (maize) cakes, a specialty of Alabama, USA.

corn salad Winter salad vegetable, *Valeriana olitoria*, also known as lamb's lettuce.

Composition/100 g: water 92.8 g, 88 kJ (21 kcal), protein 2 g, fat 0.4 g, carbohydrate 3.6 g, ash 1.2 g, Ca 38 mg, Fe 2.2 mg, Mg 13 mg, P 53 mg, K 459 mg, Na 4 mg, Zn 0.6 mg, Cu 0.1 mg, Mn 0.4 mg, Se 0.9 µg, vitamin A 355 µg RE, B_1 0.07 mg, B_2 0.09 mg, niacin 0.4 mg, B_6 0.27 mg, folate 14 µg, C 38 mg.

corn starch *See* CORNFLOUR.

corn starch hydrolysate *See* CORN SYRUP.

corn sugar *See* GLUCOSE.

corn syrup SYRUP prepared by partial hydrolysis of STARCH, a mixture of GLUCOSE and OLIGOSACCHARIDES; the higher the glucose content, the sweeter the syrup. Those containing less glucose and more oligosaccharides are used for texture in food manufacture.

See also DEXTROSE EQUIVALENT VALUE.

coronary thrombosis *See* ATHEROSCLEROSIS.

corrinoids Compounds with the corrin ring structure of VITAMIN B_{12}; some have vitamin activity.

corticosteroids Steroid HORMONES synthesised in the adrenal cortex. Two main groups: glucocorticoids (e.g. cortisol, cortisone, corticosterone) involved in glucose homeostasis, and mineralocorticoids (e.g. aldosterone) involved in salt and water balance.

cortisol   A GLUCOCORTICOID HORMONE synthesised in the adrenal cortex that acts to increase gluconeogenesis and catabolism of TRYPTOPHAN and TYROSINE in the liver; also formed in adipocytes, where it causes insulin resistance and depresses production of RESISTIN.

COSHH   Control of Substances Hazardous to Health; regulation in UK (1988); requires safety assessment by all concerned with handling of chemicals.

cossettes   Thin chips of sugar beet shredded for hot-water extraction of the sugar.

coster monger   Originally 'costard monger', late 14th century London, person selling costerd apples (the earliest cultivated variety) in the street. Now anyone selling fruit and vegetables from a barrow.

cotechino   Italian; pork sausage with white wine and spices.

cottonseed   Seed of *Gossypium* spp.; a source of cooking oil, or for margarine manufacture when hardened; the protein residue is used as animal feed. The oil is 27% saturated, 19% mono-unsaturated, 54% polyunsaturated, contains 35 mg vitamin E, 25 mg vitamin K/100 g.

coulis   Also cullis; originally the juices that run out of meat when it is cooked, now used to mean rich sauce or gravy made from meat juices, puréed shellfish, vegetables or fruit. Most usually now a sauce made from puréed and sieved fruit.

coumarin   *See* DICOUMAROL.

courgette   Variety of MARROW developed to be harvested when small; also known as Italian marrow, Italian squash or zucchini.

Composition/100 g: (edible portion 87%) water 92.7 g, 88 kJ (21 kcal), protein 2.7 g, fat 0.4 g, carbohydrate 3.1 g, fibre 1.1 g, ash 1 g, Ca 21 mg, Fe 0.8 mg, Mg 33 mg, P 93 mg, K 459 mg, Na 3 mg, Zn 0.8 mg, Cu 0.1 mg, Mn 0.2 mg, Se 0.3 µg, B_1 0.04 mg, B_2 0.04 mg, niacin 0.7 mg, B_6 0.14 mg, folate 20 µg, pantothenate 0.4 mg, C 34 mg. A 100 g serving is a source of Mg, P, a rich source of vitamin C.

Courlose™   Sodium carboxymethylcellulose, *see* CELLULOSE DERIVATIVES.

couscous   N. African; MILLET flour or fine SEMOLINA, steamed until fluffy and traditionally served with mutton stew.

Composition/100 g: water 8.6 g, 1574 kJ (376 kcal), protein 12.8 g, fat 0.6 g, carbohydrate 77.4 g, fibre 5 g, ash 0.6 g, Ca 24 mg, Fe 1.1 mg, Mg 44 mg, P 170 mg, K 166 mg, Na 10 mg, Zn 0.8 mg, Cu 0.2 mg, Mn 0.8 mg, B_1 0.16 mg, B_2 0.08 mg, niacin 3.5 mg, B_6 0.11 mg, folate 20 µg, pantothenate 1.2 mg.

cow-heel   Dish made from heel of ox or cow, stewed to a jelly; also known as neat's-foot.

cow manure factor   Obsolete name for VITAMIN B₁₂.

cow pea   *See* BEAN, BLACK EYED.

C-peptide   The linking region between the A- and B-chains of PRO-INSULIN, cleaved in the conversion of pro-insulin to INSULIN. Useful as an index of pancreatic β-islet cell function since it is cleared from the circulation more slowly than is insulin.

CpG islands   Small stretches of DNA that are comparatively rich in CpG nucleotides (i.e. cytosine followed by guanine), frequently located within the promoter region of genes. Methylation within the islands is associated with transcriptional inactivation of the gene, and is hence a mechanism of cell differentiation. Failure of methylation of CpG islands is associated with the initiation of cancer. *See also* EPIGENETICS.

crab   SHELLFISH; *Cancer* and *Carcinus* spp.; king crab is *Limulus polyphemus*.

Composition/100 g: water 79 g, 364 kJ (87 kcal), protein 18.1 g, fat 1.1 g (of which 25% saturated, 25% mono-unsaturated, 50% polyunsaturated), cholesterol 78 mg, carbohydrate 0 g, ash 1.8 g, Ca 89 mg, Fe 0.7 mg, Mg 34 mg, P 229 mg, K 329 mg, Na 293 mg, Zn 3.5 mg, Cu 0.7 mg, Mn 0.2 mg, Se 37.4 µg, vitamin A 2 µg retinol, B₁ 0.08 mg, B₂ 0.04 mg, niacin 2.7 mg, B₆ 0.15 mg, folate 44 µg, B₁₂ 9 µg, pantothenate 0.3 mg, C 3 mg. A 300 g serving (half crab) is a source of Fe, vitamin B₁, pantothenate, C, a good source of Mn, vitamin B₆, a rich source of Ca, Cu, Mg, P, Se, Zn, niacin, folate, vitamin B₁₂.

crackers   Plain thin biscuits such as water biscuits, cream crackers and wholemeal crackers, made from wheat flour, fat and bicarbonate as a raising agent.

cran   A traditional measure for herrings containing 37½ gallons (167 L) or about 800 fish.

cranberry   The fleshy, acid fruit of *Vaccinium oxycoccus* or *V. macrocarpon*, resembling a cherry; commonly used to make sauce and juice.

Composition/100 g: (edible portion 95%) water 87 g, 193 kJ (46 kcal), protein 0.4 g, fat 0.1 g, carbohydrate 12.2 g (4 g sugars), fibre 4.6 g, ash 0.2 g, Ca 8 mg, Fe 0.3 mg, Mg 6 mg, P 13 mg, K 85 mg, Na 2 mg, Zn 0.1 mg, Cu 0.1 mg, Mn 0.4 mg, Se 0.1 µg, vitamin A 3 µg RE (127 µg carotenoids), E 1.2 mg, K 5.1 mg, B₁ 0.01 mg, B₂ 0.02 mg, niacin 0.1 mg, B₆ 0.06 mg, folate 1 µg, pantothenate 0.3 mg, C 13 mg. A 110 g serving is a source of Mn, vitamin E, a good source of vitamin C.

crapaud   Edible Caribbean bull frog (*Leptodactylus pentadactylus*), also known as mountain chicken. Also (in Jersey) the name of the common toad, *Bufo bufo*.

crawfish Crustaceans (without claws), family Palinuridae, also called spiny lobster, rock lobster, sea crayfish. *See* LOBSTER.

crayfish Crustaceans; freshwater crayfish are members of the families Astacidae, Parasiticidae and Austroastacidae. Sea crayfish (CRAWFISH) are Palinuridae.

Composition/100 g: water 84 g, 301 kJ (72 kcal), protein 14.9 g, fat 1 g, cholesterol 107 mg, carbohydrate 0 g, ash 1 g, Ca 25 mg, Fe 0.6 mg, Mg 30 mg, P 218 mg, K 261 mg, Na 62 mg, Zn 1 mg, Cu 0.2 mg, Mn 0.1 mg, Se 28.4 µg, I 100 µg, vitamin A 15 µg retinol, B_1 0.05 mg, B_2 0.03 mg, niacin 1.9 mg, B_6 0.08 mg, folate 30 µg, B_{12} 2.1 µg, pantothenate 0.6 mg, C 1 mg. A 40 g serving is a source of Se, a good source of I, a rich source of vitamin B_{12}.

See also LOBSTER.

cream Fatty part of milk; 4% of ordinary milk, 4.8% of Channel Islands milk. Half cream is similar to 'top of the milk', 12% fat, cannot be whipped or frozen; single cream, 18% fat, will not whip and cannot be frozen unless included in a frozen dish; extra thick single cream is also 18% fat, but has been homogenised to a thick spoonable consistency; whipping cream, will whip to double volume, 34–37% fat; double cream, will whip and can be frozen, 48% fat; clotted, Devonshire and Cornish, 55% fat (of which 66% saturated, 30% mono-unsaturated, 4% polyunsaturated).

Soured cream is made from single cream; crème fraîche is soured double cream; 'extra thick double cream' is also 48% fat, but has been homogenised to be spoonable, and will not whip or freeze successfully.

cream, artificial A name given to:

(1) emulsion of vegetable oil, milk or milk powder, egg yolk and sugar;

(2) emulsion of water with methyl CELLULOSE, MONOGLYCERIDES, and other materials.

cream, bitty Cream on the surface of milk appears as particles of fat released from fat globules when the membrane is broken down by LECITHINASE from *Bacillus cereus*, the spores of which have resisted destruction during PASTEURISATION.

creamer, non-dairy Milk substitute used in tea and coffee (coffee whitener or creamer) made with glucose, fat and emulsifying salts. A stable product dry or as liquid. May be made with CASEIN, in which case it is not technically (or by US law) non-dairy.

creaming Beating together fat and sugar to give a fluffy mixture, for making cakes with a high fat content. The creaming quality of a fat is its ability to take up air during mixing.

cream line index The cream line or layer usually forms about 6% of the total depth of milk. The cream line index is the ratio between the percentage cream layer and the percentage of fat in the milk; in bulk pasteurised milk it is about 1.7.

cream of tartar Potassium hydrogen tartrate, used with SODIUM BICARBONATE as BAKING POWDER because it acts more slowly than TARTARIC ACID and gives a more prolonged evolution of carbon dioxide. This is tartrate baking powder. Also used to invert sugar in making boiled sweets (*see* SUGAR, INVERT).

cream, plastic A term used for a cream containing as much fat as butter (80–83%) but as an emulsion of fat in water, while butter is water in fat. Prepared by intense centrifugal treatment of cream; crumbly, not greasy, in texture; used for preparation of cream cheese and whipped cream.

cream, sleepy Cream that will not churn to butter in the normal time.

cream, synthetic *See* CREAM, ARTIFICIAL.

creatine Amino-iminomethyl-*N*-methyl glycine, important in muscle as a store of phosphate for resynthesis of ATP during muscle contraction and work.

Synthesised in the body from the AMINO ACIDS glycine and arginine, and no evidence that a dietary intake is essential; there is some evidence that additional intake may enhance muscle work output.

Meat extract contains a mixture of creatine and CREATININE derived from the creatine that was present in the fresh muscle. Creatine plus creatinine is used as an index of quality of commercial meat extract, and as a measure of meat extract present in manufactured products, such as soups.

Urinary excretion of significant amounts of creatine occurs only when there is muscle loss.

creatinine The anhydride of creatine, formed non-enzymically from CREATINE and creatine phosphate, a metabolic end-product.

Urinary excretion of creatinine can be used to estimate total muscle mass, 1 g of creatinine excreted/24 h represents 18–20 kg of fat-free muscle tissue. The creatinine:height index is the ratio of urinary creatinine excretion over 24 h/that expected for height. It provides an index of protein depletion.

creatorrhoea Excessive loss of nitrogenous compounds in faeces as a result of impaired intestinal digestion of proteins or absorption of amino acids.

creeping sickness OSTEOMALACIA in livestock due to phosphate deficiency.

crème (1) Term used for cream, custards and desserts. Crème brûlée is cream and egg custard with sugar sprinkled on top and caramelised under a hot grill; a traditional specialty of Trinity College Cambridge, and also known as burnt cream or

Cambridge cream. Crème caramel is topped with caramel. Crème Chantilly is whipped cream sweetened and flavoured with VANILLA.

(2) Various liqueurs, including: crème de bananes (banana); crème de cacao (chocolate); crème de café (coffee); crème de menthe (peppermint); crème de mûres (wild blackberries); crème de myrtilles (wild bilberries); crème de noix (green walnuts and honey); crème de violettes (violet petals).

crème fraîche   Double CREAM that has been thickened and slightly soured by lactic fermentation.

cress   Garden cress, pepper grass, *Lepidium sativum*. Seed leaves eaten raw with mustard seed leaves: mustard and cress or salad rape (*Brassica napus* var. *napus*). American or land cress is *Barbarea verna*, the leaves have a peppery flavour. Unlike WATER-CRESS it can be grown in soil without running water.

Composition/100 g: (edible portion 71%) water 89 g, 134 kJ (32 kcal), protein 2.6 g, fat 0.7 g, carbohydrate 5.5 g (4.4 g sugars), fibre 1.1 g, ash 1.8 g, Ca 81 mg, Fe 1.3 mg, Mg 38 mg, P 76 mg, K 606 mg, Na 14 mg, Zn 0.2 mg, Cu 0.2 mg, Mn 0.6 mg, Se 0.9 µg, vitamin A 346 µg RE (16650 µg carotenoids), E 0.7 mg, K 541.9 mg, B_1 0.08 mg, B_2 0.26 mg, niacin 1 mg, B_6 0.25 mg, folate 80 µg, pantothenate 0.2 mg, C 69 mg. A 50 g serving is a source of Mn, a good source of vitamin A, folate, a rich source of vitamin C.

creta praeparata   British Pharmacopoeia name for prepared chalk, made by washing and drying naturally occurring calcium carbonate. The form in which calcium is added to flour (14 oz per 280 lb sack, or approximately 3 g/kg).

cretinism   Severe underactivity of the thyroid gland (hypothyroidism) in children, resulting in poor growth, deafness and severe mental retardation. Hypothyroidism in adults is myxoedema. Commonly the result of a dietary deficiency of IODINE; may be congenital if the mother's iodine intake was severely inadequate during pregnancy.

See also THYROID HORMONES.

Crisco™   HYDROGENATED vegetable SHORTENING, first produced by Procter & Gamble in 1911.

crispbread   Name given to a flour and water wafer, originally Swedish and made from rye flour, but may be made from wheat flour. They have a much lower water content than bread and some brands are richer in protein because of added wheat GLUTEN.

crisps   *See* CHIPS; POTATO CRISPS.

cristal height   A measure of leg length taken from the floor to the summit of the iliac crest. As a proportion of height it increases with age in children, and a reduced rate of increase indicates undernutrition.

See also ANTHROPOMETRY.

critical control point (CCP)   A factor or stage in processing when a loss of control would result in an unacceptable safety or quality risk.

critical moisture content   The moisture remaining in a food at the end of a period of drying at a constant rate.

critical temperature indicator   *See* TIME–TEMPERATURE INDICATOR.

CRN   Council for Responsible Nutrition, representing the dietary supplement industry; web site http://www.crnusa.org/.

crocin   *See* SAFFRON.

Crohn's disease   Chronic inflammatory disease of the bowel, commonly the terminal ileum, of unknown aetiology, treated with antibiotics to prevent infection and anti-inflammatory agents. Sufferers may be malnourished as a result of both loss of appetite due to illness and also malabsorption. Also known as regional enteritis, since only some regions of the gut are affected.

See also GASTROINTESTINAL TRACT.

cromoglycate   1,2-Bis(2-carboxychromon-5-yloxy)-2-hydropropane, used in treatment of vomiting, colic and diarrhoea associated with food ALLERGY and IRRITABLE BOWEL SYNDROME; also used in treatment of other allergic reactions. Trade name Cromlyn.

cropadeau   Scottish; oatmeal dumpling with haddock liver in the middle.

crowdie   Scottish; soft cheese made from buttermilk or soured milk curd, also a dish of buttermilk and oatmeal.

crowdies   *See* MILK, FERMENTED.

cruciferae   Family of plants with flowers having four equal petals; most vegetables in this family belong to the genus *BRASSICA*.

crude fibre   *See* FIBRE, CRUDE.

crude protein   *See* PROTEIN, CRUDE.

crullers   DOUGHNUTS made from deep fried CHOUX PASTRY.

crumb softeners   Derivatives of mono-acylglycerols (monoglycerides) added to bread as emulsifiers to give a softer crumb and retard staling (E-430–436); also called polysorbates.

See also FAT, SUPERGLYCINERATED.

crustacea   Zoological class of hard-shelled marine arthropods (SHELLFISH) including CRAB, CRAYFISH, LOBSTER, PRAWN, SCAMPI, SHRIMP.

cryodesiccation   *See* FREEZE DRYING.

cryogen   A REFRIGERANT that absorbs latent heat and changes phase from solid or liquid to a gas, e.g. subliming or evaporating carbon dioxide or liquid nitrogen.

cryogenic freezing Freezing by use of a CRYOGEN.

Cryovac^{TM} Thermoplastic resin wrapping film that can be heat-shrunk onto foods.

cryptoxanthin Hydroxylated CAROTENOID found in a few foods such as yellow MAIZE and the seeds of CAPE GOOSEBERRY. VITAMIN A active.

crystal boiling Chinese method of cooking; food is heated in a pan of boiling water, then removed from the heat and cooking continued by the retained heat.

Crystalean^{TM} A preparation of resistant starch. *See* STARCH, RESISTANT.

crystallin The protein of the lens of the eye. Uniquely among body proteins, there is no turnover of crystallin, and while the amount increases with growth, crystallin formed before birth remains in the lens until death.

CSM Corn–soya–milk; a protein-rich baby food (20% protein) made in the USA from 68% precooked maize (corn), 25% defatted soya flour and 5% skim milk powder, with added vitamins and calcium carbonate.

CTC machine A device consisting of two contra-rotating toothed rollers that rotate at different speeds and provide a crushing, tearing and curling action, used in breaking up leaves of tea to form small particles.

CTI Critical temperature indicator, *see* TIME–TEMPERATURE INDICATOR.

cubeb Grey pepper (*Piper cubeba*) native to S.E. Asia; pungent flavour akin to camphor.

cucumber Fruit of *Cucumis sativus*, a member of the GOURD family, eaten as a salad vegetable.
  Composition/100 g: (edible portion 97%) water 95 g, 63 kJ (15 kcal), protein 0.6 g, fat 0.1 g, carbohydrate 3.6 g (1.7 g sugars), fibre 0.5 g, ash 0.4 g, Ca 16 mg, Fe 0.3 mg, Mg 13 mg, P 24 mg, K 147 mg, Na 2 mg, Zn 0.2 mg, Mn 0.1 mg, Se 0.3 µg, vitamin A 5 µg RE (105 µg carotenoids), K 16.4 mg, B_1 0.03 mg, B_2 0.03 mg, niacin 0.1 mg, B_6 0.04 mg, folate 7 µg, pantothenate 0.3 mg, C 3 mg.

cucumber, African horned *See* KIWANO.

cucurbit A term used for vegetables of the family Cucurbitaceae. *See* GOURDS.

Culinary Institute of America Founded in New Haven, Connecticut, 1946, as the New Haven Restaurant Institute, a storefront school.

cultivar Horticultural term for a cultivated variety of plant that is distinct and is uniform and stable in its characteristics when propagated.
  See also STRAIN.

cumin (cummin) Pungent herb, the seed of *Cuminum cyminum* (parsley family). Black cumin is the seed of *Nigella sativa* (fennel flower) and sweet cumin is ANISEED (*Pimpinella anisum*).

cumquat *See* KUMQUAT.

cup N. American and Australian measure for ingredients in cooking; the standard American cup contains 250 mL (8 fl oz).

curcumin Yellow pigment extracted from the rhizomes of turmeric, *Curcuma longa*.

curd, fruit Gelled emulsions of sugar, fat or oil, egg, pectin, fruit or fruit juice (commonly lemon) and colour.

curdlan A gel-forming polysaccharide used to improve water retention in meat products; produced by fermentation with the bacterium *Alcaligenes faecalis* var. *myxogenes.*

curds Clotted protein formed when milk is treated with RENNET; the fluid left is WHEY.

curd tension A measure of the toughness of the curd formed from milk by the digestive enzymes, and used as an index of the digestibility of the milk. The sample is coagulated with CHYMOSIN and the force needed to pull a knife-blade through the curd is measured under standardised conditions.

Ideal score is zero, below 20 g satisfactory; cow's milk 46; diluted with equal volume of water 20; reconstituted spray-dried milk 10; reconstituted roller-dried milk 5; EVAPORATED MILK 3; human milk 1.

curing agents *See* PICKLING.

curing, of meat *See* MEAT, CURING.

currants Fruit of *Ribes* spp.; *see* BLACKCURRANTS; REDCURRANTS.

currants, dried Made by drying the small seedless black grapes grown in Greece and Australia; usually dried in bunches on the vine or after removal from the vine on supports. The name is derived from *raisins of Corauntz* (Corinth).

See also RAISINS; SULTANAS.

curry Name given by the British (it means *sauce* in Tamil) to an Indian dish of stewed meat or vegetables. It is served with a pungent sauce whose components and pungency vary.

See also CURRY POWDER.

curry plant (curry leaves) An aromatic herb, *Murraya koenigii.*

curry powder A mixture of turmeric with spices including cardamom, cinnamon, cloves, coriander, cumin and fenugreek, made pungent with mustard, chilli and pepper. A 10 g portion can contain 7.5–10 mg iron, but much of this is probably the result of contamination during the milling of the spices.

cushion The cut nearest the udder in lamb or beef.

custard Sweet sauce, traditionally made by cooking milk with eggs; more commonly using custard powder (coloured and flavoured CORNFLOUR) and milk.

custard apple The fruit of one of a number of tropical American trees, *Anona* spp. Sour sop, *A. muricata*, has white fibrous flesh and is less sweet than the others; the fruit may weigh up to 4 kg (8 lb). The sweet sop (*A. squamosa*) is also known as the 'true' custard apple, or sugar apple. The bullock's heart (*A. reticulata*) has buff-coloured flesh.

Sweetsop, composition/100 g: (edible portion 58%) water 71.5 g, 423 kJ (101 kcal), protein 1.7 g, fat 0.6 g, carbohydrate 25.2 g, fibre 2.4 g, ash 1 g, Ca 30 mg, Fe 0.7 mg, Mg 18 mg, P 21 mg, K 382 mg, Na 4 mg, vitamin A 2 µg RE, B_1 0.08 mg, B_2 0.1 mg, niacin 0.5 mg, B_6 0.22 mg, pantothenate 0.1 mg, C 19 mg. A 110 g serving is a source of vitamin B_6 a rich source of vitamin C.

Soursop, composition/100 g: (edible portion 67%) water 81.2 g, 276 kJ (66 kcal), protein 1 g, fat 0.3 g, carbohydrate 16.8 g (13.5 g sugars), fibre 3.3 g, ash 0.7 g, Ca 14 mg, Fe 0.6 mg, Mg 21 mg, P 27 mg, K 278 mg, Na 14 mg, Zn 0.1 mg, Cu 0.1 mg, Se 0.6 µg, 1 µg carotenoids, E 0.1 mg, K 0.4 mg, B_1 0.07 mg, B_2 0.05 mg, niacin 0.9 mg, B_6 0.06 mg, folate 14 µg, pantothenate 0.3 mg, C 21 mg. A 150 g serving (quarter fruit) is a source of Cu, a rich source of vitamin C.

Cherimoya is the fruit of *A. cherimoya*. Composition/100 g: (edible portion 79%) water 79.4 g, 310 kJ (74 kcal), protein 1.6 g, fat 0.6 g, carbohydrate 17.7 g, fibre 2.3 g, ash 0.6 g, Ca 8 mg, Fe 0.3 mg, Mg 16 mg, P 26 mg, K 269 mg, Na 4 mg, Zn 0.2 mg, Cu 0.1 mg, Mn 0.1 mg, B_1 0.09 mg, B_2 0.12 mg, niacin 0.6 mg, B_6 0.21 mg, folate 18 µg, pantothenate 0.2 mg, C 12 mg. A 150 g serving (half fruit) is a source of Cu, vitamin B_2, B_6, folate, a rich source of vitamin C.

cyamopsis gum *See* GUAR GUM.

cyanocobalamin *See* VITAMIN B_{12}.

cyanogen(et)ic glycosides Organic compounds of cyanide found in a variety of plants; chemically cyanhydrin glycosides. Toxic through liberation of the cyanide when the plants are cut or chewed.

See also ALMOND; AMYGDALIN.

cycasin Methylazoxymethanol β-glucoside, a toxin in seeds of *Cycas* spp.

cyclamate Cyclohexylsulphamate, a non-nutritive SWEETENER, thirty times as sweet as sugar, used as the sodium or calcium salt; first synthesised in 1937, introduced commercially in the USA in 1950. Useful in low-calorie foods; unlike SACCHARIN, it is stable to heat and can be used in cooking. Trade name Sucaryl.

cyclitols   Cyclic SUGAR ALCOHOLS such as inositol, quercitol and tetritol.

cyclodextrins   Enzyme-modified STARCH derivatives with a hydrophilic outer surface and a hydrophobic inner cavity, used for ENCAPSULATION of flavours and other ingredients in food manufacture, and to form stable oil-in-water emulsions. Can also be used to remove CHOLESTEROL from dairy products and eggs.

Cymogran™   A protein-rich food low in PHENYLALANINE for patients with PHENYLKETONURIA.

cystathioninuria   A GENETIC DISEASE due to lack of cystathionase (EC 4.4.1.1) affecting the metabolism of the AMINO ACID METHIONINE and its conversion to CYSTEINE. May result in mental retardation if untreated. Treatment is by feeding a diet low in methionine and supplemented with cysteine, or, in some cases, by administration of high intakes of VITAMIN B_6 (about 100–500 times the normal requirement).

cysteine   A non-essential AMINO ACID, abbr Cys (C), M_r 121.2, pK_a 1.92, 8.35, 10.46 (—SH), CODONS UGPy. Nutritionally important since it is synthesised from the essential amino acid METHIONINE. In addition to its role in protein synthesis, cysteine is important as the precursor of TAURINE, in formation of COENZYME A from the VITAMIN PANTOTHENIC ACID and in formation of the tripeptide GLUTATHIONE. It is used as a dough 'improver' in baking.

   See also CYSTINE.

cysticercosis   Infection by the larval stage of TAPEWORMS caused by ingestion of their eggs in food and water contaminated by human faeces. Normally the larval form develops in the animal host, and human beings are infected with the adult form by eating undercooked infected meat.

cystic fibrosis   A GENETIC DISEASE due to a failure of the normal transport of chloride ions across cell membranes. This results in abnormally viscous mucus, affecting especially the lungs and secretion of pancreatic juice, hence impairing digestion.

cystine   The dimer of CYSTEINE produced when the sulphydryl group (—SH) is oxidised to form a disulphide (—S—S—) bridge. Such disulphide bridges are especially important in maintaining the structure of proteins, and also in the role of the tripeptide GLUTATHIONE as an ANTIOXIDANT. Hair protein (keratin) is especially rich in cystine, which accounts for about 12% of its total amino acid content.

cystinuria   A GENETIC DISEASE in which there is abnormally high excretion of the amino acids CYSTEINE and CYSTINE, resulting in the formation of kidney stones. Treatment is by feeding a diet low in the sulphur AMINO ACIDS methionine, cysteine and cystine.

cytochromes   HAEM-containing proteins. Some react with oxygen directly; others are intermediates in the oxidation of reduced COENZYMES. Unlike HAEMOGLOBIN, the iron in the haem of cytochromes undergoes oxidation and reduction.

cytochromes P450   A family of CYTOCHROMES involved in the DETOXICATION system of the body (*see* PHASE I METABOLISM). They act on a wide variety of (potentially toxic) compounds, both endogenous metabolites and foreign compounds (XENOBIOTICS), rendering them more water-soluble, and more readily conjugated for excretion in the urine.

The CYP26 group of cytochromes P450 are specific for RETINOIC ACID, leading to a variety of metabolites that may be physiologically active (especially in cell differentiation), including 4-hydroxy-, 4-oxo-, 5,6-epoxy- and 18-hydroxy-retinoic acid.

cytokines   A number of proteins secreted by cells in response to various stimuli that act to regulate proliferation and differentiation, immune and inflammatory responses, etc.

Cytokines produced by lymphocytes are sometimes known as lymphokines; those from monocytes as monokines; those secreted by adipose tissue as adipokines or adipocytokines.

cytokinins   Plant hormones derived from isopentenyl adenosine; produced by root tips, seed embryos, developing fruits and buds; they stimulate cell division (cytokinesis) and regulate development of the plant.

See also AUXINS.

cytosine   One of the PYRIMIDINE bases of NUCLEIC ACIDS.

D

D-, L- and DL-   Prefixes to chemical names for compounds that have a centre of asymmetry in the molecule, and which can therefore have two forms.

Most naturally occurring sugars have the D-conformation; apart from a few microbial proteins and some invertebrate peptides, all the naturally occurring amino acids have the L-configuration. Chemical synthesis yields a mixture of the D- and L-isomers (the racemic mixture), generally shown as DL-.

See also ISOMERS; OPTICAL ACTIVITY; *R*- AND *S*-.

***d*- and *l*-**   An obsolete way of indicating dextrorotatory and laevorotatory OPTICAL ACTIVITY, now replaced by (+) and (−).

dabberlocks   Edible seaweed, *Alaria esculenta*.

dadhi   *See* MILK, FERMENTED.

dagé   Indonesian; fermented PRESSCAKE from various oilseeds or legumes or starch crops, soaked in water and left to undergo bacterial fermentation (mainly *Bacillus* spp.) to form a glutinous mass bound by bacterial polysaccharides.

dahl *See* LEGUMES.

dahlin *See* INULIN.

daikon RADISH, large Japanese variety of *Raphanus sativus*. Often pickled in soy sauce, and an ingredient of KIMCHI.

daily value Reference amounts of energy, fat, saturated fat, carbohydrate, fibre, sodium, potassium and cholesterol, as well as protein, vitamins and minerals, introduced for food labelling in USA in 1994. The nutrient content of a food must be declared as percentage of the daily value provided by a standard serving.

Dairy-Lo™ FAT REPLACER made from protein.

Daltose™ A carbohydrate preparation consisting of maltose, glucose and dextrin for infant feeding.

damiana Leaf and stem of *Turnera diffiusa* var. *aphrodisiaca*, used as a food flavouring, reputed to have aphrodisiac and antidepressant properties.

damson Small dark purple PLUM (*Prunus damascena*); very acid, mainly used to make jam. Introduced into Europe by Crusaders returning from Damascus (early 13th century).

dandelion The leaves of the weed *Taraxacum officinale* may be eaten as a salad or cooked. In France dandelion greens are known as *pis-en-lit* because of their diuretic action.

Composition/100 g: water 86 g, 188 kJ (45 kcal), protein 2.7 g, fat 0.7 g, carbohydrate 9.2 g (3.8 g sugars), fibre 3.5 g, ash 1.8 g, Ca 187 mg, Fe 3.1 mg, Mg 36 mg, P 66 mg, K 397 mg, Na 76 mg, Zn 0.4 mg, Cu 0.2 mg, Mn 0.3 mg, Se 0.5 μg, vitamin A 247 μg RE (9607 μg carotenoids), E 4.8 mg, K 273.7 mg, B_1 0.19 mg, B_2 0.26 mg, niacin 0.8 mg, B_6 0.25 mg, folate 27 μg, pantothenate 0.1 mg, C 35 mg.

The root can be cooked as a vegetable, or may be roasted and used as a substitute for COFFEE.

Danish agar *See* FURCELLARAN.

dansyl reagent 5-Dimethylamino naphthalene sulphonic acid; reacts with amino terminal amino acid of a peptide to give a fluorescent derivative which can be identified by thin-layer CHROMATOGRAPHY after hydrolysis of the peptide.

danthron An anthroquinone stimulant LAXATIVE.

dark adaptation In the eye, the visual pigment rhodopsin is formed by reaction between VITAMIN A aldehyde (retinaldehyde) and the protein opsin, and is bleached by exposure to light, stimulating a nerve impulse (this is the basis of VISION). At an early stage of vitamin A deficiency it takes considerably longer than normal to adapt to see in dim light after exposure to normal bright light, because of the limitation of the amount of rhodopsin that can be reformed. Measuring the time taken to adapt to dim light (the dark adaptation time) provides a sensitive index of early vitamin A deficiency. More severe vitamin A deficiency results in NIGHT BLINDNESS, and eventually complete blindness.

dasheen *See* TARO.

date Fruit of date palm, *Phoenix dactylifera*. Three types: 'soft' (about 80% of the dry matter is invert sugar, *see* SUGAR, INVERT); semi-dry (about 40% invert sugar, 40% sucrose); and dry (20–40% invert sugar, 40–60% is sucrose).

Composition/100 g: (edible portion 90%) water 20.5 g, 1180 kJ (282 kcal), protein 2.5 g, fat 0.4 g, carbohydrate 75 g (63.3 g sugars), fibre 8 g, ash 1.6 g, Ca 39 mg, Fe 1 mg, Mg 43 mg, P 62 mg, K 656 mg, Na 2 mg, Zn 0.3 mg, Cu 0.2 mg, Mn 0.3 mg, Se 3 µg, 81 µg carotenoids, vitamin E 0.1 mg, K 2.7 mg, B_1 0.05 mg, B_2 0.07 mg, niacin 1.3 mg, B_6 0.17 mg, folate 19 µg, pantothenate 0.6 mg.

date, Chinese *See* JUJUBE (2).

DATEM Diacetyl tartaric esters of mono- and diglycerides used as EMULSIFIERS to strengthen bread dough and delay staling (E-472e).

date marking 'Best before' is the date up until when the food will remain in optimum condition, i.e. will not be stale. Foods with a shelf-life up to 12 weeks are marked 'best before day, month, year'; foods with a longer shelf-life are marked 'best before end of month, year'.

Perishable foods with a shelf-life of less than a month may have a 'sell by' date instead. 'Use by' date is given for foods that are microbiologically highly perishable and could become a danger to health; it is the date up to and including which the food may safely be used if stored properly.

Frozen foods and ice cream carry star markings that correspond to the star marking on freezers and frozen food compartments of refrigerators. One star (*) –4 °C (25 °F) will keep for one week; two star (**) –11 °C (12 °F), 1 month; three star (***) –18 °C (0 °F), 3 months. Corresponding times for ice cream are 1 day, 1 week, 1 month, after which they are fit to eat but the texture changes.

date plum *See* PERSIMMON.

dawadawa African; fermented dried seeds of the African locust bean *Parkia biglobosa*, usually pressed into balls; various bacteria are involved in the 3–4 day fermentation.

***db/db* mouse** Genetically OBESE mouse that is also diabetic; the defect is lack of LEPTIN receptors.

DBD process *See* DRY–BLANCH–DRY PROCESS.

DCPIP *See* DICHLOROPHENOLINDOPHENOL.

DCS Distributed control systems.

DE *See* DEXTROSE EQUIVALENT VALUE.

debranching enzymes Enzymes that hydrolyse the α-1,6 glycoside bonds that form the branch points in AMYLOPECTIN. Amyloglucosidase (EC 3.2.1.3) and glucoamylase (EC 3.2.1.20) also hydrolyse α-1,4 links; pullulanase (EC 3.2.1.41) and isoamylase (EC 3.2.1.68) hydrolyse only α-1,6 links.

See also AMYLASES; Z-ENZYME.

debrining Removal of much of the salt used in BRINING vegetables, to a level that will be acceptable in the final product. Also known as freshening.

decimal reduction time (*D* value) Term used in sterilising canned food, etc.; the duration of heat treatment required to reduce the number of micro-organisms to one-tenth of the initial value, with the temperature shown as a subscript, e.g. D_{121} is time at 121 °C.

defoamer *See* ANTIFOAMING AGENTS.

DEFRA UK Department of the Environment, Food and Rural Affairs; web site http://www.defra.gov.uk/.

defructum Roman; cooking wine that has been reduced to half its volume by boiling.

DEFT Direct Epifluorescence Filter Technique for measuring bacterial content of milk and other fluids by passing through a fine pore filter to retain bacteria that are then stained with acridine orange to permit fluorimetric quantification. A rapid and sensitive alternative to plating out a sample, culturing and counting the resultant bacterial colonies. Trade names for the equipment used include Biofoss, Bactoscan and Autotrak.

deglutition The act of swallowing.

degumming Removal of proteins, phospholipids, gum, resin, etc. in the refining of oils and fats by the addition of dilute hydrochloric or phosphoric acid, brine or alkaline phosphate solution. Permits recovery of LECITHIN from the aqueous phase.

dehydroascorbic acid The oxidised form of VITAMIN C which is readily reduced back to the active form in the body, and therefore has vitamin activity. Not measured by all methods for vitamin C estimation.

See also ASCORBIC ACID.

dehydrocanning A process in which 50% of the water is removed from a food before canning. The advantages are that the texture is retained by the partial dehydration and there is a saving in bulk and weight.

7-dehydrocholesterol Intermediate in the synthesis of CHOLESTEROL, and precursor for the synthesis of VITAMIN D in the skin.

dehydrofreezing A process for preservation of fruits and vegetables by evaporation of 50–60% of the water before freezing. The texture and flavour are claimed to be superior to those resulting from either dehydration or freezing alone, and rehydration is more rapid than with dehydrated products.

dehydroretinol An analogue of VITAMIN A found in freshwater fish, which has about half the biological activity of RETINOL. Formerly termed vitamin A$_2$.

Delaney Amendment Clause in the US Federal Food, Drug and Cosmetic Act (1958) which states that no food additive shall be deemed safe (and therefore may not be used) after it is found to induce cancer when ingested by man or animals, at any dose level.

delayed hypersensitivity An ADVERSE REACTION TO FOOD, occurring several hours after ingestion, caused by cell-mediated immune responses (activated lymphocytes) as opposed to immunoglobulin-mediated responses, which occur rapidly.

See also COELIAC DISEASE.

demerara sugar See SUGAR.

denaturation A normally irreversible change in the structure of protein by heat, acid, alkali or other agents which results in loss of solubility and COAGULATION. Denatured proteins lose biological activity (e.g. as enzymes), but not nutritional value. Indeed, digestibility is improved compared with the native structure, which is relatively resistant to enzymic hydrolysis.

denatured alcohol See ALCOHOL, DENATURED.

dendritic salt A form of ordinary table SALT, sodium chloride, with the crystals branched or star-like (dendritic) instead of the normal cubes. This is claimed to have a number of advantages: lower bulk density, more rapid solution, and an unusually high capacity to absorb moisture before becoming wet.

density, absolute Mass per unit volume of a substance; depends on temperature and pressure. For particulate matter it excludes the spaces that exist between particles, and measures only the density of the particles themselves; this is also known as solid or particulate density.

See also DENSITY, BULK.

density, bulk Mass per unit volume of particulate material, including spaces between the particles.

See also DENSITY, ABSOLUTE.

density, particulate See DENSITY, ABSOLUTE.

dental fluorosis Mottled dental enamel, see FLUORIDE.

dental plaque See PLAQUE (1).

dent corn See MAIZE.

deodorisation The removal of an undesirable flavour or odour. Fats are deodorised during refining by bubbling superheated steam through the hot oil under vacuum, when most of the flavoured substances are distilled off.

deoxycholic acid   One of the secondary BILE SALTS, formed by intestinal bacterial metabolism of CHOLIC ACID.

deoxynivalenol   Trichothecene MYCOTOXIN produced when cereals are infected with *Fusarium* spp.

4-deoxypyridixine   Antimetabolite of VITAMIN B$_6$ used in experimental studies of vitamin B$_6$ deficiency.

deoxyribonucleic acid   *See* DNA; NUCLEIC ACIDS.

deoxyuridine suppression test   *See* dUMP SUPPRESSION TEST.

depectinisation   The removal of PECTIN from fruit juice to produce a clear thin juice instead of a viscous, cloudy liquid, by enzymic hydrolysis.

depositor   Machine for depositing a precise amount of food into a mould or onto a conveyor belt.

Derby   English hard cheese, often flavoured with sage.

Derbyshire neck   *See* GOITRE.

dermatitis   A lesion or inflammation of the skin caused by outside agents (unlike eczema, which is an endogenous disease); many nutritional deficiency diseases include more or less specific skin lesions (e.g. ARIBOFLAVINOSIS, KWASHIORKOR, PELLAGRA, SCURVY), but most cases of dermatitis are not associated with nutritional deficiency, and do not respond to nutritional supplements. Dermatitis herpetiformis is an uncommon itchy and blistering rash associated with COELIAC DISEASE.

desferrioxamine   Chelating agent used in treatment of IRON overload; the iron chelate is excreted in the urine. Given by 8–12 h subcutaneous perfusion 3–7 times a week.

designer foods   Alternative name for FUNCTIONAL FOODS.

desmosine   The cross-linkage compound between chains of the CONNECTIVE TISSUE protein ELASTIN, formed by reaction of two or three lysine residues in adjacent polypeptide chains.

desmutagen   Compound acting directly on a MUTAGEN to decrease its mutagenicity.

desorption   Removal of moisture from a food.

detox diets   Weight reduction diets based on the (probably fallacious) concept that the body accumulates large amounts of toxins from food and the environment that must be cleared by a period of fasting.

detoxication   The metabolism of (potentially) toxic compounds to yield less toxic derivatives that are more soluble in water and can be excreted in the urine or BILE. A wide variety of 'foreign compounds' (i.e. compounds that are not normal metabolites in the body), sometimes referred to as xenobiotics, and some hormones and other normal body metabolites, are metabolised in the same way.

   See also CYTOCHROMES; PHASE I METABOLISM.

devils on horseback   Bacon wrapped around stoned prunes, skewered with a toothpick and then grilled.

See also ANGELS ON HORSEBACK.

devitalised gluten   *See* GLUTEN.

dewberry   A hybrid fruit, a large variety of BLACKBERRY; rather than climbing, the plant trails on the ground.

dew point   The temperature at which a mixture of water vapour in air becomes saturated if cooled at constant absolute HUMIDITY, also known as saturation temperature.

dexedrine   Anorectic (appetite suppressing, *see* APPETITE CONTROL) drug formerly used in the treatment of OBESITY.

dexfenfluramine   *See* FENFLURAMINE.

dextrins   A mixture of soluble compounds formed by the partial breakdown of STARCH by heat, acid or enzymes (AMYLASES). Formed when bread is toasted. Nutritionally equivalent to starch; industrially used as adhesives, in the sizing of paper and textiles, and as gums.

Limit dextrin is the product of enzymic hydrolysis of branched polysaccharides such as GLYCOGEN or AMYLOPECTIN, when glucose units are removed one at a time until the branch point is reached, when the DEBRANCHING ENZYME is required for further hydrolysis.

dextronic acid   *See* GLUCONIC ACID.

dextrose   Alternative name for GLUCOSE. Commercially the term 'glucose' is often used to mean CORN SYRUP (a mixture of glucose with other sugars and DEXTRINS) and pure glucose is called dextrose.

dextrose equivalent value (DE)   A term used to indicate the degree of hydrolysis of starch into GLUCOSE syrup. It is the percentage of the total solids that have been converted to reducing sugars; the higher the DE, the more sugars and fewer dextrins are present. Liquid glucoses are commercially available ranging from 2 DE to 65 DE. Complete acid hydrolysis converts all the starch into glucose but produces bitter degradation products.

Glucose syrups above 55 DE are termed 'high conversion' (of starch); 35–55, regular conversion; below 20 the products of hydrolysis are maltins or maltodextrins.

DFD   *See* MEAT, DFD.

DH   UK Department of Health; web page http://www.dh.gov.uk/.

DHA   Docosohexaenoic acid, a long chain polyunsaturated FATTY ACID (C22:6 ω3). *See* FISH OILS.

dhal   Indian term for split peas of various kinds, e.g. the pigeon pea (*Cajanus indicus*), khesari (*Lathyrus sativus*); red dhal or Massur dhal is the lentil (*Lens esculenta*).

dhanyia   *See* CORIANDER.

dhool   The name given to leaves of TEA up to the stage of drying.

DHSS   US Department of Health and Human Services; web site http://www.dhhs.gov/.

dhupa   *See* COCOA BUTTER EQUIVALENTS.

diabetes   Two distinct conditions: diabetes insipidus and diabetes mellitus. Diabetes insipidus is a metabolic disorder characterised by extreme thirst, excessive consumption of liquids and urination, due to failure of secretion of the antidiuretic hormone. HAEMOCHROMATOSIS is known as bronze diabetes.

Diabetes mellitus is a metabolic disorder involving impaired metabolism of GLUCOSE due either to failure of secretion of the HORMONE INSULIN (Type I, insulin-dependent diabetes) or impaired responses of tissues to insulin (Type II, non-insulin-dependent diabetes). If untreated, the blood concentration of glucose rises to abnormally high levels (hyperglycaemia) after a meal and glucose is excreted in the urine (glucosuria). Prolonged hyperglycaemia may damage nerves, blood vessels and kidneys, and lead to development of cataracts, so effective control of blood glucose levels is important.

Type I diabetes develops in childhood (sometimes called juvenile-onset diabetes) and is due to failure to secrete INSULIN as a result of progressive auto-immune destruction of pancreatic β-islet cells. Treatment is by injection of insulin, either purified from beef or pig pancreas, now usually, biosynthetic human insulin, together with restriction of the intake of sugars.

Type II diabetes generally arises in middle age (maturity-onset diabetes) and is due to INSULIN resistance of tissues; secretion of insulin by the pancreas is higher than normal in the early stages of the disease. It can sometimes be treated by restricting the consumption of sugars and reducing weight, or by the use of oral drugs which stimulate insulin secretion and/or enhance the insulin responsiveness of tissues (sulphonylureas and biguanides). It is also treated by injection of insulin to supplement secretion from the pancreas and overcome the resistance.

Impairment of GLUCOSE TOLERANCE similar to that seen in diabetes mellitus sometimes occurs in late pregnancy, when it is known as gestational diabetes. Sometimes pregnancy is the stress that precipitates diabetes, and commonly the condition resolves when the child is born.

Renal diabetes is the excretion of glucose in the urine without undue elevation of the blood glucose concentration. It is due to a reduction of the renal threshold, which allows the blood glucose to be excreted.

See also GLUCOKINASE; METABOLIC SYNDROME; MODY.

diabetic foods   Loose term for foods that are specially formulated to be suitable for consumption by people with DIABETES mellitus; generally low in sugars, and frequently containing SORBITOL, XYLULOSE or sugar derivatives that are slowly or incompletely absorbed.

diacetyl   Acetyl methyl carbonyl ($CH_3 \cdot CO \cdot CO \cdot CH_3$), the main flavour in butter, formed during the ripening stage by the organism *Streptococcus lactis cremoris*. Synthetic diacetyl is added to margarine as 'butter flavour'.

diafiltration   Dilution of the concentrate during reverse osmosis (*see* OSMOSIS, REVERSE) or ULTRAFILTRATION, to improve the recovery of solutes.

dialysis   A process for separating low MW solutes (e.g. salts and sugars) from larger ones (e.g. proteins) in solution. Small molecules can pass through a SEMIPERMEABLE MEMBRANE, while large molecules cannot. The membrane may be natural, such as pig bladder, or artificial, such as cellulose derivatives or collodion.

diaminopimelic acid   Intermediate in synthesis of lysine in bacteria; also important in sporulating bacteria for formation of spore coat. M_r 190.2, pK_a 1.8, 2.2, 8.8, 9.9.

diaphysis   The shaft of a long BONE.
   See also EPIPHYSIS; METAPHYSIS.

diarrhoea   Frequent passage of loose watery stools, commonly the result of intestinal infection; rarely as a result of ADVERSE REACTION TO FOODS or DISACCHARIDE INTOLERANCE. Severe diarrhoea in children can lead to dehydration and death; it is treated by feeding a solution of salt and sugar to replace fluid and electrolyte losses.

   Osmotic diarrhoea is associated with retention of water in the bowel as a result of an accumulation of nonabsorbable water-soluble compounds; especially associated with excessive intake of SORBITOL and MANNITOL. Also occurs in DISACCHARIDE INTOLERANCE.
   See also ANTIMOTILITY AGENTS.

diastase   *See* AMYLASES.

diastatic activity   A measure of the ability of flour to produce maltose from its own starch by the action of its own AMYLASE (diastase). This sugar is needed for the growth of the yeast during fermentation.
   See also AMYLOGRAPH.

diazoxide   7-Chloro-3-methyl-1,2,4-benzothiadiazone 1,1-dioxide, used in treatment of chronic hypoglycaemia associated with excessive secretion of INSULIN due to pancreatic β-islet cell hyperplasia or cancer.

dichlorophenolindophenol (DCPIP) Purple-blue dye used in titrimetric assay of VITAMIN C; reduced to a colourless leuco dye by ascorbic acid, but not by dehydroascorbate, so does not measure total vitamin C.

dicoumarol (dicoumarin, coumarin) Naturally occurring VITAMIN K antagonist, found in spoilt hay containing sweet clover (*Melilotus alba* or *M. officinalis*); leads to haemorrhagic disease in cattle as a result of impaired synthesis of prothrombin and other vitamin K-dependent blood clotting proteins.

dicyclomine *See* ATROPINE.

didronel Drug used to enhance bone mineralisation in women with post-menopausal OSTEOPOROSIS.

die A restricted opening at the discharge end of an extruder barrel.

dielectric constant The ratio of the electrical capacitance of a food to the capacitance of air or vacuum under the same conditions.

dielectric heating Similar principle to microwave heating but at lower frequencies. Food is passed between capacitor plates and high-frequency energy applied by using alternating electrostatic fields, which changes the orientation of the dipoles. The process is limited by the space between the plates; used for thawing blocks of frozen food, melting fats and drying biscuits.

See also IRRADIATION.

dietary fibre *See* FIBRE, DIETARY.

dietary folate equivalents (DFE) Method for calculating FOLIC ACID intake taking into account the lower availability of mixed folates in food compared with synthetic tetrahydrofolate used in food enrichment and supplements. 1 μg DFE = 1 μg food folate or 0.6 μg synthetic folate; total DFE = μg food folate + 1.7 × μg synthetic folate.

dietary pattern analysis Statistical technique, based on CLUSTER ANALYSIS, to analyse food consumption records in order to classify the results into predefined types of diet.

Dietary Reference Intakes (DRI) US term for DIETARY REFERENCE VALUES. In addition to average requirement and RDA, include tolerable upper levels (UL) of intake from supplements. *See* REFERENCE INTAKES.

Dietary Reference Values (DRV) A UK set of standards for the amounts of each nutrient needed to maintain good health. *See* REFERENCE INTAKES.

dietetic foods Foods prepared to meet the particular nutritional needs of people whose assimilation and metabolism of foods are modified, or for whom a particular effect is obtained by a controlled intake of foods or individual nutrients. They may be formulated for people suffering from physiological disorders or for healthy people with additional needs.

See also PARNUTS.

dietetics   The study or prescription of diets under special circumstances (e.g. metabolic or other illness) and for special physiological needs such as pregnancy, growth, weight reduction.

See also DIETITIAN.

diethylpropion   Anorectic (appetite suppressant, *see* APPETITE CONTROL) drug with amphetamine-like action, formerly used in the treatment of obesity.

diethyl pyrocarbonate   A preservative for wines, soft drinks and fruit juice at a level of 50–300 ppm; it does not inhibit the growth of moulds. It breaks down within a few days to alcohol and carbon dioxide. Also known as pyrocarbonic acid diethyl, trade name Baycovin.

diet-induced thermogenesis   The increase in heat production by the body after eating. It is due to both the metabolic energy cost of digestion (the secretion of digestive enzymes, active transport of nutrients from the gut and gut motility) and the energy cost of forming tissue reserves of fat, glycogen and protein. It can be up to 10–15% of the energy intake. Also known as the specific dynamic action (SDA), *luxus konsumption* or thermic effect of foods.

dietitian, dietician   One who applies the principles of nutrition to the feeding of individuals and groups; plans menus and special diets; supervises the preparation and serving of meals; instructs in the principles of nutrition as applied to selection of foods. In UK the training and state registration of dietitians (i.e. legal permission to practise) is controlled by law.

See also NUTRITIONIST.

differential cell count   *See* LEUCOCYTES.

differential scanning calorimetery (DSC)   Of fats; a small quantity of fat is slowly heated and compared with a reference sample at the same temperature.

See also DIFFERENTIAL THERMAL ANALYSIS.

differential thermal analysis (DTA)   Of fats; a small quantity of fat is slowly heated and its temperature compared with a reference sample.

See also DIFFERENTIAL SCANNING CALORIMETERY.

digester   *See* AUTOCLAVE.

digestibility   The proportion of a foodstuff absorbed from the digestive tract into the bloodstream; normally 90–95%. It is measured as the difference between intake and faecal output, with allowance being made for that part of the faeces that is not derived from undigested food residues (such as shed cells of the intestinal tract, bacteria, residues of digestive juices). Digestibility measured in this way is referred to as 'true digestibility', as distinct from the approximate measure 'apparent digestibility', which is simply the difference between intake and output.

digestion The breakdown of a complex compound into its constituent parts, achieved either chemically or enzymically. Most frequently refers to the digestion of food, enzymic hydrolysis of proteins to amino acids, starch to glucose, fats to glycerol and fatty acids.

See also GASTROINTESTINAL TRACT.

digestive juices The secretions of the GASTROINTESTINAL TRACT that are involved in the DIGESTION of foods: BILE, GASTRIC SECRETION, INTESTINAL JUICE, PANCREATIC JUICE, SALIVA.

digestive tract *See* GASTROINTESTINAL TRACT.

diglycerides GLYCEROL esterified with two fatty acids; an intermediate in the digestion of TRIGLYCERIDES, and used as EMULSIFIERS in food manufacture.

dihydrochalcones *See* NEOHESPERIDIN DIHYDROCHALCONE.

dihydrostreptomycin Poorly absorbed ANTIBIOTIC used in treatment of persistent bacterial DIARRHOEA and gastrointestinal infection.

dilatant Food or other material that shows an increase in VISCOSITY with increasing SHEAR STRESS.

See also PSEUDOPLASTIC; RHEOPECTIC; THIXOTROPIC.

dilatation of fats When fats melt from solids to liquid, at the same temperature, there is an increase in volume. Measurement of this increase, dilatometry, may be used to estimate the amount of solid fat present in a mixture at any given temperature. The precise measure is the difference between the volume of solid and liquid measured in millilitres per 25 g of fat.

dilatometry *See* DILATATION OF FATS.

dill The aromatic herb *Anethum graveolens* (parsley family). The dried ripe seeds are used in pickles, sauces, etc. The young leaves (dill weed) are used, fresh, dried or frozen.

dimethicone Antifoaming agent added to ANTACIDS to reduce flatulence; used alone to treat gripe, colic and wind pain in infants. Also known as simethicone.

dimethylpolysiloxane Antifoaming agent used in fats, oils and other foods. Also called methyl polysilicone or methyl silicone.

dim-sum (dim-sim) Chinese; steamed dumplings and other delicacies.

dinitrofluorobenzene *See* FLUORODINITROBENZENE.

dinitrophenol Reacts with the amino group of AMINO ACIDS; used in separation of amino acids by thin-layer CHROMATOGRAPHY. Also a potent uncoupler of mitochondrial ELECTRON TRANSPORT and

OXIDATIVE PHOSPHORYLATION; was formerly used as a slimming agent.

dinitrophenylhydrazine Reacts with many reducing sugars to form dinitrophenylhydrazones that have characteristic absorption spectra and crystal shapes. Widely used for identification of sugars before the development of modern chromatographic techniques. Also used for colorimetric determination of dehydroascorbate and total VITAMIN C after oxidation to dehydroascorbate using Cu^{2+} salts.

dipeptidases Enzymes (EC 3.4.14.x) in the intestinal mucosal brush border that hydrolyse dipeptides to their constituent amino acids.

dipeptide A PEPTIDE consisting of two amino acids.

diphenoxylate *See* ANTIDIARRHOEAL AGENTS; ANTIMOTILITY AGENTS.

diphenyl Also known as biphenyl (E-230), one of two compounds (the other is orthophenylphenol, OPP, E-231) used for the treatment of fruit after harvesting, to prevent the growth of mould.

diphenylhydantoin Anticonvulsant used in treatment of epilepsy; inhibits absorption of FOLIC ACID and can lead to folate deficiency and megaloblastic ANAEMIA.

diphosphopyridine nucleotide (DPN) Obsolete name for nicotinamide adenine dinucleotide, NAD.

diphyllobothriasis Intestinal infestation with the broad TAPEWORM *Diphyllobothrium latum* (fish tapeworm). Infection is from eating uncooked fish containing the larval stage. May cause VITAMIN B_{12} deficiency by impairing absorption.

dipsa Foods that cause thirst.

dipsesis (dipsosis) Extreme thirst, a craving for abnormal kinds of drinks.

dipsetic Tending to produce thirst.

dipsogen A thirst-provoking agent.

dipsomania An imperative morbid craving for alcoholic drinks.

direct extract *See* MEAT EXTRACT.

disaccharidases Enzymes (EC 3.2.1.x) that hydrolyse DISACCHARIDES to their constituent monosaccharides in the intestinal mucosa: sucrase (also known as INVERTASE) acts on sucrose and isomaltose, LACTASE on lactose, MALTASE on maltose and trehalase on TREHALOSE.

disaccharide Sugars composed of two monosaccharide units; the nutritionally important disaccharides are SUCROSE, LACTOSE, MALTOSE and TREHALOSE.

See also CARBOHYDRATE.

disaccharide intolerance Impaired ability to digest lactose, maltose or sucrose, owing to lack of LACTASE, MALTASE or SUCRASE in the small intestinal mucosa. The undigested sugars remain in the intestinal contents, and are fermented by bacteria in the large intestine, resulting in painful, explosive, watery DIARRHOEA. Treatment is by omitting the offending sugar from the diet.

Lack of all three enzymes is generally caused by intestinal infections, and the enzymes gradually recover after the infection has been cured. Lack of just one of the enzymes, and hence intolerance of just one of the disaccharides, is normally an inherited condition. Lactose intolerance due to loss of lactase is normal in most ethnic groups after puberty.

disc mill Machine for COMMINUTION of dry foods. In a single disc mill the food passes between a stationary casing and a rotating grooved disc; a double disc mill achieves greater shearing force by using two grooved discs rotating in opposite directions. Pin and disc mills have a single or double grooved discs with intermeshing pins to provide additional shear and impact force.

disodium guanylate, disodium inosinate Sodium salts of the PURINES, guanylic and inosinic acids, used as FLAVOUR ENHANCERS, frequently together with MONOSODIUM GLUTAMATE.

dispersed phase Droplets in an EMULSION.

dispersibility The ease with which powder particles become distributed through a liquid. Powders with good WETTABILITY and SINKABILITY have good dispersibility.

displacement analysis *See* RADIOIMMUNOASSAY.

distillers' dried solubles *See* SPENT WASH.

DIT *See* DIET-INDUCED THERMOGENESIS.

diuresis Increased production and excretion of urine; it occurs in diseases such as DIABETES, and also in response to DIURETICS.

diuretics Substances that increase the production and excretion of urine. They may be either compounds that occur naturally in foods (including CAFFEINE and ALCOHOL) or may be drugs used clinically to reduce the volume of body fluid (e.g. in the treatment of HYPERTENSION and OEDEMA).

diverticular disease Diverticulosis is the presence of pouch-like hernias (diverticula) through the muscle layer of the colon, associated with a low intake of dietary FIBRE and high intestinal pressure due to straining during defecation. Faecal matter can be trapped in these diverticula, making them inflamed, causing pain and diarrhoea, the condition of diverticulitis.

See also GASTROINTESTINAL TRACT.

djenkolic acid A sulphur-containing amino acid found in the djenkol bean, *Pithecolobium lobatum*, which grows in parts of Sumatra. It is a derivative of CYSTEINE, and is metabolised but, being relatively insoluble, unmetabolised djenkolic acid crystallises in the kidney tubules.

DNA Deoxyribonucleic acid, the genetic material in the nuclei of all cells. A polymer of deoxyribonucleotides, the PURINE bases adenine and guanine, and the PYRIMIDINE bases thymidine and cytidine, linked to deoxyribose phosphate. The sugar-phosphates form a double stranded helix, with the bases paired internally. *See also* NUCLEIC ACIDS.

DNA cloning The process of inserting the DNA containing one or more genes into a PLASMID or a bacterial virus and then growing these in bacterial (or yeast) cells.

dockage Name given to foreign material in wheat which can be removed readily by a simple cleaning procedure.

docosanoids Long-chain polyunsaturated FATTY ACIDS with 22 carbon atoms.

docosohexaenoic acid A long-chain polyunsaturated FATTY ACID (C22:6 ω3); *see* FISH OILS.

docusates *See* LAXATIVE.

dogfish A cartilaginous FISH, *Scilliorinus caniculum*, or *Squalis acanthias*, related to the sharks; sometimes called rock salmon or rock eel.

dolomite Calcium magnesium carbonate.

dolphin fish Large marine fish (about 2 m long); common dolphin fish is *Coryphaena hippurus*, pompano dolphin fish is *C. equiselis*. Both are commonly marketed as mahi-mahi.

    Composition/100 g: water 78 g, 356 kJ (85 kcal), protein 18.5 g, fat 0.7 g, cholesterol 73 mg, carbohydrate 0 g, ash 2.1 g, Ca 15 mg, Fe 1.1 mg, Mg 30 mg, P 143 mg, K 416 mg, Na 88 mg, Zn 0.5 mg, Se 36.5 µg, vitamin A 54 µg retinol, B_1 0.02 mg, B_2 0.07 mg, niacin 6.1 mg, B_6 0.4 mg, folate 5 µg, B_{12} 0.6 µg, pantothenate 0.8 mg. A 100 g serving is a source of P, pantothenate, a good source of vitamin B_6, a rich source of Se, niacin, vitamin B_{12}.

Do-Maker^{TM} **process** For continuous breadmaking. Ingredients are automatically fed into continuous dough mixer, the yeast suspension being added in a very active state.

domperidone DOPAMINE antagonist, stimulates gastric emptying and small intestinal transit; strengthens contraction of the oesophageal sphincter. Used in treatment of DYSPEPSIA and oesophageal reflux.

döner kebab *See* KEBAB.

dopa 3,4-Dihydroxyphenylalanine; a non-protein AMINO ACID, precursor of DOPAMINE, NORADRENALINE and ADRENALINE. M_r 197.2, pK_a 2.32, 8.72, 9.96, 11.79.

dopamine 3,4-Dihydroxyphenylethylamine; a neurotransmitter, and also precursor of NORADRENALINE and ADRENALINE.

dormers Victorian; chopped cooked lamb mixed with rice and suet, rolled into sausage shapes, coated in egg and breadcrumbs and fried.

dosa Indian; shallow-fried pancake made from a mixture of RICE and a LEGUME; the dough is left to undergo bacterial fermentation before cooking. The principal bacteria involved are *Leuconostoc mesenteroides* and *Streptococcus faecalis*, introduced with a starter of an earlier batch of fermented dough.

dose–response assessment The relationship between the magnitude of exposure to a (potential) toxin and the probability of adverse effects.

dosimeter Instrument to measure the dose of irradiation received by a food.

double Gloucester English hard CHEESE.

double-labelled water Dual isotopically labelled water, containing both deuterium (^2H) and ^{18}O (i.e. $^2H_2^{18}O$), used in studies of energy balance. ^2H is lost from the body only as water, while ^{18}O is lost as both water and carbon dioxide; the difference in rate of loss of the two isotopes from body water permits estimation of total carbon dioxide production, and hence energy expenditure, over a period of 7–14 days.

See also CALORIMETRY; ISOTOPES.

dough cakes A general term to include crumpets, muffins and pikelets, all made from flour, water and milk. The batter is raised with yeast and baked on a hot plate or griddle (hence sometimes known as griddle cakes). Crumpets have sodium bicarbonate added to the batter; muffins are thick and well aerated, less tough than crumpets; pikelets are made from thinned crumpet batter.

doughnuts Deep fried rings of cake dough or yeast-leavened dough.

dough strengtheners Compounds used to modify STARCH and GLUTEN, to produce a more stable dough.

Douglas bag An inflatable bag for collecting expired air to measure the consumption of oxygen and production of carbon dioxide, for the measurement of energy expenditure by indirect CALORIMETRY.

See also SPIROMETER.

Dowex An ION-EXCHANGE RESIN.

DPN (diphosphopyridine nucleotide) Obsolete name for nicotinamide adenine dinucleotide. *See* NAD.

dragée French; whole nuts with hard sugar or sugared chocolate coating. Silver dragées are coated with silver leaf.

dried solubles, distiller's *See* SPENT WASH.

dripping Unbleached and untreated fat from the adipose tissue or bones of sheep or oxen. Also the rendered fat that drips from meat as it is roasted.

drisheen Irish; blood pudding. *See* BLACK PUDDING.

dropsy Popular name for OEDEMA.

drupe Botanical term for a fleshy fruit with a single stone enclosing the seed that does not split along defined lines to liberate the seed, e.g. apricot, cherry, date, mango, olive, peach, plum.

DRV Dietary Reference Values. *See* REFERENCE INTAKES.

dry–blanch–dry process A method of drying fruit so as to retain the colour and flavour; it is faster than drying in the sun and preserves flavour and colour better than hot air drying. The material is dried to 50% water at about 82 °C, blanched for a few minutes, then dried at 68 °C over a period of 6–24 h to 15–20% water content.

dryeration A method used for drying cereal grains which involves an initial drying stage, using heated air, followed by a holding period and final drying in ambient air; relieves the stresses set up in the grain during the initial drying and reduces its brittleness compared with grain dried by conventional methods.

dry frying Frying without the use of fat by using an antistick agent (silicone or a vegetable extract).

dry ice Solid carbon dioxide, used to refrigerate foodstuffs in transit and for carbonation of liquids. It sublimes from the solid to a gas (without liquefying) at −79 °C.

drying agents Hygroscopic compounds used to absorb moisture and maintain a low HUMIDITY environment.

drying, azeotropic A method of drying food by adding a solvent that forms a low-boiling-point mixture (AZEOTROPE) with water, which can be removed under vacuum.

drying oil Any highly unsaturated oil that absorbs oxygen and, when in thin films, polymerises to form a skin. Linseed and tung oil are examples of drying oils used in paints and in the manufacture of linoleum, etc. Nutritionally they are similar to edible oils, but toxic when polymerised.

See also IODINE NUMBER.

dry weight basis (dwb) The composition of a wet food based on the mass of dry solids it contains.

DSC *See* DIFFERENTIAL SCANNING CALORIMETERY.

DTA *See* DIFFERENTIAL THERMAL ANALYSIS.

Dublin Bay prawn Scampi or Norway lobster; a shellfish. *Nephrops norvegicus. See* LOBSTER.

du Bois formula A formula for calculating BODY SURFACE AREA.

duck Water fowl, *Anas* spp.; wild duck is mallard (*A. platyrhynchos*).

Composition/100 g: (edible portion 34%) water 74 g, 553 kJ (132 kcal), protein 18.3 g, fat 5.9 g (of which 50% saturated, 33% mono-unsaturated, 17% polyunsaturated), cholesterol 77 mg, carbohydrate 0 g, ash 1.1 g, Ca 11 mg, Fe 2.4 mg, Mg 19 mg, P 203 mg, K 271 mg, Na 74 mg, Zn 1.9 mg, Cu 0.3 mg, Se 13.9 µg, vitamin A 24 µg retinol, E 0.7 mg, K 2.8 mg, B_1 0.36 mg, B_2 0.45 mg, niacin 5.3 mg, B_6 0.34 mg, folate 25 µg, B_{12} 0.4 µg, pantothenate 1.6 mg, C 6 mg. A 100 g serving is a source of Fe, Se, Zn, vitamin B_6, folate, a good source of Cu, P, vitamin B_1, B_2, niacin, pantothenate, a rich source of vitamin B_{12}.

ductless glands *See* ENDOCRINE GLANDS.

dulcin A synthetic material (*p*-phenetylurea or *p*-phenetolcarbamide, discovered in 1883) which is 250 times as sweet as sugar but is not permitted in foods. Also called sucrol and valzin.

dulcitol A six-carbon SUGAR ALCOHOL which occurs in some plants and is formed by the reduction of galactose; also known as melampyrin, dulcite or galacticol.

dulse Edible purplish-brown seaweeds, *Rhodymenia palmata* and *Dilsea carnosa*, used in soups and jellies.

dUMP suppression test Deoxyuridine suppression test, for FOLATE and VITAMIN B_{12} status. Preincubation of rapidly dividing cells with dUMP leads to a large intracellular pool of newly synthesised TMP (thymidine monophosphate), and hence little of the added [^{3}H]TMP is incorporated into DNA. In deficiency of either vitamin there is little endogenous synthesis of TMP and hence more incorporation of [^{3}H]TMP.

In folate deficiency addition of any form of folic acid will restore the suppression of incorporation of [^{3}H]TMP by dUMP, but vitamin B_{12} will have no effect. In vitamin B_{12} deficiency, addition of vitamin B_{12} or any one-carbon folate derivative other than methyl folate will be effective.

dun Brown discoloration in salted fish caused by mould growth.

Dunaliella bardawil A red marine alga discovered in 1980 in Israel, which is extremely rich in β-CAROTENE, containing 100 times more than most other natural sources.

Dunlop Scottish CHEDDAR-type CHEESE.

dunst Very fine SEMOLINA (starch from the endosperm of the wheat grain) approaching the fineness of flour. Also called break middlings (not to be confused with middlings, which is branny OFFAL).

duocrinin Peptide hormone secreted by the duodenum; increases intestinal secretion and absorption.

duodenal ulcer *See* ULCER.

duodenum First part of the small intestine, between the stomach and the jejunum; the major site of DIGESTION. Pancreatic juice and bile are secreted into the duodenum. So-called because it is about 12 finger breadths in length.

See also GASTROINTESTINAL TRACT.

durian Fruit of tree *Durio zibethinum*, grown in Malaysia and Indonesia. Each fruit weighs 2–3 kg and has a soft, cream-coloured pulp, with a smell considered disgusting by the uninitiated.

Composition/100 g: (edible portion 32%) water 65 g, 615 kJ (147 kcal), protein 1.5 g, fat 5.3 g, carbohydrate 27.1 g, fibre 3.8 g, ash 1.1 g, Ca 6 mg, Fe 0.4 mg, Mg 30 mg, P 39 mg, K 436 mg, Na 2 mg, Zn 0.3 mg, Cu 0.2 mg, Mn 0.3 mg, vitamin A 2 µg RE (29 µg carotenoids), B_1 0.37 mg, B_2 0.2 mg, niacin 1.1 mg, B_6 0.32 mg, folate 36 µg, pantothenate 0.2 mg, C 20 mg. A 150 g serving (quarter fruit) is a source of Mg, Mn, vitamin B_2, a good source of Cu, vitamin B_6, folate, a rich source of vitamin B_1, C.

durum wheat   A hard type of WHEAT, *Triticum durum* (most bread wheats are *T. vulgare*); mainly used for the production of SEMOLINA for preparation of PASTA.

Dutching   *See* COCOA, DUTCH.

Dutch oven   A semicircular metal shield which may be placed close to an open fire; fitted with shelves on which food is roasted. It may also be clamped to the fire bars.

***D* value**   *See* DECIMAL REDUCTION TIME.

dwb   *See* DRY WEIGHT BASIS.

Dynabeads^{TM}   Magnetic microspheres coated with antibodies, used in IMMUNOMAGNETIC SEPARATION.

Dyox^{TM}   Chlorine dioxide used to treat flour, *see* AGEING.

dysentery   Infection of the intestinal tract causing severe diarrhoea with blood and mucus. Amoebic dysentery is caused by *Entamoeba histolytica*, and occasionally other protozoans spread by contaminated food and water. Symptoms may develop many months after infection. Bacillary dysentery is caused by *Shigella* spp.; symptoms develop 1–6 days after infection.

dysgeusia   Distortion of the sense of taste, a common side-effect of some drugs.

See also GUSTIN; HYPOGEUSIA; PARAGEUSIA.

dyspepsia   Any pain or discomfort associated with eating; may be a symptom of gastritis, peptic ulcer, gall-bladder disease, etc.; functional dyspepsia occurs when there is no obvious structural change in the intestinal tract. Treatment includes a BLAND DIET.

See also INDIGESTION.

dysphagia   Difficulty in swallowing, commonly associated with disorders of the OESOPHAGUS. Inability to swallow is aphagia.

E

e   On food labels, before the weight or volume, to indicate that this has been notified to the regulatory authorities of the EU as a standard package size.

E   *See* E-NUMBERS and Table 7 of the Appendix.

EAA index   Essential amino acid index, an index of PROTEIN QUALITY.

earth almond   *See* TIGER NUT.

earth nut   A very small variety of TRUFFLE, *Conopodium denudatum*, also called pig nut and fairy potato. Also another name for the PEANUT.

eau de vie   Spirit distilled from fermented grape juice (sometimes other fruit juices); may be flavoured with fruits, etc.
See also MARC (1).

echoviruses   A group of RNA-containing viruses that infect the gastrointestinal tract and produce pathological changes in cells in culture, but not associated with any specific disease. Now usually classified as coxsackie viruses.
See also ENTEROVIRUSES; REOVIRUS.

Eck fistula   *See* FISTULA.

EC numbers   Systematic classification of enzymes by the class, subclass, sub-subclass and individual reaction classified, shown as EC x.x.x.x. The classes are: (1) oxidoreductases, (2) transferases, (3) hydrolases, (4) lyases, (5) isomerases, (6) ligases (synthetases).

E. coli (Escherichia coli)   Group of bacteria including both harmless COMMENSALS in the human gut and strains that cause food poisoning by production of ENTEROTOXINS (TX 3.1.2.x, 3.1.3.x, 3.1.4.x, depending on the strain) after adhering to intestinal epithelial cells. For most pathogenic strains the infective dose is 10^5–10^7 organisms, onset 16–48 h, and duration 1–3 days.

Strain O157:H7 (or VTEC) was first identified as a cause of food poisoning in the 1980s. It produces a toxin called verocytotoxin and is especially virulent; infective dose 10 organisms, onset 1–7 h and duration (if not fatal) of days or weeks.

ectomorph   Description given to a tall, thin person, possibly with underdeveloped muscles.
See also ENDOMORPH; MESOMORPH.

ecuelle   Apparatus for obtaining peel oil from citrus fruit. It consists of a shallow funnel lined with spikes on which the fruit is rolled by hand. As the oil glands are pierced, the oil and cell sap collect in the bottom of the funnel.

eddo   *See* TARO.

edema   *See* OEDEMA.

edetate   *See* EDTA.

edible portion   Used in food composition tables to indicate that the data refer to the part of the food that is usually eaten – e.g. excluding skin or pips of fruit and vegetables, bones in meat and fish.

Edifas^{TM} CELLULOSE DERIVATIVES: Edifas A is methyl ethyl cellulose (E-465); Edifas B, sodium carboxymethylcellulose (E-466).

Edman reagent Phenylisothiocyanate (PIC); reacts with amino
terminal amino acid of a protein; the basis of the Edman degradation used in sequencing proteins, and used in HPLC of amino
acids for fluorimetric detection.

Edosol^{TM} A low-sodium milk substitute, containing 43 mg
sodium/100 g, compared with dried milk at 400 mg.

EDTA Ethylene diamine tetra-acetic acid, a chelating agent that
forms stable chelation complexes with metal ions. Also called
versene, sequestrol and sequestrene. It can be used both to
remove metal ions from a solution (or at least to remove them
from activity) and also to add metal ions, for example in plant
fertilisers (E-385).

eel A long thin fish, *Anguilla* spp.; the European eel is *A. anguilla*,
the conger eel is *Conger myriaster*. Eels live in rivers but go to
sea to breed. To date, although elvers (young eels) have been
caught and raised in tanks, it has not been possible to breed them
in captivity.

Composition/100 g: water 68 g, 770 kJ (184 kcal), protein 18.4 g,
fat 11.7 g (of which 23% saturated, 69% mono-unsaturated, 9%
polyunsaturated), cholesterol 126 mg, carbohydrate 0 g, ash 1.4 g,
Ca 20 mg, Fe 0.5 mg, Mg 20 mg, P 216 mg, K 272 mg, Na 51 mg, Zn
1.6 mg, Se 6.5 µg, I 80 µg, vitamin A 1043 µg retinol, E 4 mg, B_1
0.15 mg, B_2 0.04 mg, niacin 3.5 mg, B_6 0.07 mg, folate 15 µg, B_{12}
3 µg, pantothenate 0.2 mg, C 2 mg. A 100 g serving is a source of
niacin, a good source of P, a rich source of I, vitamin A, E, B_{12}.

EFA Essential fatty acids. *See* FATTY ACIDS, ESSENTIAL.

Efamast^{TM} A preparation of γ-LINOLENIC ACID, as a dietary
supplement.

effective freezing time Time required to lower the temperature
of a food from an initial value to a predetermined final
temperature.

EFSA European Food Safety Authority; web site http://
www.efsa.eu.int/.

egg Hen eggs are graded by size. In EU, weight ranges are used:
very large eggs 73 g or over, large 63–73 g, medium 53–63 g and
small 53 g or less. In USA average weights are used: jumbo
70.0 g, extra large 63.8 g, large 56.7, g, medium 49.6 g, small 42.5 g
and peewee 35.4 g.

Composition/100 g: (edible portion 88%) water 75.8 g, 615 kJ
(147 kcal), protein 12.6 g, fat 9.9 g (of which 37% saturated, 46%
mono-unsaturated, 17% polyunsaturated), carbohydrate 0.8 g
(0.8 g sugars), ash 0.9 g, Ca 53 mg, Fe 1.8 mg, Mg 12 mg, P 191 mg,
K 134 mg, Na 140 mg, Zn 1.1 mg, Cu 0.1 mg, Se 31.7 µg, I 53 µg,

vitamin A 140 µg RE (139 µg retinol, 350 µg carotenoids), E 1 mg, K 0.3 mg, B_1 0.07 mg, B_2 0.48 mg, niacin 0.1 mg, B_6 0.14 mg, folate 47 µg, B_{12} 1.3 µg, pantothenate 1.4 mg. A 75 g serving (1 large egg) is a source of P, vitamin A, folate, pantothenate, a good source of I, vitamin B_2, a rich source of Se, vitamin B_{12}.

Duck eggs weigh around 85 g. Composition/100 g: (edible portion 88%) water 70.8 g, 774 kJ (185 kcal), protein 12.8 g, fat 13.8 g (of which 32% saturated, 57% mono-unsaturated, 11% polyunsaturated), cholesterol 884 mg, carbohydrate 1.5 g (0.9 g sugars), ash 1.1 g, Ca 64 mg, Fe 3.8 mg, Mg 17 mg, P 220 mg, K 222 mg, Na 146 mg, Zn 1.4 mg, Cu 0.1 mg, Se 36.4 µg, vitamin A 194 µg RE (192 µg retinol, 485 µg carotenoids), E 1.3 mg, K 0.4 mg, B_1 0.16 mg, B_2 0.4 mg, niacin 0.2 mg, B_6 0.25 mg, folate 80 µg, B_{12} 5.4 µg, pantothenate 1.9 mg. An 85 g serving (1 egg) is a source of vitamin E, a good source of Fe, P, vitamin A, B_2, pantothenate, a rich source of Se, folate, vitamin B_{12}.

Quail eggs weigh around 10 g. Composition/100 g: (edible portion 92%) water 74.3 g, 661 kJ (158 kcal), protein 13.1 g, fat 11.1 g (of which 39% saturated, 47% mono-unsaturated, 14% polyunsaturated), cholesterol 844 mg, carbohydrate 0.4 g (0.4 g sugars) ash 1.1 g, Ca 64 mg, Fe 3.7 mg, Mg 13 mg, P 226 mg, K 132 mg, Na 141 mg, Zn 1.5 mg, Cu 0.1 mg, Se 32 µg, vitamin A 156 µg RE (155 µg retinol, 390 µg carotenoids), E 1.1 mg, K 0.3 mg, B_1 0.13 mg, B_2 0.79 mg, niacin 0.2 mg, B_6 0.15 mg, folate 66 µg, B_{12} 1.6 µg, pantothenate 1.8 mg. A 10 g serving (1 egg) is a source of vitamin B_{12}.

egg plant *See* AUBERGINE.

egg proteins What is generally referred to as egg protein is a mixture of proteins, including ovalbumin, ovomucoid, ovoglobulin, conalbumin, vitellin and vitellenin. EGG WHITE contains 11% protein, mostly ovalbumin; yolk contains 16% protein, mainly two phosphoproteins, vitellin and vitellenin.

eggs, Chinese (or hundred year old eggs) Known as pidan, houeidan and dsaoudan, depending on variations in the method of preparation. Prepared by covering fresh duck eggs with a mixture of sodium hydroxide, burnt straw ash and slaked lime, then storing for several months (sometimes referred to as 'hundred year old eggs'). The white and yolk coagulate and become discoloured, with partial decomposition of the protein and PHOSPHOLIPIDS.

egg substitute Name formerly used for golden raising powder, a type of BAKING POWDER.

egg white The white of an egg is in three layers: an outer layer of thin white, layer of thick white, richer in ovomucin, and inner layer of thin white surrounding the yolk. The ratio of thick to thin white varies, depending on the individual hen. A higher proportion of thick white is desirable for frying and poaching, since it helps the egg to coagulate into a small firm mass instead of spreading; thin white produces a larger volume of froth when beaten than does thick.

See also EGG PROTEINS.

egg white injury BIOTIN deficiency caused by consumption of large quantities of uncooked egg white.

EGRAC Erythrocyte GLUTATHIONE REDUCTASE activation coefficient.

eicosanoids Compounds formed in the body from C20 polyunsaturated FATTY ACIDS (eicosenoic acids), including the prostaglandins, prostacyclins, thromboxanes and leukotrienes, all of which act as local hormones, and are involved in wound healing, inflammation, platelet aggregation, and a variety of other functions.

eicosapentaenoic acid (EPA) A long chain polyunsaturated FATTY ACID (C20:5 ω3). *See* FISH OILS.

eicosenoic acids Long chain polyunsaturated FATTY ACIDS with 20 carbon atoms.

einkorn A type of WHEAT, the wild form of which, *Triticum boeoticum*, was probably one of the ancestors of all cultivated wheat. Still grown in some parts of southern Europe and Middle East, usually for animal feed. The name means 'one seed', from the single seed found in each spikelet.

eiswein WINE made from grapes that have frozen on the vine, picked and processed while still frozen, so that the juice is highly concentrated and very sweet. Similar Canadian wines are known as ice wine.

elastase A proteolytic enzyme (EC 3.4.21.36) in pancreatic juice, an ENDOPEPTIDASE. Active at pH 8–11. Secreted as the inactive precursor, pro-elastase, which is activated by TRYPSIN.

elastin Insoluble protein in CONNECTIVE TISSUE; the cause of toughness in meat. Unlike COLLAGEN, it is unaffected by cooking.

elderberry Fruit of *Sambucus niger*.

Composition/100 g: water 80 g, 306 kJ (73 kcal), protein 0.7 g, fat 0.5 g, carbohydrate 18.4 g, fibre 7 g, ash 0.6 g, Ca 38 mg, Fe 1.6 mg, Mg 5 mg, P 39 mg, K 280 mg, Na 6 mg, Zn 0.1 mg, Cu 0.1 mg, Se 0.6 µg, vitamin A 30 µg RE, B_1 0.07 mg, B_2 0.06 mg, niacin 0.5 mg, B_6 0.23 mg, folate 6 µg, pantothenate 0.1 mg, C 36 mg. A 110 g serving is a source of Fe, vitamin B_6, a rich source of vitamin C.

electrodialysis Combined use of ELECTROLYSIS and ion-selective membranes to separate ELECTROLYTES and ion-selective membranes.

electrofocusing *See* ISOELECTRIC FOCUSING.

electrolysis Separation of ions in a solution by use of direct current. *See also* ELECTROLYTES.

electrolytes Salts that dissociate in solution and hence will carry an electric current; generally used to mean the inorganic ions in blood plasma and other body fluids, especially sodium, potassium, chloride, bicarbonate and phosphate.

electronic heating *See* MICROWAVE COOKING.

electron transport chain A sequence of COENZYMES and CYTOCHROMES of differing redox potential. In the MITOCHONDRIA they carry electrons from the oxidation of metabolic fuels leading to the reduction of oxygen to water, and are obligatorily linked to OXIDATIVE PHOSPHORYLATION.

electrophoresis Technique for separation of charged molecules (especially proteins and nucleic acids) by their migration in an electric field. The support medium may be a starch or polyacrylamide gel, paper or cellulose acetate.

electroporation Use of high-voltage electric pulses at low-voltage gradients to exchange genetic information between protoplast cells of micro-organisms, plants or animals. At high-voltage gradients (up to 30 kV/cm) used to sterilise or pasteurise food by permeabilisation of bacterial cell membranes.

 See also PASTEURISATION; STERILE.

electropure process A method for PASTEURISATION of milk by passing low-frequency, alternating current.

elemental diet *See* FORMULA DIET.

elements, minor *See* MINERALS, TRACE; MINERALS, ULTRATRACE.

ELISA (enzyme-linked immunosorbent assay) Sensitive and specific analytical technique for determination of analytes present at very low concentrations in biological samples, in which either the tracer analyte or the antibody is bound to an enzyme; the product of the enzyme may be measured directly, or may be a catalyst or coenzyme for a second enzyme, giving considerable amplification, and hence permitting high sensitivity without the use of radioactive tracers.

 See also FLUORESCENCE IMMUNOASSAY; RADIOIMMUNOASSAY.

elixir Alcoholic extract (tincture) of a naturally occurring substance; originally devised by medieval alchemists (the elixir of life), now used for a variety of medicines, liqueurs and BITTERS.

elute To wash off or remove. Specifically applied to removal of adsorbed compounds in chromatography.

 See also ION-EXCHANGE RESIN.

elutriation Technique for separating fine and coarse particles by suspending the mixture in water and decanting the upper layer while it still contains the finer particles.

elver   Young EEL, about 5 cm in length.

EM   Electron microscope or microscopy, *see* MICROSCOPE, ELECTRON.

emaciation   Extreme thinness and wasting, caused by disease or undernutrition.

   See also CACHEXIA; MARASMUS; PROTEIN–ENERGY MALNUTRITION.

Embden groats   *See* GROATS.

emblic   Berry of the S.E. Asian malacca tree, *Emblica officinalis*, similar in appearance to the gooseberry. Also known as the Indian gooseberry. An exceptionally rich source of vitamin C, 600 mg/100 g.

embolism   Blockage of a blood vessel caused by a foreign object (embolus) such as a quantity of air or gas, a piece of tissue or tumour, a blood clot (THROMBUS) or fatty tissue derived from ATHEROMA, in the circulation.

embolus   *See* EMBOLISM.

emetic   Substance that causes vomiting.

Emmental   Swiss hard CHEESE, used in FONDUE.

emmer   A type of WHEAT known to have been used more than 8000 years ago. Wild emmer is *Triticum dicoccoides* and true emmer is *T. dicoccum*. Nowadays grown mainly for animal feed.

Emprote™   A dried milk and cereal preparation consumed as a beverage, containing 33% protein.

EMS   *See* EOSINOPHILIA MYALGIA SYNDROME.

emu   Flightless Australian bird, *Dromaius novaehollandiae*, weighing 50–60 kg, farmed as a source of low-fat meat.

   Composition/100 g: water 75 g, 431 kJ (103 kcal), protein 22.5 g, fat 0.8 g, cholesterol 71 mg, carbohydrate 0 g, ash 1.1 g, Ca 3 mg, Fe 4.5 mg, Mg 42 mg, P 236 mg, K 300 mg, Na 120 mg, Zn 3.5 mg, Cu 0.2 mg, Se 32.5 µg, vitamin E 0.2 mg, B_1 0.27 mg, B_2 0.45 mg, niacin 7.4 mg, B_6 0.63 mg, folate 13 µg, B_{12} 6.7 µg, pantothenate 2.7 mg. A 100 g serving is a source of Cu, Mg, vitamin B_1, a good source of P, Zn, vitamin B_2, a rich source of Fe, Se, niacin, vitamin B_6, B_{12}, pantothenate.

emulsification   Reduction in droplet size of immiscible liquids to achieve a stable EMULSION. Also known as HOMOGENISATION.

emulsifiers (emulsifying agents)   Substances that are soluble in both fat and water; enable fat to be uniformly dispersed in water as an EMULSION. STABILISERS maintain emulsions in a stable form. Emulsifying agents are also used in baking to aid the smooth incorporation of fat into the dough and to keep the crumb soft. Emulsifying agents used in foods include AGAR, ALBUMIN, ALGINATES, CASEIN, egg yolk, GLYCERYL MONOSTEARATE, GUMS, IRISH MOSS, LECITHIN, soaps. *See* Table 7 of the Appendix.

emulsifying salts Sodium citrate, sodium phosphates and sodium tartrate, used in the manufacture of milk powder, evaporated milk, sterilised cream and processed cheese.

emulsin A mixture of enzymes (mainly β-glycosidase, EC 3.2.1.21) in bitter ALMOND that hydrolyse the glucoside AMYGDALIN to benzaldehyde, glucose and cyanide.

emulsion Colloidal suspension (*see* COLLOID) of one liquid (the dispersed phase) in another (the continuous phase). Common food emulsions are either oil-in-water or water-in-oil.

See also EMULSIFICATION; EMULSIFIERS; HOMOGENISATION; HOMOGENISERS; STOKE'S LAW.

emulsoids *See* COLLOID.

encapsulation Core material, which may be liquid or powder, is encased in an outer shell or case, to protect it, or permit release in response to a given environmental change (e.g. temperature, pH). When the encapsulated particles are less the 50 μm in diameter the process is known as microencapsulation.

encopresis Faecal incontinence.

endemic The usual cases of a particular illness in a community.

endergonic Used of chemical reactions that require an input of energy (usually as heat or light) such as the synthesis of complex molecules.

endive Curly serrated green leaves of *Cichorium endivia*. Called chicory in US and chicorée frisée in France.

Composition/100 g: (edible portion 86%) water 94 g, 71 kJ (17 kcal), protein 1.3 g, fat 0.2 g, carbohydrate 3.3 g (0.3 g sugars), fibre 3.1 g, ash 1.4 g, Ca 52 mg, Fe 0.8 mg, Mg 15 mg, P 28 mg, K 314 mg, Na 22 mg, Zn 0.8 mg, Cu 0.1 mg, Mn 0.4 mg, Se 0.2 μg, vitamin A 108 μg RE (1300 μg carotenoids), E 0.4 mg, K 231 mg, B_1 0.08 mg, B_2 0.08 mg, niacin 0.4 mg, B_6 0.02 mg, folate 142 μg, pantothenate 0.9 mg, C 7 mg.

endocrine glands Those (ductless) glands that produce and secrete HORMONES, including the THYROID gland (secreting thyroxine and tri-iodothyronine), PANCREAS (INSULIN and GLUCAGON), ADRENAL GLANDS (ADRENALINE, GLUCOCORTICOIDS, MINERALOCORTICOIDS), ovary and testes (sex steroids). Some endocrine glands respond directly to chemical changes in the bloodstream; others are controlled by hormones secreted by the pituitary gland, under control of the hypothalamus.

endomorph In relation to body build, means short and stocky.

See also ECTOMORPH; MESOMORPH.

endomysium *See* MUSCLE.

endopeptidases Enzymes that hydrolyse proteins (i.e. proteinases or peptidases), by cleaving PEPTIDE bonds inside protein molecules, as opposed to EXOPEPTIDASES, which remove amino acids from the end of the protein chain. The main endopeptidases in DIGESTION are chymotrypsin, elastase, pepsin and trypsin.

endosperm The inner part of cereal grains; in wheat it constitutes about 83% of the grain. Mainly starch, and the source of SEMOLINA. Contains only about 10% of the vitamin B_1, 35% of the vitamin B_2, 40% of the niacin and 50% of the vitamin B_6 and pantothenic acid of the whole grain.

See also FLOUR, EXTRACTION RATE.

endothelium-derived relaxation factor *See* NITRIC OXIDE.

endotoxins Toxins produced by bacteria as an integral part of the cell, so cannot be separated by filtration; unlike EXOTOXINS, they do not usually stimulate antitoxin formation but the antibodies that they induce act directly on the bacteria. They are relatively stable to heat compared with exotoxins.

See also TX NUMBERS.

Energen rolls™ A light BREAD roll of wheat flour plus added GLUTEN.

energy The ability to do work. The SI unit of energy is the Joule, and nutritionally relevant amounts of energy are kilojoules (kJ, 1000 J) and megajoules (MJ, 1 000 000 J). The CALORIE is still widely used in nutrition; 1 cal = 4.186 J (approximated to 4.2).

While it is usual to speak of the calorie or joule content of a food it is more correct to refer to the energy content or yield. The total chemical energy in a food, as released by complete combustion (in the bomb CALORIMETER) is gross energy. Allowing for the losses of unabsorbed food in the faeces gives digestible energy. Allowing for loss in the urine due to incomplete combustion in the body (e.g. urea from the incomplete combustion of proteins) gives metabolisable energy. Allowing for the loss due to DIET-INDUCED THERMOGENESIS gives net energy, i.e. the actual amount available for use in the body.

See also ENERGY CONVERSION FACTORS.

energy balance The difference between intake of ENERGY from foods and ENERGY EXPENDITURE for BASAL METABOLIC RATE and physical activity. Positive energy balance leads to increased body tissue, the normal process of growth. In adults, positive energy balance leads to creation of body reserves of fat, resulting in overweight and OBESITY. Negative energy balance leads to utilisation of body reserves of fat and protein, resulting in wasting and undernutrition.

energy conversion factors Various factors are used to calculate the energy yields of foodstuffs:

The complete heats of combustion (gross energy) as determined by CALORIMETRY are: protein 23.9 kJ (5.7 kcal), fat 39.5 kJ (9.4 kcal); carbohydrate 17.2 kJ (4.1 kcal)/g.

The Rubner conversion factors for metabolic energy yield are: protein 17 kJ (4.1 kcal); fat 39 kJ (9.3 kcal); carbohydrate 17 kJ (4.1 kcal)/g.

The Atwater factors also allow for losses in digestion and incomplete oxidation of the nitrogen of proteins: protein 16.8 kJ (4 kcal); fat 37.8 kJ (9 kcal); carbohydrate 16.8 kJ (4 kcal)/g.

The following factors are generally used: carbohydrate 17 kJ (4 kcal); fat 38 kJ (9 kcal); carbohydrate (as monosaccharides) 17 kJ (4 kcal); alcohol 29 kJ (7 kcal); sugar alcohols 10 kJ (2.4 kcal); organic acids 13 kJ (3 kcal)/g.

energy drinks Beverages containing glucose, vitamins, minerals, herb extracts and caffeine, and sometimes other ingredients, claimed to provide energy and to promote alertness and well-being. Some now contain artificial sweeteners instead of glucose, so negating the claims to be a source of (metabolisable) energy.

energy expenditure The total energy cost of maintaining constant conditions in the body, i.e. homeostasis (BASAL METABOLIC RATE, BMR) plus the energy cost of physical activities. The average total energy expenditure in western countries is about 1.4 × BMR; a desirable level of physical activity is 1.7 × BMR.

energy, kinetic Energy due to the motion of an object.

energy, potential Energy due to the position of an object.

energy requirements Energy requirements are calculated from estimated BASAL METABOLIC RATE and physical activity. Average energy requirements for adults are 8 MJ (1900 kcal)/day for women and 10 MJ (2400 kcal)/day for men, but obviously vary widely with physical activity.

energy-rich bonds An outdated and chemically incorrect concept in ENERGY metabolism, which suggested that the bond between ADP and phosphate in ATP, and between CREATINE and phosphate in creatine phosphate, which have a high chemical free energy of hydrolysis, somehow differ from 'ordinary' chemical bonds.

enfleurage A method of extracting ESSENTIAL OILS from flowers by placing them on glass trays covered with purified LARD or other fat, which eventually becomes saturated with the oil.

enocianina Desugared grape extract used to colour fruit flavours. Prepared by acid extraction of the skins of black grapes; it is blue in neutral conditions and red in acid.

eNose™ An array of sensors attached to a gas chromatograph simulating the human olfactory response, used to profile flavours – an 'electronic nose'.

See also ZNOSE.

en papillote   French method of cooking in a closed container, a parchment paper or aluminium foil case.

See also SOUS VIDE.

enrichment   The addition of nutrients to foods. Although often used interchangeably, the term FORTIFICATION is used of mandatory (legally imposed) additions, and enrichment means the voluntary addition of nutrients beyond the levels originally present.

See also NUTRIFICATION; RESTORATION.

enrobing   In confectionery manufacture, the process of coating a product with chocolate, or other materials.

ensete   *See* BANANA, FALSE.

Entamoeba   Genus of protozoa, some of which are parasitic in the human gut. *Entamoeba coli* is harmless; *E. histolytica* causes amoebic DYSENTERY; *E. gingivalis* is found in spaces between the teeth and is associated with PERIODONTAL disease.

enteral foods   *See* MEDICAL FOODS.

enteral nutrition   Provision of supplementary feeding by direct intubation into the stomach or small intestine, as opposed to PARENTERAL NUTRITION.

See also GASTROSTOMY FEEDING; NASOGASTRIC TUBE; PARENTERAL NUTRITION; RECTAL FEEDING.

enteritis   Inflammation of the mucosal lining of the small intestine, usually resulting from infection. Regional enteritis is CROHN'S DISEASE.

enterobiasis   Infestation of the large intestine with PINWORM.

Enterococcus faecium   *See* PROBIOTICS.

enterocolitis   Inflammation of the mucosal lining of the small and large intestine, usually resulting from infection.

enterocrinin   Peptide hormone secreted by the upper small intestine; increases intestinal secretion and absorption.

enterocytes   Cells of the small or large intestinal mucosa.

enterogastrone   Peptide hormone secreted by the stomach and duodenum; decreases gastric secretion and motility. Its secretion is stimulated by fat; hence, fat in the diet inhibits gastric activity.

enteroglucagon   Peptide hormone secreted by the ileum and colon; increases gut motility and mucosal growth.

enterohepatic circulation   Excretion of metabolites in BILE, followed by reabsorption from the intestine, possibly after further metabolism by intestinal bacteria. Total flux through the gut may be several-fold higher than dietary intake or faecal excretion. Especially important with respect to the BILE SALTS, CHOLESTEROL, FOLIC ACID, VITAMIN B_{12} and STEROID hormones.

enterokinase   Obsolete name for ENTEROPEPTIDASE.

enterolith   Stone within the intestine, commonly builds up around a GALLSTONE or swallowed fruit stone.

entero-oxyntin   Peptide hormone secreted by the upper small intestine; increases gastric secretion.

enteropathy   Any disease or disorder of the intestinal tract.

enteropeptidase   An enzyme (EC 3.4.21.9) secreted by the small intestinal mucosa which activates trypsinogen (from the pancreatic juice) to the active proteolytic enzyme TRYPSIN. Sometimes known by the obsolete name of enterokinase.

enterostatin   A pentapeptide released from the amino terminal of the precursor protein of pancreatic COLIPASE during fat ingestion; it selectively suppresses the intake of dietary fat.

enterotoxin   Substances more or less specifically toxic to the cells of the intestinal mucosa, normally produced by bacteria; they may be present in the food (e.g. *BACILLUS CEREUS*, *CLOSTRIDIUM BOTULINUM*, *STAPHYLOCOCCUS AUREUS*) or may be produced by the bacteria in the gut (e.g. *CLOSTRIDIUM PERFRINGENS*, *VIBRIO CHOLERA*, *AEROMONAS* SPP., pathogenic *E. COLI*).

   See also TX NUMBERS.

enteroviruses   Viruses that multiply mainly in the intestinal tract, and commonly invade the central nervous system, including coxsackie virus and poliovirus.

enthalpy   The sum of the internal energy and the product of the pressure and volume of a substance.

entoleter   A machine used to disinfest cereals and other foods. The material is fed to the centre of a high-speed rotating disc carrying studs so that it is thrown against the studs; the impact kills insects and destroys their eggs.

entrainment   Loss of oil droplets with steam in frying, or loss of concentrated product during evaporation by boiling.

entropy   A measure of the degree of disorder in a system.

E-numbers   Within the EU, food additives may be listed on labels either by name or by their number in the EU list of permitted additives. *See* Table 7 of the Appendix.

enzyme   A PROTEIN that catalyses a metabolic reaction. Enzymes are specific for both the compounds acted on (the substrates) and the reactions carried out. Because of this, enzymes extracted from plant or animal sources, micro-organisms or those produced by GENETIC MODIFICATION are widely used in the chemical, pharmaceutical and food industries (e.g. CHYMOSIN in cheese-making, MALTASE in beer production, synthesis of VITAMIN C and CITRIC ACID), as well as in washing powders.

   Because they are proteins, enzymes are permanently inactivated by heat, strong acid or alkali and other conditions that cause DENATURATION of proteins.

Many enzymes contain non-protein components which are essential for their function. These are known as prosthetic groups, COENZYMES or cofactors and may be metal ions, metal ions in organic complexes (e.g. haem in HAEMOGLOBIN and CYTOCHROMES) or a variety of organic compounds, many of which are derived from VITAMINS. The (inactive) protein without its prosthetic group is known as the apo-enzyme, and the active assembly of protein plus prosthetic group is the holo-enzyme.

See also EC NUMBERS; ENZYME ACTIVATION ASSAYS; TENDERISERS.

enzyme activation assays   Used to assess the nutritional status of an individual with respect to VITAMINS B_1, B_2 and B_6. A sample of red blood cells is tested for activity of the relevant enzyme before and after adding the vitamin-derived coenzyme; enhancement of enzyme activity beyond a certain level serves as a biochemical index of deficiency of the vitamin in question. The enzymes involved are TRANSKETOLASE for vitamin B_1, GLUTATHIONE REDUCTASE for vitamin B_2 and either aspartate or alanine TRANSAMINASE for vitamin B_6.

enzyme electrodes   An immobilised enzyme plus an electrochemical sensor, enclosed in a probe, used in food analysis and clinical chemistry, e.g. glucose oxidase (EC 1.1.3.4) produces hydrogen peroxide, which can be measured polarographically; lysine decarboxylase (EC 4.1.1.18) produces carbon dioxide which can be measured electrochemically.

enzyme, immobilized   Enzyme bound physically to glass, plastic or other support, so permitting continuous flow processes, or recovery and re-utilisation of enzymes in batch processes.

enzyme induction   Synthesis of new enzyme protein in response to a stimulus, commonly a hormone, but sometimes a metabolic intermediate or other compound (e.g. a drug or food additive).

enzyme inhibition   A number of compounds reduce the activity of enzymes; sometimes this is a part of normal metabolic regulation and integration (e.g. the responses to HORMONES), and sometimes it is the action of drugs. Some inhibitors are reversible, others act irreversibly on the enzymes, and therefore have a longer duration of action (the activity of the enzyme remains low until more has been synthesised).

enzyme precursors   *See* ZYMOGENS.

enzyme repression   Reduction in synthesis of enzyme protein in response to a stimulus such as a hormone or the presence of large amounts of the end-product of a pathway.

eosinophilia myalgia syndrome   Often lethal blood and muscle disorder reported in 1989 among people using supplements of the amino acid TRYPTOPHAN, as a result of which tryptophan supplements were withdrawn in most countries. Subsequently shown to be associated mainly (or perhaps solely) with contamination of a single batch of tryptophan from one manufacturer with ethylidene *bis*-tryptophan, but doubts remain about the safety of tryptophan supplements.

EPA Eicosapentaenoic acid, a long-chain polyunsaturated fatty acid (C20:5 ω3). *See* FISH OILS.

epazote Herb (*Chenopodium ambriosiodes*) used in Mexican cooking and to make a herb tea. Also known as Mexican tea, wormseed, goosefoot, pigweed, Jerusalem oak.

Composition/100 g: water 89 g, 134 kJ (32 kcal), protein 0.3 g, fat 0.5 g, carbohydrate 7.4 g, fibre 3.8 g, ash 2.5 g, Ca 275 mg, Fe 1.9 mg, Mg 121 mg, P 86 mg, K 633 mg, Na 43 mg, Zn 1.1 mg, Cu 0.2 mg, Mn 3.1 mg, Se 0.9 µg, vitamin A 3 µg RE (38 µg carotenoids), B_1 0.03 mg, B_2 0.35 mg, niacin 0.6 mg, B_6 0.15 mg, folate 215 µg, pantothenate 0.2 mg, C 4 mg.

epicarp *See* FLAVEDO.

epidemic Sudden outbreak of a disease affecting a large number of people.

epidemiology The study of patterns of diseases and their causative agents in a population.

epigenetics The study of the processes involved in the development of an organism, including gene silencing during tissue diferentiation. Also the study of heritable changes in gene function that occur without a change in the sequence of DNA – the way in which environmental factors (including nutrition) affecting a parent can result in changes in the way genes are expressed in the offspring.

See also CPG ISLANDS; PROGRAMMING.

epinephrine *See* ADRENALINE.

epiphysis The end of a long BONE; it develops separately from the shaft (DIAPHYSIS) and later undergoes fusion to form the complete bone. This fusion is impaired in RICKETS.

Epogam^{TM} A preparation of γ-LINOLENIC ACID, for treatment of eczema.

Epopa^{TM} Mixed plant and fish oils, rich in ω3 and ω6 polyunsaturated FATTY ACIDS.

EPSL Edible protective superficial coating.

Epsom salts Magnesium sulphate, originally found in a mineral spring in Epsom, Surrey, UK; acts as a LAXATIVE because the OSMOTIC PRESSURE of the solution causes it to retain water in the intestine and so increase the bulk and moisture content of the faeces.

Equal^{TM} *See* ASPARTAME.

equilibrium moisture content   The moisture content of a wet material which is in equilibrium with its surrounding atmosphere.

equilibrium, nitrogen   *See* NITROGEN BALANCE.

equilibrium relative humidity   The relative HUMIDITY of the atmosphere which is in equilibrium with a wet material with a specified moisture content and at a specified temperature.

ercalciol   *See* VITAMIN D.

erepsin   Obsolete name for a mixture of enzymes contained in INTESTINAL JUICE, including aminopeptidases and dipeptidases.

ergocalciferol   *See* VITAMIN D.

ergosterol   A sterol isolated from yeast; when subjected to ultraviolet irradiation, it is converted to ercalciol (ergocalciferol, vitamin D_2). The main source of manufactured VITAMIN D.

ergot   A fungus that grows on grasses and cereal grains; the ergot of medical importance is *Claviceps purpurea*, which grows on RYE. The consumption of infected rye is harmful, causing the disease known as St Anthony's Fire (ergotism), and can be fatal.

   The active principles in ergot are ALKALOIDS (ergotinine, ergotoxine, ergotamine, ergometrine, etc.), which yield lysergic acid (the active component) on hydrolysis. Its effect is to increase the tone and contraction of smooth muscle, particularly of the pregnant uterus. For this reason ergot has been used in obstetrics, but pure ergonovine maleate and ergotonine tartrate are preferable.

   Ergotism is poisoning by ergot infection of rye which occurs from time to time among people eating rye bread. The last outbreak in the UK was in Manchester in 1925, when there were 200 cases. Symptoms appear when as little as 1% of ergot-infected rye is included in the flour.

eriodictin   A FLAVONOID (flavonone) found in citrus pith.

erucic acid   A mono-unsaturated FATTY ACID, *cis*-13-docosenoic acid (C22:1 ω9) found in RAPE seed (*Brassica napus*) and mustard seed (*B. junca* and *B. nigra*) oils; it may constitute 30–50% of the oil in some varieties. Causes fatty infiltration of heart muscle in experimental animals; low erucic acid varieties of rape seed have been developed for food use (CANBRA OIL).

   See also CANOLA.

eructation   Belching, the act of bringing up air from the stomach, with a characteristic sound.

erythorbic acid   The D-isomer of ASCORBIC ACID, also called D-araboascorbic acid and *iso*-ascorbic acid; only slight VITAMIN C activity. Used in food processing as an antioxidant.

erythritol   A SUGAR ALCOHOL, used as a bulk SWEETENER (derived from the four-carbon sugar erythrose), manufactured by fermentation of glucose; 60–70% as sweet as sucrose.

erythroamylose Obsolete name for AMYLOPECTIN.

erythrocytes *See* BLOOD CELLS.

erythropoiesis The formation and development of the red BLOOD CELLS in the bone marrow.

erythrosine BS Red colour permitted in foods in most countries (E-127, Red number 3 in USA; the sodium or potassium salt of 2,4,5,7-tetraiodofluorescein). Used in preserved cherries, sausages and meat and fish pastes; it is unstable to light and heat.

esculin *See* AESCULIN.

ESPEN European Society for Parenteral and Enteral Nutrition and Metabolism, now called European Society for Clinical Nutrition and Metabolism; web site http://www.espen.org/.

ESR Electron spin resonance.

essential amino acid index An index of PROTEIN QUALITY.

essential amino acid pattern The quantities of essential AMINO ACIDS considered desirable in the diet.

essential amino acids *See* AMINO ACIDS.

essential fatty acids *See* FATTY ACIDS, ESSENTIAL.

essential nutrients Those nutrients that are required by the body and cannot be synthesised in the body in adequate amounts to meet requirements, so must be provided by the diet, includes the essential amino acids and fatty acids, vitamins and minerals. Really a tautology, since by definition nutrients are essential dietary constituents.

essential oils Volatile, aromatic or odoriferous oils found in plants and used for flavouring foods; prepared by distillation. Chemically distinct from the edible oils, since they are not glycerol esters.

See also OLEORESINS; TERPENES.

ester Compound formed by condensation between an acid and an alcohol. FATS are esters of the alcohol glycerol and long-chain FATTY ACIDS. Many esters are used as synthetic flavours (see FLAVOURS, SYNTHETIC).

esterases Enzymes (EC 3.1.x.x) that hydrolyse ESTERS to yield free acid and alcohol. Those that hydrolyse the ester linkages of fats are generally known as LIPASES, and those that hydrolyse PHOSPHOLIPIDS as phospholipases.

ester value *See* SAPONIFICATION.

ethane Hydrocarbon gas (C_2H_6) formed in small amounts by metabolism of oxidised LINOLENIC acid and exhaled on the breath; used as an index of oxygen radical damage to tissue lipids, and indirectly as an index of ANTIOXIDANT status.

See also FATTY ACIDS; PENTANE.

ethanolamine 2-Amino-ethanol, one of the water-soluble bases of PHOSPHOLIPIDS. Used as softening agent for hides, as dispersing agent for agricultural chemicals and to peel fruits and vegetables.

ethene Or ethylene, a hydrocarbon gas ($CH_2{=}CH_2$), produced by the oxidation of METHIONINE in CLIMACTERIC fruits as a hormone to speed ripening, the climacteric increase in respiration. This explains why some fruits ripen faster when stored in plastic bags. Used commercially in very small amounts (1 ppm) to speed fruit ripening after harvesting.

ethionine A toxic amino acid, the ethyl analogue of METHIONINE.

ethyl alcohol *See* ALCOHOL.

ethyl carbamate *See* URETHANE.

ethylene *See* ETHENE.

ethylene diamine tetra-acetic acid *See* EDTA.

ethylene scavengers A variety of compounds that will adsorb ethylene (ETHENE) in packed fruits and vegetables, and so slow ripening during storage. When potassium permanganate is used, it changes colour from purple to brown, so indicating the remaining capacity to scavenge ethylene.

ethyl formate Used as a fumigant against insects such as raisin moth, dried fruit beetle, and fig moth, and as a flavour; an ingredient of artificial lemon, strawberry and rum flavours.

ethylmethylcellulose *See* CELLULOSE DERIVATIVES.

ethyl vanillin *See* VANILLA.

EUFIC European Food Information Council; web site http://www.eufic.org/.

eugenol Flavouring obtained from clove oil and also found in carnation and cinnamon leaves.

euglobulin The name given to the fraction of serum GLOBULIN that is precipitated by dialysis of blood serum against distilled water. The name implies that this fraction is a typical globulin by reason of its insolubility in water.

eukeratins *See* KERATIN.

eutectic ice The solid formed when a mixture of 76.7% water and 23.3% salt (by weight) is frozen. It melts at −21 °C. It has about three times the refrigerant effect of solid carbon dioxide (DRY ICE), and is especially useful for icing fish on board trawlers.

eutectic mixture Mixture of two compounds showing a sharp melting point, the EUTECTIC TEMPERATURE.

eutectic temperature In freezing, the temperature at which a crystal of an individual solute exists in equilibrium with the unfrozen liquor and ice. The final eutectic temperature is the lowest eutectic temperature of solutes in equilibrium with unfrozen liquor and ice.

eutrophia Normal nutrition.

evaporation, falling film *See* CALANDRIA.

evaporation, flash   A short, rapid application of heat so that a small volume (about 1% of the total) is quickly distilled off, carrying with it the greater part of the volatile components. The flash distillate is collected separately from the later distillate and is added back to the concentrate to restore the flavour; applied to the concentration of products such as fruit juices.

evening primrose   *Oenothera biennis.* The oil from the seeds is a rich source of γ-LINOLENIC ACID, which may account for 8% of total FATTY ACIDS. Used as a dietary supplement and claimed to have beneficial effects in a number of conditions, with some evidence of efficacy.

exchange list   List of portions of foods in which energy yield, fat, carbohydrate and/or protein content are equivalent, so simplifying meal and diet planning for people with special needs.

exclusion diet   A limited diet excluding foods known possibly to cause food intolerance (*see* ADVERSE REACTIONS TO FOODS), to which foods are added in turn to test for intolerance.

exergonic   Chemical reactions that proceed with the output of energy, usually as heat (then sometimes known as exothermic reactions) or light. The reactions involved in the oxidation of foodstuffs are generally exergonic.

exhausting   Removal of air from a container before processing.

exon   A region of DNA within a gene that contains information coding for the protein that is retained during the post-transcriptional modification of mRNA.
   See also INTRON.

exopeptidases   Proteolytic enzymes that hydrolyse the peptide bonds of the terminal amino acids of proteins or peptides, as opposed to ENDOPEPTIDASES, which cleave at sites in the middle of a peptide chain. There are two groups: aminopeptidases (EC 3.4.11.x) which remove the amino acid at the amino terminal of the protein, and carboxypeptidases (EC 3.4.16.x and 3.4.17.x), which remove the amino acid at the carboxyl terminal.

exophthalmus   Protrusion of the eyeballs from the sockets, commonly associated with hyperthyroid GOITRE.

exotoxins   Toxic substances produced by bacteria, which diffuse out of the cells and stimulate the production of antibodies which specifically neutralise them (antitoxins). They are generally heat-labile and inactivated in about 1 h at 60 °C. Exotoxins include those produced by the organisms responsible for BOTULISM, tetanus and diphtheria.
   See also ENDOTOXINS; TX NUMBERS.

expansion rings   In relation to cans, the concentric rings stamped into the ends of the can to allow bulging during heat processing without straining the seams.

expeller A horizontal barrel, containing a helical screw, used to extract oil from seeds or nuts.

expeller cake The residue from oilseeds after most of the oil has been removed by pressing; a valuable source of protein for animal feeding.

explosion puffing Technique used to create a porous structure in partially dried, diced fruit or vegetable pieces to accelerate the drying process, or cereal grains to produce breakfast cereals, by heating in a sealed vessel (a puffing gun) then unsealing to reduce the pressure rapidly.

expression The extraction or separation of liquids from solids by pressure, especially juices from fruit and oil from olives and oil seeds. Various types of press are used; either batch or continuous presses. Batch presses may be either a simple tank or a slatted cage in which the material is pressed; continuous presses may use a belt pressed between rollers, a screw EXPELLER or fluted metal rollers.

extensograph (extensometer) An instrument for measuring the stretching strength of dough as an index of its baking quality.

extraction rate *See* FLOUR, EXTRACTION RATE.

extremophiles Micro-organisms that can grow under extreme conditions of heat (THERMOPHILES and extreme thermophiles, some of which live in hot springs at 100 °C), cold (PSYCHROPHILES), high concentrations of salt (HALOPHILES), high pressure or extremes of acid or alkali.

extrinsic factor *See* ANAEMIA, PERNICIOUS; VITAMIN B_{12}.

extruder *See* EXTRUSION.

extrusion Process in which the raw materials are mixed, kneaded, sheared, shaped and extruded; essentially a screw press that forces the product through a restricted opening. When the food is also heated the process is termed extrusion cooking, a high-temperature short-time procedure.

Extruders can be classified as: autogenous, in which temperature increases as a result of pressure and flow; isothermal, in which temperature is kept constant; and polytropic, operating between these two extremes. Alternatively, they may be classified by the way in which pressure is developed: direct or positive displacement (ram or piston-type extruders and the intermeshing counter-rotating twin-screw extruders) and indirect or viscous drag (roller, single screw, intermeshing co-rotating twin-screw and non-intermeshing multiple-screw extruders).

extrusion cooking Ingredients are heated under pressure, then extruded through fine pores, when the superheated water evaporates rapidly, leaving a porous textured product.

exudative diathesis   Vascular disease of VITAMIN E-deficient chicks, characterised by accumulation of greenish fluid under the skin of the breast and abdomen.

F

FAD   *See* FLAVIN ADENINE DINUCLEOTIDE.

faeces   Composed of undigested food residues, remains of digestive secretions that have not been reabsorbed, bacteria from the intestinal tract, cells, cell debris and mucus from the intestinal lining, substances excreted into the intestinal tract (mainly in the BILE). The average amount is about 100 g/day, but varies widely depending on the intake of dietary FIBRE.

faecolith   Small hard mass of faeces, found especially in the vermiform APPENDIX.

faggot   (1) Traditional British meatball made from pig OFFAL and meat.

(2) Bundle of herbs, *see* BOUQUET GARNI.

fair maids   Cornish name for PILCHARDS (thought to be a corruption of the Spanish *fumade* = smoked).

fairy potato   *See* EARTH NUT.

famotidine   *See* HISTAMINE RECEPTOR ANTAGONISTS.

FANSA   The Food and Nutrition Science Alliance, a partnership of the American Dietetic Association, the American Society for Clinical Nutrition, the American Society for Nutritional Sciences and the Institute of Food Technologists.

FAO   Food and Agriculture Organization of the United Nations, founded in 1943; headquarters in Rome. Its goal is to achieve freedom from hunger worldwide. According to its constitution the specific objectives are 'raising the levels of nutrition and standards of living . . . and securing improvements in the efficiency of production and distribution of all food and agricultural products.' Web site http://www.fao.org/.

Farex™   A cereal food for infants.

farfals   *See* PASTA.

farina   General term for starch. In UK specifically POTATO STARCH; in the USA starch obtained from wheat other than DURUM WHEAT; starch from the latter is SEMOLINA. Farina dolce is Italian flour made from dried chestnuts.

farinaceous   Starchy.

farinograph   An instrument for measuring the physical properties of a dough.

farl   Scottish; triangular oatmeal cake.

fascioliasis   Infestation of the bile ducts and liver with the liver FLUKE *Fasciola hepatica*, commonly acquired by eating wild

WATERCRESS on which the larval stage of the parasite is present.

fasciolopsiasis Infestation of the intestinal tract with the FLUKE *Fasciolopsis buski*, commonly acquired by eating uncooked water chestnuts contaminated with the larval stage of the parasite.

fast foods (fast service foods) General term used for a limited menu of foods that lend themselves to production line techniques; suppliers tend to specialise in products such as HAMBURGERS, PIZZAS, chicken or SANDWICHES.

fasting Going without food. The metabolic fasting state begins some 4 h after a meal, when the digestion and absorption of food are complete and body reserves of fat and GLYCOGEN begin to be mobilised. In more prolonged fasting the blood concentration of KETONE BODIES rises, as they are exported from the liver for use by muscle and other tissues as a metabolic fuel.

fasting-induced adipocyte factor Circulating protein that inhibits ADIPOSE TISSUE lipoprotein LIPASE, and so inhibits deposition of lipid in adipose tissue.

fat (1) Chemically, fats (or lipids) are substances that are insoluble in water but soluble in organic solvents such as ether, chloroform and benzene, and are actual or potential esters of FATTY ACIDS. The term includes TRIACYLGLYCEROLS (triglycerides), PHOSPHOLIPIDS, WAXES and STEROIDS.

(2) In more general use the term 'fats' refers to the neutral fats, which are esters of fatty acids with GLYCEROL (triacylglycerols or triglycerides).

fat, blood *See* LIPIDS, PLASMA; LIPOPROTEINS, PLASMA.

fat, brown *See* ADIPOSE TISSUE, BROWN.

fat-extenders *See* FAT, SUPERGLYCINERATED.

fat free EU regulations restrict use of the term 'fat free' to foods that contain less than 0.15 g of fat/100 g; in the USA low-fat foods must state the percentage of fat; thus a product described as 95% fat free contains only 5 g of fat/100 g.

fat, high-ratio *See* FAT, SUPERGLYCINERATED.

fat mouse Genetically obese mouse that secretes pro-insulin because of a defect in the gene for the pro-insulin converting enzyme, CARBOXYPEPTIDASE E. The same enzyme is also involved in the post-synthetic modification of other peptide hormone precursors, including PRO-OPIOMELANOCORTIN.

fat, neutral FATS that are chemically TRIACYLGLYCEROLS (triglycerides).

fat, non-saponifiable, saponifiable *See* SAPONIFICATION.

fat, polymorphic One that can crystallise in more than one form.

fat replacers   Substances that provide a creamy, fat-like texture used to replace or partly replace the fat in a recipe food. Made from a variety of substances, e.g. Slendid is the trade name for a product derived from pectin, Olestra is SUCROSE POLYESTER which is not absorbed by the body, Simplesse is a protein product, N-oil is made from tapioca.

fat, saturated   FATS containing only or mainly saturated FATTY ACIDS.

fat-soluble vitamins   VITAMINS A, D, E and K; they occur in food dissolved in the fats and are stored in the body to a greater extent than the water-soluble vitamins.

fat, superglycerinated   Neutral fats are triacylglycerols, i.e. with three molecules of fatty acid to each molecule of glycerol. Mono- and diacylglycerols (sometimes called mono- and diglycerides) are known as superglycerinated high-ratio fats or fat extenders (E-471).

Glyceryl monostearate (GMS) is solid at room temperature, flexible and non-greasy; used as a protective coating for foods, as a plasticiser for softening the crumb of bread, to reduce spattering in frying fats, as emulsifier and stabiliser. Glyceryl mono-oleate (GMO) is semiliquid at room temperature.

fatty acids   Organic ACIDS consisting of carbon chains with a terminal carboxyl group. The nutritionally important fatty acids have an even number of carbon atoms, commonly between 12 and 22. Saturated fatty acids are those in which there are only single bonds between adjacent carbon atoms. It is recommended that intake should not exceed about 10% of food energy intake, since they increase levels of low-density lipoprotein CHOLESTEROL (a major risk factor in heart disease).

Unsaturated fatty acids have one or more carbon–carbon double bonds in the molecule. These double bonds can be reduced (saturated) with hydrogen, the process of HYDROGENATION, forming saturated fatty acids. Fatty acids with only one double bond are termed mono-unsaturated; OLEIC ACID is the main one found in fats and oils. Fatty acids with two or more double bonds are termed polyunsaturated fatty acids, often abbreviated to PUFA.

Unsaturated fatty acids reduce the concentration of LDL cholesterol in the blood. In general, fats from animal sources are high in saturated and relatively low in unsaturated fatty acids; vegetable and fish oils are generally higher in unsaturated and lower in saturated fatty acids.

In addition to their systematic and trivial names, fatty acids can be named by a shorthand giving the number of carbon atoms in the molecule (e.g. C18), then a colon and the number of double bonds (e.g. C18:2), followed by the position of the first double bond from the methyl end of the molecule as *n*- or ω (e.g. C18:2 *n*-6, or C18:2 ω6). *See* Table 8 of the Appendix.

fatty acids, essential (EFA) FATTY ACIDS that cannot be made in the body and are therefore dietary essentials – two polyunsaturated fatty acids: linoleic (C18:2 ω6) and α-linolenic (C18:3 ω3).

Several other fatty acids have some EFA activity in that they cure some, but not all, of the signs of (experimental) EFA deficiency. Arachidonic (C20:4 ω6), eicosapentaenoic (EPA C20:5 ω3) and docosahexaenoic (DHA C22:6 ω3) acids are physiologically important, although they are not dietary essentials since they can be formed from linoleic and α-linolenic acids.

Estimated average requirement for ω6 PUFA is 1% of total energy intake (260 mg/MJ) and for ω3 PUFA is 0.2% (50 mg/MJ), with a recommendation that total PUFA intakes should not be more than 10–15% of total energy; a desirable intake, and the basis of REFERENCE INTAKES, is 8–10% of energy intake, about 2–2.6 g/MJ.

fatty acids, free (FFA) or non-esterified (NEFA) Fatty acids may be liberated from triacylglycerols (triglycerides) either by enzymic hydrolysis (when they are generally known as non-esterified fatty acids, NEFA, or unesterified fatty acids, UFA) or as a result of hydrolytic rancidity of the fat. Determination of NEFA is therefore an index of the quality of fats.

Free fatty acids circulate in the bloodstream, bound to albumin. They are released from ADIPOSE TISSUE in the FASTING state, as a fuel for muscle and other tissues. The normal concentration in plasma is between 0.5 and 2 μmol/L, increasing with fasting and exercise.

fatty acids, polyunsaturated Long-chain fatty acids containing two or more double bonds, separated by methylene bridges: $- CH_2 - CH = CH - CH_2 - CH = CH - CH_2 -$.

fatty acids, unesterified, non-esterified (NEFA) *See* FATTY ACIDS, FREE.

fatty acids, volatile Short-chain fatty acids, acetic, propionic and butyric, which, apart from their presence in some foods, are produced by bacteria in the human intestine and rumen of cattle from undigested starch and dietary FIBRE. To some extent they can be absorbed and used as a source of energy. Butyric acid formed in the colon may have some anticarcinogenic action, and is a significant metabolic fuel for colonic ENTEROCYTES.

fat, unsaturated FATS containing a high proportion of unsaturated FATTY ACIDS.

fat, yellow *See* SPREAD, FAT.

favism   Acute haemolytic ANAEMIA induced in genetically sensitive people by eating broad beans, *Vicia faba*, or in response to various drugs, including especially antimalarials. The disease is due to a deficiency of the enzyme glucose6-phosphate dehydrogenase (EC 1.1.1.19) in red blood cells, which are then vulnerable to the toxins, vicine and convicine, in the beans. The condition affects some 100 million people worldwide, and is commonest in people of Mediterranean and Afro-Caribbean descent.

FDA   US Food and Drug Administration, government regulatory agency; web site http://www.fda.gov/; web site for FDA consumer magazine http://www.fda.gov/fdac/.

FD&C   USA; abbreviation for synthetic colours permitted for use in food, drugs and cosmetics.

FDF   Food and Drink Federation, organisation speaking for the UK food and drink manufacturing industry; web site http://www.fdf.org.uk/.

FDNB   *See* FLUORODINITROBENZENE.

fecula (fécule)   Foods that are almost solely starch, prepared from roots and stems by grating, e.g. TAPIOCA, SAGO and ARROWROOT. Starchy powder from rice, potatoes, etc.

feedback control   Control of a process using information from sensors to adjust the conditions.

Fehling's reagent   Alkaline cupric tartrate solution used for detection and semi-quantitative determination of glucose and other reducing sugars.

   See also BENEDICT'S REAGENT, SOMOGYI–NELSON REAGENT.

feijoa   Fruit of S American tree *Acca sellowiana* (formerly *Feijoa sellowiana*), also known as pineapple guava, guavasteen; mainly grown in New Zealand.

   Composition/100g: (edible portion 75%) water 87g, 205kJ (49kcal), protein 1.2g, fat 0.8g, carbohydrate 10.6g, ash 0.7g, Ca 17mg, Fe 0.1mg, Mg 9mg, P 20mg, K 155mg, Na 3mg, Cu 0.1mg, Mn 0.1mg, vitamin B_1 0.01mg, B_2 0.03mg, niacin 0.3mg, B_6 0.05mg, folate 38μg, pantothenate 0.2mg, C 20mg. A 50g serving (1 fruit without refuse) is a source of vitamin C.

feijoa beans   *See* BEAN, ADZUKI.

Feingold diet   Exclusion of foods containing synthetic colours, flavours and preservatives and limitation of intake of fruits and vegetables such as oranges, apricots, peaches, tomatoes and cucumbers; intended to treat hyperactive children. There is little evidence either that these foods are a cause of hyperactivity or that the exclusion diet is beneficial.

felafel   Middle Eastern; deep fried balls of CHICKPEA batter.

FEMA   US Flavor and Extract Manufacturers' Association, web site http://www.femaflavor.org/.

fenelar Norwegian; leg of mutton dry-brined with salt, saltpetre and sugar, then in a sweet pickle, smoked and air dried.

fenfluramine An anorectic (appetite suppressant, *see* APPETITE CONTROL) drug with amphetamine-like actions formerly used in the treatment of obesity; withdrawn in 1995 in response to reports of heart valve damage (in the combined preparation with phentermine, FEN-PHEN). Only the D-isomer is active (dexfenfluramine).

fennel (1) Aromatic seeds and feathery green leaves of the perennial plant *Foeniculum vulgare*, used to flavour a variety of dishes.

(2) *Foeniculum dulce* (or *F. vulgare* var. *azoricum*). Annual plant, also called Florence fennel or finnochio; the swollen bases of the leaves are eaten as a vegetable, raw or cooked. The seeds are also used as flavouring.

Composition/100 g: (edible portion 72%) water 90.2 g, 130 kJ (31 kcal), protein 1.2 g, fat 0.2 g, carbohydrate 7.3 g, fibre 3.1 g, ash 1 g, Ca 49 mg, Fe 0.7 mg, Mg 17 mg, P 50 mg, K 414 mg, Na 52 mg, Zn 0.2 mg, Cu 0.1 mg, Mn 0.2 mg, Se 0.7 µg, vitamin A 7 µg RE B_1 0.01 mg, B_2 0.03 mg, niacin 0.6 mg, B_6 0.05 mg, folate 27 µg, pantothenate 0.2 mg, C 12 mg. A 110 g serving (half bulb) is a source of folate, a good source of vitamin C.

fen-phen The combination of FENFLURAMINE and PHENTERMINE, formerly used as an appetite suppressant (APPETITE CONTROL) drug in the treatment of obesity; withdrawn in 1995 in response to reports of heart valve damage.

fenugreek *Trigonella feonumgraecum*, a leguminous plant eaten as a vegetable; the seeds are used for flavouring. Traditionally eaten by women in Asia to help gain weight.

fermentation Anaerobic METABOLISM. Used generally of alcoholic fermentation of sugars, also production of acetic, lactic, and citric acids by micro-organisms in pickling and manufacture of VINEGAR.

fermentation, secondary In WINE making; may be addition of further sugar and yeast to produce carbon dioxide for sparkling wines, or a malo-lactic fermentation using *Lactobacillus* spp. to convert sharp-tasting malic acid to the milder lactic acid; again this produces carbon dioxide, characteristic of pétillant (lightly sparkling) wines.

See also VINEGAR.

fermented milk *See* MILK, FERMENTED.

fermentograph An instrument for measuring the gas-producing power of a dough. The fermenting dough is contained in a balloon immersed in water and as gas is produced the balloon expands and rises in the water, the rise being measured continuously.

ferric ammonium citrate The form in which IRON is sometimes added to foods. Occurs as brown-red scales (16.5–18.5% iron) and as green scales (14.5–16% iron).

ferritin The main IRON storage protein in tissues; also found in serum, where the concentration reflects the total amount of storage iron in the body, and therefore permits assessment of iron status over the range from deficiency, through normal to overload. Although it provides the most sensitive index of iron depletion, its synthesis is also significantly reduced in response to trauma and infection.

See also ACUTE PHASE PROTEINS; TRANSFERRIN RECEPTOR.

ferrous gluconate IRON salt of GLUCONIC ACID, used in iron supplements and as a colouring agent in olives.

ferrum redactum *See* IRON, REDUCED.

FFA Free fatty acids, *see* FATTY ACIDS, FREE.

FIAF *See* FASTING-INDUCED ADIPOCYTE FACTOR.

fibre, crude The term given to indigestible part of foods, defined in the UK Fertiliser and Feedingstuffs Act of 1932 as the residue left after successive extraction under closely specified conditions with petroleum ether, 1.25% sulphuric acid and 1.25% sodium hydroxide, minus ash. No relationship to dietary fibre (*see* FIBRE, DIETARY).

fibre, dietary Material mostly derived from plant cell walls which is not digested by human digestive enzymes but is partially broken down by intestinal bacteria to volatile FATTY ACIDS that can be used as a source of energy. A large proportion consists of NON-STARCH POLYSACCHARIDES; these include soluble fibre that reduces levels of blood cholesterol and increases the viscosity of the intestinal contents and insoluble fibre (cellulose and cell walls) that acts as a LAXATIVE. Earlier known as roughage or bulk.

fibre, insoluble The part of dietary FIBRE (or NON-STARCH POLY-SACCHARIDE) that is not soluble in water – CELLULOSE, hemicelluloses and lignin. These increase the bulk of the intestinal contents.

fibre, soluble The plant GUMS and small oligosaccharides in dietary FIBRE (or NON-STARCH POLYSACCHARIDE) that are soluble in water, forming viscous gels.

fibric acids A variety of analogues of clofibric acid (chlorophenoxy-isobutyrate), including bezafibrate, clofibrate (the ethyl ester), fenofibrate and gemfibrozil (which is not halogenated), used in treatment of HYPERLIPIDAEMIA. They lower VLDL and LDL, and raise HDL, by stimulation of lipoprotein LIPASE (EC 3.1.1.34).

fibrin *See* FIBRINOGEN.

fibrinogen One of the proteins of the blood plasma responsible for COAGULATION. When PROTHROMBIN is activated to thrombin in response to injury, it hydrolyses fibrinogen to fibrin, which is deposited as strands that trap red cells and platelets, forming the clot.

fibronectin A plasma protein that has a very rapid rate of turnover, and can be used as an index of undernutrition.

fibrous proteins *See* ALBUMINOIDS.

ficin (ficain) Proteolytic enzyme (EC 3.4.22.3) from the FIG.

fiddleheads *See* BRACKEN.

field egg *See* AUBERGINE.

field mushroom *Agaricus campestris*, *A. vaporarius*, *see* MUSHROOMS.

fig The fruit of *Ficus carica*; eaten fresh or dried. Figs have mild laxative properties, e.g. syrup of figs is a medicinal preparation.

Composition/100 g: (edible portion 99%) water 79.1 g, 310 kJ (74 kcal), protein 0.8 g, fat 0.3 g, carbohydrate 19.2 g (16.3 g sugars), fibre 2.9 g, ash 0.7 g, Ca 35 mg, Fe 0.4 mg, Mg 17 mg, P 14 mg, K 232 mg, Na 1 mg, Zn 0.2 mg, Cu 0.1 mg, Mn 0.1 mg, Se 0.2 µg, vitamin A 7 µg RE (94 µg carotenoids), E 0.1 mg, K 4.7 mg, B_1 0.06 mg, B_2 0.05 mg, niacin 0.4 mg, B_6 0.11 mg, folate 6 µg, pantothenate 0.3 mg, C 2 mg.

fig, Adam's *See* PLANTAIN.

fig, berberry or Indian *See* PRICKLY PEAR.

FIGLU test For FOLIC ACID status. Measurement of urinary excretion of formiminoglutamate (FIGLU) after a test dose of 2–5 g of HISTIDINE. FIGLU formiminotransferase (EC 2.1.2.5) is a folate-dependent enzyme.

See also ANAEMIA, MEGALOBLASTIC.

filbert *See* HAZEL NUT.

filé powder Dried powdered young leaves of the sassafras tree (*Sassafras albidum*); very aromatic, an ingredient of GUMBO.

filo pastry *See* PHYLLO PASTRY.

filter cake Solid matter retained after FILTRATION of a liquid.

filter mat drying Partially spray-dried material (about 20% moisture) is allowed to fall onto a perforated belt through which air is passed to complete the drying process.

Filtermat™ process For AGGLOMERATION of dried foods; the product is partially dried by spray drying, then deposited onto a perforated belt and dried further. There is sufficient moisture in the intermediate product for agglomerates to form on the belt.

filter medium *See* FILTRATION.

filth test Name given to a test that originated in the USA for determining the contamination of a food with rodent hairs and insect fragments as an index of hygienic handling.

filtrate The liquid that passes through a filter; *see* FILTRATION.

filtrate factor Obsolete name for PANTOTHENIC ACID.

filtration The separation of solids from liquids by passing the mixture through a bed of porous material (the filter medium), either under gravity and hydrostatic pressure alone or using pressure above, or vacuum below, to force the liquid through the filter bed.

> *See also* FILTER CAKE; FILTRATE.

fines herbes Mixture of chopped parsley, tarragon, chives, chervil, marjoram and sometimes watercress.

fingerware Edible seaweed, *Laminaria digitata*.

fining agents Substances used to clarify liquids by precipitation, e.g. egg albumin, casein, bentonite, ISINGLASS, GELATINE.

finnan haddock Smoke-cured haddock (named after Findon in Scotland).

> *See also* ARBROATH SMOKIE.

finocchio Variety of FENNEL with swollen leaf base; *Foeniculum vulgare* var. *azoricum*.

fire point The temperature at which a frying oil will sustain combustion; between 340 and 360 °C for most fats.

> *See also* FLASH POINT; SMOKE POINT.

fireless cooker *See* HAYBOX COOKING.

firkin A quarter of a barrel of beer, 9 Imperial gallons (40 L); also 56 lb (25.5 kg) of butter.

firming agents Fresh fruits contain insoluble PECTIN as a gel around the fibrous tissues which keeps the fruit firm. Breakdown of cell structure allows conversion of pectin to pectic acid, with loss of firmness. The addition of calcium salts (chloride or carbonate) forms a calcium pectate gel which protects the fruit against softening; these are known as firming agents. Alum (aluminium potassium sulphate) is sometimes used to firm pickles.

FISH Fluorescent *in situ* hybridisation, a technique for locating specific regions of DNA in a chromosome using a fluorescently labelled DNA probe.

fish days Historical; days on which fish, but not meat, could be eaten. Originally decreed by the Church (Fridays, fast days and throughout Lent); more were decreed in England during the 16th century, both to encourage ship building and the training of mariners, and also, because of the shortage of meat, to permit an increase in the numbers of cattle. The Vatican rescinded the rule forbidding Catholics to eat meat on Fridays in 1966.

fish, demersal Fish species living on or near the sea bed – the white (non-oily) fish such as COD, HADDOCK, HALIBUT, plaice, sole and whiting. Caught by trawls which are dragged along the bottom of the sea, or seine nets. Known in USA as ground fish. *See also* FISH, WHITE.

fish, fatty *See* FISH, OILY.

fish flour *See* FISH PROTEIN CONCENTRATE.

fish ham Japanese product made from a red fish such as TUNA or marlin, pickled with salt and nitrite, mixed with whale meat and pork fat and stuffed into a large sausage-type casing.

fish meal Surplus fish, waste from filleting (fish-house waste) and fish unsuitable for human consumption are dried and powdered. The resultant meal is a valuable source of protein for animal feedingstuff, or, after deodorisation, as human food since it contains about 70% protein. Meal made from white fish is termed white fish meal, distinct from the oily type which is sometimes of very poor quality and is used mainly as fertiliser.

fish odour syndrome *See* TRIMETHYLAMINE.

fish oils These contain long-chain polyunsaturated FATTY ACIDS which offer some protection against heart disease. The two main ones are eicosapentaenoic acid (EPA C20:5 ω3) and docosohexaenoic acid (DHA C22:6 ω3). Fish oil concentrates containing these fatty acids are sold as pharmaceutical preparations.

    See also COD LIVER OIL; HALIBUT; MENHADEN.

fish, oily ANCHOVY, HERRING, MACKEREL, PILCHARD, SALMON, SARDINE, TROUT, TUNA, WHITEBAIT, containing about 15% fat (varying from 5 to 20% through the year) and containing 10–40 µg vitamin D per 100 g, as distinct from white fish, which contain 1–2% fat and only a trace of vitamin D.

    See also FISH, PELAGIC.

fish paste A spread made from ground fish and cereal. In UK, legally contains not less than 70% fish.

fish, pelagic Literally 'of or pertaining to the ocean' – fish normally caught at or near the surface of the sea. Mainly the migratory, shoaling, seasonal fish; oily fish (*see* FISH, OILY) such as HERRING, MACKEREL, PILCHARD and TUNA.

fish protein concentrate Deodorised, decolorised, defatted FISH MEAL, also known as fish flour.

fish solubles *See* STICKWATER.

fish tester Instrument for assessing the freshness of fish by measuring dielectric properties of skin and muscle, developed as the GR Torrymeter by the (now disestablished) Torry Research Station in Scotland.

fish, white Non-oily fish, e.g. COD, DOGFISH, HADDOCK, HALIBUT, PLAICE, SAITHE, SKATE, SOLE, WHITING. *See* FISH, DEMERSAL.

fistula An abnormal connection between two hollow organs, or between a hollow organ and the external environment; may occur as a result of infection, injury or surgery.

five-spice powder   Chinese; a mixture of star ANISE, anise pepper, FENNEL, CLOVES and CINNAMON, and sometimes powdered dried orange peel.

flabelliferins   SAPONINS of β-SITOSTEROL from the fruit pulp of the palmyrah palm, *Borassus flabillefer*, that have hypocholestero-laemic action.

Flash 18   A method of canning foods (Swift & Co, USA) under pressure (126 kPa = 18 psi above atmospheric). The food is ster-ilised at 121 °C and then canned at that temperature, not requir-ing further heat. The process is claimed to give improved taste and texture compared with conventional canning, and the possi-bility of using large containers without overheating the food.

flash evaporation   *See* EVAPORATION, FLASH.

flash pasteurisation   *See* PASTEURISATION.

flash point   With reference to frying oils, the temperature at which the decomposition products can be ignited, but will not support combustion; ranges between 290 and 330 °C.

  See also FIRE POINT; SMOKE POINT.

flatfish   Fish with a flattened shape, including dab, flounder, halibut, plaice, sole and turbot.

  Composition/100 g: water 79 g, 381 kJ (91 kcal), protein 18.8 g, fat 1.2 g (of which 38% saturated, 25% mono-unsaturated, 38% polyunsaturated), cholesterol 48 mg, carbohydrate 0 g, ash 1.2 g, Ca 18 mg, Fe 0.4 mg, Mg 31 mg, P 184 mg, K 361 mg, Na 81 mg, Zn 0.4 mg, Se 32.7 μg, I 25 μg, vitamin A 10 μg retinol, E 0.5 mg, K 0.1 mg, B_1 0.09 mg, B_2 0.08 mg, niacin 2.9 mg, B_6 0.21 mg, folate 8 μg, B_{12} 1.5 μg, pantothenate 0.5 mg, C 2 mg. A 100 g serving is a source of I, niacin, a good source of P, a rich source of Se, vitamin B_{12}.

flatogens   Substances that cause gas production, FLATULENCE, in the intestine, by providing fermentable substrate for intestinal bacteria.

flat sours   Bacteria such as *Bacillus stearothermophilus* render canned food sour by fermenting carbohydrates to lactic, formic and acetic acids, without gas production. This means that the ends of the can are not swelled out but remain flat. Economically they are the most important of the thermophilic spoilage agents (THERMOPHILES); some species can grow slowly at 25 °C and thus spoil products after long storage periods.

flatulence (flatus)   Production of gas in the intestine – hydrogen, carbon dioxide and methane. May be caused by a variety of foods that contain FLATOGENS.

flavanols, flavanones   Alternative name for FLAVONOIDS.

flavedo   The coloured outer peel layer of citrus fruits, also called the epicarp or zest. It contains the oil sacs, and hence the aromatic oils, and numerous plastids which are green and contain chlorophyll in the unripe fruit, turning yellow or orange in the ripe fruit, when they contain carotene and xanthophyll.

flavin The group of compounds containing the iso-alloxazine ring structure, as in riboflavin (VITAMIN B_2); a general term for riboflavin derivatives.

flavin adenine dinucleotide (FAD) A COENZYME in oxidation reactions, derived from VITAMIN B_2, phosphate, ribose and adenine.

flavin mononucleotide (FMN) A COENZYME in oxidation reactions, chemically the phosphate of VITAMIN B_2 (riboflavin).

flavone *See* FLAVONOIDS.

flavonoids (bioflavonoids) Polyphenolic compounds widely distributed in plants where they are responsible for colour, taste and smell as well as attracting or repelling insects and micro-organisms. Some 4000 have been identified, with a wide range of chemical properties. They occur as glycosides in which the sugar moiety is usually glucose or rhamnose.

FLAVONOIDS

At one time a mixture of flavonoids was shown to decrease capillary permeability and fragility in human beings and was named vitamin P, but later, 1950, when it was found that they are not dietary essentials, the name was dropped.

More recently there has been epidemiological evidence from observations in population groups with a high intake of fruits and vegetables that flavonoids may have a role in protection against some forms of cancer. Some are antioxidants and may help to prevent atherosclerosis; others have weak OESTROGEN activity (PHYTOESTROGENS) and have been associated with lower incidence of breast, uterus and prostate cancer.

Total dietary intake is around 1 g per day (650 mg when calculated as aglycones), a large part of which comes from tea, red wine, berries and onions.

flavonols Alternative name for FLAVONOIDS.

flavoproteins Enzymes that contain the vitamin RIBOFLAVIN, or a derivative such as flavin adenine dinucleotide or riboflavin phosphate, as the PROSTHETIC GROUP. Mainly involved in oxidation reactions in METABOLISM.

flavour *See* TASTE; ORGANOLEPTIC.

flavour enhancer A substance that enhances or potentiates the flavours of other substances without itself imparting any characteristic flavour of its own, e.g. MONOSODIUM GLUTAMATE, RIBOTIDE, as well as small quantities of sugar, salt and vinegar.

flavour potentiator *See* FLAVOUR ENHANCER.

flavour profile A method of judging the flavour of foods by examination of a list of the separate factors into which the flavour can be analysed, the so-called character notes.

flavour scalping The adsorption of food flavours by packaging materials; may result in undesirable loss of flavour, or may be used to remove unwanted flavours in storage.

See also PACKAGING, ACTIVE.

flavours, biogenetic Flavours naturally present in a food.

flavours, synthetic Mostly mixtures of ESTERS, e.g. banana oil is ethyl butyrate and amyl acetate; apple oil is ethyl butyrate, ethyl valerianate, ethyl salicylate, amyl butyrate, glycerol, chloroform and alcohol; pineapple oil is ethyl and amyl butyrates, acetaldehyde, chloroform, glycerol, alcohol.

flavours, thermogenetic Flavours formed by heat treatment during food processing and cooking.

Flavr Savr^{TM} The first genetically modified tomato; approved by the US Food and Drug Administration in 1994, but not a commercial success.

flaxseed Seeds of *Linum usitatissimum*; also called linseed. Grown mainly as an oilseed (and for the fibre for textile use), but the seeds are also a rich source of PHYTOESTROGENS.

Composition/100 g: water 8.8 g, 2060 kJ (492 kcal), protein 19.5 g, fat 34 g (of which 10% saturated, 21% mono-unsaturated, 69% polyunsaturated), carbohydrate 34.3 g (1 g sugars), fibre 27.9 g, ash 3.5 g, Ca 199 mg, Fe 6.2 mg, Mg 362 mg, P 498 mg, K 681 mg, Na 34 mg, Zn 4.2 mg, Cu 1 mg, Mn 3.3 mg, Se 5.5 µg, 651 µg carotenoids, vitamin E 0.3 mg, B_1 0.17 mg, B_2 0.16 mg, niacin 1.4 mg, B_6 0.93 mg, folate 278 µg, pantothenate 1.5 mg, C 1 mg. A 10 g serving is a source of Mg, Mn, folate.

flea seed *See* PSYLLIUM.

fleishig   Jewish term for dishes containing meat, which cannot be served with or before milk dishes.

See also MILCHIG; PAREVE.

flint corn   See MAIZE.

flippers   See SWELLS.

floridean starch   A branched polysaccharide of glucose obtained from red algae (*Florideae* spp.).

florigens   See PHYTOCHROMES.

flounder   Small FLATFISH, *Platichthys* spp., also called fluke.

flour   Most commonly refers to ground wheat, although also used for other cereals and applied to powdered dried matter such as FISH FLOUR, potato flour, etc.

See also BREAD; FLOUR, EXTRACTION RATE.

flour, ageing and bleaching   See AGEING.

flour, agglomerated   A dispersible form, easily wetted, produced by agglomerating the fine particles in steam; particles are greater than 100 μm in diameter, so the flour is dust-free.

flour, air classified   Sieving cannot separate particles smaller than 80 μm, and for production of FLOUR with more precisely defined particle size it is subjected to centrifugation against an air current.

flour enrichment   The addition of vitamins and minerals to flour, to contain not less than: (UK) vitamin B_1 0.24 mg, niacin 1.6 mg, iron 1.65 mg, calcium 120 mg/100 g; (USA) vitamin B_1 0.44–0.56 mg, vitamin B_2 0.2–0.33 mg, niacin 3.6–4.4 mg, folic acid 140 μg, iron 2.9–3.7 mg/100 g; calcium not specified.

flour, enzyme inactivated   Flour in which the enzyme α-AMYLASE has been inactivated by heat to prevent degradation when the flour is used as a thickening agent in gravies, soups, etc.

flour, extraction rate   The yield of flour obtained from wheat in the milling process. 100% extraction (or straight-run flour) is wholemeal flour containing all of the grain; lower extraction rates are the whiter flours from which progressively more of the BRAN and GERM (and thus B vitamins and iron) have been removed, down to a figure of 72% extraction, which is normal white flour. 'Patent' flours are of lower extraction rate, 30–50%, and so comprise mostly the ENDOSPERM of the grain.

Wholemeal, composition/100 g: water 10.3 g, 1419 kJ (339 kcal), protein 13.7 g, fat 1.9 g (of which 23% saturated, 15% mono-unsaturated, 62% polyunsaturated), carbohydrate 72.6 g (0.4 g sugars), fibre 12.2 g, ash 1.6 g, Ca 34 mg, Fe 3.9 mg, Mg 138 mg, P 346 mg, K 405 mg, Na 5 mg, Zn 2.9 mg, Cu 0.4 mg, Mn 3.8 mg, Se 70.7 μg, 225 μg carotenoids, E 0.8 mg, K 1.9 mg, B_1 0.45 mg, B_2 0.22 mg, niacin 6.4 mg, B_6 0.34 mg, folate 44 μg, pantothenate 1 mg.

White, composition/100 g: water 11.9 g, 1524 kJ (364 kcal), protein 10.3 g, fat 1 g, carbohydrate 76.3 g (0.3 g sugars), fibre 2.7 g, ash 0.5 g, Ca 15 mg, Fe 4.6 mg, Mg 22 mg, P 108 mg, K 107 mg, Na 2 mg, Zn 0.7 mg, Cu 0.1 mg, Mn 0.7 mg, Se 33.9 µg, 18 µg carotenoids, E 0.1 mg, K 0.3 mg, B_1 0.79 mg, B_2 0.49 mg, niacin 5.9 mg, B_6 0.04 mg, folate 183 µg (if enriched), pantothenate 0.4 mg.

See also BREAD.

flour, high-ratio Flour of very fine, uniform particle size, treated with chlorine to reduce the GLUTEN strength. Used for making cakes, since it is possible to add up to 140 parts sugar to 100 parts of this flour, whereas only half this quantity of sugar can be incorporated into ordinary flour. *See* FLOUR STRENGTH.

flour improvers *See* AGEING.

flour, national *See* FLOUR, WHEATMEAL.

flour, patent *See* FLOUR, EXTRACTION RATE.

flour, self-raising Wheat flour to which BAKING POWDER has been added to produce carbon dioxide in the presence of water and heat; the dough is thus aerated without prolonged fermentation. Usually 'weaker' flours are used (*see* FLOUR STRENGTH). Legally, self-raising flour must contain not less than 0.4% available carbon dioxide.

flour strength A property of the flour proteins enabling the dough to retain gas during fermentation to give a 'bold' loaf. 'Strong' flour is higher in protein, has greater elasticity and resistance to extension, and greater ability to absorb water. A 'weak' flour gives a loaf that lacks volume.

See also EXTENSOMETER; FARINOGRAPH.

flour, wheatmeal Name given to 85% extraction flour (*see* FLOUR, EXTRACTION RATE) when introduced in the UK in February 1941; later called national flour. The term has been obsolete, and replaced by 'brown', since 1956.

flour, wholemeal Flour made from the entire grain of wheat, i.e. 100% extraction rate (*see* FLOUR, EXTRACTION RATE).

flow, streamline (or laminar) Flow of liquids in layers without significant mixing between layers.

fluence Energy imparted to the surface of a material by light.

fluid balance *See* WATER BALANCE.

fluid bed dryer A bed of solid particles supported on a cushion of hot air jets (fluidised); the material may be conveyed this way, while being dried. The method achieves mixing without mechanical damage; applied to cereals, tableting granules, salt, coffee and dried vegetables.

fluke (1) Small FLATFISH, *Platichthys* spp., also called FLOUNDER.

(2) Parasitic flatworms of the order Trematoda.

flummery Old English pudding made by boiling down the water from soaked oatmeal until it becomes thick and gelatinous. Similar to FRUMENTY. Dutch flummery is made with gelatine or isinglass and egg yolk; Spanish flummery with cream, rice flour and cinnamon.

Fluon *See* PTFE.

fluorescence The ability to absorb light at one wavelength and emit at another within 10–100 ns.

See also FLUORIMETRY.

fluorescence immunoassay Sensitive and specific analytical technique for determination of analytes present at very low concentrations in biological samples; the ANTIBODY is labelled with a substrate that yields a fluorescent product, but in such a way that it does not act as a substrate for the enzyme when the antigen (analyte) is bound. Therefore only free antibody will yield the fluorescent product when the enzyme is added. Unlike RADIO-IMMUNOASSAY, does not require separation of bound and free antigen.

See also ELISA.

fluoridation The addition of FLUORIDE to drinking water.

fluoride The ion of the element fluorine. Although it occurs in small amounts in plants and animals, and has effects on the formation of dental enamel and bones, it is not considered to be a dietary essential and no deficiency signs are known.

Drinking water containing about 1 part per million of fluoride protects teeth from decay, and in some areas fluoride is added to drinking water to achieve this level. Naturally, the fluoride content of water ranges between 0.05 and 14 ppm.

Water containing more than about 12 ppm fluoride can lead to chalky white patches on the surface of the teeth, known as mottled enamel. At higher levels there is strong brown mottling of the teeth and inappropriate deposition of fluoride in bones, fluorosis.

fluorimetry (fluorometry) Sensitive and relatively specific analytical technique dependent on emission of light more or less immediately (within 10–100 ns) after absorption of light by a compound in solution. Both the exciting and emitted wavelengths are characteristic of the analyte, and the intensity of fluorescence is proportional to the concentration of analyte present.

fluorodinitrobenzene (FDNB, dinitrofluorobenzene) Reacts with free amino groups; commonly used to determine free ε-amino groups of LYSINE (and hence AVAILABLE LYSINE) in proteins.

fluorosis Damage to teeth (brown mottling of the enamel) and bones caused by an excessive intake of FLUORIDE.

fluoxetine   An antidepressant acting to stimulate serotoninergic activity (a SEROTONIN-specific reuptake inhibitor); also has anorectic activity, and is used in treatment of OBESITY and BULIMIA NERVOSA. Trade name Prozac.

FMN   *See* FLAVIN MONONUCLEOTIDE.

FNIC   Food and Nutrition Information Center, located at the National Agricultural Library, part of the US Department of Agriculture; web site http://www.nal.usda.gov/fnic/.

FOAD   Fetal origins of adult disease, *see* EPIGENETICS; PROGRAMMING.

foam   Colloidal suspension (*see* COLLOID) of gas bubbles in a liquid or semi-liquid phase. Most so-called aerosol foams (e.g. whipped cream) are correctly foams, since an aerosol is a colloidal suspension of liquid droplets in a gas phase. Formation of foams can be a problem in manufacturing processes, and can be prevented by use of ANTIFOAMING AGENTS or mechanical means of eliminating the foam, such as heating, centrifuging, spraying or ultrasonic vibration.

foam cells   Macrophages that have accumulated very large amounts of CHOLESTEROL and other lipids as a result of uptake of (chemically modified) low-density LIPOPROTEIN. They infiltrate the arterial wall and lead to the development of fatty streaks, and eventually ATHEROSCLEROSIS.

foam-mat drying   A method of drying food. The liquid concentrate is whipped to a foam with the aid of a foaming agent, spread on a tray and dried in a stream of warm air. It can be reconstituted very rapidly with water because of the fine structure of the foam.

foie gras   (French, *fat liver*). The liver of goose or duck that has been force fed and fattened; may be cooked whole or used as the basis of PÂTÉ de foie gras, the most highly prized of the pâtés.

folacin, folate   *See* FOLIC ACID.

folate equivalents   *See* DIETARY FOLATE EQUIVALENTS.

folic acid   A VITAMIN that functions as a carrier of one-carbon units in a variety of metabolic reactions. Essential for the synthesis of purines and pyrimidines (and so for NUCLEIC ACID synthesis and hence cell division); the principal deficiency disease is megaloblastic ANAEMIA, due to failure of the normal maturation of red BLOOD CELLS, with release into the circulation of immature precursors of red blood cells.

Occurs in foods as a variety of one-carbon substituted derivatives, and with a varying number of γ-glutamyl residues. Mixed food folate is about 50% as biologically active as synthetic tetrahydrofolic acid used in enrichment and supplements.

Supplements of 400μg free folic acid/day begun before conception reduce the incidence of spina bifida and other neural

198

tube defects in babies; it is unlikely that ordinary foods could provide this much folate, so supplements are advised. In many countries flour is fortified with folate.

See also DIETARY FOLATE EQUIVALENTS; dUMP SUPPRESSION TEST; FIGLU TEST; HOMOCYSTEINE; METHYLENE TETRAHYDROFOLATE REDUCTASE.

FOLIC ACID

folinic acid 5-Formyl FOLIC ACID, more stable to oxidation than folic acid itself, and commonly used in pharmaceutical preparations. The synthetic (racemic) compound is known as leucovorin.

fondant Minute sugar crystals in a saturated sugar syrup; used as the creamy filling in chocolates and biscuits and for decorating cakes. Prepared by boiling sugar solution with the addition of GLUCOSE syrup or an inverting agent (*see* SUGAR, INVERT) and cooling rapidly while stirring.

fondue Swiss; cheese melted with wine and herbs, eaten by dipping small squares of bread into the hot mixture. Fondue bourguignonne is small cubes of marinated meat, cooked on a long fork in a vessel of hot oil at the table.

food Any solid or liquid material consumed by a living organism to supply ENERGY, build and replace tissue or participate in such reactions. Defined by the FAO/WHO CODEX ALIMENTARIUS Commission as a substance, whether processed, semiprocessed or raw, that is intended for human consumption and includes drink, chewing gum and any substance that has been used in the manufacture, preparation or treatment of food, but does not include cosmetics, tobacco or substances used only as drugs.

food balance A national account of the annual production of food, changes in stocks, imports and exports, and distribution of food over various uses in the country. Permits estimation of *per capita* food availability, but not consumption.

foodborne disease Infectious or toxic disease caused by agents that enter the body through the consumption of food. The causative agents may be present in food as a result of infection of animals from which food is prepared or contamination at source or during manufacture, storage and preparation.

Three main categories:

(1) diseases caused by micro-organisms (including parasites) that invade and multiply in the body;
(2) diseases caused by toxins produced by micro-organisms growing in the gastrointestinal tract;
(3) disease caused by the ingestion of food contaminated with poisonous chemicals or containing natural toxins or the toxins produced by micro-organisms in the food.

See also FOOD POISONING.

foodborne outbreak The consumption of contaminated food from one source by a number people who later become ill.

food combining *See* HAY DIET.

food composition tables Tables of the chemical composition and energy and nutrient yield of foods, based on chemical analysis. First American tables 'Chemical Composition of American Food Materials' published by USDA in 1896; first UK tables 'The Chemical Composition of Foods' by R A McCance and E M Widdowson published in 1940. Although the analyses are performed with great precision, they are, of necessity, only performed on a few samples of each type of food. There is considerable variation, especially in the content of vitamins and minerals, between different samples of the same food. Therefore, calculation of energy and nutrient intakes based on use of food composition tables, even when intake has been weighed, can be considered to be accurate to within only about ±10%, at best.

food intolerance *See* ADVERSE REACTIONS TO FOOD.

food intoxication Illness due to ingestion of toxic compounds naturally present in foods, resulting from chemical contamination or formed by micro-organisms.

See also ADVERSE REACTIONS TO FOOD; FOOD POISONING.

food phosphate factor Term applied to the resistance of bacteria to thermal destruction; defined as the ratio of the resistance to heat when present in a food to that when in phosphate buffer (at pH 6.98). The protective action of the ingredients of food renders the bacteria more resistant than when it is in the buffer.

food poisoning May be due to:

(1) contamination with harmful bacteria or other micro-organisms – the commonest bacterial contamination is due to *AEROMONAS* spp., *BACILLUS CEREUS*, *CAMPYLOBACTER* spp., *CLOSTRIDIUM* spp., *E. COLI*, *LISTERIA* spp., *SALMONELLA* spp., *SHIGELLA* spp., *STAPHYLOCOCCUS AUREUS*, *YERSINIA ENTEROCOLITICA*;

    (2) toxic chemicals, either naturally present or the result of contamination;

    (3) ADVERSE REACTIONS to certain proteins or other natural constituents of foods.

    See also DYSENTERY; ENTEROTOXINS; TX NUMBERS.

food pyramid A way of showing a healthy diet graphically, by grouping foods and the amounts of each group that should be eaten each day, based on dietary guidelines. Originally developed in the USA in 1992, and now adopted in many countries, with differences to allow for different national patterns of diet.

food science The study of the basic chemical, physical, biochemical and biophysical properties of foods and their constituents, and of changes that these may undergo during handling, preservation, processing, storage, distribution and preparation for consumption. Hence food scientist.

food technology The application of science and technology to the treatment, processing, preservation and distribution of foods. Hence food technologist.

food yeast *See* YEAST.

forcemeat A highly seasoned stuffing made from chopped minced veal, pork or sausage meat mixed with onion and range of herbs (Fr. *farce* = stuff).

formiminoglutamic acid *See* FIGLU TEST.

forming Moulding of dough and other materials into different shapes.

formula diet Composed of simple substances that do not require digestion, are readily absorbed and leave minimum residue in the intestine: glucose, amino acids or peptides, mono- and diglycerides rather than starch, proteins and fats.

formulation aids Compounds used to produce a desired physical state or texture in food, such as binders, fillers, plasticisers.

fortification The deliberate addition of specific nutrients to foods in order to increase their content, sometimes to a higher level than normal, as a means of providing the population with an increased level of intake. Generally synonymous with enrichment, supplementation and restoration; in the USA enrichment is used to mean the addition to foods of nutrients that they do not normally contain, while fortification is the restoration of nutrients lost in processing.

    See also WINE, FORTIFIED.

FOSHU Japanese term for FUNCTIONAL FOODS – Foods for Specified Health Use; processed foods containing ingredients that aid specific bodily functions, as well as being nutritious.

fouling Deposits of food or limescale on surfaces of heat exchangers.

four ale BEER originally sold at four pence per quart. The four ale bar is the public bar.

fovantini *See* PASTA.

FPLC (fast protein liquid chromatography) Modification of HPLC for separation of proteins under denaturing conditions.

fractional test meal A method of examining the secretion of gastric juices; the stomach contents are sampled at intervals after a test meal of gruel, and acidity (and sometimes also PEPSIN activity) is measured.

frangipane (frangipani) Originally a jasmine perfume which gave its name to an almond cream flavoured with the perfume. The term is used for a cake filling made from eggs, milk and flour with flavouring, and also for a pastry filled with an almond flavoured mixture.

frappé (1) Iced, frozen or chilled.

(2) Egg-white and sugar syrup whipped until so aerated that the density reaches 5 lb per gallon (100 g in 200 mL).

freedom food UK, animals maintained under relatively extensive conditions (but not FREE RANGE), with high standard of animal welfare monitored by the Royal Society for the Prevention of Cruelty to Animals.

free flow agents Alternative name for ANTICAKING AGENTS.

free from For a food label or advertising to bear a claim that it is free from fat, saturates, cholesterol, sodium or alcohol it must contain no more than a specified (low) amount. The precise levels at which such claims are permitted differ from one country to another. In the USA the food so described must contain only a trivial or physiologically insignificant amount of the specified nutrient.

free radical A highly reactive molecular species with an unpaired electron.

See also ANTIOXIDANT.

free range Applied to laying hens kept at no more than 1000 birds to the hectare with free access to open air and grass during daylight.

freeze concentration Concentration of a liquid by freezing out pure ice, leaving a more concentrated solution; it requires less input of energy, and causes less loss of flavour, than concentration by evaporation. Used especially in the concentration of fruit juices, VINEGAR and BEER.

See also APPLE JACK.

freeze drying Also known as lyophilisation. A method of drying in which the material is frozen and subjected to high vacuum.

The ice sublimes off as water vapour without melting. Freeze-dried food is very porous, since it occupies the same volume as the original and so rehydrates rapidly. There is less loss of flavour, texture and nutrients than with most other methods of drying. Controlled heat may be applied to the process without melting the frozen material; this is accelerated freeze drying.

freezerburn A change in the texture of frozen meat, fish and poultry during storage due to the sublimation of ice.

freezer, cryogenic Freezer using evaporating solid carbon dioxide or liquid nitrogen directly in contact with the food; the latent heat of sublimation or vaporisation comes from the food being treated.

freezer temperatures For long-term storage of frozen foods (up to 2–3 months), domestic freezers run at −18 °C (0 °F); in UK this is a three star rated deep freeze. A freezing compartment of a refrigerator (for short-term storage of frozen foods) is between −11 °C (12 °F), two star rated, for storage up to four weeks and −4 °C (25 °F), one star rated, for storage up to a week. A three star deep freeze with a snowflake symbol is one that is suitable for freezing foods, as opposed to storing ready-frozen food; it has a higher cooling capacity than a simple storage cabinet.

See also DATE MARKING.

freezing In blast freezing the food is frozen by a blast of cold air; small particle foods may be frozen as a fluidised bed, when it is supported on an upwards blast of cold air. Plate freezing involves contact of the food with vertical or horizontal plates of refrigerant-cooled metal. Cryogenic freezing involves direct contact of the food with the refrigerant, which is commonly liquid nitrogen or solid carbon dioxide.

freezing agents Compounds that reduce the temperature of foods through direct contact.

freezing plateau The period during freezing when the temperature of a food remains almost constant as the latent heat of crystallisation is removed and ice is formed.

freezing time, effective Time required to lower the temperature of the centre of a food to a predetermined final temperature.

frenching Breaking up the fibres of meat by cutting, usually diagonally or in a criss-cross pattern.

fresh For food labelling and advertising purposes, the US Food and Drug Administration has defined fresh to mean a food that is raw, has never been frozen or heated and contains no preservatives. (IRRADIATION at low levels is permitted.) 'Fresh frozen' and 'frozen fresh' may be used for foods that are quickly frozen while still fresh, and BLANCHING before freezing is permitted.

freshening *See* DEBRINING.

friability The hardness of a food and its tendency to crack.

frigi-canning A process of preserving food by controlled heating, sufficient to destroy the vegetative form of micro-organisms (and possibly to damage spores sufficiently to prevent germination) followed by sealing aseptically and storing at a low temperature, but above freezing point.

frijole bean *Phaseolus acutifolius*, also known as Mexican haricot bean, tepary or pinto. Able to withstand drought.

frijoles Mexican dish based on boiled fava or lima (butter) beans that have been left to cool, then fried. Also known as refried beans.

fromage frais (fromage blanc) French 'fresh cheese', soft, unripened CHEESE, 80% water, made from skim milk or semi-skim milk and may include added cream.
See also QUARK.

fructan (or fructosan) A general name for POLYSACCHARIDES of FRUCTOSE, such as INULIN. Not digested, and hence a part of dietary FIBRE or NON-STARCH POLYSACCHARIDES.

fructo-oligosaccharide A FRUCTAN, manufactured by the partial enzymic hydrolysis of INULIN. Used as a PREBIOTIC, as a soluble non-starch polysaccharide, to increase calcium absorption and as a bulk SWEETENER.
See also OLIGOSACCHARIDES.

fructose Also known as fruit sugar or laevulose. A six-carbon monosaccharide SUGAR (hexose) with a keto group on carbon-2. Found as the free sugar in fruits and honey, and as a constituent of the DISACCHARIDE SUCROSE. 1.7-times sweeter than sucrose.
See also CARBOHYDRATES; SUGAR, INVERT.

fruit Botanically, the part of a plant containing seeds; other parts of the plant are vegetables. In general usage, fruits are sweet or eaten sweetened (and hence include RHUBARB, which is leaf stalks, and hence a vegetable), while vegetables are savoury or eaten with salt (and hence include TOMATOES, which are fruits).
See also HERBS.

fruitarian A person who eats only fruits, nuts and seeds; an extreme form of VEGETARIAN.

fruit juice Legally defined in the UK as 100% pure fruit juices made from fresh fruit or fruit concentrates. Only the flesh may be used, not the pith or peel.

fruit leather Extruded mixtures of dried fruit purees and other ingredients (sugar, starch, glucose, acid and pectin), as a snack food.

frumenty An old English pudding made from whole wheat stewed in water for 24 h until the grains have burst and set in a thick jelly, then boiled with milk. Similar to FLUMMERY.

frying Cooking foods with oil at temperatures well above the boiling point of water. In shallow frying (or contact frying) the food is in direct contact with the hot surface of the pan and HEAT TRANSFER is mainly by conduction. In deep-fat frying, in which the food is completely covered with oil, heat transfer is by convection of the hot oil, and may reach a temperature around 185 °C. Nutrient losses are less than in roasting, about 10–20% thiamin, 10–15% riboflavin and niacin from meat; about 20% thiamin from fish.

FSA UK Food Standards Agency; web site http://www.food.gov. uk/.

fudge CARAMEL in which crystallisation of the sugar (graining) is deliberately induced by the addition of FONDANT (saturated SYRUP containing sugar crystals).

fugu The Japanese puffer fish, *Fuga* spp., responsible for TETRODONTIN POISONING.

fuki A herb, *Petasites japonicus*, also known as Japanese butterbur, sweet coltsfoot.

Composition/100 g: (edible portion 88%) water 94.5 g, 59 kJ (14 kcal), protein 0.4 g, fat 0 g, carbohydrate 3.6 g, ash 1.5 g, Ca 103 mg, Fe 0.1 mg, Mg 14 mg, P 12 mg, K 655 mg, Na 7 mg, Zn 0.2 mg, Cu 0.1 mg, Mn 0.3 mg, Se 0.9 μg, vitamin A 3 μg RE, B_1 0.02 mg, B_2 0.02 mg, niacin 0.2 mg, B_6 0.1 mg, folate 10 μg, C 32 mg.

fula W African; dumplings made from millet that has been steeped in water overnight, to undergo a bacterial lactic acid fermentation, then boiled.

fuller's earth An adsorbent clay, calcium montmorillonite, or bentonite; adsorbs both by physical means and by ion exchange. Used to bleach oils, clarify liquids and absorb grease.

fumaric acid Unsaturated dicarboxylic acid, used as an ACIDULANT.

fumeol Refined smoke with the bitter principles removed; used for preparing 'liquid' smokes for dipping foods such as fish to give them a smoked flavour.

See also SMOKING.

fumigants Volatile compounds used for controlling insects or pests.

fumonisins A group of carcinogenic MYCOTOXINS from *Fusarium* spp. growing on cereals; inhibits synthesis of ceramides by inhibition of sphingosine *N*-acetyltransferase (EC 2.3.1.24).

functional foods Foods eaten for specified health purposes, because of their (rich) content of one or more nutrients or non-nutrient substances which may confer health benefits.

fungal protein *See* MYCOPROTEIN.

fungi Subdivision of Thallophyta, plants without differentiation into root, stem and leaf; cannot photosynthesise, all are parasites or saprophytes. Microfungi are MOULDS, as opposed to larger fungi, which are mushrooms and toadstools. YEASTS are sometimes classed with fungi. Mycorrhizal fungi form symbiotic associations with tree roots.

Species of moulds such as *Penicillium*, *Aspergillus*, etc. are important causes of food spoilage in the presence of oxygen and relatively high humidity. Those that produce toxins (MYCOTOXINS) are especially problematical.

On the other hand, species of *Penicillium* such as *P. cambertii* and *P. rocquefortii* are desirable and essential in the ripening of some types of CHEESE.

A number of larger fungi (MUSHROOMS) are cultivated, and other wild species are harvested for their delicate flavour. The mycelium of smaller fungi (including *Graphium*, *Fusarium* and *Rhizopus* spp.) are grown commercially on waste carbohydrate as a rich source of protein (MYCOPROTEIN) for food manufacture.

furans Derivatives of five-membered heterocyclic compounds (C_4H_4O), associated with caramel-like, sweet, fruity, nutty and meaty flavours in foods; formed in foods by the MAILLARD REACTION and thermal degradation of carbohydrates.

furcellaran Danish agar; an anionic, sulphated polysaccharide extracted from the red alga, *Furcellaria fastigiata*, structurally similar to CARRAGEENAN; used as a gelling agent.

fusel oil Alcoholic fermentation produces about 95% alcohol and 5% fusel oil, a mixture of organic acids, higher alcohols (propyl, butyl and amyl), aldehydes and esters, known collectively as CONGENERS. Present in low concentration in wines and beer, and high concentration in pot-still spirit. On maturation of the liquor fusel oil changes and imparts the special flavour to the spirit. Many of the symptoms of HANGOVER can be attributed to fusel oil in alcoholic beverages.

fussol Monofluoroacetamide, a systemic insecticide for treating fruit.

F value The time required to destroy a given percentage of microorganisms at a specified reference temperature and Z VALUE.

G

gaffelbitar Semi-preserved HERRING in which microbial growth is checked by the addition of 10–12% salt and sometimes BENZOIC ACID.

galactans POLYSACCHARIDES composed of GALACTOSE derivatives; a major constituent of CARAGEENAN.

galacticol *See* DULCITOL.

Galactomin™ A preparation free from lactose and galactose, for people suffering from lactose intolerance.

galacto-oligosaccharides Small OLIGOSACCHARIDES consisting of glucosyl-(galactose)$_{2-5}$, formed from LACTOSE by galactosyl transfer catalysed by LACTASE (EC 3.2.1.23). Considered to be a PREBIOTIC.

galactorrhoea Abnormal secretion of milk, due to excessive secretion of PROLACTIN.

galactosaemia Congenital lack of UDP-glucose galactosyltransferase (EC 2.7.7.12), or more rarely galactokinase (EC 2.7.1.6) leading to elevated blood concentration of GALACTOSE, and hence non-enzymic GLYCATION of proteins, and the development of cataract and neurological damage; subjects suffer mental retardation, growth failure, vomiting and jaundice, with enlargement of liver and spleen. Treatment is by severe restriction of LACTOSE intake, since this is the only significant source of galactose.

galactose A six-carbon monosaccharide (hexose), differing from GLUCOSE in orientation of the hydroxyl group on carbon-4. About one-third as sweet as sucrose. The main dietary source is the disaccharide LACTOSE in milk, important in formation of the galactolipids (cerebrosides) of nerve tissue.

See also CARBOHYDRATES; GALACTOSAEMIA.

β-galactosidase Enzyme (EC 3.2.1.23) that hydrolyses β-galactans in NON-STARCH POLYSACCHARIDES; responsible for loss of firmness during ripening and storage of fruits.

galangal Root spices (*Alpinia galanga, A. officinarum*) related to ginger, but with a faint flavour of camphor.

Galanol™ BORAGE seed oil, a rich source of γ-LINOLENIC ACID, as a dietary supplement.

galenicals Crude drugs; infusions, decoctions and tinctures prepared from medicinal plants.

gallates Salts and esters of gallic acid, found in many plants. Used in making dyes and inks, and medicinally as an astringent. Propyl, octyl and dodecyl gallates are legally permitted antioxidants in foods (E-310–312).

gall bladder The gland in the liver that stores the BILE before secretion into the small intestine.

See also GALLSTONES; GASTROINTESTINAL TRACT.

gallon A unit of volume. The Imperial gallon is 4.546 litres, and the US (or Queen Anne) gallon is 3.7853 litres; therefore 1 Imperial gallon = 1.2 US gallons.

gallstones (cholelithiasis) Crystals of cholesterol, bile salts and calcium salts, formed in the bile duct of the GALL BLADDER when the bile becomes supersaturated.

game Non-domesticated (i.e. wild) animals and birds shot for sport and eaten. RABBIT and PIGEON may be shot at any time, but other game species, such as GROUSE, HARE, PARTRIDGE, PHEASANT, QUAIL, deer (VENISON) and wild DUCK, may not be shot during the closed season, to protect breeding stocks. Game birds are generally raised on farms to provide sport, rather than being hunted in the wild, and increasingly game species are farmed and killed in conventional ways to provide food. Traditionally, game is hung for several days to soften the meat, when it develops a strong flavour.

gammelost Norwegian dark brown cheese with mould growth on the rind that is pressed into the paste while it is ripening.

gammon *See* BACON.

gangliosides Glycolipids, structurally similar to cerebrosides, but with a charged polar oligosaccharide head region.

garam masala A mixture of aromatic spices widely used in Indian cooking; contains powdered black pepper, cumin, cinnamon, cloves, mace, cardamom seeds and sometimes also coriander and/or bay leaf.

garbanzo *See* CHICKPEA.

garbellers 15th century; people appointed by the Grocers' Company of London to inspect spices and other groceries, and destroy adulterated products.

gari Fermented CASSAVA meal. Cassava is grated, soaked in water and left to undergo bacterial fermentation for 2–5 days in permeable sacks so that liquid drains out; the resulting solid mass is sieved and lightly toasted or fried (garified).

garlic The bulb of *Allium sativum* with a pungent odour when crushed, widely used to flavour foods. There is some evidence that garlic has a beneficial effect in lowering blood CHOLESTEROL.

Composition/100 g: (edible portion 87%) water 58.6 g, 624 kJ (149 kcal), protein 6.4 g, fat 0.5 g, carbohydrate 33.1 g (1 g sugars), fibre 2.1 g, ash 1.5 g, Ca 181 mg, Fe 1.7 mg, Mg 25 mg, P 153 mg, K 401 mg, Na 17 mg, Zn 1.2 mg, Cu 0.3 mg, Mn 1.7 mg, Se 14.2 µg, 26 µg carotenoids, vitamin K 1.4 mg, B_1 0.2 mg, B_2 0.11 mg, niacin 0.7 mg, B_6 1.24 mg, folate 3 µg, pantothenate 0.6 mg, C 31 mg.

garlic mustard A common wild plant of hedgerows and woodland (*Alliaria petiolata*); the leaves have a garlic-like flavour and can be used in salads or cooked as a vegetable.

gas storage, controlled (modified) *See* PACKAGING, MODIFIED ATMOSPHERE.

gastrectomy Surgical removal of part or all of the stomach.

gastric inhibitory peptide Peptide HORMONE secreted by the mucosa of the duodenum and jejunum in response to absorbed fat and carbohydrate; stimulates the pancreas to secrete INSULIN. Also known as glucose-dependent insulinotropic polypeptide.

gastric secretion   Gastric juice contains the enzymes CHYMOSIN (EC 3.4.23.4), LIPASE (EC 3.1.1.3), pepsinogen (the inactive precursor of PEPSIN, EC 3.4.23.1), INTRINSIC FACTOR, MUCIN and hydrochloric acid.

The acid is secreted by the parietal (oxyntic) cells at a strength of 0.16 mol/L (0.5–0.6% acid); the same cells also secrete INTRINSIC FACTOR, and failure of acid secretion (ACHLORHYDRIA) is associated with pernicious ANAEMIA due to failure of VITAMIN B_{12} absorption.

Pepsinogen is secreted by the chief cells of the gastric mucosa, and is activated to pepsin by either gastric acid or the action of existing pepsin; it is a proteolytic enzyme (*see* PROTEOLYSIS).

See also ANAEMIA, PERNICIOUS; PROTON PUMP.

gastric ulcer   *See* ULCER.

gastrin   Peptide hormone secreted by G-cells of the antrum of the stomach; stimulates PARIETAL CELLS to secrete acid.

gastroenteritis   Inflammation of the mucosal lining of the stomach (gastritis) and/or small or large intestine, normally resulting from infection, or, in the case of gastritis, from excessive alcohol consumption.

gastroenterology   The study and treatment of diseases of the GASTROINTESTINAL TRACT.

gastrointestinal tract   (*see* p. 209) A term for the whole of the digestive tract, from the mouth to the anus. Average length 4.5 m (15 feet).

gastrolith   Stone in the stomach, usually builds up around a BEZOAR.

gastroplasty   Surgical alteration of the shape of the stomach without removing any part. Has been used to reduce the physical capacity of the stomach as a treatment for severe OBESITY.

gastrostomy feeding   Feeding a liquid diet directly into the stomach through a tube that has been surgically introduced through the abdominal wall.

See also ENTERAL NUTRITION; NASOGASTRIC TUBE.

Gatorade™   A sports drink containing mineral salts in approximately the proportions they are lost in sweat.

gavage   The process of feeding liquids by stomach tube. Also feeding an excessive amount (hyperalimentation).

GC-MS   Gas CHROMATOGRAPHY linked to a mass spectrometer as the detection system.

gean   Scottish name for the fruit of *Prunus avium*; also known as wild cherry, sweet cherry and mazzard.

gefilte fish (gefilte, gefültte)   German for stuffed fish; of Russian or Polish origin, where it is commonly referred to as Jewish fish.

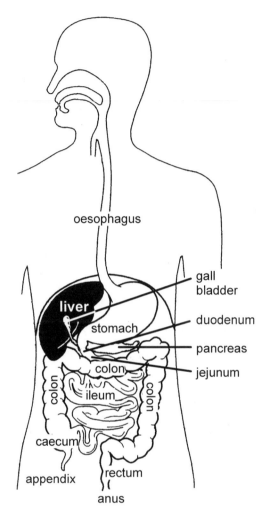

oesophagus

gall
bladder

liver

duodenum

stomach

pancreas

jejunum

colon

colon

colon

ileum

caecum

appendix

rectum

anus

GASTROINTESTINAL TRACT

The whole fish is served and the filleted portion chopped and stuffed back between the skin and the backbone. More frequently today, the fish is simply chopped and made into balls, which are either fried or boiled. In the UK has been referred to legally as 'fish cutlets in fish sauce' instead of a fish cake.

gel Colloidal suspension (*see* COLLOID) consisting of a continuous phase (commonly water) and a dispersed phase (the gelling agent); the water molecules are held in a three-dimensional network of the gelling agent. Examples include plant GUMS, GELATINE, PECTIN.

gelatine   A soluble protein prepared from COLLAGEN or bones by boiling. Type A is prepared by acid treatment of collagen and has an isoionic point of 7–9. Type B is prepared by alkaline treatment and has an isoionic point of 4.8–5.2 because of loss of the amide groups of glutamine and asparagine. Used for sugar confectionery, in canned meats, for table jellies and in pharmaceutical capsules. Gelatine from fish (especially the swim bladder) is ISINGLASS. Gelatine has an unusual amino acid composition: 14% hydroxyproline, 16% proline and 26% glycine; of poor nutritional value, since it lacks TRYPTOPHAN. Chinese gelatine is AGAR.

gelatine sugar   Obsolete name for GLYCINE.

gelatinisation   Formation of a water-retentive gel by expansion of starch granules when heated in moist conditions.
    See also STALING.

gelation   The formation of the PECTIN gel that gives fruit preserves and jams their texture; dependent on the pectin, sugar, acid and water content of the fruit.

gellan gum   A POLYSACCHARIDE produced by fermentation of the bacterium *Sphingomonas elodea* (*Pseudomonas elodea*), used in some foods.

gelograph   Instrument for measuring the VISCOSITY or gel strength of a protein (or other) solution using an oscillating needle.

gelometer   *See* BLOOM GELOMETER.

gemfibrizol   *See* FIBRIC ACIDS.

generic descriptor   The name used to cover the different chemical forms of a VITAMIN that have the same biological activity.

genetic diseases   Also known as inborn errors of metabolism. Diseases due to a single defective gene, with a characteristic pattern of inheritance in families. Many affect the ability to metabolise individual amino acids or carbohydrates and can be treated by dietary restriction.
    See also AMINO ACID DISORDERS; DISACCHARIDE INTOLERANCE.

genetic modification   A change in the genes of a living organism, as occurs in nature, and which has been used for many years in selective breeding, or, more quickly and specifically, in the laboratory, when genes from another organism may be introduced (sometimes known as genetic engineering).
    See also GM FOODS; SUBSTANTIAL EQUIVALENCE.

genome   The complete genetic sequence of an organism, hence the science of genomics.

genomics, nutritional   General term to include both NUTRIGENETICS and NUTRIGENOMICS.

gentiobiose   A disaccharide consisting of two molecules of glucose joined β-1,6.

Gentleman's relish™   A paste of anchovies, butter, cereal, salt and spices developed in the UK in the 19th century; also called patum peperium.

geophagia   Eating of dirt or soil.

See also PICA.

geosmin   Dimethyl-bicyclodecanol; microbial metabolite that can cause earthy or musty off-flavour in fish and drinking water.

GEP   Gas exchange preservation, *see* PACKAGING, MODIFIED ATMOSPHERE.

Gerber test   For fat (CREAM) in milk. The milk is mixed with sulphuric acid (or detergent) and amyl alcohol; the protein and carbohydrate are dissolved, and the fat separates out. The reaction is carried out in a Gerber bottle with a thin graduated neck, in which the fat collects for measurement after centrifugation.

germ, wheat   The embryo or sprouting portion of the WHEAT berry, comprising about 2.5% of the seed. Contains 64% of the vitamin B_1, 26% of the vitamin B_2, 21% of the vitamin B_6 and most of the fat of the grain. It is discarded, with the bran, when the grain is milled to white FLOUR.

Wheat germ oil is 20% saturated, 16% mono-unsaturated, 65% polyunsaturated, contains 149 mg vitamin E, 25 mg vitamin K/100 g.

See also FLOUR, EXTRACTION RATE.

geuse (gueuze)   *See* BEER.

GFP   *See* GREEN FLUORESCENT PROTEIN.

ghatti gum   Or Indian gum, polysaccharide exudate of the tree *Anogeissus latifolia*. The gum is formed as a protective sealant when the bark. Used in the same way as GUM ARABIC.

ghee (or ghrt)   Clarified BUTTER fat; may also be made from vegetable oils.

Composition/100 g: water 0.2 g, 3667 kJ (876 kcal), protein 0.3 g, fat 99.5 g (of which 66% saturated, 30% mono-unsaturated, 4% polyunsaturated), cholesterol 256 mg, carbohydrate 0 g, Ca 4 mg, P 3 mg, K 5 mg, Na 2 mg, vitamin A 840 µg RE (824 µg retinol, 193 µg carotenoids), E 2.8 mg, K 8.6 mg.

gherkin   Young green CUCUMBER of a small variety (*Cucumis anguira*), used mainly for pickling.

ghrelin   A peptide HORMONE secreted by cells in the gastrointestinal tract that both stimulates the secretion of growth hormone and regulates feeding behaviour and energy balance by acting on the hypothalamus. Secretion is increased in the fasting state and under conditions of negative energy balance, and decreased under conditions of positive energy balance. Secretion is increased in anorexia and is low in the fasting state in obese people.

ghrt *See* GHEE.

giardiasis Intestinal inflammation and DIARRHOEA caused by infection with the protozoan parasite *Giardia lamblia*.

gibberellins Plant growth substances derived from gibberellic acid, originally found in the fungus *Gibberella fujikori* growing on rice. About 30 gibberellins are known; they cause stem extension and allow mutant dwarf forms of plants to revert to normal size, induce flower formation and break bud dormancy. Used in horticulture to control flowering and fruit maturation, also to induce α-AMYLASE in malting (*see* MALT) of barley.

giblets The edible part of the entrails of a bird; gizzard, liver, heart and neck.

gigot French; leg of lamb or mutton. In Ireland gigot chops are neck chops used for stewing.

gill Obsolete British measure of liquid, 5 or 10 fl oz ($\frac{1}{4}$ or $\frac{1}{2}$ pint), varying regionally.

gin Alcoholic drink made by distilling fermented starch or other carbohydrate, flavoured mainly with juniper berries together with coriander seeds, angelica, cinnamon, orange and lemon peel. Distillate is diluted to 40% ALCOHOL by volume, 925 kJ (220 kcal)/100 mL. Name derived from French *genièvre* (juniper); originally known as geneva, schiedam or hollands, since it is Dutch in origin.

There are two types of English gin: Plymouth gin with a fuller flavour, and London gin. Plymouth gin has a protected designation and legally may only be distilled in Plymouth; it is made by adding the botanicals to the still, while for London gin they are added to the distilled liquor.

Dutch and German gins are more strongly flavoured than English or American; steinhäger and schinkenhäger are distilled from a mash of wheat, barley and juniper berries; wacholder is made from neutral spirit flavoured with juniper. Dutch gin may be *jonge* (young) or *oude* (aged, matured).

gingelly (gingili) *See* SESAME.

ginger The rhizome of *Zingiber officinale*, used as a spice. Preserved ginger is made from young fleshy rhizomes boiled with sugar and either packed in syrup or crystallised.

Fresh ginger, composition/100 g: (edible portion 93%) water 78.9 g, 335 kJ (80 kcal), protein 1.8 g, fat 0.8 g, carbohydrate 17.8 g (1.7 g sugars), fibre 2 g, ash 0.8 g, Ca 16 mg, Fe 0.6 mg, Mg 43 mg, P 34 mg, K 415 mg, Na 13 mg, Zn 0.3 mg, Cu 0.2 mg, Mn 0.2 mg, Se 0.7 µg, E 0.3 mg, K 0.1 mg, B_1 0.03 mg, B_2 0.03 mg, niacin 0.8 mg, B_6 0.16 mg, folate 11 µg, pantothenate 0.2 mg, C 5 mg.

ginger beer Alcoholic beverage made by fermenting a sugar solution flavoured with GINGER.

ginger paralysis   *See* JAMAICA GINGER PARALYSIS.

gingivitis   Inflammation, swelling and bleeding of the gums; may be due to SCURVY, but most commonly the result of poor oral hygiene.

gingko   The maidenhair tree, *Gingko biloba*. The seeds are edible when roasted but may be toxic when raw. Extracts from the leaves are used as a herbal remedy; they contain potentially active FLAVONOIDS and TERPENES, but there is limited evidence of efficacy.

gin-nan   Food poisoning associated with excessive consumption of GINGKO seeds, especially if uncooked.

ginseng   Herbal products from the roots of three species; Korean or Chinese ginseng is *Panax ginseng*, Siberian is *Eleutherococcus senticosus*; American is *P. quinquefolius*. Reported to have an immunostimulant action and act as a tonic, with limited evidence of efficacy.

GIP   Glucose-dependent insulinotropic peptide, originally thought to act as inhibitor of gastric acid secretion based and named Gastric Inhibitory Peptide. Like GLP-1, it stimulates INSULIN secretion (hence the higher insulin response to oral than to intravenous glucose).

   See also INCRETINS.

gipping (of fish)   Partial evisceration to remove intestines but not pyloric caeca, which contain the enzymes responsible for the characteristic flavour of HERRING when it is subsequently salted.

gjetost   Norwegian sweet, semi-caramelised hard cheese made from whey. Normally goat milk; mysost is similar, made from cow milk.

   Composition/100 g: water 13.4 g, 1951 kJ (466 kcal), protein 9.6 g, fat 29.5 g (of which 69% saturated, 28% mono-unsaturated, 3% polyunsaturated), cholesterol 94 mg, carbohydrate 42.7 g, ash 4.8 g, Ca 400 mg, Fe 0.5 mg, Mg 70 mg, P 444 mg, K 1409 mg, Na 600 mg, Zn 1.1 mg, Cu 0.1 mg, Se 14.5 µg, vitamin A 334 µg retinol, B_1 0.31 mg, B_2 1.38 mg, niacin 0.8 mg, B_6 0.27 mg, folate 5 µg, B_{12} 2.4 µg, pantothenate 3.4 mg. A 40 g serving is a source of vitamin A, a good source of Ca, P, pantothenate, a rich source of vitamin B_2, B_{12}.

Glamorgan sausage   Welsh; dish based on Caerphilly cheese, breadcrumbs and egg, fried in sausage shape.

Glanolin™   BLACKCURRANT seed oil, a rich source of γ-LINOLENIC ACID, as a dietary supplement.

Glasgow magistrate   *See* RED HERRING.

glass transition temperature   In sugar confectionery, the temperature at which a rubbery gel becomes a clear glass, a change that does not involve latent heat.

gliadin A PROLAMIN, one of the proteins that make up wheat GLUTEN. Allergy to, or intolerance of, gliadin is COELIAC DISEASE.

globins PROTEINS that are rich in the AMINO ACID HISTIDINE (and hence basic), relatively deficient in ISOLEUCINE. Often found as the protein part of conjugated proteins such as haemoglobin.

globulins Class of PROTEINS that are heat-coagulatable and soluble in dilute solutions of salts; they differ from ALBUMINS in being relatively insoluble in water. They occur in blood (serum globulins), milk (lactoglobulins) and some plants, e.g. edestin from hemp seed and amandin from almonds.

glossitis Inflammation of the tongue; may be one of the signs of RIBOFLAVIN deficiency.

GLP-1 Glucagon-like peptide-1, a peptide HORMONE secreted by cells of the distal ileum in response to food intake; formed by post-synthetic modification of PROGLUCAGON. Like GIP it stimulates INSULIN secretion (hence the higher insulin response to oral than to intravenous glucose).

> *See also* INCRETINS.

glucagon Peptide HORMONE secreted by the α-islet cells of the PANCREAS. Elevates blood glucose by increasing the breakdown of liver GLYCOGEN and stimulating GLUCONEOGENESIS.

glucagon-like peptide Peptide hormone secreted by the terminal ileum; increases secretion of INSULIN and decreases that of GLUCAGON.

glucans Soluble undigested polysaccharides of glucose; found particularly in OATS, BARLEY and RYE.

> *See also* FIBRE, SOLUBLE; NON-STARCH POLYSACCHARIDES.

glucaric acid Or saccharic acid, the dicarboxylic acid derived from glucose.

glucide (gluside) Name occasionally used for SACCHARIN.

glucitol Obsolete name for SORBITOL.

glucoamylase *See* AMYLASE; DEBRANCHING ENZYME.

glucocorticoids The STEROID HORMONES secreted by the adrenal cortex (*see* ADRENAL GLANDS), which regulate carbohydrate metabolism.

> *See also* CORTICOSTEROIDS.

glucokinase An isoenzyme of HEXOKINASE (EC 2.7.1.1), with a high K_m, found only in liver and β-islet cells of the pancreas. One type of a rare form of DIABETES mellitus (MODY, maturity onset diabetes of the young) is due to a genetic defect in glucokinase.

glucomannan A polysaccharide consisting of glucose and mannose.

gluconeogenesis The synthesis of glucose from non-carbohydrate precursors, such as lactate, pyruvate, glycerol and glucogenic AMINO ACIDS.

gluconic acid   The acid formed by oxidation of the hydroxyl group on carbon-1 of glucose to a carboxylic acid group. Also termed dextronic acid, maltonic acid and glycogenic acid.

glucono-δ-lactone   GLUCONIC ACID lactone; liberates acid slowly, and used in chemically leavened (aerated) BREAD to form carbon dioxide from bicarbonate.

glucosaccharic acid   *See* SACCHARIC ACID.

glucosamine   The amino derivative of GLUCOSE, a constituent of a variety of complex POLYSACCHARIDES.

glucosan   A general term for polysaccharides of GLUCOSE, such as STARCH, CELLULOSE and GLYCOGEN.

glucose   A six-carbon monosaccharide sugar (hexose), with the chemical formula $C_6H_{12}O_6$, occurring free in plant and animal tissues and formed by the hydrolysis of STARCH and GLYCOGEN. Also known as dextrose, grape sugar and blood sugar.

The CARBOHYDRATE in blood is glucose; normal concentration is between 4.5 and 5.5 mmol/L (80–100 mg/100 mL). In the fed state, glucose is used for the synthesis of GLYCOGEN in liver and muscle, as well as for synthesis of fats; in the fasting state, glycogen is hydrolysed as a source of glucose to maintain the blood concentration.

Used in the manufacture of SUGAR CONFECTIONERY when it is sometimes known as DEXTROSE. The mixture with FRUCTOSE prevents sucrose from crystallising. It is 74% as sweet as sucrose.

glucose, confectioners'   Glucose SYRUPS are known as glucose in confectionery making (GLUCOSE is referred to as DEXTROSE).

glucose isomerase   Bacterial enzyme (EC 5.3.1.5) that catalyses isomerisation of glucose to fructose. Used in the production of FRUCTOSE syrups. Main commercial source is *Streptomyces* spp.

glucose metabolism   Series of reactions in which glucose is oxidised to carbon dioxide and water as a metabolic fuel (i.e. to provide energy). The overall reaction is: $C_6H_{12}O_6 + 6O_2 \rightarrow 6CO_2 + 6H_2O$, yielding 16.4 kJ (3.9 kcal)/g, or 2.88 MJ (686 kcal)/mol.

The first sequence of reactions does not require oxygen and is referred to as (anaerobic) glycolysis or glucose fermentation, yielding two molecules of the three-carbon compound pyruvate. Under anaerobic conditions this can be reduced to LACTIC ACID. Pyruvate is normally oxidised to acetyl CoA, which is then oxidised to carbon dioxide and water via the citric acid or Krebs cycle. Both glycolysis and the citric acid cycle are linked to the formation of ATP from ADP and phosphate, as a metabolically usable energy source.

An alternative to part of glycolysis, the pentose phosphate pathway or hexose monophosphate shunt, is important in the formation of reduced NADPH for FATTY ACID synthesis.

glucose oxidase   Enzyme (EC 1.1.3.4) that oxidises glucose to gluconic acid, with the formation of hydrogen peroxide. Used for specific quantitative determination of glucose, including urine and blood glucose, and to remove traces of glucose from foodstuffs (e.g. from dried egg to prevent the MAILLARD REACTION during storage). Also used to remove traces of oxygen from products such as beer, wine, fruit juices and mayonnaise to prevent oxidative rancidity. Originally isolated from *Penicillium notatum* and called notatin; main commercial source is *Aspergillus niger*.

glucose6-phosphate dehydrogenase deficiency   *See* FAVISM.

glucose syrups   *See* SYRUP; DEXTROSE EQUIVALENT VALUE.

glucose tolerance   The ability of the body to deal with a relatively large dose of glucose is used as a test for DIABETES mellitus. The fasting subject ingests 50 or 75 g of glucose (sometimes calculated as 1 g/kg body weight) and the concentration of blood glucose is measured at intervals. In normal subjects the fasting glucose concentration is between 4.5 and 5.5 mmol/L, and rises to about 7.5 mmol/L, returning to the starting level within $1-1\frac{1}{2}$ h. In diabetes, it rises considerably higher and takes longer to return to the baseline value. The graph of the results forms a glucose tolerance curve.

glucose tolerance factor (GTF)   Organic chelate of CHROMIUM, M_r around 1500, variously reported to contain NICOTINIC ACID (see NIACIN), GLUTATHIONE and other amino acid derivatives. Potentiates the action of INSULIN, but has no activity in the absence of insulin. Acts by increasing the protein kinase activity of the insulin receptor when insulin is bound.

glucosides   *See* GLYCOSIDES.

glucosinolates   Substances occurring widely in *Brassica* spp. (e.g. Brussels sprouts, cabbage, watercress, radishes); broken down by the enzyme myrosinase (thioglucosidase, EC 3.2.3.1) to yield, among other products, the mustard oils which are responsible for the pungent flavour (especially in mustard and horseradish).

Several of the glucosinolates that are thioesters interfere with the metabolism of IODINE by the thyroid gland (*see* THYROID HORMONES), and hence are GOITROGENS. There is evidence that the various glucosinolates in vegetables may have useful anticancer activity, since they increase the rate at which a variety of potentially toxic and carcinogenic compounds are conjugated and excreted (PHASE II METABOLISM).

glucostatic mechanism   A theory that appetite depends on the difference between arterial and venous concentrations of glucose; when the difference falls, the hunger centres in the hypothalamus are stimulated.

glucosuria (also glycosuria)   Appearance of GLUCOSE in the urine, as in DIABETES and after the administration of drugs that lower the renal threshold.

glucuronic acid   The acid derived from glucose by the oxidation of the hydroxyl group on carbon-6. Many substances, including hormones and potentially toxic ingested substances, are excreted as conjugates with glucuronic acid, known as glucuronides. It is present in various complex polysaccharides.

glucuronides   A variety of compounds are metabolised by conjugation with GLUCURONIC ACID to yield water-soluble derivatives for excretion from the body (*see* PHASE II METABOLISM).

glutamic acid   A non-essential AMINO ACID; abbr Glu (E), M_r 147.1, pK_a 2.10, 4.07, 9.47, CODONS GAPu. Acidic since it has two carboxylic acid groups; the amide is GLUTAMINE.

See also MONOSODIUM GLUTAMATE.

glutamine   A non-essential amino acid, abbr Gln (Q), M_r 146.1, pK_a 2.17, 9.13, CODONS CAPu. The amide of GLUTAMIC ACID.

glutathione   A tripeptide, γ-glutamyl-cysteinyl-glycine (GSH). Important in protection against oxidative damage, since it can be oxidised to the disulphide compound (GSSG), which can then be reduced back to active glutathione. Also important in PHASE II METABOLISM of foreign compounds, yielding mercapturic acids as a result of *S*-conjugation, and in the transport of amino acids into cells.

glutathione peroxidase   SELENIUM-containing enzyme (EC 1.11.1.9) that protects tissues from oxidative damage by removing peroxides resulting from free radical action, linked to oxidation of GLUTATHIONE; part of the body's ANTIOXIDANT protection. Low activity in red blood cells indicates selenium deficiency, but not useful as an index of marginal status.

glutathione reductase   Enzyme (EC 1.6.4.2) that catalyses the reduction of oxidised GLUTATHIONE (GSSG) to glutathione (GSH), and hence an important antioxidant system. Activation of this enzyme *in vitro* by added cofactor (flavin adenine dinucleotide, derived from vitamin B_2) provides a means of assessing VITAMIN B_2 nutritional status, sometimes known as the erythrocyte glutathione reductase activation coefficient (EGRAC) test. An activation coefficient above 1.7 indicates deficiency.

See also ENZYME ACTIVATION ASSAYS.

glutelins   Proteins insoluble in water and neutral salt solutions but soluble in dilute acids and alkalis, e.g. wheat glutenin.

gluten The protein complex in WHEAT, and to a lesser extent RYE, which gives dough the viscid property that holds gas when it rises. None in OATS, BARLEY, MAIZE. It is a mixture of two proteins, gliadin and glutelin. Allergy to, or intolerance of, the gliadin fraction of gluten is COELIAC DISEASE (gluten-sensitive enteropathy). In the undamaged state with extensible properties it is termed vital gluten; when overheated, these properties are lost and the product is termed devitalised gluten, used for protein enrichment of foods.

gluten-free foods Formulated without any WHEAT or RYE protein (although the starch may be used) for people suffering from COELIAC DISEASE.

gluten-sensitive enteropathy *See* COELIAC DISEASE.

glutose A six-carbon sugar (hexose) with a keto group on carbon-3; not metabolised and non-fermentable.

glycaemic index The increase in blood glucose after a test dose of a carbohydrate, relative to that in response to an equivalent amount of glucose. A measure of the rate and extent of small intestinal digestion of the carbohydrate.

See also STARCH, RESISTANT.

glycation Non-enzymic reaction between glucose (or other carbohydrates) and amino groups in proteins, resulting in formation of a glycoprotein. Glycation of collagen, crystallin and other proteins is the basis of many of the adverse effects of poor glycaemic control in DIABETES.

See also GLYCOSYLATION; HAEMOGLOBIN, GLYCATED; MAILLARD REACTION.

glycerides Esters of GLYCEROL with FATTY ACIDS. *See* TRIACYLGLYCEROL; FAT, SUPERGLYCERINATED.

glycerine (glycerin) *See* GLYCEROL.

glycerol (glycerine) 1,2,3-Propane triol (CH_2OH—CHOH—CH_2OH), a trihydric alcohol. Simple or neutral FATS are esters of glycerol with three molecules of FATTY ACID, i.e. triacylglycerols, sometimes known as triglycerides. Glycerol is a clear, colourless, odourless, viscous liquid, sweet to taste; it is made from fats by alkaline hydrolysis (SAPONIFICATION). Used as a solvent for flavours, as a humectant to keep foods moist, and in cake batters to improve texture and slow staling.

glycerose Glyceraldehyde, a three-carbon sugar (CHO—CHOH—CH_2OH) derived from GLYCEROL.

glyceryl lactostearate Or lactostearin. Formed by glycerolysis of hydrogenated soya bean oil followed by esterification with lactic acid, resulting in a mixture of mono- and diacylglycerols and their lactic mono-esters. Used as an emulsifier in shortenings (E-472b).

glyceryl monostearate *See* FAT, SUPERGLYCERINATED.

glycine A non-essential AMINO ACID, abbr Gly (G), M_r 75.1, pK_a 2.35, 9.78, CODONS CGNu. It has a sweet taste (70% of the sweetness of sucrose) and is sometimes used mixed with SACCHARIN as a sweetener. Known at one time as collagen sugar.

glycinin A GLOBULIN in soya bean.

glycitols *See* SUGAR ALCOHOLS. Glycitol was used at one time as an alternative name for SORBITOL.

glycochenodeoxycholic acid The GLYCINE conjugate of CHENODEOXYCHOLIC ACID, one of the BILE acids.

glycocholic acid The GLYCINE conjugate of CHOLIC ACID, one of the BILE acids.

glycogen The storage carbohydrate in the liver and muscles, a branched polymer of GLUCOSE units, with the same structure as AMYLOPECTIN, and sometimes referred to as animal starch. In an adult there are about 250 g of glycogen in the muscles and 100 g in the liver in the fed state. Since glycogen is rapidly broken down to glucose after an animal is killed, meat and animal liver do not contain glycogen; the only dietary sources are oysters and other shellfish that are eaten virtually alive and contain about 5% glycogen.

glycogenesis The synthesis of glycogen from glucose in liver and muscle after a meal, stimulated by the hormone INSULIN.

glycogenic acid *See* GLUCONIC ACID.

glycogenolysis The breakdown of GLYCOGEN to GLUCOSE for use as a metabolic fuel and to maintain the concentration of blood glucose in the fasting state. Stimulated by the hormones ADRENALINE and GLUCAGON.

glycogen storage diseases A group of rare GENETIC DISEASES caused by a defect of one or another of the various enzymes involved in glycogen synthesis and mobilisation, characterised by excessive accumulation of GLYCOGEN in liver and/or muscle and, in some forms, profound fasting HYPOGLYCAEMIA. Treatment is by feeding small frequent meals, rich in carbohydrate.

glycolysis The first sequence of reactions in GLUCOSE metabolism, leading to the formation of two molecules of pyruvate from each glucose molecule.

glycoproteins Also known as proteoglycans; polysaccharides covalently bound to a protein, commonly via *N*- or *O*-acylglucosamine linkage to the hydroxyl group of SERINE or THREONINE.

See also MUCOPOLYSACCHARIDES; MUCOPROTEINS.

glycosides Compounds of a sugar attached to another molecule; called glucosides when glucose is the sugar.

glycosuria *See* GLUCOSURIA.

glycosylation   Chemical reaction leading to the substitution of one or more glycosyl groups into a compound; GLYCATION is a general term for any reaction leading to incorporation of glucose into a protein.

glycyrrhizin   Triterpenoid glycoside extracted from LIQUORICE root *Glycyrrhiza glabra*; 50–100 times as sweet as sucrose but with liquorice flavour. Used to flavour tobacco and pharmaceutical preparations, and as a foaming agent in some non-alcoholic beverages.

glyoxylate (sometimes also glyoxalate)   The keto-acid of GLYCINE. *See also* HYPEROXALURIA; OXALIC ACID.

GM foods   Produced by GENETIC MODIFICATION of the plant or animal. EU legislation requires that all foods containing genetically modified protein or DNA, including those sold in catering outlets, must be so labelled, unless there is less than 0.9% GM material in the food (this limit is subject to negotiation at the time of publication). Products made from GM crops, but highly purified, so that no GM protein or DNA is present (SUBSTANTIAL EQUIVALENCE), were exempt from labelling, but new legislation will require that they be labelled. Foods manufactured using products of GM organisms (e.g. cheese made using GM chymosin) and meat, milk and eggs from animals fed on GM crops need not be labelled as containing GM material.

GMP   *See* GOOD MANUFACTURING PRACTICE.

GMS   Glyceryl monostearate, *see* FAT, SUPERGLYCERINATED.

goat   Ruminant, *Capra* spp. Young is kid.

Composition/100 g: water 76 g, 456 kJ (109 kcal), protein 20.6 g, fat 2.3 g (of which 37% saturated, 53% mono-unsaturated, 11% polyunsaturated), cholesterol 57 mg, carbohydrate 0 g, ash 1.1 g, Ca 13 mg, Fe 2.8 mg, P 180 mg, K 385 mg, Na 82 mg, Zn 4 mg, Cu 0.3 mg, Se 8.8 µg, B_1 0.11 mg, B_2 0.49 mg, niacin 3.8 mg, folate 5 µg, B_{12} 1.1 µg, A 100 g serving is a source of Se, a good source of Cu, Fe, P, Zn, niacin, a rich source of vitamin B_2, B_{12}.

goblet cell   Secretory cell in the intestinal mucosa which secretes the major constituents of MUCUS.

gobo   *See* BURDOCK.

goitre   Enlargement of the thyroid gland, seen as a swelling in the neck, commonly due to deficiency of IODINE in the diet or to the presence of GOITROGENS in foods. In such cases there is commonly underproduction of the THYROID HORMONES, i.e. hypothyroid goitre. Euthyroid goitre is a condition in which the enlargement of the thyroid gland is sufficient to compensate for a deficiency of iodine and permit normal production of thyroid hormones. In infancy, iodine deficiency can also lead to severe mental retardation, goitrous cretinism, with deafness. Supplementation with iodide often prevents the condition, hence the use of iodised SALT.

Hyperthyroid goitre (THYROTOXICOSIS) is due to excessive stimulation of the thyroid gland, with overproduction of the thyroid hormones.

goitrogens Compounds in foods (especially *Brassica* spp., groundnuts, cassava and soya bean) that inhibit either synthesis of THYROID HORMONES (GLUCOSINOLATES) or uptake of iodide into the thyroid gland (thiocyanates), and hence can cause GOITRE, especially when the dietary intake of iodine is marginal.

golden berry *See* CAPE GOOSEBERRY.

golden syrup Light coloured SYRUP made by evaporation of cane sugar juice.

See also TREACLE; SUGAR.

Gomez classification One of the earliest systems for classifying PROTEIN–ENERGY MALNUTRITION in children, based on percentage of expected weight for age: over 90% is normal, 76–90% is mild (first degree), 61–75% is moderate (second degree) and less than 60% is severe (third degree) malnutrition.

good manufacturing practice (GMP) Part of a food and drink control operation aimed at ensuring that products are consistently manufactured to a quality appropriate to their intended use (detailed in Food and Drink Good Manufacturing Practice, IFST 1998).

goose Domesticated water-fowl, *Anser anser*.

Composition/100 g: (edible portion 47%) water 68 g, 674 kJ (161 kcal), protein 22.8 g, fat 7.1 g (of which 50% saturated, 34% mono-unsaturated, 16% polyunsaturated), cholesterol 84 mg, carbohydrate 0 g, ash 1.1 g, Ca 13 mg, Fe 2.6 mg, Mg 24 mg, P 312 mg, K 420 mg, Na 87 mg, Zn 2.3 mg, Cu 0.3 mg, Se 16.8 µg, vitamin A 12 µg retinol, B_1 0.13 mg, B_2 0.38 mg, niacin 4.3 mg, B_6 0.64 mg, folate 31 µg, B_{12} 0.5 µg, pantothenate 2 mg, C 7 mg. A 100 g serving is a source of Fe, Zn, vitamin folate, C, a good source of Cu, Se, vitamin B_2, niacin, a rich source of P, vitamin B_6, B_{12}, pantothenate.

gooseberry Berry of the shrub *Ribes grossularia*. The British National Fruit Collection contains 155 varieties.

Composition/100 g: water 88 g, 184 kJ (44 kcal), protein 0.9 g, fat 0.6 g, carbohydrate 10.2 g, fibre 4.3 g, ash 0.5 g, Ca 25 mg, Fe 0.3 mg, Mg 10 mg, P 27 mg, K 198 mg, Na 1 mg, Zn 0.1 mg, Cu 0.1 mg, Mn 0.1 mg, Se 0.6 µg, I 2 µg, vitamin A 15 µg RE, E 0.4 mg, B_1 0.04 mg, B_2 0.03 mg, niacin 0.3 mg, B_6 0.08 mg, folate 6 µg, pantothenate 0.3 mg, C 28 mg. A 110 g serving a rich source of vitamin C.

gooseberry, Indian *See* EMBLIC.

goosefoot *See* EPAZOTE.

gossypol Yellow toxic pigment found in some varieties of cottonseed. When included in chicken feed, it causes discoloration of the yolk, but has not been found to be toxic to human beings, and has been investigated as a possible male contraceptive agent. Chemically a dialdehyde, it reacts with the ε-amino group of lysine, thus reducing available lysine and PROTEIN QUALITY.

gossypose *See* RAFFINOSE.

goujon Small deep fried pieces of FISH. The name is derived from gudgeon, a small freshwater fish. Now also used for small pieces of chicken breast.

gourds Vegetables of the family Cucurbitaceae, including calabash or bottle gourd (*Lagenaria vulgaris*), ash gourd (*Benincasa hispida*), snake gourd (*Trichosanthes anguina*), CUCUMBER (*Cucumis sativus*), vegetable MARROW (*Cucurbita pepo*), PUMPKIN (*Cucurbita moschata*), SQUASH (*Cucurbita maxima*), coocha or chayote (*Sechium edule*), cantaloupe MELON (*Cucumis melo*), WATERMELON (*Citrullus vulgaris*). The hedged gourd is KIWANO.

Calabash gourd, composition/100g: (edible portion 70%) water 95.5g, 59kJ (14kcal), protein 0.6g, fat 0g, carbohydrate 3.4g, ash 0.4g, Ca 26mg, Fe 0.2mg, Mg 11mg, P 13mg, K 150mg, Na 2mg, Zn 0.7mg, Mn 0.1mg, Se 0.2µg, vitamin A 1µg RE, B_1 0.03mg, B_2 0.02mg, niacin 0.3mg, B_6 0.04mg, folate 6µg, pantothenate 0.2mg, C 10mg.

Chayote, composition/100g: (edible portion 99%) water 95g, 71kJ (17kcal), protein 0.8g, fat 0.1g, carbohydrate 3.9g (1.9g sugars), fibre 1.7g, ash 0.3g, Ca 17mg, Fe 0.3mg, Mg 12mg, P 18mg, K 125mg, Na 2mg, Zn 0.7mg, Cu 0.1mg, Mn 0.2mg, Se 0.2µg, vitamin E 0.1mg, K 4.6mg, B_1 0.03mg, B_2 0.03mg, niacin 0.5mg, B_6 0.08mg, folate 93µg, pantothenate 0.2mg, C 8mg. A 100g serving (half fruit) is a source of vitamin C, a rich source of folate.

Wax gourd, composition/100g: (edible portion 71%) water 96.1g, 54kJ (13kcal), protein 0.4g, fat 0.2g, carbohydrate 3g, fibre 2.9g, ash 0.3g, Ca 19mg, Fe 0.4mg, Mg 10mg, P 19mg, K 6mg, Na 111mg, Zn 0.6mg, Mn 0.1mg, Se 0.2µg, vitamin B_1 0.04mg, B_2 0.11mg, niacin 0.4mg, B_6 0.04mg, folate 5µg, pantothenate 0.1mg, C 13mg.

gout Painful disease caused by accumulation of crystals of URIC ACID in the synovial fluid of joints; may be due to excessive synthesis and metabolism of PURINES, which are metabolised to uric acid, or to impaired excretion of uric acid. Traditionally associated with a rich diet; both ALCOHOL and FRUCTOSE increase purine synthesis.

G proteins Guanine nucleotide binding proteins. Part of a transmembrane signalling mechanism in response to HORMONES, etc., that bind to cell surface receptors, leading to activation of enzymes that form intracellular SECOND MESSENGERS.

Gracilaria Genus of red algae, widely cultivated as a source of AGAR, now also cultivated to feed farmed ABALONE.

graddan Hebrides, historical; cereal grains dehusked by holding ears of corn over flames until the husk is burnt, but before the grain is charred.

grading Assessment of the overall quality of a food by a number of criteria (e.g. size, colour, flavour, texture, laboratory analysis).

Graham bread Wholewheat bread in which the bran is very finely ground. Graham cakes are made from wholemeal flour and milk. The name is that of a miller of wholemeal flour who advocated its use in the USA (*Treatise on Bread and Bread Making*, 1837). *See also* ALLINSON BREAD.

graining Crystallisation of refined sugar when boiled. Prevented by adding glucose or cream of tartar as SUGAR DOCTORS.

grains of paradise *See* PEPPER, MELEGUETA.

Gram-negative, Gram-positive A method of classifying bacteria depending on whether or not they retain crystal-violet dye (Gram stain). Named after the Danish botanist H. C. J. Gram (1858–1938).

grams, Indian Various small dried peas (LEGUMES), e.g. green gram (*Phaseolus aureus*), black gram (*Phaseolus mungo*), red gram (*Cajanus indicus*), Bengal gram or CHICKPEA (*Cicer aretinum*).

grana Hard dry grating cheeses such as PARMESAN.

granadilla *See* PASSION FRUIT.

grape Fruit of a large number of varieties of *Vitis vinifera*. One of the oldest cultivated plants; three main groups: dessert grapes, WINE grapes and varieties that are used for drying to produce raisins, currants and sultanas. Of the many varieties of grape that are grown for WINE making, nine are considered classic varieties: Cabernet Sauvignon, Chardonnay, Chenin Blanc, Merlot, Pinot Noir, Riesling, Sauvignon Blanc, Sémillon, Syrah.

Composition/100 g: (edible portion 96%) water 81 g, 289 kJ (69 kcal), protein 0.7 g, fat 0.2 g, carbohydrate 18.1 g (15.5 g sugars), fibre 0.9 g, ash 0.5 g, Ca 10 mg, Fe 0.4 mg, Mg 7 mg, P 20 mg, K 191 mg, Na 2 mg, Zn 0.1 mg, Cu 0.1 mg, Mn 0.1 mg, Se 0.1 µg, I 1 µg, vitamin A 3 µg RE (112 µg carotenoids), E 0.2 mg, K 14.6 mg, B_1 0.07 mg, B_2 0.07 mg, niacin 0.2 mg, B_6 0.09 mg, folate 2 µg, pantothenate 0.1 mg, C 11 mg.

Grapeseed oil is 10% saturated, 17% mono-unsaturated, 73% polyunsaturated, contains 28.8 mg vitamin E/100 g.

grapefruit Fruit of *Citrus paradisi*; thought to have arisen as sport of the POMELO or shaddock (*Citrus grandis*), a coarser CITRUS fruit, or as a hybrid between pomelo and sweet orange. The pith contains NARINGIN, which is very bitter. Name said to have arisen because the fruit is borne on the tree in clusters (like grapes). Ruby grapefruit, with red flesh, was discovered as a sport in Texas in 1929.

Composition/100 g: (edible portion 50%) water 90.9 g, 134 kJ (32 kcal), protein 0.6 g, fat 0.1 g, carbohydrate 8.1 g (7 g sugars), fibre 1.1 g, ash 0.3 g, Ca 12 mg, Fe 0.1 mg, Mg 8 mg, P 8 mg, K 139 mg, Zn 0.1 mg, Se 0.3 µg, vitamin A 46 µg RE (1703 µg carotenoids), E 0.1 mg, B_1 0.04 mg, B_2 0.02 mg, niacin 0.3 mg, B_6 0.04 mg, folate 10 µg, pantothenate 0.3 mg, C 34 mg. A 170 g serving (half fruit) is a rich source of vitamin C.

grape sugar   *See* GLUCOSE.

grappa   *See* MARC.

GRAS (generally regarded as safe)   Designation given to food additives when further evidence is required before the substance can be classified more precisely (US usage).

grass tetany   MAGNESIUM deficiency in cattle.

gratin   (1) A fireproof dish.

(2) Also gratiné, French term for the thin brown crust formed on top of foods that have been covered with butter and bread-crumbs, then heated under the grill or in the oven. Au gratin when cheese is also used.

grattons (gratterons)   French; crispy remains of melted fat tissue of poultry or pork. German equivalent is gribbens.

Grau-Hamm press   For determination of the water binding or water holding capacity of meat (*see* MEAT, WATER BINDING CAPAC-ITY; MEAT, WATER HOLDING CAPACITY).

gravadlax (gravlaks, gravlax)   Originally Scandinavian; pickled or marinated raw salmon.

Graves' disease   *See* THYROTOXICOSIS.

gravity, original   The concentration of solids in the WORT from which BEER is made.

gray (Gy)   The SI unit for ionising radiation (= 100 rad). 1 Gy = 1 J/kg.

great millet   *See* SORGHUM.

green butter   *See* VEGETABLE BUTTERS.

green fluorescent protein (GFP)   A protein from the jellyfish *Aequorea victoria* that emits green fluorescence when excited by UV light. The *GFP* gene is widely used as a REPORTER GENE in genetic engineering.

greengage   Green variety of PLUM introduced into England in the early 18th century by Sir William Gage.

green S   Food COLOUR, also known as Wool green S and Brilliant acid green BS, E-142.

green sickness 17th century name for IRON deficiency ANAEMIA, especially in young women, and sometimes described as one of the signs of 'love melancholy'.

grey body A concept used to take account of the fact that materials are not perfect absorbers or radiators of heat (which would be the case with a theoretical black body).

gribbens (greben, gribbenes) *See* GRATTONS.

griddle Also girdle; iron plate used for baking scones, etc. on top of stove.

grilse Young SALMON that has returned to fresh water after one year in the sea.

grinding, cryogenic Mixing liquid nitrogen or solid carbon dioxide with food to cool it during grinding.

griskin CHINE of pork, also used for a thin piece of loin.

grissini Italian 'finger rolls' or stick bread 15–45 cm (6–18 in) long, and normally crisp and dry.

grist Cereal for grinding.

gristle The CONNECTIVE TISSUE of the meat, consisting mainly of the insoluble proteins COLLAGEN and ELASTIN. Usually inedible and accounts for the toughness of some cuts of meat. Prolonged slow cooking converts collagen to GELATINE, but has no effect on elastin.

grits, corn *See* HOMINY.

groats Oats from which the husk has been entirely removed; when crushed, Embden groats result. Used to make gruel and porridge.

grog British naval drink; sugared rum mixed with hot water. Named after Admiral Edward Vernon (1684–1757), who was nicknamed 'Old Grog' because of his grosgrain (heavy corded silk) coat.

ground cherry *See* CAPE GOOSEBERRY.

ground fish *See* FISH, DEMERSAL.

groundnut *See* PEANUT.

ground tomato *See* CAPE GOOSEBERRY.

grouse GAME bird, *Lagopus lagopus*. Shooting period in UK 12 August to 10 December; eaten fresh or after being hung for 2–4 days to develop flavour. The whole bird weighs about 700 g.

growth hormone *See* SOMATOTROPHIN.

gruel Thin porridge made from oatmeal, barley or other cereal.

Gruyère Swiss hard cheese, used in fondue.

GTF *See* GLUCOSE TOLERANCE FACTOR.

guanine One of the PURINES.

guarana Dried paste from the seeds of a climbing shrub, *Paullina cupana*, native of the Amazon region. It contains caffeine and related compounds; used in the UK as an ingredient of drinks, chewing gum, a powder to be sprinkled on food and capsules and tablets.

guar gum   Cyamopsis GUM; from the cluster bean, *Cyamopsis tetragonolobus*. Member of Leguminosae, used in India as livestock feed. The gum is a water-soluble galactomannan; used in 'slimming' preparations, since it is not digested by digestive enzymes, and experimentally in the treatment of DIABETES, since it slows the absorption of glucose after a meal.

guava   Fruit of the central and south American tropical shrub *Psidium guajava*.

Composition/100 g: (edible portion 78%) water 81 g, 285 kJ (68 kcal), protein 2.5 g, fat 0.9 g, carbohydrate 14.3 g (8.9 g sugars), fibre 5.4 g, ash 1.4 g, Ca 18 mg, Fe 0.3 mg, Mg 22 mg, P 40 mg, K 417 mg, Na 2 mg, Zn 0.2 mg, Cu 0.2 mg, Mn 0.2 mg, Se 0.6 µg, vitamin A 31 µg RE (5578 µg carotenoids), E 0.7 mg, K 2.6 mg, B_1 0.07 mg, B_2 0.04 mg, niacin 1.1 mg, B_6 0.11 mg, folate 49 µg, pantothenate 0.5 mg, C 228 mg. A 55 g serving (1 fruit without refuse) is a source of folate, a rich source of vitamin C.

guinea corn   *See* SORGHUM.

guinea fowl   Game bird, now farmed, *Numida meleagris*, not seasonal.

Composition/100 g: (edible portion 64%) water 74 g, 460 kJ (110 kcal), protein 20.6 g, fat 2.5 g (of which 32% saturated, 37% mono-unsaturated, 32% polyunsaturated), cholesterol 63 mg, carbohydrate 0 g, ash 1.3 g, Ca 11 mg, Fe 0.8 mg, Mg 24 mg, P 169 mg, K 220 mg, Na 69 mg, Zn 1.2 mg, Se 17.5 µg, vitamin A 12 µg retinol, B_1 0.07 mg, B_2 0.11 mg, niacin 8.8 mg, B_6 0.47 mg, folate 6 µg, B_{12} 0.4 µg, pantothenate 0.9 mg, C 2 mg. A 100 g serving is a source of pantothenate, a good source of P, Se, vitamin B_6, a rich source of niacin, vitamin B_{12}.

guinea pepper   *See* PEPPER, MELEGUETA.

gum   Carbohydrate polymers that can disperse in water to form a viscous mucilaginous mass. Used in food processing to stabilise emulsions, as a thickening agent and in sugar confectionery. Most (apart from dextrans) are not digested and have no food value, although they contribute to the intake of NON-STARCH POLYSACCHARIDES.

Exudate gums: karaya (sterculia) from *Sterculia arens*, partially acetylated high molecular weight heteropolymers of rhamnose, galactose and galacturonic acid; tragacanth from *Astralagus* spp. a neutral arabinogalactan; ghatti from *Anageissus latifolia*.

Seed gums: guar from *Cyamopsis tetragonolobus*; locust bean is *Ceratonia siliqua*; psyllium *Plantago* spp. esp. *P. ovata*; quince seed *Cydonia vulgaris* and *C. oblongata*.

Dextran gums: α-D-glucose polymers produced by *Leuconostoc mesenteroides*. Xanthan gum produced by *Xanthomonas campestris*.

gum arabic (gum acacia)   Exudate from the stems of *Acacia* spp.; the best product comes from *A. senegal*. Used as thickening agent, as stabiliser, often in combination with other gums, in gum drops and soft jelly gums and to prevent crystallisation in sugar confectionery.

gumbo   (1) American (Creole); soup or stew made from okra, onions, celery and pepper, flavoured with filé powder (powdered dried SASSAFRAS leaves), and containing chicken, meat, fish or shellfish.

(2) *See* OKRA.

gum, British   Partly hydrolysed starch, DEXTRIN.

gum, chewing   *See* CHEWING GUM.

gum drops (fruit gums)   SUGAR CONFECTIONERY based on SUCROSE and GLUCOSE with GUM ARABIC (hard gums) or a mixture of GELATINE and GUM ARABIC (soft gums).

gum tragacanth   Obtained from the trees of *Astralagus* spp., used as a stabiliser.

gur   Mixture of sugar crystals and syrup, brown and toffee-like, made by evaporation of juice of sugar cane; also called jaggery.

gustin   ZINC-containing protein associated with taste acuity.

See also HYPOGEUSIA; DYSGEUSIA.

gut   *See* GASTROINTESTINAL TRACT.

Guthrie test   Test for a number of GENETIC DISEASES (especially PHENYLKETONURIA) based on measuring the concentrations of AMINO ACIDS in a small sample of blood taken by pricking the heel of the child a few days after birth, by biological assay using mutated bacteria for which the amino acid is a growth factor. Now largely superseded by chromatographic methods.

gut sweetbread   *See* PANCREAS.

GYE   Guinness yeast extract, *see* YEAST EXTRACT.

gyle   ALCOHOL solution formed in the first stage of VINEGAR production, 6–9% alcohol. Subsequent fermentation with *Acetobacter* spp. converts the alcohol to ACETIC ACID.

H

HACCP   Hazard analysis of critical control points. A technique for identification of stages in a process (e.g. in food manufacture) where there are risks that can be anticipated, assigning a degree of seriousness and identifying control mechanisms.

hachis   Minced or chopped mixture of meat and herbs.

haddock   White FISH, *Melanogrammus aeglefinus*.

Composition /100 g: water 79.9 g, 364 kJ (87 kcal), protein 18.9 g, fat 0.7 g, cholesterol 57 mg, carbohydrate 0 g, ash 1.2 g, Ca 33 mg, Fe 1 mg, Mg 39 mg, P 188 mg, K 311 mg, Na 68 mg, Zn 0.4 mg, Se 30.2 µg, I 250 µg, vitamin A 17 µg RE (17 µg retinal), E 0.4 mg, K 0.1 mg, B_1 0.04 mg, B_2 0.04 mg, niacin 3.8 mg, B_6 0.3 mg, folate 12 µg, B_{12} 1.2 µg, pantothenate 0.1 mg. A 100 g serving is a source of Mg, vitamin B_6, a good source of P, niacin, a rich source of I, Se, vitamin B_{12}.

haem (heme)   The iron-containing PORPHYRIN that, in combination with the protein globin, forms HAEMOGLOBIN and MYOGLOBIN. It is also part of a wide variety of other proteins, collectively known as haem proteins, including the CYTOCHROMES.

See also PROTOPORPHYRIN.

haemagglutinins (hemagglutinins)   *See* LECTINS.

haematemesis (hematemesis)   Vomiting bright red blood, due to bleeding in the upper GASTROINTESTINAL TRACT.

haematin (hematin)   Formed by the oxidation of HAEM; the iron is oxidised from the ferrous (Fe^{2+}) to the ferric (Fe^{3+}) state.

haematinic (hematinic)   General term for those nutrients, including IRON, FOLIC ACID, VITAMIN B_{12}, required for the formation and development of blood cells in bone marrow (the process of haematopoiesis), deficiency of which may result in ANAEMIA.

haematocrit (hematocrit)   Packed volume of red blood cells, expressed as fraction of the total volume of blood; determined by centrifugation in calibrated capillary tube (haematocrit tube), as an index of ANAEMIA, and especially microcytic and MEGALOBLASTIC ANAEMIAS. Not a sensitive index of IRON status, because it only falls after HAEMOGLOBIN synthesis has been impaired.

haemin (hemin)   The hydrochloride of HAEMATIN, derived from HAEMOGLOBIN. The crystals are readily recognisable under the microscope and used as a test for blood.

haemochromatosis   IRON overload; excessive absorption and storage of iron in the body, commonly the result of a GENETIC DISEASE, leading to tissue damage (including DIABETES) and bronze coloration of the skin. Sometimes called bronze diabetes.

haemoglobin (hemoglobin)   The HAEM-containing protein in red blood cells, responsible for the transport of oxygen and carbon dioxide in the bloodstream.

See also ANAEMIA; IRON.

haemoglobin, glycated   Also known as glycosylated haemoglobin or haemoglobin A_{1c}. The result of non-enzymic reaction between GLUCOSE and ε-amino groups of LYSINE. Measurement of glycated haemoglobin is used as an index of glycaemic control in DIABETES mellitus over the preceding 2–3 months; normally 3–6% of haemoglobin is glycated, but when there has been prolonged HYPERGLYCAEMIA as much as 20% may be glycated.

See also GLYCATION; MAILLARD REACTION.

haemoglobinometer (hemoglobinometer) Instrument to measure the amount of haemoglobin in blood by colorimetry.

haemolysis (hemolysis) Destruction of red blood cells by lysis of the cell membrane; may occur in a variety of pathological conditions, as a result of incorrectly matched blood transfusion or in VITAMIN E deficiency.

See also ANAEMIA, HAEMOLYTIC; FAVISM.

haemorrhagic (hemorrhagic) disease of the newborn Excessive bleeding due to VITAMIN K deficiency; in most countries infants are given vitamin K by injection shortly after birth to prevent this rare but serious (potentially fatal) condition.

haemorrhoids (hemorrhoids) Or piles. Varicosity in the lower rectum or anus due to congestion of the veins, caused or exacerbated by a low-FIBRE diet and consequent straining to defecate.

haemosiderin (hemosiderin) *See* IRON STORAGE.

Hagberg falling number Measure of α-AMYLASE (EC 3.2.1.1) activity of flour based on the change in viscosity of flour paste.

haggis Traditional Scottish dish made from sheep's heart, liver and lungs cooked and chopped with suet, onions, oatmeal and seasoning, stuffed into a sheep's stomach. Said to have been originated by the Romans when campaigning in Scotland; when breaking camp in an emergency, the food was wrapped in the sheep's stomach. A similar Norman-French dish was afronchemoyle.

hair analysis Measurement of various minerals, including CHROMIUM, SELENIUM and ZINC in hair has been proposed as an index of status, but interpretation of the results is confounded by adsorption of minerals onto the hair from shampoo, etc.

hake A white FISH, *Merluccius bilinearis*.

hakka muggies Shetland; seasoned cod liver and oatmeal boiled in the stomach (muggie) of a fish.

See also HAGGIS.

halal Food conforming to the Islamic (Muslim) dietary laws. Meat from permitted animals (in general grazing animals with cloven hooves, and thus excluding pig meat) and birds (excluding birds of prey). The animals are killed under religious supervision by cutting the throat to allow removal of all blood from the carcass, without prior stunning. Food that is not halal is haram.

haldi *See* TURMERIC.

half-life (1) The time taken for half of a given PROTEIN to be replaced. Proteins are continuously being degraded and replaced even in the mature adult, and the half-life is used as a quantitative measure of this dynamic equilibrium. The values of half-life of different proteins range from a few minutes or hours for enzymes which control the rate of metabolic pathways, to almost a year for structural proteins such as collagen. The average half-life of human liver and serum proteins is 10 days, and of the total body protein is 80 days.

(2) Of radioactive ISOTOPES, the time in which half of the original material undergoes radioactive decay.

half-products *See* PREFORMS.

halibut A white FISH, *Hippoglossus* spp.

Composition /100 g: water 70 g, 779 kJ (186 kcal), protein 14.4 g, fat 13.8 g (of which 20% saturated, 69% mono-unsaturated, 11% polyunsaturated), cholesterol 46 mg, carbohydrate 0 g, ash 1 g, Ca 3 mg, Fe 0.7 mg, Mg 26 mg, P 164 mg, K 268 mg, Na 80 mg, Zn 0.4 mg, Se 36.5 µg, I 47 µg, vitamin A 17 µg retinol, E 0.9 mg, K 0.1 mg, B_1 0.06 mg, B_2 0.08 mg, niacin 1.5 mg, B_6 0.42 mg, folate 1 µg, B_{12} 1 µg, pantothenate 0.3 mg. A 100 g serving is a source of vitamin a good source of P, vitamin B_6, a rich source of I, Se, vitamin B_{12}.

Halibut liver oil is one of the richest natural sources of vitamins A and D, containing 50 mg vitamin A and 80 µg vitamin D per gram.

halophiles (halophilic bacteria) Able to grow at up to 25% salt. The growth of colonic bacteria is inhibited at 8–9% salt, *Clostridia* at 7–10%, food poisoning staphylococci at 15–20% and *Penicillium* at 20%. Film-forming YEASTS can grow in 24% salt.

Halphen test For the presence of cottonseed oil in other oils and fats.

halvah (halva, halwa, halawa, chalva) (1) A sweetmeat composed of an aerated mixture of glucose, sugar and crushed sesame seeds; because of the seeds, the sweet contains 25% fat.

(2) Indian desserts of various types, made from carrot, pumpkin or banana, sweetened and flavoured.

halverine Name sometimes given to low-fat spreads with less than the statutory amount of fat in a MARGARINE.

ham The whole hind leg of the pig, removed from the carcass and cured individually. Hams cured or smoked in different ways have different flavours. Green ham has been cured but not smoked.

Composition /100 g: water 67 g, 682 kJ (163 kcal), protein 16.6 g, fat 8.6 g (of which 36% saturated, 54% mono-unsaturated, 10% polyunsaturated), cholesterol 57 mg, carbohydrate 3.8 g, fibre 1.3 g, ash 3.7 g, Ca 24 mg, Fe 1 mg, Mg 22 mg, P 153 mg, K 287 mg,

Na 1304 mg, Zn 1.4 mg, Cu 0.1 mg, Mn 0.6 mg, Se 20.7 µg, I 7 µg, vitamin E 0.1 mg, B_1 0.63 mg, B_2 0.18 mg, niacin 2.9 mg, B_6 0.33 mg, folate 7 µg, B_{12} 0.4 µg, pantothenate 0.4 mg, C 4 mg. A 60 g serving (2 slices) is a source of Mn, P, Se, a good source of vitamin B_1, B_{12}.

hamburger   Or Hamburg steak, also known as beefburger. A flat patty made from ground (minced) BEEF, seasoned with salt, pepper and herbs, and bound with egg and flour. Commercial beefburgers are usually 80–100% meat, but must by law (in UK) contain 52% lean meat, of which 80% must be beef. Cereal, cereal fibre or bean fibre may be added as filler or 'meat extender'.

Hammarsten's casein   *See* CASEIN.

hammer mill   Continuous process mill in which material is powdered by impact from a set of hammers. A modified hammer mill using knives instead of hammers is used to shred food.

hand of pork   The foreleg of PORK; usually salted and boiled.

hangover   Headache and feeling of malaise resulting from excessive consumption of ALCOHOLIC BEVERAGES. The severity differs with different beverages and is not due to the toxic effects of alcohol alone, but to the presence of higher alcohols and esters (collectively known as CONGENERS or FUSEL OIL), the substances that give different beverages their distinctive flavours.

Hansa can   An all-aluminium can (developed in Germany) with easily opened ends.

Hansa herring   Salted HERRING, dating from 13th century, prepared by the fishermen of the Hanseatic League, the ports of the Baltic and north German rivers, after the fish had been landed, as opposed to fish salted at sea.

haram   Food forbidden by Islamic law. *See also* HALAL.

harasume   Japanese; transparent noodles made from mung bean paste.

hardening of oils   *See* HYDROGENATION.

hardness of water   *See* WATER HARDNESS.

hare   Game animal, similar to RABBIT but larger; caught wild but not farmed commercially. *Lepus europaeus* is the common hare; some 20 *Lepus* spp. occur in Europe.

Hartnup disease   Rare genetic defect of tryptophan transport, leading to development of PELLAGRA.

Harvard standards   Tables of height and weight for age used as reference values for the assessment of growth and nutritional status in children, based on data collected in the USA in the 1930s. Now replaced by the NCHS (US National Center for Health Statistics) standards.

See also NCHS STANDARDS; TANNER STANDARDS.

HarvestPlus International research initiative coordinated by the International Center for Tropical Agriculture and the International Food Policy Research Institute to develop micronutrient-rich dietary staples (initially BEANS, CASSAVA, MAIZE, RICE, sweet potatoes and WHEAT) by conventional plant breeding techniques. Web site http://www.harvestplus.org/.

hash Dish of cooked meat reheated in highly flavoured sauce. In the USA canned CORNED BEEF is known as corned beef hash.

haslet (harslet) Old English country dish made from pig's offal (heart, liver, lungs and sweetbreads) cooked in small pieces with seasoning and flour. Also known as pig's fry.

hasty pudding English, 16th century; made from flour, milk, butter and spices, which since they were usually readily available, could be quickly made into the pudding for unexpected visitors. Made in the USA with maize (corn) flour instead of wheat flour.

Hausa groundnut LEGUME grown in West Africa, *Kerslingiella geocarpa.*

haybox cooking The food is cooked for only a short time, then placed in a well-lagged container, the haybox, where it remains hot for many hours, so cooking continues without further use of fuel. Also known as the fireless cooker.

Hay diet A system of eating based on the concept that carbohydrates and proteins should not be eaten at the same meal, for which there is no scientific basis, originally proposed by William Hay in 1936. It ignores the fact that almost all carbohydrate-rich foods also contain significant amounts of protein. In any case, in the absence of adequate carbohydrate, protein is oxidised as a metabolic fuel and therefore not available for tissue building. Also called combining diet or food combining.

hazard analysis The identification of potentially hazardous ingredients, storage conditions, packaging, critical process points and relevant human factors which may affect product safety or quality.

haze Term in brewing to indicate cloudiness of BEER. Chill haze appears at $0\,°C$ and disappears at $20\,°C$; permanent haze remains at $20\,°C$ but there is no fundamental difference. Caused by GUMS derived from the barley, leucoanthocyanins and tannins from the malt and hops, and glucose, pentoses and amino acids.
See also CHILLPROOFING.

hazel nut Fruit of the tree *Corylus avellana*; cultivated varieties include Barcelona nut, cob nut and filbert (*C. maxima*).
Composition /100 g: (edible portion 46%) water 5.3 g, 2629 kJ (628 kcal), protein 14.9 g, fat 60.8 g (of which 8% saturated, 79% mono-unsaturated, 14% polyunsaturated), carbohydrate 16.7 g (4.3 g sugars), fibre 9.7 g, ash 2.3 g, Ca 114 mg, Fe 4.7 mg, Mg

163 mg, P 290 mg, K 680 mg, Zn 2.5 mg, Cu 1.7 mg, Mn 6.2 mg, Se 2.4 μg, vitamin A 1 μg RE (106 μg carotenoids), E 15 mg, K 14.2 mg, B_1 0.64 mg, B_2 0.11 mg, niacin 1.8 mg, B_6 0.56 mg, folate 113 μg, pantothenate 0.9 mg, C 6 mg. A 10 g serving (10 nuts) is a source of Cu, vitamin E, a good source of Mn.

Hazelnut oil is 8% saturated, 82% mono-unsaturated, 11% polyunsaturated; contains 47.2 mg vitamin E /100 g.

HCFCs Hydrochlorofluorocarbons, *see* REFRIGERANTS.

HDL High-density lipoprotein, *see* LIPOPROTEINS, PLASMA.

headcheese Mock BRAWN.

headspace The space between the surface of a food and the underside of the lid in a container.

health foods Substances whose consumption is advocated by various reform movements, including vegetable foods, whole grain cereals, food processed without chemical additives, food grown on organic compost, 'magic' foods (bees' ROYAL JELLY, KELP, LECITHIN, SEAWEED, etc.) and pills and potions. Numerous health claims are made but rarely is there any evidence to support these claims.

healthy US legislation permits a claim of 'healthy' for a food that is LOW IN fat and saturated fat, and contains no more than 480 mg of sodium and 60 mg of cholesterol per serving.

heart Both lamb and ox hearts are eaten.

Lamb, composition /100 g: (edible portion 78%) water 77 g, 511 kJ (122 kcal), protein 16.5 g, fat 5.7 g (of which 51% saturated, 36% mono-unsaturated, 13% polyunsaturated), cholesterol 135 mg, carbohydrate 0.2 g, ash 0.9 g, Ca 6 mg, Fe 4.6 mg, Mg 17 mg, P 175 mg, K 316 mg, Na 89 mg, Zn 1.9 mg, Cu 0.4 mg, Se 32 μg, vitamin B_1 0.37 mg, B_2 0.99 mg, niacin 6.1 mg, B_6 0.39 mg, folate 2 μg, B_{12} 10.3 μg, pantothenate 2.6 mg, C 5 mg. A 100 g serving is a source of Zn, vitamin B_6, a good source of P, vitamin B_1, a rich source of Cu, Fe, Se, vitamin B_2, niacin, B_{12}, pantothenate.

Ox, composition /100 g: (edible portion 71%) water 77 g, 469 kJ (112 kcal), protein 17.7 g, fat 3.9 g (of which 47% saturated, 37% mono-unsaturated, 17% polyunsaturated), cholesterol 124 mg, carbohydrate 0.1 g, ash 1.1 g, Ca 7 mg, Fe 4.3 mg, Mg 21 mg, P 212 mg, K 287 mg, Na 98 mg, Zn 1.7 mg, Cu 0.4 mg, Se 21.8 μg, vitamin E 0.2 mg, B_1 0.24 mg, B_2 0.91 mg, niacin 7.5 mg, B_6 0.28 mg, folate 3 μg, B_{12} 8.6 μg, pantothenate 1.8 mg, C 2 mg. A 100 g serving is a source of Mg, vitamin a good source of Zn, vitamin B_6, a rich source of Cu, Fe, P, Se, vitamin B_1, B_2, niacin, B_{12}, pantothenate.

heartburn A burning sensation in the chest usually caused by reflux (regurgitation) of acid digestive juices from the stomach, into the oesophagus. A common form of INDIGESTION, treated by ANTACIDS.

heart of palm   Edible inner part of the stem of CABBAGE PALM.
   Composition /100 g: water 69.5 g, 481 kJ (115 kcal), protein 2.7 g, fat 0.2 g, carbohydrate 25.6 g (17.2 g sugars), fibre 1.5 g, ash 2 g, Ca 18 mg, Fe 1.7 mg, Mg 10 mg, P 140 mg, K 1806 mg, Na 14 mg, Zn 3.7 mg, Cu 0.6 mg, Se 0.7 µg, vitamin A 3 µg RE (41 µg carotenoids), E 0.5 mg, B_1 0.05 mg, B_2 0.18 mg, niacin 0.9 mg, B_6 0.81 mg, folate 24 µg, C 8 mg.

heart sugar   Obsolete name for INOSITOL.

heat capacity (or thermal capacity)   The ratio of heat supplied to, or removed from, a substance and its change in temperature. Specific heat capacity is expressed per unit mass; molar heat capacity per mol.

heat exchanger   Equipment for heating or cooling liquids rapidly by providing a large surface area for the rapid and efficient transfer of heat. Used, e.g., for continuous PASTEURISATION and subsequent cooling.

heath hen   GAME bird, *Tympanuchus cupido cupido*, native to New England.

heating, direct   Processes in which the heat (and products of combustion) from burning fuel come into direct contact with the food, as in baking ovens and kiln driers.

heating, indirect   Processes in which there is a HEAT EXCHANGER (e.g. metal plates, steam or hot water in pipes) between the burning fuel and the food.

heat, latent   The amount of heat necessary to change a given mass of a substance from one state to another (i.e. melting of a solid or boiling of a liquid to yield vapour), without a change in its temperature.

heat of combustion   ENERGY released by complete combustion, as for example, in the bomb CALORIMETER. *See* ENERGY CONVERSION FACTORS.

heat pump   System of producing heat or cold by compression or expansion of air, also known as Joule cycle or air cycle. Modern systems can produce temperatures as low as −80 °C or as high as 200 °C and are being introduced as an environmentally friendly method of refrigeration, replacing fluorocarbon and chlorofluorocarbon REFRIGERANTS.

heat, sensible   Heat used to raise the temperature of a food or removed during cooling, without a change in phase.

heat, specific   The amount of heat that accompanies a unit change in temperature by a unit mass of material.

heat transfer   Occurs in three ways: radiation (transfer by infrared electromagnetic waves), conduction (movement of heat through a solid material) and convection (transfer by movement of molecules through a fluid as a result of lower density at higher temperatures).

heat transfer, steady-state Heating or cooling when there is no change in temperature at any specific location.

heat transfer, unsteady-state Heating or cooling where the temperature of the food and/or the heating or cooling medium are constantly changing.

hedonic scale Term used in tasting panels where the judges indicate the extent of their like or dislike for the food.

heel-prick test *See* GUTHRIE TEST.

Hegsted score Method of expressing the lipid content of a diet, calculated as $2.16 \times$ % energy from saturated fat $-1.65 \times$ % energy from polyunsaturated fat $-0.0677 \times$ mg cholesterol. *See also* KEYS SCORE.

Helicobacter pylori Bacterium commonly infecting the gastric mucosa. The underlying cause of ULCERS, and implicated in the development of gastric cancer. Formerly classified as *CAMPYLOBACTER*.

helminths Various parasitic worms, including FLUKES, TAPEWORMS and nematodes.

hemicelluloses Complex CARBOHYDRATES included as DIETARY FIBRE, composed of polyuronic acids combined with xylose, glucose, mannose and arabinose. Found together with cellulose and lignin in plant cell walls; most GUMS and mucilages are hemicelluloses.

hemoglobin American spelling of HAEMOGLOBIN; similarly, hematin = haematin, heme = haem, hemosiderin = haemosiderin.

hemp seed Fruits of *Cannabis sativa*, eaten toasted in China, as a condiment in Japan; the oil is added to salad dressings and dips, but is not suitable for cooking. The seed contains little or no cannabinoids.

HEPA filter *See* HIGH EFFICIENCY PARTICULATE AIR FILTER.

heparin Complex carbohydrate (glycosaminoglycan) from mast cells in liver, lung, muscle, heart and blood which prevents blood coagulation by activating antithrombin III, and so inhibiting the conversion of prothrombin to thrombin. *In vivo* cleared rapidly from the bloodstream, but *in vitro* 10 mg prevents the coagulation of 100 mL of blood.

hepatic encephalopathy Impairment of brain function, leading to coma, as a result of liver disease.

hepatitis Inflammatory liver disease, characterised by jaundice, abdominal pain and anorexia. May be due to bacterial or viral infection, alcohol abuse or various toxins. Treatment is usually conservative, with a very low fat diet (secretion of BILE is impaired) and complete abstinence from alcohol. Even after recovery, people may continue to be carriers of the virus, especially for hepatitis B and C, which are transmitted through blood and other body fluids. Liver cancer and cirrhosis are more common among people who have suffered from hepatitis B or C.

hepatoflavin   Name given to a substance isolated from liver, later shown to be RIBOFLAVIN.

hepatolenticular degeneration   *See* WILSON'S DISEASE.

hepatomegaly   Enlargement of the liver as a result of congestion (e.g. in heart failure), inflammation or fatty infiltration (as in KWASHIORKOR).

herbs   Soft-stemmed aromatic plants used fresh or dried to flavour and garnish dishes, and sometimes for medicinal effects. Not clearly distinguished from SPICES, except that herbs are usually the leaves or the whole of the plant, while spices are only part of the plant, commonly the seeds, or sometimes the roots or rhizomes.

herb tea   *See* TISANE.

Hermesetas™   *See* SACCHARIN.

hermetically sealed container   A package that is designed to be secure against entry of micro-organisms and maintain the commercial sterility of its contents after processing.

herring   Oily FISH, *Clupea harengus*; young herrings are sild. Sprat is *Clupea sprattus*; young are brislings. Pilchard is *Clupea pilchardus*; young are sardines. Kippers, bloaters and red herrings are salted and smoked herrings; bucklings are hot-smoked herrings. GAFFELBITAR are preserved herring.

Composition /100 g: water 72 g, 661 kJ (158 kcal), protein 18 g, fat 9 g (of which 26% saturated, 47% mono-unsaturated, 27% polyunsaturated), cholesterol 60 mg, carbohydrate 0 g, ash 1.5 g, Ca 57 mg, Fe 1.1 mg, Mg 32 mg, P 236 mg, K 327 mg, Na 90 mg, Zn 1 mg, Cu 0.1 mg, Se 36.5 µg, I 29 µg, vitamin A 28 µg retinol, E 1.1 mg, K 0.1 mg, B_1 0.09 mg, B_2 0.23 mg, niacin 3.2 mg, B_6 0.3 mg, folate 10 µg, B_{12} 13.7 µg, pantothenate 0.6 mg, C 1 mg. A 100 g serving is a source of I, vitamin E, B_2, niacin, B_6, a good source of P, a rich source of Se, vitamin B_{12}.

herring, liquefied   HERRING reduced to liquid state by enzyme action at slightly acid pH; used as protein concentrate for animal feed.

hesperidin   A FLAVONOID found in the pith of unripe citrus fruits; a glucorhamnisode of the flavonone hesperin. At one time called VITAMIN P, since it affects the fragility of the capillary walls, although there is no evidence that it is a dietary essential.

Hess test   A test for capillary fragility in SCURVY. A slight pressure is applied to the arm for 5 min when a shower of petechiae (small blood spots) appear on the skin below the area of application in vitamin C deficient subjects.

heterofermentative Of micro-organisms, producing more than one main metabolic product. *See also* HOMOFERMENTATIVE.

heterophysiasis Intestinal infestation with the parasitic FLUKE *Heterophyes heterophyes* after consumption of raw fish containing the larval stage.

heteropolysaccharide POLYSACCHARIDE containing more than one type of MONOSACCHARIDE.

heterosides *See* HOLOSIDES.

heterotrophes *See* AUTOTROPHES.

hexamethylene tetramine Preservative (fungicide), E-239. Also known as hexamine.

hexamic acid Cyclohexyl sulphamic acid, the free acid of CYCLAMATE.

hexamine *See* HEXAMETHYLENE TETRAMINE.

hexokinase The enzyme (EC 2.7.1.1) that catalyses the phosphorylation of GLUCOSE to glucose 6-phosphate. *See also* GLUCOKINASE.

hexosans POLYSACCHARIDES of HEXOSE sugars, including STARCH, GLYCOGEN, CELLULOSE and HEMICELLULOSE.

hexose monophosphate shunt The pentose phosphate pathway of GLUCOSE metabolism.

hexoses Six-carbon monosaccharide SUGARS such as GLUCOSE or FRUCTOSE.

hexuronic acid The acid derived from a hexose SUGAR by oxidation of the hydroxyl group on carbon-6. Originally proposed as a name for ASCORBIC ACID. The hexuronic acid derived from glucose is glucuronic acid.

HFAs Hydrofluoroalkanes, *see* REFRIGERANTS.

HFCs Hydrofluorocarbons, *see* REFRIGERANTS.

HFCS High-fructose corn syrup, *see* SYRUP, FRUCTOSE.

HF heating High-frequency heating, *see* MICROWAVE COOKING.

HFN *See* HAGBERG FALLING NUMBER.

HGH Human growth hormone (SOMATOTROPHIN).

HHP High hydrostatic pressure, a technology proposed for preservation of foods by inactivation of ENZYMES without heating; requires pressures of the order of 8–900 MPa.

hiatus hernia Protrusion of a part of the stomach upwards through the diaphragm. The condition occurs in about 40% of the population, most people suffering no ill effects; in a small number of people there is reflux of stomach contents into the oesophagus, causing HEARTBURN.

See also GASTROINTESTINAL TRACT.

hickory nut North American walnut, *Carya* spp.

Composition /100 g: (edible portion 32%) water 2.7 g, 2750 kJ (657 kcal), protein 12.7 g, fat 64.4 g (of which 11% saturated, 53% mono-unsaturated, 36% polyunsaturated), carbohydrate 18.3 g, fibre 6.4 g, ash 2 g, Ca 61 mg, Fe 2.1 mg, Mg 173 mg, P 336 mg, K 436 mg, Na 1 mg, Zn 4.3 mg, Cu 0.7 mg, Mn 4.6 mg, Se 8.1 μg, vitamin A 7 μg RE, B_1 0.87 mg, B_2 0.13 mg, niacin 0.9 mg, B_6 0.19 mg, folate 40 μg, pantothenate 1.7 mg, C 2 mg. An 18 g serving (3 nuts) is a source of vitamin B_1, a rich source of Mn.

high-density lipoproteins (HDL) One of the classes of plasma LIPIDS.

high-efficiency particulate air (HEPA) filter A filter of unwoven fibrous material to remove micro-organisms from air or other gases.

high-frequency heating *See* MICROWAVE COOKING.

high-fructose corn syrup *See* SYRUP, FRUCTOSE.

high in EU legislation states that for a food label or advertising to bear a claim that it is 'high in' a nutrient it must contain 50% more of the claimed nutrient than a similar product for which no claim is made. Claims may also be made for foods containing more than 12 g of protein, 6 g of dietary fibre or more than 30% of the labelling reference amount of a vitamin or mineral /100 g (*see* Table 2 of the Appendix).

US legislation permits a claim of 'high in' for foods containing more than 20% of the daily value for a particular nutrient in a serving. For a claim that a food is 'higher in' a nutrient it must contain at least 25% more of the claimed nutrient than a similar food for which no claim is made.

high-performance (high-pressure) liquid chromatography, HPLC An extremely sensitive analytical technique, typically able to separate and measure nanogram or smaller amounts of compounds in 10–100 μL samples.

high-pressure processing Use of pressures of the order of 300–400 MPa (45000 to 60000 psi), causing irreversible denaturation of proteins, and hence inactivation of micro-organisms and insects and their eggs, without the changes in flavour and texture of the food associated with heat treatment.

high-ratio fats, shortenings *See* FAT, SUPERGLYCERINATED.

high-ratio flour *See* FLOUR, HIGH-RATIO.

high-temperature short-time treatment (HTST) Sterilisation by heat for times ranging from a few seconds to minutes; usually applied to flow sterilisation, in which the process time is less than about 1 min; based on the fact that at higher temperatures bacteria are destroyed more rapidly than damage occurs to nutrients and texture.

hindle wakes Old English (14th century) method of cooking chicken, stuffed with fruit and spices, including prunes. Possibly a corruption of *hen de la wake* (feast).

HIPEF High-intensity pulsed electric field processing for non-thermal destruction of micro-organisms and inactivation of enzymes by rapid discharge of a high-voltage electric field.

Hirschsprung's disease Congenital failure of development of the nerve network of the lower colon or rectum, so that it neither expands nor conducts the contents of the bowel, which therefore accumulate in, and distend, the upper colon.

Hi-soy™ Full-fat SOYA FLOUR.

histamine The amine formed by decarboxylation of the amino acid HISTIDINE, found in cheese, beer, chocolate, sauerkraut and wine. Excessive release of histamine from mast cells is responsible for many of the symptoms of allergic reactions. Stimulates secretion of gastric acid, and administration of histamine is used as test for ACHLORHYDRIA.

histamine receptor antagonists Inhibitors of the histamine H_2 receptor, including cimetidine, ranitidine, famotidine and nisatidine, are used in treatment of gastric ULCERS; they act to reduce secretion of gastric acid in response to hormone or nerve stimulation.

histidinaemia GENETIC DISEASE due to a lack of histidase (EC 4.3.1.3), leading to impaired metabolism of the AMINO ACID HISTIDINE. If untreated leads to mental retardation and nervous system abnormalities. Treatment is by feeding a diet very low in histidine.

histidine An essential amino acid, abbr His (H), M_r 155.2, pK_a 1.80, 6.04 (imidazole), 9.76, CODONS CAPy.

histidine load test *See* FIGLU TEST.

histones Proteins rich in arginine and lysine, soluble in water but not dilute ammonia. They occur mainly in the cell nucleus and are concerned with the super-coiling and regulation of DNA.

HLB value *See* HYDROPHILE–LIPOPHILE BALANCE.

HMG CoA reductase Hydroxymethylglutaryl CoA reductase (EC 1.1.1.34), the first and rate-limiting enzyme of CHOLESTEROL synthesis. The STATINS are a family of HMG CoA reductase inhibitors used to treat HYPERCHOLESTEROLAEMIA.

HMT *See* HEXAMETHYLENE TETRAMINE.

Hobart mixer First electric mixing machine for bakeries, patented in 1918 by Herbert Johnston, working for Hobart Manufacturing Co.

hochoshi Japanese; cutting specialists, groups of people with their own secret methods of cutting fish, meat and vegetables. During the 12th century ceremonial cutting of food became a spectacle for Japanese nobility.

hock (1) Generic term for white wines from the Rhine region of Germany, known in USA as Rhine wines; bottled in brown glass, to distinguish from Moselle wines (in green glass).

(2) The knuckle of PORK; also used in USA for foreleg pork shank.

hodge podge Victorian; stew made from left-over cooked meat with vegetables.

hogget One-year-old sheep. *See* LAMB.

hogshead A traditional UK measure of volume or size of barrel: for beer or cider contains 54 gallons (243 L); for wine contains 52½ gallons (236 L).

hoki A white FISH (*Macruronus novaezealandiae*); New Zealand's most abundant commercial fish species. Also known as whiptail, blue hake or blue grenadier.

holocellulose Mixture of CELLULOSE and HEMICELLULOSE in wood, the fibrous residue that remains after the removal of lignin and minerals.

holoenzyme An enzyme protein together with its COENZYME or PROSTHETIC GROUP.

See also ENZYME ACTIVATION ASSAYS.

holosides Complex carbohydrates that yield only sugars on hydrolysis, as distinct from heterosides, which yield other substances as well as sugars on hydrolysis, e.g. tannins, anthocyanins, nucleosides.

hominy Prepared MAIZE kernels, also known as samp. Lye hominy – pericarp and germ removed by soaking in caustic soda. Pearled hominy – degermed hulled maize. Corn grits are ground hominy.

homocysteine An amino acid formed as an intermediate in the metabolism of METHIONINE; demethylated methionine; M_r 117.2, pK_a 2.22, 8.87, 10.86 (—SH). Does not occur in foods to any significant extent, and not generally considered to be of nutritional importance.

High blood homocysteine (possibly a result of poor FOLIC ACID, VITAMIN B_2, B_6 and B_{12} status) has been implicated in the development of ATHEROSCLEROSIS and heart disease, associated with a genetic polymorphism in METHYLENE TETRAHYDROFOLATE REDUCTASE, EC 1.7.99.5).

homocystinuria A GENETIC DISEASE caused by lack of cystathionine synthetase (EC 4.2.1.22), leading to impaired conversion of the AMINO ACID methionine to cysteine, characterised by excretion of HOMOCYSTEINE and its derivatives. May result in mental retardation and early death from ATHEROSCLEROSIS and coronary thrombosis if untreated, as well as fractures of bones and dislocation of the lens of the eye. Treatment (which must be continued throughout life) is either by feeding a diet low in methionine and supplemented with cysteine or, in some cases, by administration of high intakes of VITAMIN B$_6$ (about 100–500 times the normal requirement).

homofermentative Of micro-organisms, producing only one main metabolic product.

  See also HETEROFERMENTATIVE.

homogenisation EMULSIONS usually consist of a suspension of globules of varying size. Homogenisation reduces these globules to a smaller and more uniform size. In homogenised milk the smaller globules adsorb more protein, which acts as a stabiliser, and the cream does not rise to the top.

homogenisers Equipment for preparation and refinement of EMULSIONS; five main types. High-speed mixers rely on shearing forces developed by rotating blades. Pressure homogenisers force the mixture of liquids through a narrow aperture under high pressure to induce shear forces by turbulence. Colloid mills are DISC MILLS with a very narrow clearance between the discs. Ultrasonic homogenisers use high-frequency sound waves (18–20 kHz) giving a cavitation force of 10 tonnes/cm^2 causing alternate cycles of compression and tension, forming emulsions of droplet size 1–2 μm. The mixture is pumped through the homogeniser at a pressure of 340–1400 kPa. Hydroshear homogenisers and microfluidisers feed the liquid mixture into a double cone shaped chamber at high speed to create shear forces.

homopantothenic acid Pantoyl-γ-aminobutyric acid, a homologue of PANTOTHENIC ACID, reported to enhance cholinergic function in the central nervous system, and used to improve cognitive function in Alzheimer's disease.

honey Syrupy liquid made by bees (the honey bee is *Apis mellifera*) from the nectar of flowers (which is essentially sucrose). The flavour and colour depend on the flowers from which the nectar was obtained and the composition varies with the source. If the ratio of fructose:glucose is high, there is a tendency for the honey to crystallise. Comb honey is stored by bees in cells of freshly built broodless combs and sold in the comb; drained honey is drained from decapped combs.

honey berry Variety of RASPBERRY.

honeydew honey During periods of prolonged drought, bees may supplement their nectar supplies with honeydew, the sweet fluid excreted on leaves by leaf-sucking insects. The resultant HONEY is dark, with an unpleasant taste.

honeydew melon *See* MELON.

honeyware *See* BADDERLOCKS.

hontarako   Japanese; salted and dried cod ROE.

hookworm   Intestinal parasitic nematodes (*Ancyclostoma duodenale* and *Necator americanus*); infestation causes severe damage to the intestinal wall, leading to blood loss, and is a common cause of IRON deficiency and ANAEMIA.

hopanthate   *See* HOMOPANTOTHENIC ACID.

hopper   Indian; steamed batter cake made from rice flour mixed with coconut water and allowed to undergo lactic acid bacterial and yeast fermentation overnight.

hops   Perennial climbing plant, *Humulus lupulus*; the dried female flowers contain bitter aromatic acids (HUMULONES and isohumulones) and ESSENTIAL OILS, and are added to beer both to preserve it and enhance the flavour. The tender shoots may be eaten as a vegetable.

hordein   A protein in BARLEY; one of the PROLAMINS.

hordenin   Alkaloid found in germinated BARLEY, SORGHUM and MILLET which can cause HYPERTENSION and respiratory inhibition.

Horlicks™   A preparation of malted dried milk, for consumption as a beverage when added to milk.

hormesis   The dose response to a toxin or nutrient that shows a stimulation or beneficial effect at low levels and inhibition or an adverse effect at higher levels.

hormones   Compounds produced in ENDOCRINE GLANDS, and released into the bloodstream, where they act as chemical messengers to affect other tissues and organs.

hormones, human   Originally the hormones extracted from human tissues, used therapeutically; now applied to proteins such as INSULIN and GROWTH HORMONE produced in micro-organisms into which the human gene has been introduced; correctly known as recombinant human hormones.

hormones, sex   Male hormones, or androgens, include testosterone, dihydrotestosterone and androsterone; female hormones, or OESTROGENS, include oestradiol, oestrone and progesterone. Chemically, all are STEROIDS, derived from CHOLESTEROL. The synthetic female hormones stilboestrol and hexoestrol have similar biological activities to the oestrogens, but are quite different chemically. Apart from clinical use, oestrogens have been used for chemical caponisation (*see* CAPON) of cockerels and to enhance the growth rate of cattle.

horse bread   Medieval English; bread made with any cereal to hand, as well as peas and beans.

horseradish   The root of *Armoracia lapathifolia*. Pungency is caused by volatile oils. Used as a condiment, usually as a creamed sauce or grated and mixed with beetroot.

horseradish tree   *See* MORINGA.

Hortvet freezing test   *See* MILK, FREEZING-POINT TEST.

hot break   Coagulation and precipitation of high molecular weight proteins during the boiling of WORT for BEER production. Also known as trub.

Hot Springs Conference   International Conference held in 1943 at which the Food and Agriculture Organisation (FAO) of the United Nations originated.

Hovis™   A mixture of brown flour and wheat germ; from Latin *hominis vis*, strength of man; originally, in the 1880s, called Smith's Old Patent Germ Bread. Now a trade name for various types of bread and flour.

Howard mould count   Standardised microscope technique for measuring mould contamination.

howtowdie   Scottish; boiled chicken with poached egg and spinach.

HPLC   *See*   HIGH-PERFORMANCE   (HIGH-PRESSURE)   LIQUID CHROMATOGRAPHY.

hrisa   North African condiment, a mixture of PEPPER and CUMIN.

HSH   Hydrogenated   starch   hydrolysates,   *see*   SYRUP, HYDROGENATED.

5HT   *See* 5-HYDROXYTRYPTAMINE.

HTST   *See* HIGH-TEMPERATURE SHORT-TIME TREATMENT.

huckleberry   Wild north American berry, the fruit of *Gaylussacia baccata* and other species, named after the French chemist Gay-Lussac (1778–1850).

huff paste   Northern British name for pastry made from SUET, flour and water, used to enclose meat, fish or poultry while baking.

hull   *See* HUSK.

humble pie   *See* UMBLES.

humectants   Substances such as GLYCEROL, SORBITOL, invert sugar (*see* SUGAR, INVERT), HONEY which prevent loss of moisture from foods, especially flour confectionery, which would make them unappetising; also prevent sugar crystallising and prevent growth of ice crystals in frozen foods. Also used in other products such as tobacco, inks and glues.

humidification   The process of increasing the water vapour content (HUMIDITY) of air.

humidity   The water content of air. The weight of water per unit weight of air is the absolute or specific humidity. Saturation humidity is the absolute humidity of air that is saturated with water vapour at a given temperature. Relative humidity is the degree of saturation: the ratio of water vapour pressure in the atmosphere to water vapour pressure that would be exerted by pure water at the same temperature.

humidity, absolute (or specific) The water vapour content of moist air, usually expressed on a dry-weight basis, e.g. kilograms of water vapour per kilogram of dry air. Sometimes expressed on a volume basis, e.g. kilograms of water vapour per cubic metre of dry air.

humid volume The volume of moist air containing unit mass of dry air at a pressure of one atmosphere and a specified temperature.

hummus Middle Eastern hors d'oeuvre; a purée of CHICKPEAS and TAHINI with garlic, oil and lemon juice.

humulones Bitter aromatic acids (humulone, cohumulone and adhumulone) in HOPS, used to flavour and preserve BEER. Converted to isohumulones during boiling of the WORT. Also known as α-acids, to distinguish them from the lupulones (β-acids).

hurdle technology The concept of mild but effective food preservation based on considering all the different factors that inhibit (or act as hurdles to) the growth of spoilage organisms.

hursting mill Horizontal stone grinders formerly used for grain milling.

husk (or hull) The outer woody CELLULOSE covering of seeds and grains. In wheat it is loosely attached and removed during threshing; in rice it is firmly attached. High in fibre content and of limited use as animal feed.

HVP Hydrolysed vegetable protein; used as a flavour enhancer.

hyaluronidase Enzyme that catalyses random cleavage of 1,4 links (EC 3.2.1.35) or 1,3 links (EC 3.2.1.36) between glucuronic acid and N-acetylglucosamine in hyaluronic acid. Injected under the skin of poultry before slaughter to enhance tenderness and flavour.

> *See also* TENDERISERS.

hydrocooling Vegetables are washed in cold water, then subjected to vacuum while still wet. The evaporation of the water chills the vegetables for transport. Also applied to vegetables washed in ice-water without vacuum treatment.

hydrodyne process Method of tenderising meat in which it is subjected to supersonic shock waves generated under water by a small explosive charge to shatter the fibres without affecting its other properties; faster than other methods.

hydrogen Formed in small amounts by intestinal bacterial fermentation; measurement of exhaled hydrogen on the breath provides a sensitive way of diagnosing DISACCHARIDE intolerance.

hydrogenation Conversion of liquid oils to semi-hard fats by the addition of hydrogen across carbon–carbon double bonds; used for margarines and shortenings intended for bakery products. *See* FATTY ACIDS, UNSATURATED.

hydrogen peroxide Antimicrobial agent, H_2O_2. Readily loses active oxygen, the effective sterilising agent, forming water. Can be used at 0.1% to preserve milk (Buddeised milk, not permitted in the UK), but destroys vitamin C, methionine and tryptophan.

hydrogen swells *See* SWELLS.

hydrolyse To split a complex compound into its constituent parts by the action of water, either enzymically or catalysed by the addition of acid or alkali. Hence hydrolysis.

hydropathy Of proteins, their relative preferences for aqueous versus non-polar environments; the extent to which they are HYDROPHILIC or HYDROPHOBIC.

hydrophile–lipophile balance (HLB value) The ratio of HYDROPHILIC to HYDROPHOBIC groups on the molecules of an EMULSIFIER.

hydrophilic A solute that will dissolve in water and other polar solvents.

hydrophobic A solute that will dissolve in non-polar solvents, but not in water.

hydroponics The practice of growing plants without soil in a solution of inorganic salts.

hydrostatic steriliser Continuous steriliser in which the process is carried out under sufficient depth of water to maintain the required pressure. Used for continuous sterilisation of canned foods on a large scale.

hydrotalcite Aluminium magnesium carbonate/hydroxide hydrate; used as an ANTACID.

hydroxocobalamin *See* VITAMIN B_{12}.

hydroxyapatite Calcium orthophosphate hydroxide, the main mineral of bones, $Ca_{10}(PO_4)_6(OH)_2$.

hydroxybenzoic acid esters *See* PARABENS.

hydroxycholecalciferol *See* VITAMIN D.

hydroxylysine Amino acid found only in CONNECTIVE TISSUE proteins (collagen and elastin); incorporated into the protein as LYSINE and then hydroxylated in a vitamin C-dependent reaction; abbr Hyl, M_r 162.2, pK_a 2.13, 8.62, 9.67.

hydroxyproline Amino acid found mainly in CONNECTIVE TISSUE proteins (collagen and elastin); incorporated into the protein as PROLINE and then hydroxylated in a vitamin C-dependent reaction; abbr Hyp, M_r 131.1, pK_a 1.82, 9.66. Peptides of hydroxyproline are excreted in the urine and the output is increased when collagen turnover is high, as in rapid growth or resorption of tissue. Excretion is significantly lower than normal in children whose growth is impaired by PROTEIN–ENERGY MALNUTRITION. Measurement of hydroxyproline in meat products permits determination of the connective tissue content of the product

hydroxyproline index   The ratio of urinary hydroxyproline: creatinine/kg body weight; low in malnourished children.

5-hydroxytryptamine (5HT)   Also called serotonin. A neurotransmitter amine synthesised from the AMINO ACID TRYPTOPHAN, also formed in blood platelets; it acts as a vasoconstrictor. Found in PLANTAINS and some other foods, but metabolised in the intestinal mucosa by MONOAMINE OXIDASE.

Hyfoama^{TM} Hydrolysed milk and wheat protein used to prepare stable foams for confectionery manufacture that, unlike egg albumin foams, do not denature and cannot be overwhipped.

hygrometer   Instrument for measuring HUMIDITY and/or WATER ACTIVITY. Also known as a psychrometer.

hygroscopic   Readily absorbing water, as when table salt becomes damp. Materials such as calcium chloride and silica gel absorb water very readily and are used as drying agents. Hygroscopic foods are those in which the partial pressure of water vapour varies with the moisture content, so that they take up moisture from the atmosphere.

Hy-Lite^{TM} *See* BIOLUMINESCENCE.

hyoscine   *See* ATROPINE.

hyperalimentation   Provision of unusually large amounts of energy, either intravenously (PARENTERAL NUTRITION) or by NASOGASTRIC TUBE or GASTROSTOSTOMY tube (*see* ENTERAL NUTRITION).

hyperammonaemia   High blood ammonia concentration (normal <80 μmol/L), especially after protein intake, leading to coma, convulsions and possibly death. May be due to a variety of GENETIC DISEASES (*see* AMINO ACID DISORDERS) or liver failure. Treatment is normally by severe restriction of protein intake.

hypercalcaemia   Elevated plasma calcium believed to be due to hypersensitivity of some children to VITAMIN D toxicity. There is excessive absorption of calcium, with loss of appetite, vomiting, constipation, flabby muscles and calcinosis, deposition of calcium in the tissues. It can be fatal in infants.

hyperchlorhydria   Excess secretion of hydrochloric acid in the stomach due to secretion of a greater volume of gastric juice (GASTRIC SECRETION) rather than to a higher concentration.

hypercholesterolaemia   Abnormally high concentrations of CHOLESTEROL in the blood; normal total plasma cholesterol is below 5.2 mmol/L; above 6.5 mmol/L is considered abnormal and indicative of the need for intervention. Generally considered to be a sign of high risk for ATHEROSCLEROSIS and ISCHAEMIC HEART DISEASE. Treatment is by restriction of fat (especially saturated fat, *see* FAT, SATURATED) and cholesterol intake and a high intake of non-starch polysaccharides, which increase the excretion of cholesterol and its metabolites (the BILE SALTS) in the faeces.

In severe cases, drugs (HMG COA REDUCTASE inhibitors) may be given to inhibit the synthesis of cholesterol in the body, or ION-EXCHANGE RESINS may be fed, to increase the excretion of bile salts. Familial hypercholesterolaemia is a GENETIC DISEASE in which affected individuals have extremely high blood concentrations of cholesterol, frequently dying from ischaemic heart disease in early adulthood; treatment is as for other forms of hypercholesterolaemia, but more rigorous.

See also LIPOPROTEINS, PLASMA.

hyperfiltration *See* OSMOSIS, REVERSE.

hyperglycaemia High blood glucose (normal is 3.5–5.5 mmol/L), caused by a failure of the normal hormonal mechanisms of blood glucose control.

See also DIABETES; GLUCOSE TOLERANCE; INSULIN.

hyperinsulinaemia (hyperinsulinism) Excessive secretion of INSULIN, either as a result of an INSULINOMA, or due to HYPER-GLYCAEMIA resulting from INSULIN RESISTANCE.

hyperkalaemia Excessively high blood concentration of POTASSIUM.

hyperkinetic syndrome (hyperkinesis) Mental disorder of children, characterised by excessive activity and impaired attention and learning ability. Has been attributed to ADVERSE REACTIONS TO FOOD additives, but there is little evidence.

hyperlipidaemia (hyperlipoproteinaemia) A variety of conditions in which there are increased concentrations of LIPIDS in plasma, PHOSPHOLIPIDS, TRIGLYCERIDES, free and esterified CHOLESTEROL or free FATTY ACIDS.

See also HYPERCHOLESTEROLAEMIA; LIPOPROTEINS, PLASMA.

hyperoxaluria GENETIC DISEASE leading to excessive formation of OXALIC ACID, which causes the formation of kidney stones. Treatment includes a diet low in those fruits and vegetables that are sources of oxalic acid and in some cases supplements of VITAMIN B_6 some 50–100 times greater than normal requirements.

hyperphosphataemia Excessively high blood concentration of PHOSPHATE.

hypersalivation Excessive flow of SALIVA.

hypertension High BLOOD PRESSURE; a risk factor for ischaemic heart disease, stroke and kidney disease. May be due to increased sensitivity to SALT (correctly, sensitivity to SODIUM), and treated by restriction of salt intake, together with drugs; increased intake of fruits and vegetables (as a safe source of potassium) is recommended.

See also SALT-FREE DIETS.

hyperthyroidism   *See* THYROTOXICOSIS.

hypertonic   A solution more concentrated than the body fluids; *see* ISOTONIC.

hypervitaminosis   Overdosage with vitamins, leading to toxic effects. A problem with high levels of intake of VITAMINS A, D, B₆ and NIACIN, normally at levels of intake from supplements considerably higher than might be obtained from foods, although hypervitaminosis A and D may result from (enriched) foods.

    See also HORMESIS; HYPERCALCAEMIA; REFERENCE INTAKES; UL.

hypobaric storage   Of fruits and vegetables, storage below atmospheric pressure to enhance loss of CO_2 and ethylene, so slowing ripening.

    See also PACKAGING, MODIFIED ATMOSPHERE.

hypocalcaemia   Low blood CALCIUM, leading to tetany (uncontrollable twitching of muscles) if severe; may be due to underactivity of the parathyroid gland, kidney failure or VITAMIN D deficiency.

hypochlorhydria   Partial deficiency of hydrochloric acid secretion in the gastric juice.

    See also ACHLORHYDRIA; ANAEMIA, PERNICIOUS; GASTRIC SECRETION.

hypogeusia   Diminished sense of taste. An early sign of marginal zinc deficiency, and potentially useful as an index of zinc status.

    See also DYSGEUSIA; GUSTIN; PARAGEUSIA.

hypoglycaemia   Abnormally low blood glucose; (normal is 3.5–5.5 mmol/L); may result in loss of consciousness, hypoglycaemic coma.

hypoglycaemic agents   Three groups of compounds are used as oral hypoglycaemic agents for treatment of non-insulin-dependent DIABETES mellitus: the sulphonylureas (chlorpropamide, glibenclamide, glicazide, glimepiride, glipizide, gliquidone, tolazamide, tolbutamide) act to enhance secretion of INSULIN; buformin, metformin and phenformin are biguanides that act to decrease GLUCONEOGENESIS and increase peripheral utilisation of glucose; thiazolidinediones activate the PPARγ receptor, so decreasing insulin resistance, modifying adipocyte differentiation and decreasing LEPTIN secretion.

hypokalaemia   Abnormally low plasma potassium.

hypophosphataemia   Abnormally low plasma PHOSPHATE.

hypoproteinaemia   Abnormally low total plasma protein concentration.

hyposite   Little used word, from Greek, for low-energy food.

hypothermia   Low body temperature (normal is around 37 °C). Occurs among elderly people far more readily than in younger adults, often with fatal results. Also used in connection with deliberate reduction of body temperature to 28 °C to permit heart and brain surgery.

hypothyroidism Underactivity of the thyroid gland, leading to reduced secretion of THYROID HORMONES and a reduction in BASAL METABOLIC RATE. Commonly associated with GOITRE due to IODINE deficiency. In hypothyroid adults there is a characteristic moon-faced appearance, lethargy and dull mental apathy. In infants, hypothyroidism can lead to severe mental retardation, CRETINISM. *See also* THYROTOXICOSIS.

hypotonic A solution more dilute than the body fluids, *See* ISOTONIC.

hypovitaminosis VITAMIN deficiency.

hypoxanthine A PURINE, an intermediate in the metabolism of ADENINE and GUANINE to URIC ACID.

hyssop Pungent aromatic herb, *Hyssopus officinalis*, used in salads, soups and in making liqueurs.

I

iatrogenic A condition caused by medical intervention or drug treatment; iatrogenic nutrient deficiency is caused by drug–nutrient interactions.

IBC Intermediate bulk container.

iberian moss *See* CARRAGEENAN.

ice cream A frozen confection made from fat, milk solids and sugar. Some European countries permit the use of non-milk fat and term the product ice cream, while if milk fat is used, it is termed dairy ice cream. According to UK regulations, contains not less than 5% fat and 7% other milk solids. In the USA the minimum butterfat content is 10% with at least 20% total milk solids. Reduced fat ice cream contains 25% less fat, and light ice cream 50% less fat, or one-third less energy (and less than 50% of energy from fat). Low-fat ice cream contains not more than 3 g, and non-fat ice cream less than 0.5 g milk fat per serving. Stabilisers such as carboxymethylcellulose, GUMS and ALGINATES are included, and emulsifiers such as polysorbate and monoglycerides. Mono- and diglycerides bind the looser globules of water and are added in 'non-drip' ice cream.

ice, eutectic *See* EUTECTIC ICE.

Iceland moss A lichen, *Cetraria islandica*, that can be boiled to make a jelly.

ichthyosarcotoxins Toxins in fish.

IDDM Insulin-dependent DIABETES mellitus.

idi Indian, Sri Lankan; steamed bread made from rice and legume flour. The dough is left to undergo bacterial fermentation overnight; the main organisms are *Leuconostoc mesenteroides* and *Streptococcus faecalis*.

idiopathic A condition of unknown origin or cause.

idiosyncrasy Unusual and unexpected sensitivity or reaction to a drug or food.

IDL Intermediate-density lipoprotein; *see* LIPOPROTEINS, PLASMA.

idli S.E. Asian; small cakes made from a mixture of cooked rice and black gram, fermented with the aid of mould.

IHD Ischaemic heart disease.

ileitis Inflammation of the ILEUM.

ileocolitis Inflammation of the ILEUM and COLON.

ileostomy Surgical formation of an opening of the ileum on the abdominal wall, performed to treat severe ulcerative COLITIS; *see* GASTROINTESTINAL TRACT.

ileotomy Surgical removal of (part of) the ILEUM.

ileum Last portion of the small intestine, between the jejunum and the colon (large intestine), *see* GASTROINTESTINAL TRACT.

ileus Obstruction of the intestines, *see* GASTROINTESTINAL TRACT.

illipe butter *See* COCOA BUTTER EQUIVALENTS.

IMF *See* INTERMEDIATE MOISTURE FOODS.

immune system Series of defence mechanisms of the body. There are two major parts: humoral, mediated through antibodies secreted into the circulation (IMMUNOGLOBULINS); and cell-mediated. Lymphocytes produce antibodies against, and bind to, the antigens of foreign cells, leading to death of the invading organisms; other white blood cells are phagocytic and engulf the invading organisms.

immunoassay A variety of analytical techniques with very high specificity and sensitivity using antibodies raised against the analyte, coupled with an enzyme, fluorescent dye or radioactive material as a detection system.

 See also ELISA; FLUORESCENCE IMMUNOASSAY; RADIOIMMUNOASSAY.

immunoglobulins Specific antibodies produced in the blood in response to foreign proteins or other ANTIGENS. Five classes, IgA, IgE, IgG, IgM and IgI; present in circulating blood as a result of previous exposure to the antigens, and also present in breast milk to confer passive immunity.

immunomagnetic separation Technique for rapid isolation of food-borne pathogens using magnetic microspheres coated with ANTIBODIES.

IMP (1) *See* INTEGRATING MOTOR PNEUMOTACHOGRAPH.

 (2) Inosine monophosphate, one of the PURINE nucleotides.

impingement drying   Hot air is blown against the surface of the food through nozzles; used mainly to remove surface moisture from thin sheets of food.

improvers, flour   *See* AGEING.

IMS   *See* IMMUNOMAGNETIC SEPARATION.

inanition   Exhaustion and wasting due to complete lack or non-assimilation of food; a state of starvation.

inborn errors of metabolism   *See* GENETIC DISEASE.

incaparina   A number of protein-rich dietary supplements developed by the Institute of Nutrition of Central America and Panama (INCAP), based on cottonseed flour, or soya and vegetables, with various nutrient supplements, containing 27.5% protein.

incidence rate   Measure of morbidity based on the number of new episodes of a disease arising in a population over a given period of time.

   See also PREVALENCE RATE.

incretins   Hormones that increase the amount of INSULIN secreted in response to glucose, reduce GLUCAGON secretion and delay gastric emptying. They may also have actions to improve insulin sensitivity, and they may increase the formation of pancreatic β-islet cells.

   See also GIP; GLP-1; OREXINS.

index of nutritional quality (INQ)   An attempt to provide an overall figure for the nutrient content of a food or diet. The ratio of the amount of the nutrient/1000 kcal: the REFERENCE INTAKE/1000 kcal.

Indian corn   *See* MAIZE.

Indian fig   *See* PRICKLY PEAR.

Indian gum   Ghatti GUM, polysaccharide exudate from the stems of *Anogeissus latifolia*.

Indian rice grass   Perennial, growing wild in the USA, *Oryzopsis hymenoides*; tolerant to drought. The seeds resemble MILLET, small, round, dark in colour, covered with white hairs. Traditionally used by native Americans for flour, now almost exclusively for forage.

indigestion   Discomfort and distension of the stomach after a meal, also known as dyspepsia, including HEARTBURN. Persistent indigestion may be a symptom of a digestive disorder such as HIATUS HERNIA or peptic ULCER.

indigo carmine   Blue food colour (E-132), derivative of indigotin, which comes from tropical leguminous plants *Indigofera* spp.

induction   Of enzymes; an increase in the total amount of the enzyme protein in a cell as a result of increased TRANSCRIPTION of DNA, leading to an increased amount of mRNA.

   See also REPRESSION.

induction period   The lag period during which a fat or oil shows stability to oxidation because of its content of natural or added ANTIOXIDANTS, which are oxidised preferentially. After this there is a sudden and large consumption of oxygen and the fat becomes rancid.

infarction   Death of an area of tissue because its blood supply has been stopped.

INFOODS   International Network of Food Data Systems, created to develop standards and guidelines for collection of food composition data, and standardised terminology and nomenclature. Web site http://*www.fao.org/infood/*.

infuse (infusion)   To extract the flavour from herbs, spices, etc., by steeping them in a liquid, usually by pouring on boiling liquid, covering and leaving to stand without further cooking, as in making tea.

injera   Ethiopean; flat bread made from TEFF flour fermented for 30–72 hours with a starter from a previous batch; the main organism is the yeast *Candida guilliermondii*.

inorganic   Materials of MINERAL, as distinct from animal or vegetable, origin. Apart from carbonates and cyanides, inorganic chemicals are those that contain no carbon.

inositol   A carbohydrate derivative which is an essential nutrient for micro-organisms and many animals and sometimes classified as a vitamin, although there is no evidence that it is a dietary essential for human beings. Deficiency causes alopecia in mice and 'spectacle eye' (denudation around the eye) in rats. Obsolete names inosite and meat sugar.

Chemically, hexahydrocyclohexane $(CHOH)_6$; there are nine isomers, but only one, *meso-* or *myo*-inositol, is of physiological importance. It is a constituent of many PHOSPHOLIPIDS (phosphatidyl inositols) involved in membrane structure and as part of the signalling mechanism for HORMONES which act at the cell surface. The insecticide gammexane is hexachlorocyclohexane, and appears to function by competing with inositol. Inositol hexaphosphate is PHYTIC ACID.

INQ   *See* INDEX OF NUTRITIONAL QUALITY.

in silico   Experiments conducted by computer simulation, by analogy with *IN VITRO* and *IN VIVO*.

instant foods   Dried foods that reconstitute rapidly when water is added, e.g. tea, coffee, milk, soups, precooked cereal products, potatoes. The dried powders may be agglomerated to control particle size and improve solubility. 'Instant puddings' are formulated with pregelatinised starch and disperse rapidly in cold milk.

insulin   Peptide HORMONE secreted by the β-islet cells of the PAN-CREAS; controls GLUCOSE METABOLISM. DIABETES mellitus is the result of inadequate supply of insulin or tissue resistance to its action. Since insulin is a protein it would be digested if taken by mouth so must be injected. Originally the hormone was prepared from beef or pork pancreas, but these differ slightly in structure from human insulin, and lead to antibody formation after pro-longed use. Most insulin for therapeutic use is now human insulin, the product of biosynthesis from the human insulin gene.

   See also DIABETES; GLUCOSE TOLERANCE; HYPOGLYCAEMIC AGENTS; METABOLIC SYNDROME.

insulinaemic index   The rise in blood insulin elicited by a test dose (usually 50 g) of a carbohydrate food compared with that after an equivalent dose of glucose.

   See also GLYCAEMIC INDEX.

insulin-like growth factors   *See* SOMATOMEDINS.

insulinoma   INSULIN-secreting tumour of the β-islet cells of the PANCREAS.

insulin resistance   Resistance of target tissues to the actions of INSULIN, leading to HYPERINSULINAEMIA and HYPERGLYCAEMIA, commonly associated with abdominal adipose tissue. Only the metabolic actions of insulin are affected; the slower actions medi-ated via MAP KINASES are unaffected, so there is an exaggerated mitotic response to insulin, causing increased proliferation of vascular smooth muscle, leading to ATHEROSCLEROSIS and HYPERTENSION.

   See also METABOLIC SYNDROME.

integrating motor pneumotachograph (IMP)   Apparatus for mea-suring ENERGY EXPENDITURE indirectly from oxygen consumption. It meters the expired air and removes a proportion for analysis.

   See also SPIROMETER.

intense sweeteners   *See* SWEETENERS, INTENSE.

interesterification   Exchange of FATTY ACIDS between TRIACYL-GLYCEROLS in order to modify the properties of the fat; may be achieved by heat treatment or using fungal LIPASE.

interferon   A family of proteins that are secreted by macrophages (IFN-α), fibroblasts (IFN-β) and lymphocytes (IFN-γ) in response to viral, bacterial or LECTIN stimulation. They have potent antiviral activity, acting by inhibiting TRANSLATION of viral RNA, and inhibit proliferation of cancer cells.

interleukins   A family of CYTOKINES that act as signalling mole-cules between leukocytes.

intermediate moisture foods   These are semimoist with about 25% (15–50%) moisture but with some of the water bound (and so unavailable to MICRO-ORGANISMS) by the addition of glycerol, sorbitol, salt or certain organic acids, so preventing the growth of micro-organisms.

international units (IU)   Used as a measure of the potency or biological activity of substances such as vitamins and hormones, before chemical measurement was possible. Still sometimes used (3.33 IU VITAMIN A = 1 µg; 40 IU VITAMIN D = 1 µg; 1 IU VITAMIN E = 1 mg).

intervention study   Comparison of an outcome (e.g. morbidity or mortality) between two groups of people deliberately subjected to different dietary, drug or other regimes.

intestinal flora   Bacteria and other micro-organisms that are normally present in the GASTROINTESTINAL TRACT.

intestinal juice   Also called succus entericus. Digestive juice secreted by the intestinal glands lining the small intestine. It contains a variety of enzymes, including ENTEROPEPTIDASE, the enzyme that converts trypsinogen to active TRYPSIN, AMINOPEPTIDASE, nucleases and nucleotidases.

See also GASTROINTESTINAL TRACT.

intestine   The GASTROINTESTINAL TRACT; the small intestine (duodenum, jejunum and ileum) where the greater part of digestion and absorption take place, and the large intestine.

intolerance (to foods)   See ADVERSE REACTIONS TO FOODS.

intravenous nutrition   See PARENTERAL NUTRITION.

intrinsic factor   A protein secreted in the gastric juice by the parietal (oxyntic) cells of the gastric mucosa; essential for the absorption of VITAMIN B$_{12}$; impaired secretion results in pernicious ANAEMIA.

See also ACHLORHYDRIA; dUMP SUPPRESSION TEST; SCHILLING TEST.

intron   A region of DNA within a gene that does not contain information coding for the protein and is spliced out during the post-transcriptional modification of mRNA.

See also EXON.

intussusception   Telescoping or invagination of one part of the bowel into another.

inulin   Soluble undigested polymer of FRUCTOSE found in root vegetables, especially Jerusalem ARTICHOKE. Included with NON-STARCH POLYSACCHARIDES (DIETARY FIBRE). Also called dahlin and alant starch. Filtered by the kidney and not reabsorbed, so used clinically to measure glomerular filtration rate and kidney function.

inversion   Applied to SUCROSE, meaning its hydrolysis to glucose and fructose (see SUGAR, INVERT).

invertase   Also known as sucrase or saccharase; either of two enzymes, glucohydrolase (EC 3.2.1.20) or fructohydrolase (EC 3.2.1.26), with differing specificity, that hydrolyse SUCROSE to yield glucose and fructose. Used in the manufacture of invert sugar (*see* SUGAR, INVERT) and in chocolate confectionery to hydrolyse crystalline sucrose to a liquid syrup. The bifunctional sucrase–isomaltase of the intestinal mucosa is glucohydrolase.

invert sugar   *See* SUGAR, INVERT.

in vitro   Literally 'in glass'; used to indicate an observation made experimentally in the test tube, as distinct from the natural living conditions, *IN VIVO*.

in vivo   In the living state, as distinct from *IN VITRO*.

iodine   An essential mineral, a TRACE ELEMENT; reference intakes are about 140 µg per day. Iodine is required for synthesis of the THYROID HORMONES, which are iodotyrosine derivatives. A prolonged deficiency of iodine in the diet leads to GOITRE. It is plentifully supplied by sea foods and by vegetables grown in soil containing iodide. In areas where the soil is deficient in iodide, locally grown vegetables are iodine deficient, and hence goitre occurs in defined geographical regions, especially inland upland areas over limestone soil. Where deficiency is a problem, salt may be iodised (*see* IODISED SALT) to increase iodide intake.

iodine number (iodine value)   Measurement of the degree of unsaturation of FATTY ACIDS by iodination of the carbon–carbon double bonds. The Wijs method uses iodine chloride, Hanus iodine bromide, and Rosenmund–Kuhnhenn a pyridine sulphate/bromine reagent.

iodine, protein-bound   The THYROID HORMONES, tri-iodothyronine and thyroxine, are transported in the bloodstream bound to proteins; measurement of protein-bound iodine, as opposed to total plasma iodine, was used as an index of thyroid gland activity before more specific methods of measuring the hormones were developed.

iodised oil   Oil intended for administration either by injection or orally in regions of severe IODINE deficiency; prepared by treating vegetable oils with iodine, which adds across double bonds. Oils used include poppyseed, peanut and rape seed oils; injections provide protection for 2–4 years, oral administration about 1 year.

iodised salt   In areas of mild IODINE deficiency, salt is often enriched with iodate at levels of 10–25 mg iodate/kg; in areas of moderate deficiency to levels of 25–40 mg/kg. Where there is severe deficiency, IODISED OIL is used. In some areas all salt is enriched, in others it is optional. In some countries bread must be made with iodised salt.

iodopsin   *See* RHODOPSIN.

IoM   Institute of Medicine of the US National Academies; web site http://www.iom.edu/.

ion   An atom or molecule that has lost or gained one or more electrons, and thus has an electric charge. Positively charged ions are known as cations, because they migrate towards the cathode (negative pole) in solution, while negatively charged ions migrate towards the positive pole (anode) and hence are known as anions.

ion-exchange resin   An organic compound that will adsorb ions under some conditions and release them under other conditions. The best-known example is in water softening, where calcium ions are removed from the water by binding to the resin, displacing sodium ions. The resin is then regenerated by washing with a concentrated solution of salt, when the sodium ions displace the calcium ions. Ion-exchange resins are used for purification of chemicals, metal recovery, a variety of analytical techniques and treatment of HYPERCHOLESTEROLAEMIA.

ionisation   The process whereby the positive and negative IONS of a salt or other compound separate when dissolved in water. The degree of ionisation of an acid or alkali determines its strength (*see* pH).

ionising radiation   *See* IRRADIATION.

IQB (individual quick blanch)   Steam BLANCHING method in which all particles receive the same heat treatment, unlike conventional steam blanching where particles at the periphery of the bed are overheated when those in the centre are adequately treated.

IQF   Individual quick frozen or freezing.

Irish moss   A red seaweed, *Chondrus crispus*; source of the polysaccharide CARRAGEENAN.

Composition/100 g: water 81 g, 205 kJ (49 kcal), protein 1.5 g, fat 0.2 g, carbohydrate 12.3 g (0.6 g sugars), fibre 1.3 g, ash 4.7 g, Ca 72 mg, Fe 8.9 mg, Mg 144 mg, P 157 mg, K 63 mg, Na 67 mg, Zn 2 mg, Cu 0.1 mg, Mn 0.4 mg, Se 0.7 µg, vitamin A 6 µg RE (71 µg carotenoids), E 0.9 mg, K 66.9 mg, B_1 0.01 mg, B_2 0.47 mg, niacin 0.6 mg, B_6 0.07 mg, folate 182 µg, pantothenate 0.2 mg, C 3 mg.

iron   An essential MINERAL. The average adult has 4–5 g of iron, of which 60–70% is present in the blood as haem in the circulating HAEMOGLOBIN, and the remainder present in MYOGLOBIN in muscles, a variety of enzymes and tissue stores. Iron is stored in the liver in ferritin, in other tissues in haemosiderin, and in the blood transport protein transferrin.

Iron balance: losses in faeces 0.3–0.5 mg per day, in sweat and skin cells 0.5 mg, traces in hair and urine, total loss 0.5–1.5 mg per day. Blood loss leads to a considerable loss of iron. The average diet contains 10–15 mg, of which 0.5–1.5 mg is absorbed. The haem iron of meat and fish is considerably better absorbed than the inorganic iron of vegetable foods. Absorption of iron is enhanced by VITAMIN C taken at the same time as iron-containing foods, and reduced by phosphate, CALCIUM and PHYTIC ACID.

    See also ANAEMIA; FERRITIN; HAEMOCHROMATOSIS; IRON STORAGE; TRANSFERRIN.

iron ammonium citrate   *See* FERRIC AMMONIUM CITRATE.

iron binding capacity, total   *See* TRANSFERRIN.

iron chink   Machine designed in 1903 by US inventor A. K. Smith to behead, split and gut salmon in a continuous operation; so-called because it replaced Chinese labour in canneries.

iron ration   Heat-resistant high-energy chocolate ration enriched with vitamins and minerals devised for US Army by Capt. Paul Logan and first produced by Hershey Chocolate in 1937, as the Logan Bar Ration D (for daily). Heat-resistant because it did not contain COCOA BUTTER.

iron, reduced   Metallic iron in finely divided form, produced by reduction of iron oxide. The form in which iron is sometimes added to foods, such as bread. Also known by its Latin name *ferrum redactum*.

iron storage   FERRITIN is the iron storage protein in the intestinal mucosa, liver, spleen and bone marrow. It is a ferric hydroxide–phosphate–protein complex containing 23% iron. Haemosiderin is a long-term reserve of iron in tissues; colloidal iron hydroxide combined with protein and phosphate, probably formed by agglomeration of FERRITIN, the short-term storage form. Abnormally high levels of haemosiderin occur in SIDEROSIS.

irradiation   IONISING RADIATION (X-rays or γ-rays) kills micro-organisms and insects, so is used for sterilisation of foods; also inhibits sprouting of potatoes.

    See also MICROWAVE COOKING; RADAPPERTISATION; RADICIDATION; RADURISATION; ULTRAVIOLET RADIATION.

IRRI   International Rice Research Institute, Los Baños, Philippines. Web site http://www.irri.org/.

irritable bowel syndrome   Also known as spastic colon or mucous colitis. Abnormally increased motility of the large and small intestines, leading to pain and alternating diarrhoea and constipation; often precipitated by emotional stress.

isaño   Edible tubers of the Andean plant *Tropaeolum tuberosum*.

ischaemia   Inadequate blood supply to a tissue.

ischaemic heart disease   Or coronary heart disease. Group of syndromes arising from failure of the coronary arteries to supply sufficient blood to heart muscles; associated with ATHEROSCLERO-SIS of coronary arteries.

isinglass GELATINE prepared from the swim bladder of fish (especially sturgeon). Used commercially to clear wine and beer, and sometimes in jellies and ice cream. Japanese isinglass is AGAR.

islets of Langerhans The ENDOCRINE parts of the PANCREAS; GLUCAGON is secreted by the α-cells, INSULIN by the β-cells and GASTRIN by the γ-cells of the islets.

ISO 9000 Quality Standard The international standard for the management of quality, widely used in the food industry, catering and food distribution, but developed originally for the engineering industry. ISO 9001 covers the specification for design, manufacture and installation; ISO 9002 the specification for manufacture and installation; ISO 9003 the specification for final inspection and test.

isoacids Obsolete term for isomers of unsaturated FATTY ACIDS (including *trans*-isomers) formed during HYDROGENATION of oils.

isoamylase *See* DEBRANCHING ENZYMES.

isoascorbic acid *See* ERYTHORBIC ACID.

isobaric Processes in which the pressure is held constant and volume varies with temperature.
> *See also* ADIABATIC; ISOTHERMAL.

isodesmosine *See* DESMOSINE.

isoelectric focusing (electrofocusing) A technique for separating proteins, etc., by ELECTROPHORESIS on a support medium that provides a pH gradient, so that each comes to rest at a position determined by its ISOELECTRIC POINT.

isoelectric point The pH at which an ionised molecule (e.g. a protein or amino acid) has no net charge.

isoenzymes Enzymes that have the same catalytic activity, but different structures, properties and/or tissue distribution.

isoflavones *See* FLAVONOIDS.

isohumulones *See* HUMULONES.

isoleucine An essential amino acid, abbr Ile (I), M_r 131.2, pK_a 2.32, 9.76, CODONS AUA, AUPu. Rarely limiting in food. It is one of the branched-chain amino acids, together with leucine and valine.

isomalt A bulk SWEETENER, about half as sweet as sucrose, consisting of a mixture of two disaccharide POLYOLS, glucosorbitol and glucomannitol. About 50% metabolised, yielding 9 kJ (2.4 kcal)/gram. Thought to be less laxative than SORBITOL or MANNITOL, and does not encourage tooth decay, so is used in TOOTH-FRIENDLY SWEETS. It absorbs very little water, so products are less sticky than those made with sucrose and have a longer shelf-life.

isomalto-oligosaccharides *See* OLIGOSACCHARIDES.

isomaltose A disaccharide of glucose linked α-1,6 (MALTOSE is linked α-1,4); not fermentable. It arises from the branch points of STARCH following hydrolysis by AMYLASE, and is hydrolysed in the small intestinal mucosal brush border by sucrase-isomaltase. Also known as brachyose.

Isomerose[TM] High-fructose corn syrup (*see* SYRUPS, FRUCTOSE): 70–72% solids, 42% fructose, 55% glucose, 3% polysaccharides.

isomers Molecules containing the same atoms but differently arranged, so that the chemical and biochemical properties differ.

(1) In positional isomers the functional groups are on different carbon atoms; e.g. leucine and isoleucine, citric and isocitric acids.

(2) D- and L-isomerism refers to the spatial arrangement of four different chemical groups on the same carbon atom (stereoisomerism or optical isomerism). *R*- and *S*-isomerism is the same, but determined by systematic chemical rules. *See* D-, L- AND DL-.

(3) *Cis*- and *trans*-isomerism refers to the arrangement of groups adjacent to a carbon–carbon double bond; in the *cis*-isomer the groups are on the same side of the double bond, while on the *trans*-isomer they are on opposite sides.

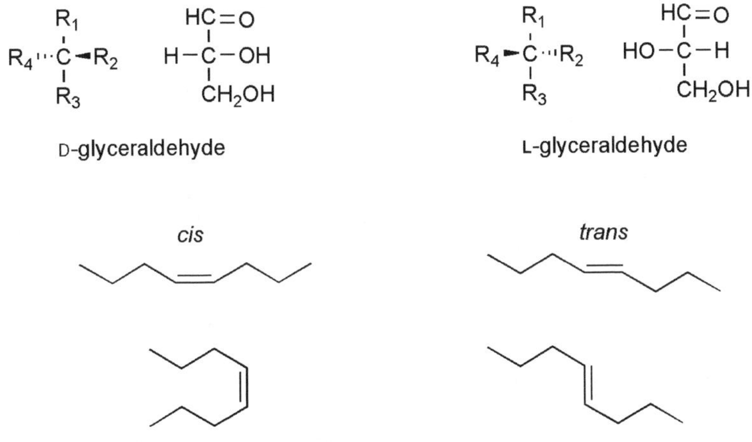

D-glyceraldehyde
L-glyceraldehyde

cis
trans

DL- AND *CIS–TRANS* ISOMERISM

isoniazid Isonicotinic acid hydrazide, used in the treatment of tuberculosis. Separately from its antimycobacterial action, forms an inactive adduct with pyridoxal, leading to depletion of VITAMIN B_6, and secondary PELLAGRA as a result of impaired synthesis of NIACIN from TRYPTOPHAN.

isopropyl citrate   Ester of isopropyl alcohol and citric acid, used to chelate metal ions that might otherwise cause rancidity in oils. *See* CHELATING AGENTS.

isostatic   Uniform pressure throughout a food or other material.

isosyrups   *See* SYRUPS, HIGH FRUCTOSE.

isothermal   Processes in which the temperature is held constant and volume varies with pressure.
See also ADIABATIC; ISOBARIC.

isotonic   Solutions with the same OSMOTIC PRESSURE (concentration of solutes); often refers to a solution with the same osmotic pressure as body fluids. Hypertonic and hypotonic refer to solutions that are respectively more and less concentrated.

isotopes   Forms of elements with the same chemical properties, differing in atomic mass because of differing numbers of neutrons in the nucleus. Thus, hydrogen has three isotopes, of atomic masses 1, 2 and 3, generally written as ^1H (the most abundant isotope of hydrogen), ^2H (deuterium) and ^3H (tritium). The incorporation of isotopes into compounds (labelled compounds or tracers) permits the metabolic fates of those compounds in the body to be followed easily.

Stable isotopes can be detected only by their atomic mass. Since they emit no radiation, they are considered completely safe for use in labelled compounds given to human beings. Examples of stable isotopes commonly used in nutrition research include ^2H, ^{13}C, ^{15}N and ^{18}O.

Unstable isotopes decay to stable elements, emitting radiation in the process. This may be α-particles, β-radiation (electrons), γ-radiation or X-rays, depending on the particular isotope. Radioactive isotopes can readily be detected by the radiation emitted. The time taken for half the radioactive isotope to decay is the HALF-LIFE (2) of the isotope, and can vary from a fraction of a second, through several days to years (e.g. the half-life of ^3H is 12.5 years, that of ^{14}C is 5200 years).

isotretinoin   13-*Cis* retinoic acid, a RETINOID used in the treatment of severe acne.

isozymes   *See* ISOENZYMES.

ispaghula   Polysaccharide GUM derived from the seed husks of *Plantago ovata*. Used as a thickening agent in foods and as a LAXATIVE.

itai-itai disease   *See* CADMIUM.

iu   *See* INTERNATIONAL UNITS.

IUFoST   International Union of Food Science and Technology; web site http://www.iufost.org/.

IUNS   International Union of Nutritional Sciences; web site http://www.iuns.org/.

jaboticaba Fruit of the tree *Myrciaria cauliflora* with purple astringent skin and sweet white pulp; the fruits grow straight from the trunk.

jack fruit Large fruit, up to 30 kg, from tropical tree *Artocarpus* spp., related to BREADFRUIT. Both pulp and seeds are eaten.

Composition/100 g: (edible portion 28%) water 73.2 g, 393 kJ (94 kcal), protein 1.5 g, fat 0.3 g, carbohydrate 24 g, fibre 1.6 g, ash 1 g, Ca 34 mg, Fe 0.6 mg, Mg 37 mg, P 36 mg, K 303 mg, Na 3 mg, Zn 0.4 mg, Cu 0.2 mg, Mn 0.2 mg, Se 0.6 µg, vitamin A 15 µg RE, B_1 0.03 mg, B_2 0.11 mg, niacin 0.4 mg, B_6 0.11 mg, folate 14 µg, C 7 mg. A 110 g serving is a source of Cu, Mg, vitamin C.

jaggery (1) Coarse dark sugar made from the sap of the coconut palm.

(2) Raw sugar cane juice, used in India as sweetening agent, also known as gur.

jaguar gum *See* GUAR GUM.

jake paralysis *See* JAMAICA GINGER PARALYSIS.

jam A conserve of fruit boiled to a pulp with sugar; sets to a PECTIN jelly on cooling (known in the USA as jelly). Standard jam, with certain exceptions, contains a minimum of 35 g of fruit per 100 g; extra jam, with certain exceptions, contains 45 g.

Jamaica ginger paralysis Polyneuritis caused by poisoning from an extract of Jamaica ginger ('jake') due to triorthocresyl phosphate.

Jamaican pepper *See* ALLSPICE.

jambolan Fruit of *Syzygium cumini* (*S. jambolanum*), also known as Indian blackberry, Java, Portuguese, Malabar, black or purple plum.

Composition/100 g: (edible portion 81%) water 83.1 g, 251 kJ (60 kcal), protein 0.7 g, fat 0.2 g, carbohydrate 15.6 g, ash 0.4 g, Ca 19 mg, Fe 0.2 mg, Mg 15 mg, P 17 mg, K 79 mg, Na 14 mg, vitamin B_1 0.01 mg, B_2 0.01 mg, niacin 0.3 mg, B_6 0.04 mg, C 14 mg.

Japanese isinglass *See* AGAR.

jasmine tea A perfumed or scented TEA made by adding petals of jasmine flowers to Chinese tea.

jejuno–ileostomy Surgical procedure in which the terminal JEJUNUM or proximal ILEUM is removed or by-passed. Has been used as a treatment for severe OBESITY.

jejunostomy feeding *See* ENTERAL NUTRITION.

jejunum Part of the small intestine, between the duodenum and the ileum; *see* GASTROINTESTINAL TRACT.

jelly (1) Clear JAM made from strained fruit juice by boiling with sugar. Also used in this sense in N. America to mean any jam.

(2) Table jelly is a dessert made from GELATINE, sweetened and flavoured; known in N. America as jello.

(3) Savoury gelatine jelly made from calf's foot or gelatinous stock; *see* ASPIC.

jellyfish seaweed   South-east Asian; strips of dried and salted jellyfish.

jelutong-pontianank   The latex of the jelutong tree (*Dyera costulata*) grown in Malaysia and Indonesia, used as a partial replacement for CHICLE in the manufacture of CHEWING GUM.

jerked beef, jerky   *See* CHARQUI.

Jerusalem oak   *See* EPAZOTE.

Job's tears   *See* ADLAY.

jodbasedow   *See* THYROTOXICOSIS.

jojoba oil   Liquid wax of long-chain FATTY ACIDS (eicosenoic and docosenoic (erucic) acids) esterified with long-chain alcohols (eicosanol and docosanol) from seeds of the shrub *Simmondsia chinensis*. Of interest in cosmetics as a replacement for sperm whale oil but also has food applications, e.g. coating agent for dried fruits.

jonathan   Calcined, ground oat chaff, used in 19th century as adulterant for maize and other cereals.

joule   The SI unit of ENERGY; used to express energy content of foods and energy expenditure of human and other animals. Gradually adopted as a replacement for the CALORIE from about 1970; 4.2 (precisely 4.186) kilojoules (kJ) is equal to 1 kilocalorie (kcal).

Joule cycle   *See* HEAT PUMP.

jowar   Indian name for SORGHUM (*Sorghum vulgare*), also known as great millet, kaffir corn, guinea corn.

jujube   (1) Sweet made from gum and sugar.

(2) Chinese date, Indian plum, fruit of the shrub *Zisiphus mauritania* or *Z. jujuba*, important fruit crop in India; the fruit is reddish-brown up to 2 cm in diameter with a single stone.

Composition/100 g: (edible portion 93%) water 77.9 g, 331 kJ (79 kcal), protein 1.2 g, fat 0.2 g, carbohydrate 20.2 g, ash 0.5 g, Ca 21 mg, Fe 0.5 mg, Mg 10 mg, P 23 mg, K 250 mg, Na 3 mg, Zn 0.1 mg, Cu 0.1 mg, Mn 0.1 mg, vitamin A 2 µg RE, B_1 0.02 mg, B_2 0.04 mg, niacin 0.9 mg, B_6 0.08 mg, C 69 mg.

jumbals   17th century British; biscuits made from caraway flavoured dough, twisted into knots or plaits before baking.

juniper   The ripened berries of the bush *Juniperis communis*, used as a flavouring in GIN.

junket   Dessert made from milk by treating with RENNET to curdle the protein.

K

kaffir beer   African BEER brewed from MILLET.

kaffir corn   *See* SORGHUM.

kaffir manna corn   *See* MILLET.

kahweol   Diterpene in COFFEE oil, potentially anticarcinogenic by enhancement of PHASE II METABOLISM of foreign compounds, but unlike CAFESTOL, probably not associated with HYPERCHOLES-TEROLAEMIA and hypertriglyceridaemia. Only released into the beverage when coffee is boiled for a prolonged period of time.

kaki   *See* PERSIMMON.

kale   Scottish name for any type of CABBAGE; in England means specifically open-headed varieties with curly leaves, also known as curly kale or borecole. Distinct from sea kale or SWISS CHARD.

   Composition/100 g: (edible portion 61%) water 84.5 g, 209 kJ (50 kcal), protein 3.3 g, fat 0.7 g, carbohydrate 10 g, fibre 2 g, ash 1.5 g, Ca 135 mg, Fe 1.7 mg, Mg 34 mg, P 56 mg, K 447 mg, Na 43 mg, Zn 0.4 mg, Cu 0.3 mg, Mn 0.8 mg, Se 0.9 µg, vitamin A 769 µg RE (48 776 µg carotenoids), K 817 mg, B_1 0.11 mg, B_2 0.13 mg, niacin 1 mg, B_6 0.27 mg, folate 29 µg, pantothenate 0.1 mg, C 120 mg. An 85 g serving is a source of Ca, vitamin B_6, folate, a good source of Cu, Mn, a rich source of vitamin A, C.

kamaboko   Japanese; foods prepared from SURIMI, but generally excluding more recently developed seafood analogues. Strictly, kamaboko is steamed or grilled on a wooden plate.

kamut   Variety of DURUM WHEAT (*Triticum durum*). The flour is claimed to be higher in protein, and to cause fewer allergic reactions, than ordinary wheat.

kanga-kopuwai   New Zealand (Maori); MAIZE gruel prepared by allowing whole maize cobs to ferment under water for 3 months, then removing the kernels, grinding into a paste and boiling.

kanji   Indian; alcoholic beverage made by fermentation of carrot or beetroot juice.

kaolin   Adsorbent clay used to treat diarrhoea and vomiting.

karasumi   Japanese; preserved ROE of grey mullet or tuna.

karat   Variety of BANANA growing in Micronesia that is an especially rich source of β-CAROTENE.

karaya gum   Obtained from the Indian tree *Sterculia arens*. Used as stabiliser, e.g. in frozen water ices; also used in combination with other stabilisers; sometimes used as laxative. Also called sterculia gum (E-416).

Karl Fischer method   For determination of the moisture content of dehydrated foods. Water is extracted from the sample into anhydrous methanol, then titrated against the Karl Fischer reagent (sulphur dioxide, pyridine and iodine in anhydrous methanol) with electrometric determination of the end-point.

Karo Syrup™   A mixture of dextrin, maltose, glucose and sucrose (dextromaltose) prepared from maize starch, used as carbohydrate modifier in milk preparations for infant feeding.

kasha   *See* BUCKWHEAT.

Kashin–Beck syndrome   Osteo-articular disorder that is endemic in regions of China where there is severe SELENIUM deficiency, and responds to selenium supplementation.
>   *See also* KESHAN DISEASE.

kasnudln   Austrian; egg and flour dough with sweet or savoury filling, a type of ravioli.

katadyn process   *See* MATZKA PROCESS; OLIGODYNAMIC.

katemfe   An intensely sweet African fruit, *Thaumatococcus daniellii*, called katemfe in Sierra Leone and miraculous fruit of Sudan (not the same as MIRACLE BERRY). The active principle is the protein THAUMATIN.

kathepsins   *See* CATHEPSINS.

katsuobushi   East Asian, Indian; TUNA dried and fermented with the mould *Aspergillus repens*; may also be smoked.

kava   Polynesian; a non-alcoholic stimulant beverage made from the roots of *Piper methysticum*; there is some evidence that herbal products (kava kava) are effective in treatment of anxiety, but excessive consumption can cause unconsciousness.

kawal   Sudanese; balls of paste from the leaves of the legume *Cassia obtusifolia*, fermented for 12–15 days in a sealed earthenware vessel (zeer) then sun-dried. The main organisms are *Bacillus subtilis* and *Propionobacterium* spp. Used in soups and stews.

kb   Kilobase, a measure of the size of DNA and RNA by the number of thousands of bases in the sequence under consideration.

kcal   Abbreviation for kilocalorie (1000 CALORIES), sometimes shown as Cal.

kebab   Turkish for roast meat. Shishkebab is small pieces of mutton rubbed with salt, pepper, etc. and roasted on a skewer (*shish* in Turkish) sometimes interspaced with vegetables. Shashlik is a Georgian version. Döner kebab is a Turkish specialty consisting of marinated mutton or lamb packed into a cylindrical mass and grilled on a vertical rotating spit (*showarma* in Arabic).

kedgeree   Indian; dish of rice and pulses. Modified to Victorian breakfast dish of flaked fish with egg and rice.

kefalotyri   Greek hard cheese; the curds are cut and heated before being pressed into moulds.

kefir   *See* MILK, FERMENTED.

kelor *See* MORINGA.

kelp Large brown seaweeds, *Laminaria* spp. Occasionally used as food or food ingredient but mostly the ash is used as a source of alkali and iodine. Sometimes claimed as a HEALTH FOOD with unspecified properties. 55% of the dry weight is LAMINARIN, a NON-STARCH POLYSACCHARIDE.

Composition/100 g: water 82 g, 180 kJ (43 kcal), protein 1.7 g, fat 0.6 g, carbohydrate 9.6 g (0.6 g sugars), fibre 1.3 g, ash 6.6 g, Ca 168 mg, Fe 2.8 mg, Mg 121 mg, P 42 mg, K 89 mg, Na 233 mg, Zn 1.2 mg, Cu 0.1 mg, Mn 0.2 mg, Se 0.7 μg, vitamin A 6 μg RE (70 μg carotenoids), E 0.9 mg, K 66 mg, B_1 0.05 mg, B_2 0.15 mg, niacin 0.5 mg, folate 180 μg, pantothenate 0.6 mg, C 3 mg.

kelvin SI unit of temperature; $K = °C - 273.15$. *See* TEMPERATURE, ABSOLUTE.

kenima North Indian, Nepali; fried SOY bean cake; the beans are soaked in water and allowed to undergo lactic acid bacterial fermentation before cooking.

kenkey Ghanaian; MAIZE dumplings, wrapped in leaves or maize cob sheaths and steamed. The dough is left to undergo lactic acid bacterial fermentation, a portion is then boiled to produce AFLATA, which is then mixed with the remainder before cooking. Madidi is similar.

kephalins Or cephalins; PHOSPHOLIPIDS containing ethanolamine, hence PHOSPHATIDYLETHANOLAMINES. Found especially in brain and nerve tissue.

Kepler extract of malt Trade name for one of the earliest of the MALT EXTRACTS, intended as a dietary supplement to aid digestion, since it was rich in DIASTASE.

keratin The insoluble protein of hair, horn, hoof, feathers and nails. Not hydrolysed by digestive enzymes, and therefore nutritionally useless. Used as fertiliser, since it is slowly broken down by soil bacteria. Steamed feather meal is used to some extent as a supplement for RUMINANTS.

keratinisation Process by which epithelial cells become horny due to deposition of KERATIN; may occur excessively and inappropriately in VITAMIN A deficiency.

keratomalacia Dryness and ulceration of the cornea as a result of VITAMIN A deficiency. Blindness is usually inevitable unless the deficiency is corrected at an early stage.

kermes A red colourant derived from the insect *Kermes ilicis* found on several species of oak, particularly *Quercus coccifera*. The pigment is kermesic acid. *See also* COCHINEAL.

kermesic acid *See* COCHINEAL; KERMES.

kesari dhal A LEGUME, *Lathyris sativus*.

See also LATHYRISM.

Keshan disease Cardiomyopathy that is endemic in regions of China where there is severe SELENIUM deficiency, and responds to selenium supplementation, although other factors, including coxsackie virus and the MYCOTOXIN MONILIFORMIN, may also be involved.

See also KASHIN–BECK SYNDROME.

keshi yena Caribbean (Curaçao); hollowed out Dutch cheese filled with meat, rice and currants.

Kesp™ Texture vegetable protein made by a spinning process.

ketchup (catsup or catchup) From the Chinese *koechap* or *kitsiap*, originally meaning brine of pickled fish. Now used for spicy sauce or condiment made with juice of fruit or vegetables, vinegar and spices.

ketoacidosis (or ketonaemia) High concentrations of KETONE BODIES in the blood, so far in excess of the capacity for their metabolism that the blood level rises sufficiently to affect pH. May occur in patients with insulin-dependent DIABETES mellitus, but rare in those with non-insulin-dependent diabetes.

ketogenic amino acids *See* AMINO ACIDS, KETOGENIC.

ketogenic diet A diet poor in carbohydrate (20–30 g) and rich in fat; causes accumulation of KETONE BODIES in tissue; formerly used in the treatment of epilepsy. *See also* ATKINS DIET.

ketonaemia *See* KETOACIDOSIS.

ketone bodies Acetone, acetoacetate and β-hydroxybutyric acid (not chemically a ketone) synthesised in liver from acetyl CoA (the product of β-oxidation of fatty acids), especially in the fasting state, and exported for use by other tissues as a metabolic fuel. When production exceeds the rate of utilisation the plasma concentration may rise high enough to cause significant KETOACIDOSIS (especially in uncontrolled insulin-dependent DIABETES mellitus), and significant amounts may be excreted in the urine (ketonuria).

ketones Chemical compounds containing a carbonyl group (C=O), with two alkyl groups attached to the same carbon; the simplest ketone is ACETONE (dimethylketone, $(CH_3)_2$—C=O).

ketonic rancidity Moulds of *Penicillium* and *Aspergillus* spp. attack fats containing short-chain fatty acids and produce KETONES with a characteristic odour and taste, so-called ketonic rancidity. Fats such as butter, coconut and palm kernel are most susceptible.

Ketonil™ A protein-rich food low in PHENYLALANINE for patients with PHENYLKETONURIA.

ketonuria Excretion of KETONE BODIES in the urine.

ketosis High concentrations of KETONE BODIES in the blood.

Keys score Method of expressing the lipid content of a diet, calculated as $1.35 \times (2 \times \%$ energy from saturated fat $-\%$ energy from polyunsaturated fat$) + 1.5 \times \sqrt{}$ (mg cholesterol/1000 kcal).

See also HEGSTED SCORE.

khushkhash *See* ORANGE, BITTER.

kibble To grind or chop coarsely.

Kick's law Equation to calculate the energy cost of reducing particle size, based on the log of the initial:final size.

See also BOND'S LAW; COMMINUTION; RITTINGER'S LAW.

kid Young goat (*Capra aegragus*) usually under three months old; similar to LAMB, but with a stronger flavour.

kidney Usually from lamb, ox, pig.

Lamb, composition/100 g: (edible portion 97%) water 79 g, 406 kJ (97 kcal), protein 15.7 g, fat 3 g (of which 45% saturated, 27% mono-unsaturated, 27% polyunsaturated), cholesterol 337 mg, carbohydrate 0.8 g, ash 1.3 g, Ca 13 mg, Fe 6.4 mg, Mg 17 mg, P 246 mg, K 277 mg, Na 156 mg, Zn 2.2 mg, Cu 0.4 mg, Mn 0.1 mg, Se 126.9 µg, vitamin A 95 µg retinol, B_1 0.62 mg, B_2 2.24 mg, niacin 7.5 mg, B_6 0.22 mg, folate 28 µg, B_{12} 52.4 µg, pantothenate 4.2 mg, C 11 mg. A 100 g serving is a source of Zn, vitamin A, B_6, folate, C, a rich source of Cu, Fe, P, Se, vitamin B_1, B_2, niacin, B_{12}, pantothenate.

Ox, composition/100 g: (edible portion 84%) water 77 g, 431 kJ (103 kcal), protein 17.4 g, fat 3.1 g (of which 45% saturated, 30% mono-unsaturated, 25% polyunsaturated), cholesterol 411 mg, carbohydrate 0.3 g, ash 1.3 g, Ca 13 mg, Fe 4.6 mg, Mg 17 mg, P 257 mg, K 262 mg, Na 182 mg, Zn 1.9 mg, Cu 0.4 mg, Mn 0.1 mg, Se 141 µg, vitamin A 419 µg RE (419 µg retinol, 20 µg carotenoids), E 0.2 mg, B_1 0.36 mg, B_2 2.84 mg, niacin 8 mg, B_6 0.67 mg, folate 98 µg, B_{12} 27.5 µg, pantothenate 4 mg, C 9 mg. A 100 g serving is a source of Zn, vitamin C, a good source of vitamin B_1, a rich source of Cu, Fe, P, Se, vitamin A, B_2, niacin, B_6, folate, B_{12}, pantothenate.

kielbasa Polish; seasoned pork and beef sausage, may be smoked.

kieves Irish name for MASH TUNS.

kilderkin Cask for beer (18 gallons = 80.1 L) and ale (16 gallons = 71.2 L).

Kiliani reaction Colorimetric reaction for CHOLESTEROL; the development of a purple colour on reaction with ferric chloride.

kimbu Japanese; dried seaweed (*see* KELP).

kimchi Korean; dish based on fermented cabbage with garlic, red peppers and pimientos, often with the addition of fish and other foods.

kinky hair syndrome *See* MENKES SYNDROME.

kipfel (kipfl) Austrian; crescent shaped roll created to celebrate the lifting of the siege of Vienna (1683). Reputedly the precursor of the croissant, believed to have been introduced to France by Marie Antoinette.

kipper   HERRING that has been lightly salted and smoked, invented by John Woodger, a fish curer of Seahouses, Northumberland, 1843. Dried to 60% water.

Kirschner number   Measure of the water-soluble fatty acids up to and including butyric acid in a lipid.

See also POLENSKE NUMBER; REICHERT–MEISSL NUMBER; STEAM DISTILLATION.

kishk   North African, Middle Eastern, East Asian; YOGURT or fermented milk mixed with parboiled or crushed wheat or flour and left to ferment for 2–3 days, then shaped into small balls and dried. Used in soups.

kisra   Sudanese; thin flat bread made from SORGHUM. The batter is mixed with a starter from a previous batch and left to undergo lactic acid bacterial and yeast fermentation overnight, then poured onto heated plate to bake for about 1 minute.

kitul   *See* TODDY PALM.

kiwano   Fruit of *Cucumis metuliferus*, originally from arid regions of southern and central Africa, now grown commercially in Australia and New Zealand, but with a limited market because of its bland flavour. Also known as melano, African horned cucumber, jelly melon, hedged gourd, horned melon, English tomato.

kiwi   Fruit of *Actinidia sinensis*, originally native of China and also known as Chinese gooseberry.

Composition/100 g: (edible portion 86%) water 83 g, 255 kJ (61 kcal), protein 1.1 g, fat 0.5 g, carbohydrate 14.7 g (9 g sugars), fibre 3 g, ash 0.6 g, Ca 34 mg, Fe 0.3 mg, Mg 17 mg, P 34 mg, K 312 mg, Na 3 mg, Zn 0.1 mg, Cu 0.1 mg, Mn 0.1 mg, Se 0.2 µg, vitamin A 4 µg RE (174 µg carotenoids), E 1.5 mg, K 40.3 mg, B_1 0.03 mg, B_2 0.03 mg, niacin 0.3 mg, B_6 0.06 mg, folate 25 µg, pantothenate 0.2 mg, C 93 mg. A 60 g serving is a rich source of vitamin C.

Kjeldahl determination   Widely used method of determining total nitrogen in a substance by digesting with sulphuric acid and a catalyst first described in 1883; the nitrogen is reduced to ammonia which is then measured. In foodstuffs most of the nitrogen is PROTEIN, and the term crude protein is the total 'Kjeldahl nitrogen' multiplied by factor 6.25 (since most proteins contain 16% nitrogen).

See also NITROGEN CONVERSION FACTOR.

Klim^{TM} Dried milk powder.

klipfish   Salted and dried cod, mainly produced in Norway, also known as bacalao or bacalau. The fish is boned, stored in salt for a month, washed and dried slowly.

See also STOCKFISH.

K_m The Michaelis constant of an enzyme. A measure of the affinity of the enzyme for its substrate, equal to the concentration of substrate at which the enzyme achieves half its maximum rate of activity.

kneading   To work dough by stretching and folding until it achieves the required consistency.

knee height   Distance from the heel to the anterior surface of the thigh, proximal to the patella. Highly correlated with stature, and used as a surrogate measure of height in people with severe spinal curvature or those who are unable to stand.

knocked corn   Orkneys, historical; threshed BARLEY lightly bruised in a mortar with warm water; the husks were floated off and the grains boiled.

kohlrabi   Swollen stem of *Brassica oleracea gongylodes* (turnip-rooted cabbage, kale turnip); green and purple varieties.

Composition/100g: (edible portion 46%) water 91g, 113kJ (27kcal), protein 1.7g, fat 0.1g, carbohydrate 6.2g (2.6g sugars), fibre 3.6g, ash 1g, Ca 24mg, Fe 0.4mg, Mg 19mg, P 46mg, K 350mg, Na 20mg, Cu 0.1mg, Mn 0.1mg, Se 0.7µg, vitamin A 2µg RE (22µg carotenoids), E 0.5mg, K 0.1mg, B_1 0.05mg, B_2 0.02mg, niacin 0.4mg, B_6 0.15mg, folate 16µg, pantothenate 0.2mg, C 62mg. A 30g serving is a rich source of vitamin C.

koilonychia   Development of (brittle) concave fingernails, commonly associated with IRON deficiency ANAEMIA.

koji   Japanese; koji mould (*Aspergillus oryzae*) grown on roasted cereal to provide a starter for fermentation to produce NATTO and MIRIN.

See also MISO.

koko   West and central African; sour cereal porridge made from maize, millet or sorghum that has been soaked and left to undergo lactic acid bacterial fermentation for 24 hours, then boiled.

kokoh   In the Zen macrobiotic diet this is a mixture of ground seeds and cereals fed to young infants; it is deficient in a number of nutrients and can result in growth retardation unless supplemented.

kokum   *See* COCOA BUTTER EQUIVALENTS.

kola nut   The seed of *Cola nitida* or other *Cola* species. The nut contains approximately 1.5% caffeine and is used in beverages and as an adjunct with other flavours.

kolatchen   Eastern European; sour cream biscuit made with flour, butter, sour cream and yeast, served warm.

kolbasa   Russian; garlicky well-seasoned pork and beef sausage; may be smoked.

konjac GUM derived from tubers of *Amorphophallus konjac*; eaten in Japan as a firm jelly.

konnyaku Chinese, Japanese; flour made from tubers of the devil's tongue plant, *Amorphallus rivieri*.

Korsakoff's psychosis Failure of recent memory, although events from the past are recalled, with CONFABULATION; associated with VITAMIN B₁ deficiency, especially in alcoholics.

See also WERNICKE–KORSAKOFF SYNDROME.

kosher The selection and preparation of foods in accordance with traditional Jewish ritual and dietary laws. Foods that are not kosher are traife. The only kosher meat is from animals that chew the cud and have cloven hooves, such as cattle, sheep, goats and deer; the hindquarters must not be eaten. The only fish permitted are those with fins and scales; birds of prey and scavengers are not kosher. Moreover, the animals must be slaughtered according to ritual before the meat can be considered kosher.

See also HALAL; FLEISHIG; MILCHIG; PAREVE.

koumiss See MILK, FERMENTED.

kpokpoi West African; small (2–3 mm) steamed balls of fermented maize or yam flour; similar to COUSCOUS (which is not fermented).

Krebs' cycle Or citric acid cycle, a central pathway for the METABOLISM of fats, carbohydrates and amino acids. Named for Sir Hans Krebs (1900–81), who first described the pathway.

krill Term that refers to many species of planktonic crustaceans but mostly the SHRIMP *Euphausia superba*. This is the main food of whales, and some penguins and other seabirds; occurs in shoals in the Antarctic, containing up to 12 kg/m³. Collected in limited quantities for use as human food.

kryptoxanthin See CRYPTOXANTHIN.

kuban See MILK, FERMENTED.

kudzu See KUZU.

kumiss See MILK, FERMENTED.

kumquat A CITRUS fruit *Fortunella* spp.; widely distributed in S. China and now cultivated elsewhere; resembles other citrus fruits, but very small, ovoid shape, with acid pulp, and sweet, edible skin.

Composition/100 g: (edible portion 93%) water 81 g, 297 kJ (71 kcal), protein 1.9 g, fat 0.9 g, carbohydrate 15.9 g (9.4 g sugars), fibre 6.5 g, ash 0.5 g, Ca 62 mg, Fe 0.9 mg, Mg 20 mg, P 19 mg, K 186 mg, Na 10 mg, Zn 0.2 mg, Cu 0.1 mg, Mn 0.1 mg, vitamin A 15 µg RE (477 µg carotenoids), E 0.2 mg, B₁ 0.04 mg, B₂ 0.09 mg, niacin 0.4 mg, B₆ 0.04 mg, folate 17 µg, pantothenate 0.2 mg, C 44 mg. A 30 g serving (4 fruits) is a good source of vitamin C.

kuru Or trembling disease; progressive degeneration of central nervous system cells, associated with cannibalism in Papua-New Guinea, and believed to be caused by a PRION. More or less eradicated since ritual cannibalism was abolished.

kurut North African, Middle Eastern, East Asian; hard dried balls of fermented milk or milk curds.

kushuk Iraqi; parboiled wheat and turnip allowed to undergo lactic acid bacterial fermentation for 4–10 days; liquid used as soup and the solid eaten as porridge or mixed with vegetables. Also an alternative name for KISHK.

kuzu Starch from the tubers of the kuzu (or kudzu) vine (*Pueraria lobata* or *P. thunbergiana*) used as a thickening agent in Chinese and Japanese cuisine.

kwashiorkor *See* PROTEIN–ENERGY MALNUTRITION.

kyphosis Excessive outward curvature of the spine, causing hunching of the back. May result from collapse of the vertebrae in OSTEOPOROSIS.

L

L- *See* D, L- AND DL-.

lac A red colourant (a complex mixture of anthraquinones) obtained from the insect *Laccifera lacca* (*Coccus lacca*) found on the trees *Schleichera oleosa, Ziziphus mauritiana* and *Butea monosperma*, which grow in India and Malaysia. The lac insects are also the source of shellac.

laccase *See* PHENOL OXIDASES.

lacquer With reference to canned foods (*see* CANNING), a layer of synthetic resin is coated onto the tinplate and hardened with heat. The layer of lacquer protects the tin lining from attack by acid fruit juices.

lactalbumin One of the proteins of milk. Unlike CASEIN, not precipitated from acid solution; hence, during cheese-making the WHEY contains lactalbumin and lactoglobulin. They are precipitated by heat and a whey CHEESE can be made in this way.

lactase The enzyme (β-galactosidase, EC 3.2.1.23) that hydrolyses LACTOSE to glucose and galactose; present in the brush border of the intestinal mucosal cells. Deficiency of lactase (ALACTASIA) is common in most ethnic groups after adolescence, leading to lactose intolerance. Fungal lactase is used to produce lactose-free MILK for people suffering from alactasia.

See also DISACCHARIDE INTOLERANCE.

lactic acid The acid produced by the anaerobic metabolism of glucose. Originally discovered in sour milk, it is responsible for the flavour of fermented MILK and for the precipitation of the CASEIN curd in cottage CHEESE. Also produced by fermentation in silage, PICKLING, SAUERKRAUT, COCOA, tobacco; its value here is in suppressing the growth of unwanted organisms.

It is formed in mammalian muscle under conditions of maximum exertion (*see* GLUCOSE METABOLISM) and by metabolism of glycogen in meat immediately after death of the animal. Lactic acid in muscle was at one time known as sarcolactic acid.

Used as an acidulant in sugar confectionery, soft drinks, pickles and sauces. (E-270; salts of lactic acid are E-325–327.)

lactic acid, buffered   A mixture of LACTIC ACID and sodium lactate used in sugar confectionery to provide an acid taste without INVERSION of the sugar, which occurs at lower pH.

lactitol   SUGAR ALCOHOL derived from LACTULOSE. Not digested by digestive enzymes but fermented by intestinal bacteria to short-chain fatty acids, some of which are absorbed; it yields about 8 kJ (2 kcal)/g and hence has a potential use as a low-calorie bulk sweetener; also retards crystallisation and improves moisture retention in foods (E-966). Because of bacterial fermentation in the colon, it is also used as an osmotic LAXATIVE. Also known as lactit, lactositol, lactobiosit.

Lactobacillus   Genus of bacteria capable of growth in acidic medium, and producing LACTIC ACID by fermentation of carbohydrates. Responsible for souring of MILK, and production of flavour in YOGURT and other fermented milk products.

See also PROBIOTICS.

***Lactobacillus casei* factor**   Obsolete name for FOLIC ACID.

lactobiose   *See* LACTOSE.

lactobiosit   *See* LACTITOL.

lactochrome   Obsolete name for riboflavin (VITAMIN B_2).

lactoferrin   Iron–protein complex in human milk (only a trace in cow's milk), only partly saturated with iron; has a role inhibiting the growth of *E. coli* and other potentially pathogenic organisms.

lactoflavin   Obsolete name for riboflavin (VITAMIN B_2), so named because it was isolated from milk.

lactogen   A drug or other substance that increases the production and secretion of milk. Lactogenic hormone is PROLACTIN.

lactoglobulin   *See* LACTALBUMIN.

lactometer   Floating device used to measure the specific gravity of milk (1.027–1.035).

Lac-tone[TM]   Protein-rich baby food (26% protein) made in India from peanut flour, skim milk powder, wheat flour and barley flour with added vitamins and calcium.

lacto-ovo-vegetarian   One whose diet excludes animal foods (i.e. flesh) but permits milk and eggs.

lactose   Milk sugar, the CARBOHYDRATE of milk; a DISACCHARIDE, β-1,4-glucosyl-galactose. Used pharmaceutically as a tablet filler and as a medium for growth of micro-organisms. The fermentation of lactose to LACTIC ACID by bacteria is responsible for the souring of milk. Ordinary lactose is α-lactose, which is 16% as sweet as sucrose; if crystallised above 93 °C, it is isomerised to the β-form which is more soluble and sweeter.

    See also DISACCHARIDE INTOLERANCE; LACTASE.

lacto-serum   *See* WHEY.

lactositol   *See* LACTITOL.

lactostearin   *See* GLYCERYL LACTOSTEARATE.

lactosucrose   A   trisaccharide   (galactosyl-glucosyl-fructose) formed from sucrose and lactose by fructosyl transfer catalysed by INVERTASE (EC 3.2.1.6). Considered to be a PREBIOTIC.

lactulose   A DISACCHARIDE, β-1,4-fructosyl-galactose, which does not occur naturally but is formed in heated or stored milk by isomerisation of LACTOSE. About half as sweet as sucrose. Not hydrolysed by human digestive enzymes but fermented by intestinal bacteria to form LACTIC ACID and PYRUVIC ACID. Thought to promote the growth of *Lactobacillus bifidus* and so added to some infant formulae. Because of bacterial fermentation in the colon it is an osmotic LAXATIVE.

ladies' fingers   *See* OKRA; also a short kind of banana.

laetrile   *See* AMYGDALIN.

laevorotatory   *See* OPTICAL ACTIVITY.

laevulose   *See* FRUCTOSE.

lafun   West and East African; flour made from yam, cassava or plantain that has been soaked in water and allowed to undergo lactic acid bacterial fermentation for 2–5 days, then sun-dried and pounded into flour.

lamb   Meat from sheep (*Ovis aries*) younger than 12–14 months.

    Composition/100 g (varying according to joint): (edible portion 79%) water 61–64 g, 960–1100 kJ (230–260 kcal), protein 17–18 g, fat 17–21 g (of which 47% saturated, 44% mono-unsaturated, 9% polyunsaturated), cholesterol 70 mg, ash 0.9 g, Ca 9–16 mg, Fe 1.5–1.7 mg, Mg 21–23 mg, P 160–170 mg, K 230–250 mg, Na 60 mg, Zn 3–4 mg, Cu 0.1 mg, Se 20 μg, vitamin E 0.2 mg, B_1 0.1 mg, B_2 0.2 mg, niacin 6 mg, B_6 0.14 mg, folate 19 μg, B_{12} 2.5 μg, pantothenate 0.7 mg. A 100 g serving is a source of Fe, vitamin B_2, pantothenate, a good source of P, Se, Zn, a rich source of niacin, vitamin B_{12}.

lamb's lettuce   Or corn salad. Hardy annual plant, *Valerianella locusta* or *V. olitoria*, traditionally used in salads in winter and early spring.

lamb's wool Old English drink made by pouring hot ale over pulped roasted apples and adding sugar and spices.

laminarin A NON-STARCH POLYSACCHARIDE from KELP (*Laminaria* spp.); a short polymer of glucose linked β(1–3) with β(1–6) branch points.

lamination Bonding together of two or more packaging films, papers or foods.

lamprey (lampern) Cartilaginous fish resembling eel; sea lamprey is *Petromyzon marinus*, river lamprey or lampern is *Lampetra fluviatilis*.

Lancashire English hard CHEESE with a crumbly texture.

landrace Variety of plant or animal, highly adapted to local conditions, often associated with traditional agriculture.

Lanepa^{TM} Capsules of fish oil rich in ω3 polyunsaturated fatty acids.

langouste SHELLFISH, *Palinurus vulgaris*; *see* LOBSTER.

lanolin The fat from wool. Consists of a mixture of cholesterol oleate, palmitate and stearate, not useful as food; used in various cosmetics.

lansoprazole *See* PROTON PUMP.

lao-chao South-east Asian; sweet slightly alcoholic glutinous rice. Boiled rice is inoculated with a starter (RAGI), which introduces various amylase-producing moulds, including *Rhizopus* spp., and fermented for 2–3 days.

larch gum A POLYSACCHARIDE of galactose and arabinose (ratio 1:6), found in the aqueous extract of the Western larch tree (*Larix occidentalis*); a potential substitute for GUM ARABIC, since it is readily dispersed in water.

lard Originally rendered fat from pig carcass (sheep and cattle also used). The best quality is from the fat surrounding the kidneys; neutral lard is the highest quality, prepared by agitating the minced fat with water at a temperature below 50 °C; kidney fat provides No. 1 quality; back fat provides No. 2 quality. Leaf lard is made from the residue of kidney and back fat after the preparation of neutral lard by heating with water above 100 °C in an autoclave. Prime steam lard is fat from any part of the carcass, rendered in the autoclave. Fatty acids 41% saturated, 47% mono-unsaturated, 12% polyunsaturated. Lard used to be stored in pig's bladder, hence the expression 'bladder of lard' for a grossly obese person.

See also LARD COMPOUNDS; LARD SUBSTITUTES.

lard compounds Blends of animal fats, such as oleostearin or PREMIER JUS, with vegetable oils, to produce products similar to LARD in consistency and texture.

See also LARD SUBSTITUTES.

lardine   *See* MARGARINE.

lard substitutes   Vegetable shortenings made from mixtures of partially hardened vegetable fats with the consistency of LARD.
See also LARD COMPOUNDS.

lardy cake   West of England; made from bread dough, lard, sugar and dried fruit.

lasagne   Wide ribbons of PASTA; *lasagne verdi* is flavoured with spinach. Narrow ribbons are lasagnette.

lathyrism   The effect of consuming *Lathyrus* spp. peas (chickling vetch, flat-podded vetch, Spanish vetchling, Indian vetch), which contain the neurotoxin oxalyl-diaminopropionic acid. Although growing *Lathyrus* spp. has been banned in many countries, lathyrism continues to be a public health problem in India since kesari dhal, *Lathyrus sativa*, is a hardy crop that survives adverse conditions and can become a large part of the diet in times of drought.
See also ODORATISM.

lauric acid   A medium-chain length saturated FATTY ACID (C12:0) in butter, coconut oil and palm oil.

lauter tun   Vertical cylindrical tank for extracting and clarifying WORT and separating it from spent grain in malting and brewing.

Laval separator   Centrifuge for separating cream from milk, invented by Swedish engineer Carl Gustaf Patrik de Laval, 1877.

laver   Edible seaweed, *Porphyra* spp. Laver bread is made by boiling in salted water and mincing to a gelatinous mass. It is made into a cake with oatmeal or fried. Locally known in S. Wales as bara lawr.

Composition/100 g: water 85 g, 147 kJ (35 kcal), protein 5.8 g, fat 0.3 g, carbohydrate 5.1 g (0.5 g sugars), fibre 0.3 g, ash 3.8 g, Ca 70 mg, Fe 1.8 mg, Mg 2 mg, P 58 mg, K 356 mg, Na 48 mg, Zn 1 mg, Cu 0.3 mg, Mn 1 mg, Se 0.7 µg, vitamin A 260 µg RE (3121 µg carotenoids), E 1 mg, K 4 mg, B_1 0.1 mg, B_2 0.45 mg, niacin 1.5 mg, B_6 0.16 mg, folate 146 µg, pantothenate 0.5 mg, C 39 mg.

lax   Scandinavian name for SALMON.
See also GRAVADLAX; LOX.

laxarinic acid   *See* MALTOL.

laxatives   Compounds used to treat CONSTIPATION. Bulk-forming laxatives include various preparations of non-starch polysaccharide.

Stimulant or contact laxatives include senna and cascara (*Rhamnus purshianus, Frangula purshiana*) in which the active ingredients are anthroquinones, aloe vera extract, bisacodyl (a diphenylmethene derivative), phenolphthalein and sodium picosulphate.

Osmotic laxatives include magnesium salts (EPSOM SALTS), LACTITOL and LACTULOSE.

Emollient laxatives (faecal softeners) include liquid paraffin and docusates (which act as detergents to permit penetration of water into the faecal mass).

A number of drugs are used to increase intestinal motility.

lazybed Narrow strip of land, about 500–800 m in length, used traditionally in the Andes for growing potatoes, and adopted in Ireland about 1640; one lazybed will provide enough potatoes for a family for a year.

LC-MS Liquid CHROMATOGRAPHY linked to a mass spectrometer as the detection system.

LD$_{50}$ An index of acute toxicity (lethal dose 50%); the amount of the substance that kills 50% of the test population of experimental animals when administered as a single dose.

LDL Low-density lipoprotein, *see* LIPOPROTEINS, PLASMA.

leaching The process of extracting soluble compounds from a food with water or another solvent; may be deliberate (as, e.g., in water extraction of SUGAR from beet, or solvent extraction of oil from oilseeds), or accidental, when vitamins and minerals leach into cooking water and are lost.

lead A mineral of no nutritional interest, since it is not known to have any function in the body. It is toxic and its effects are cumulative. May be present in food from traces naturally present in the soil, as contamination of vegetables grown near main roads, which absorb volatile lead compounds formerly used as a petrol additive, from shellfish that have absorbed it from seawater, from lead glazes on cooking vessels and in drinking water where lead pipes are used. Traces are excreted in the urine.

lean body mass Measure of body composition excluding adipose tissue, i.e. cells, extracellular fluid and skeleton.

Lean Cuisine^{TM} A range of frozen meals prepared to a specified energy content.

leathers, fruit Fruit purées dried in air in thin layers, 4–5 mm thick, then built up into thicker preparations.

leaven YEAST, or a piece of dough kept to ferment the next batch.

leavening Baked goods may be leavened mechanically by air incorporated in dough mixing, or steam produced in baking; chemically using a BAKING POWDER (sodium, potassium or ammonium bicarbonate together with an acid); or biologically by YEAST fermentation.

leben *See* MILK, FERMENTED.

Lecigran^{TM} SOYA bean LECITHIN preparation, claimed to lower blood CHOLESTEROL.

lecithin   Chemically lecithin is phosphatidyl choline; a PHOSPHO-
LIPID containing CHOLINE. Commercial lecithin, prepared from
soya bean, peanut and maize, is a mixture of phospholipids in
which phosphatidyl choline predominates.

Used in food processing as an EMULSIFIER, e.g. in salad dressing, processed cheese and chocolate, and as an antispattering
agent in frying oils. Is plentiful in the diet and not a dietary
essential.

lecithinase   Any of a number of PHOSPHOLIPASES that hydrolyse
LECITHIN.

lectin   One of a series of proteins found especially in LEGUME
seeds that are mitogenic, stimulating cell division, and also act
to agglutinate cells (especially red blood cells, hence the old
names haemagglutinin and phytoagglutinin). Lectins may be a
cause of serious non-bacterial food poisoning, after consumption
of raw or undercooked beans of some varieties of *Phaseolus
vulgaris* (red kidney beans) causing vomiting and diarrhoea
within 2 h, and severe damage to the intestinal mucosa; they
are denatured, and hence inactivated, only by boiling for about
10 min.

leek   *Allium ampeloprasum*; a member of the onion family which
has been known as a food for over 4000 years. The lower part is
usually blanched by planting in trenches or earthing up, and
eaten along with the upper long green leaves.

Composition/100 g: (edible portion 44%) water 83 g, 255 kJ
(61 kcal), protein 1.5 g, fat 0.3 g, carbohydrate 14.1 g (3.9 g sugars),
fibre 1.8 g, ash 1 g, Ca 59 mg, Fe 2.1 mg, Mg 28 mg, P 35 mg, K
180 mg, Na 20 mg, Zn 0.1 mg, Cu 0.1 mg, Mn 0.5 mg, Se 1 µg,
vitamin A 83 µg RE (2900 µg carotenoids), E 0.9 mg, K 47 mg,
B_1 0.06 mg, B_2 0.03 mg, niacin 0.4 mg, B_6 0.23 mg, folate 64 µg,
pantothenate 0.1 mg, C 12 mg. An 80 g serving is a source of Fe,
Mn, vitamin C, a good source of folate.

leghaemoglobin   Haem-containing protein in the root nodules of
leguminous plants that binds O_2 for transport within the root,
and so permits the growth of obligate anaerobic nitrogen-fixing
micro-organisms, *Rhizobium* spp.

See also NITROGENASE.

legumes   Food seeds of members of the leguminosae family. Consumed in the immature green state in the pod or as the dried
mature seed (grain legumes and pulses) after boiling; a 100 g
cooked portion contains approximately 50 g of the dried product.

Include ground nut, *Arachis hypogea*, and soya bean, *Glycine
max*, and African yam bean, *Sphenostylis stenocarpa*, grown for
their edible tubers as well as seeds.

Phaseolus vulgaris Navy, Boston, pinto, string, snapbean (USA); haricot, kidney and when unripe, French, wax bean (UK); flageolet (yellow variety).

P. coccineus (*P. multiflora*) runner, scarlet runner, multiflora bean.

P. acutifolius (var. *latifolius*) tepary, rice haricot bean, Texan bean (USA).

P. lunatus (*lumensis, inamoensus*) Lima bean (USA), butter, Madagascar butter, Rangoon, Burma, Sieva bean.

Cajanus cajan (*C. indicus*) pigeon, Angola, non-eye pea, Congo bean or pea, red gram, yellow dhal.

Vigna umbellata (*P. calcaratus*) rice bean, red bean (also used for adzuki bean). *Vigna mango* (*P. mungo*) urd bean, black gram, mash. *V.* or *P. angularis* adzuki bean.

Vigna unguiculata (or *V. sesquipedalis* or *sinensis*, systematics confused) cow pea, black-eyed bean or pea, China pea, cowgram, catjang, southern pea. *Vigna unguiculata sesquipedalis* (L) asparagus bean, pea bean, yard-long bean.

V. aconitifolia (*P. aconitifolia*) moth, mat bean, Turkish gram. *V. radiata* (*P. aureus, P. radiatus*) mung bean, green or golden gram. *Lablab purpureus* (*Dolichos lablab*) bonavista, dolichos, Egyptian kidney, Indian butter, lablab, tonga, hyacinth bean.

Canavalia ensiformis jack, overlook, sword bean. *Lens culinaris* (*esculenta*) lentil, red dhal, masur dhal, split pea.

Pisum sativa garden, green pea. *Pisum aevense* field pea. *Voandzeia subterranea* bambar(r)a groundnut, earth pea, ground bean, Kaffir pea, Madagascar groundnut.

Cicer aretinum chickpea, Bengal gram.

Cyamopsis tetragonoloba cluster bean. *Lathyrus sativus* grass, lathyrus, chickling pea, Indian vetch, khesari dhal. *Macrotyloma uniflorum* (*Dolichos uniflorus*) horse gram, horse grain, kulthi bean, Madras gram. *Macuna pruriens* velvet bean. *Psophocarpus tetragonolobus* winged bean, asparagus bean or pea, four-cornered, Goa, Manila, Mauritius bean. *Vicia faba* broad bean, faba, field, horse, pigeon, trick, windsor bean.

legumin Globulin protein in legumes.

Leicester English hard CHEESE coloured with ANNATTO.

lemon Sour fruit of *Citrus limon*.

Composition/100 g: (edible portion 53%) water 89 g, 121 kJ (29 kcal), protein 1.1 g, fat 0.3 g, carbohydrate 9.3 g (2.5 g sugars), fibre 2.8 g, ash 0.3 g, Ca 26 mg, Fe 0.6 mg, Mg 8 mg, P 16 mg, K 138 mg, Na 2 mg, Zn 0.1 mg, Se 0.4 µg, vitamin A 1 µg RE (35 µg carotenoids), E 0.2 mg, B_1 0.04 mg, B_2 0.02 mg, niacin 0.1 mg, B_6 0.08 mg, folate 11 µg, pantothenate 0.2 mg, C 53 mg. An 80 g serving is a rich source of vitamin C.

lemon grass   Herb, *Cymbopogon* spp., with lemon flavour, used in South-east Asian cuisine; dried leaves are sereh powder.

lemon verbena   South American herb, *Lippia citriodora*, used to flavour drinks and salads.

lentils   LEGUMES; dried seeds of many varieties of *Lens esculenta*, they may be green, yellow or orange-red.

Composition/100g: water 11.2g, 1415kJ (338kcal), protein 28.1g, fat 1g, carbohydrate 57.1g (5.4g sugars), fibre 30.5g, ash 2.7g, Ca 51mg, Fe 9mg, Mg 107mg, P 454mg, K 905mg, Na 10 mg, Zn 3.6mg, Cu 0.9mg, Mn 1.4mg, Se 8.2µg, vitamin A 2µg RE (23µg carotenoids), E 0.3mg, K 5mg, B_1 0.47mg, B_2 0.25mg, niacin 2.6mg, B_6 0.54mg, folate 433µg, pantothenate 1.8mg, C 6 mg. An 85g serving is a source of vitamin B_2, niacin, a good source of Zn, vitamin B_1, B_6, pantothenate, a rich source of Cu, Fe, Mg, Mn, P, folate.

leptin   A peptide hormone synthesised in adipose tissue which acts to regulate appetite in response to the adequacy or otherwise of body fat reserves. Its crystal structure suggests that it is a member of the CYTOKINE family. The *ob* gene (defective in the *ob/ob* genetically obese mouse) codes for leptin; the *db* gene (defective in the *db/db* genetically obese diabetic mice) codes for the hypothalamic leptin receptor.

lettuce   Leaves of the plant *Lactuca sativa*; many varieties are grown commercially.

Composition/100g: (edible portion 94%) water 95g, 71kJ (17kcal), protein 1.2g, fat 0.3g, carbohydrate 3.3g (1.2g sugars), fibre 2.1g, ash 0.6g, Ca 33mg, Fe 1mg, Mg 14mg, P 30mg, K 247 mg, Na 8mg, Zn 0.2mg, Mn 0.2mg, Se 0.4µg, vitamin A 290µg RE (5796µg carotenoids), E 0.1mg, K 102.5mg, B_1 0.07mg, B_2 0.07mg, niacin 0.3mg, B_6 0.07mg, folate 136µg, pantothenate 0.1mg, C 24mg. A 20g serving is a source of folate.

leucine   An essential amino acid; rarely limiting in foods; abbr Leu (L), M_r 131.2, pK_a 2.33, 9.74, CODONS UUPu, CUNu. Chemically, amino-isocaproic acid.

leucocytes   White blood cells, normally 5000–9000/mL; includes polymorphonuclear neutrophils, lymphocytes, monocytes, polymorphonuclear eosinophils and polymorphonuclear basophils. A 'white cell count' determines the total; a differential cell count estimates the numbers of each type. Fever, haemorrhage and violent exercise cause an increase (leucocytosis); starvation and debilitating conditions a decrease (leucopenia).

leucocytosis   Increase in the number of LEUCOCYTES in the blood.

leucopenia   Decrease in the number of LEUCOCYTES in the blood.

leucosin   One of the water-soluble proteins of wheat flour.

leucovorin   *See* FOLINIC ACID.

levans Polymers of FRUCTOSE (the main one is INULIN) that occur in tubers and some grasses.

levitin One of the proteins of egg yolk; about 20% of the total, the remainder being vitellin. Rich in sulphur, accounting for half of the sulphur in the yolk.

Leyden Dutch semi-hard CHEESE containing caraway and cumin seeds.

Leyden hutsput Dutch; hotpot made from (stale) beef and root vegetables, traditionally served on 3 October, together with white bread and herrings, to celebrate the relief of the siege of Leyden (1574).

licorice *See* LIQUORICE.

Lieberkühn, crypts of Glands lining the small intestine which secrete the intestinal juice.

Liebermann–Burchard reaction Colorimetric reaction for CHOLESTEROL; the development of a blue colour on reaction with acetic anhydride and sulphuric acid.

light (or lite) As applied to foods usually indicates:

(1) a lower content of fat compared with the standard product (e.g. BREADSPREADS, sausages);

(2) sodium chloride substitutes lower in SODIUM (*see* SALT, LIGHT);

(3) low-alcohol BEER or WINE.

US legislation restricts the term light to modified foods that contain one-third less energy or half the fat of a reference unmodified food, or to those where the sodium content of a low-fat, low-calorie food has been reduced by half.

See also FAT FREE; FREE FROM; LOW IN; REDUCED.

lights Butchers' term for the lungs of an animal.

lignans Naturally occurring compounds in various foods that have both oestrogenic and antioestrogenic activity (*see* PHYTOESTROGENS); may provide some protection against breast and uterine cancer, and have activity in menopausal hormone replacement therapy.

lignin (lignocellulose) A polymer of aromatic alcohols, in plant cell walls; included in measurement of DIETARY FIBRE, but not of NON-STARCH POLYSACCHARIDE.

limb fat area Cross-sectional area of arm or leg fat, calculated from SKINFOLD THICKNESS and limb circumference, as an index of total body fat.

See also ANTHROPOMETRY.

Limburger Originally Belgian, strong flavoured soft cheese.

lime The fruit of *Citrus aurantifolia*, cultivated almost solely in the tropics, since it is not as hardy as other CITRUS fruits. Used to prevent scurvy in the British Navy (replacing, at the time, lemon juice) and so giving rise to the nickname of 'Limeys' for British sailors and for British people in general.

Composition/100 g: (edible portion 84%) water 88 g, 126 kJ (30 kcal), protein 0.7 g, fat 0.2 g, carbohydrate 10.5 g (1.7 g sugars), fibre 2.8 g, ash 0.3 g, Ca 33 mg, Fe 0.6 mg, Mg 6 mg, P 18 mg, K 102 mg, Na 2 mg, Zn 0.1 mg, Cu 0.1 mg, Se 0.4 µg, vitamin A 2 µg RE (30 µg carotenoids), E 0.2 mg, K 0.6 mg, B_1 0.03 mg, B_2 0.02 mg, niacin 0.2 mg, B_6 0.04 mg, folate 8 µg, pantothenate 0.2 mg, C 29 mg. A 60 g serving is a good source of vitamin C.

limit dextrin *See* DEXTRINS.

Limmisax™ *See* SACCHARIN.

Limmits™ A 'slimming' preparation composed of wholemeal biscuits with a methyl cellulose mixture as filling, containing some vitamins and minerals; intended as a meal replacement.

limonin The bitter principle in the albedo of the Valencia orange. Isolimonin in the navel orange. Both are present as a non-bitter precursor which is liberated into the juice during extraction and is slowly hydrolysed, making the juice bitter.

limonoids Family of highly oxygenated triterpene derivatives found as aglycones in citrus seeds and peel oil, and as glucosides in juice; responsible for delayed bitterness of the fruit, and potentially protective against cancer.

limosis Abnormal hunger or excessive desire for food.

linamarin Cyanogenic (cyanide forming) GLUCOSIDE found in CASSAVA (manioc) which may be a cause of neuropathies in areas where cassava is major food; the cyanide is removed in traditional processing by grating and exposing to air.

ling Bottom-dwelling (demersal) FISH (*Geypterus blacodes*), a member of the cusk eel family; mainly caught around New Zealand.

Composition/100 g: water 79.6 g, 364 kJ (87 kcal), protein 19 g, fat 0.6 g, cholesterol 40 mg, carbohydrate 0 g, ash 1.4 g, Ca 34 mg, Fe 0.6 mg, Mg 63 mg, P 198 mg, K 379 mg, Na 135 mg, Zn 0.8 mg, Cu 0.1 mg, Se 36.5 µg, vitamin A 30 µg RE (30 µg retinol, B_1 0.11 mg, B_2 0.19 mg, niacin 2.3 mg, B_6 0.3 mg, folate 7 µg, B_{12} 0.6 µg, pantothenate 0.3 mg. A 100 g serving is a source of vitamin B_2, niacin, B_6, a good source of Mg, P, a rich source of Se, vitamin B_{12}.

linguic Portuguese; pork sausage seasoned with garlic, cinnamon and cumin, cured in brine.

linguini *See* PASTA.

linoleic acid An essential polyunsaturated FATTY ACID (C18:2 ω6), predominant in most edible vegetable oils.

linoleic acid, conjugated   Isomers of linoleic acid in which two or more of the double bonds are conjugated (i.e. alternating with single bonds) rather than separated by a methylene bridge.

α-linolenic acid   An essential polyunsaturated FATTY ACID (C18:3 ω3).

γ-linolenic acid   A non-essential polyunsaturated FATTY ACID (C18:3 ω6), which has some pharmacological actions. Found in oils from the seeds of evening primrose, borage and blackcurrant.

linseed   *See* FLAXSEED.

liothyronine   Obsolete name for the THYROID HORMONE tri-iodothyronine (T3).

lipaemia   Increase in blood lipids, as occurs normally after a meal.

lipase   Enzyme (EC 3.1.1.x) that hydrolyses triacylglycerols to free fatty acids and 2-mono-acylglycerol. Lipase secreted by the tongue and in gastric and pancreatic juice is EC 3.1.1.3; lipases are also present in many seeds and grains. Final hydrolysis to yield glycerol is catalysed by acylglycerol lipase (EC 3.1.1.23).

Most lipases have low specificity and will hydrolyse any triacylglycerol. Sometimes responsible for the development of (hydrolytic) RANCIDITY in stored foods, and the development of flavour in cheese.

See also ACID NUMBER; INTERESTERIFICATION.

lipase, clearing factor   *See* LIPASE, LIPOPROTEIN.

lipase, hormone-sensitive   LIPASE in ADIPOSE TISSUE that is activated in response to ADRENALINE, and inactivated in response to insulin, so controlling release of free fatty acids as a metabolic fuel.

lipase, lipoprotein   LIPASE (EC 3.1.1.34) in muscle and ADIPOSE TISSUE that is responsible for the uptake of free fatty acids from triacylglycerols in LIPOPROTEINS. Also known as clearing factor lipase, since it removes triacylglycerol from chylomicrons after a meal, resulting in reduction in their size, and clearing of the milky appearance of chylomicron-rich plasma.

lipectomy   Surgical removal of subcutaneous fat.

lipidema   Condition in which fat deposits accumulate in the lower extremities, from hips to ankles, with tenderness of the affected parts.

lipids   (also sometimes lipides, lipins) A general term for fats and oils (chemically TRIACYLGLYCEROLS), WAXES, PHOSPHOLIPIDS, STEROIDS and TERPENES. Their common property is insolubility in water and solubility in hydrocarbons, chloroform and alcohols. Fats are solid at room temperature, while oils are liquids.

Non-saponifiable lipids are not hydrolysed by treatment with sodium or potassium hydroxide and therefore cannot be extracted into an aqueous medium: CHOLESTEROL and other sterols, SQUALENE, CAROTENOIDS and VITAMINS A, D, E and K. The saponifiable lipids are triacylglycerols (and mono- and diacylglycerols) and phospholipids, which can be extracted into an aqueous medium after alkaline hydrolysis (SAPONIFICATION).

lipids, plasma   Total blood lipid concentration in the fasting state is about 590 mg per 100 mL plasma: 150 mg TRIACYLGLYCEROLS, 160 mg (4 mmol) cholesterol, 200 mg phospholipids, mainly in the plasma LIPOPROTEINS. After a meal the total fat increases, as a result of the CHYLOMICRONS containing the recently absorbed dietary fat.

See also LIPOPROTEINS, PLASMA.

lipochromes   Plant pigments soluble in lipids and organic solvents, e.g. chlorophyll, carotenoids.

lipodystrophy   Abnormality in the metabolism or deposition of fats; abnormal pattern of subcutaneous fat deposits.

lipofuscin   A group of pigments that accumulate in several body tissues, particularly the myocardium, during life and are consequently associated with the ageing process.

lipoic acid   1,2-Dithiolane-3-valeric acid (6,8-thioctic acid), coenzyme in the oxidative decarboxylation of pyruvate, α-ketoglutarate and branched-chain keto-acids. Not a dietary essential.

lipolysis   Hydrolysis of triacylglycerols to mono- and diacylglycerols, glycerol and free fatty acids, catalysed by LIPASE.

lipolytic rancidity   Spoilage of foods as a result of HYDROLYSIS of fats to free fatty acids on storage (by the action of LIPASE, either bacterial lipase or the enzyme naturally present in the food). Since the enzyme is inactivated by heat, occurs only in uncooked foods.

See also ACID NUMBER.

lipoprotein [a] (Lp[a])   Complex of low-density lipoprotein in which an additional protein, apo-a, is bound to apo-protein B-100 by a disulphide bridge. It is genetically determined and there is a strong association between Lp[a] and coronary artery disease.

lipoproteins, plasma   Lipids, encased in protein, in the blood plasma.

Chylomicrons are assembled in the intestinal mucosa, and contain the products of digestion of dietary fat. They are absorbed into the lymphatic circulation, and enter the bloodstream at the thoracic duct. Triacylglycerol is hydrolysed by lipoprotein LIPASE in ADIPOSE TISSUE and muscle, and the chylomicron remnants are cleared by the liver.

Very low-density lipoproteins are secreted by the liver, containing newly synthesised triacylglycerol and that from chylomicron remnants, and cholesterol; hydrolysis by lipoprotein LIPASE in muscle and ADIPOSE TISSUE yields progressively intermediate density and then low-density lipoprotein (LDL). LDL is normally cleared by the liver, but oxidative damage may prevent uptake by the liver, when macrophages scavenge LDL, leading to the formation of foam cells and the development of atherosclerotic plaque.

High-density lipoprotein is secreted by the liver as the apo-protein, and accumulates cholesterol from tissues, which is normally transferred to LDL for clearance by the liver.

liposis *See* ADIPOSIS.

liposuction Procedure for removal of subcutaneous ADIPOSE TISSUE in obese people using a tube inserted through the skin at different locations.

lipotropes (lipotrophic factors) Compounds such as CHOLINE, BETAINE and METHIONINE that act as methyl donors; deficiency may result in fatty infiltration of the liver.

lipovitellenin A lipoprotein complex in egg comprising about 15% of the solids of the yolk.

lipoxygenase Enzyme (EC 1.13.11.12) that catalyses the oxidation of polyunsaturated FATTY ACIDS to *trans*-hydroperoxides (an intermediate step in PROSTAGLANDIN synthesis); in plant oils may be important in the development of oxidative RANCIDITY. Lipoxygenase from soya or fava bean flour is used in breadmaking to improve mixing tolerance and dough stability; it also bleaches carotenoids and other lipid pigments in the flour.

liptauer Hungarian; cheese spread made from sheep and cow milk.

liqueurs Distilled, flavoured and sweetened alcoholic liquors, normally 20–40% alcohol by volume.

liquid oleo *See* PREMIER JUS.

liquid paraffin *See* MEDICINAL PARAFFIN.

liquorice Used in confectionery and to flavour medicines; liquorice root and extract are obtained from the plant *Glycyrrhiza glabra*; stick liquorice is the crude evaporated extract of the root. The plant has been grown in the Pontefract district of Yorkshire since the 16th century; hence the name Pontefract cakes for the sugar confection of liquorice.

See also GLYCYRRHIZIN.

Listeria A genus of bacteria commonly found in soil, of which the commonest is *Listeria monocytogenes*. They can cause FOOD POISONING (listeriosis). *Listeria* spp. are especially found in unwashed vegetables and some soft cheeses; they resist cold and the presence of salt and can multiply in a refrigerator. Symptoms of listeriosis are flu-like, with high fever and dizziness. Pregnant women, babies and the elderly are especially at risk. *L. monocytogenes* causes systemic infection; minimum infective dose not known; onset within days, duration weeks.

listeriosis *See* LISTERIA.

Lita™ FAT REPLACER made from protein.

litchi *See* LYCHEE.

lite *See* LIGHT.

lithium Metal not known to have any physiological function, although it occurs in food and water; lithium salts are used in the treatment of bipolar manic-depressive disease.

lithocholic acid One of the secondary BILE SALTS, formed by intestinal bacterial metabolism of CHENODEOXYCHOLIC ACID.

liver Usually from calf, pig, ox, lamb, chicken, duck or goose.

Composition/100 g (depending on source, beef, calf, lamb or poultry): water 71–76 g, 500–570 kJ (120–140 kcal), protein 16–20 g, fat 4–5 g (of which: beef liver 55% saturated, 23% mono-unsaturated, 23% polyunsaturated; calf liver 47% saturated, 29% mono-unsaturated, 24% polyunsaturated; chicken liver 44% saturated, 33% mono-unsaturated, 22% polyunsaturated; duck liver 52% saturated, 26% mono-unsaturated, 22% polyunsaturated; goose liver 59% saturated, 30% mono-unsaturated, 11% polyunsaturated), cholesterol 275–515 mg, carbohydrate 3–6 g, ash 1.1–1.3 g, Ca 5–43 mg, Fe 5–30 mg, Mg 18–24 mg, P 260–380 mg, K 230–310 mg, Na 70–140 mg, Zn 3–12 mg, Cu 3–12 mg, Mn 0.3 mg, Se 20–70 µg, vitamin A 5000–12 000 µg retinol, E 0.4 mg, K 1–3 mg, B_1 0.2–0.6 mg, B_2 0.9–2.8 mg, niacin 7–13 mg, B_6 0.8–1 mg, folate 125–740 µg, B_{12} 17–60 µg, pantothenate 6–7 mg, C 1–18 mg. A 100 g serving is a source of Mn, vitamin B_1, a good source of Zn, a rich source of Cu, Fe, P, Se, vitamin A, B_2, niacin, B_6, folate, B_{12}, pantothenate.

The vitamin A content of liver is high enough for it to pose a possible hazard to unborn children, and pregnant women have been advised not to eat liver. *See* VITAMIN A TOXICITY.

Fish liver is a particularly rich source of vitamins A and D, as well as long-chain polyunsaturated fatty acids, and fish liver oils (especially COD and HALIBUT) are used as sources of these vitamins as nutritional supplements.

livetin A water-soluble protein in egg yolk.

lobster Crustacean, *Homarus vulgaris*.

Composition/100 g: water 77 g, 377 kJ (90 kcal), protein 18.8 g, fat 0.9 g, cholesterol 95 mg, carbohydrate 0.5 g, ash 2.2 g, Ca 48 mg, Fe 0.3 mg, Mg 27 mg, P 144 mg, K 275 mg, Na 296 mg, Zn 3 mg, Cu 1.7 mg, Mn 0.1 mg, Se 41.4 µg, I 100 µg, vitamin A 21 µg RE (21 µg retinol), E 1.5 mg, K 0.1 mg, B_1 0.01 mg, B_2 0.05 mg, niacin 1.5 mg, B_6 0.06 mg, folate 9 µg, B_{12} 0.9 µg, pantothenate 1.6 mg, A 250 g serving is a source of Ca, folate, a good source of Mg, niacin, a rich source of Cu, I, P, Se, Zn, vitamin E, B_{12}, pantothenate.

lobster, rock or spiny *See* CRAWFISH.

Locasol™ A low-calcium milk substitute.

locksoy Chinese fine-drawn rice macaroni.

locoweed *Astralagus* and *Oxytropus* spp., common in arid areas of western USA. Toxic to cattle, causing locoism: neurological damage, abortion and birth defects. Apparently caused by an alkaloid, swainsonine, which is also found in mouldy hay.

locust bean (1) CAROB seed. (2) African locust bean, *Parkia* spp.

Loeb membrane Thin layer of membrane used in reverse osmosis (*see* OSMOSIS, REVERSE) supported on thicker layer of porous support material.

Lofenalac™ Food low in PHENYLALANINE for treatment of PHENYLKETONURIA.

Logan Bar Ration D *See* IRON RATION.

loganberry Cross between European raspberry and Californian blackberry, *Rubus ursinus* var. *loganobaccus*, named after James Harvey Logan, Californian judge, 1881.

Composition/100 g: water 84.6 g, 230 kJ (55 kcal), protein 1.5 g, fat 0.3 g, carbohydrate 13 g (7.7 g sugars), fibre 5.3 g, ash 0.5 g, Ca 26 mg, Fe 0.6 mg, Mg 21 mg, P 26 mg, K 145 mg, Na 1 mg, Zn 0.3 mg, Cu 0.1 mg, Mn 1.2 mg, Se 0.2 µg, vitamin A 2 µg RE (139 µg carotenoids), E 0.9 mg, K 7.8 mg, B_1 0.05 mg, B_2 0.03 mg, niacin 0.8 mg, B_6 0.06 mg, folate 26 µg, pantothenate 0.2 mg, C 15 mg. A 110 g serving is a source of folate, a good source of vitamin C, a rich source of Mn.

logarithmic phase The most rapid period of bacterial growth, when the numbers increase in geometric progression. Under ideal conditions bacteria can double in number every 20 min.

lo han kuo *See* MOGROSIDE.

Lonalac™ A milk preparation free from SODIUM.

London broil American name for steak, broiled or grilled and sliced thinly against the grain.

longan Fruit of the tree *Euphoria longan*, native of China, related to the LYCHEE.

Composition/100 g: (edible portion 53%) water 83 g, 251 kJ (60 kcal), protein 1.3 g, fat 0.1 g, carbohydrate 15.1 g, fibre 1.1 g, ash 0.7 g, Ca 1 mg, Fe 0.1 mg, Mg 10 mg, P 21 mg, K 266 mg, Zn 0.1 mg, Cu 0.2 mg, Mn 0.1 mg, B_1 0.03 mg, B_2 0.14 mg, niacin 0.3 mg, C 84 mg.

loofah Young fruit of the curcubit *Luffa acutangula* is edible, but becomes too bitter as it matures.

loonzein Rice from which the husk has been removed; also known as brown rice, hulled rice and cargo rice.

loperamide   *See* ANTIDIARRHOEAL AGENTS; ANTIMOTILITY AGENTS.

loquat   The small pear-shaped fruit of *Eriobotyra japonica*, a member of the apple family, also known as Japanese medlar or plum.

Composition/100 g: (edible portion 65%) water 86.7 g, 197 kJ (47 kcal), protein 0.4 g, fat 0.2 g, carbohydrate 12.1 g, fibre 1.7 g, ash 0.5 g, Ca 16 mg, Fe 0.3 mg, Mg 13 mg, P 27 mg, K 266 mg, Na 1 mg, Zn 0.1 mg, Mn 0.1 mg, Se 0.6 µg, vitamin A 76 µg RE, B_1 0.02 mg, B_2 0.02 mg, niacin 0.2 mg, B_6 0.1 mg, folate 14 µg, C 1 mg.

loss factor   A measure of the amount of energy that a material will dissipate when subjected to an alternating electric field (in microwave and dielectric heating). Also termed the 'dielectric loss' or 'loss tangent'.

lotus   The sacred lotus of India and China, *Nelumbium nuciferum*, a water plant whose rhizomes and seeds are eaten.

Rhizome, composition/100 g: (edible portion 79%) water 79 g, 310 kJ (74 kcal), protein 2.6 g, fat 0.1 g, carbohydrate 17.2 g, fibre 4.9 g, ash 1 g, Ca 45 mg, Fe 1.2 mg, Mg 23 mg, P 100 mg, K 556 mg, Na 40 mg, Zn 0.4 mg, Cu 0.3 mg, Mn 0.3 mg, Se 0.7 µg, B_1 0.16 mg, B_2 0.22 mg, niacin 0.4 mg, B_6 0.26 mg, folate 13 µg, pantothenate 0.4 mg, C 44 mg.

Seeds, composition/100 g: water 14.2 g, 1390 kJ (332 kcal), protein 15.4 g, fat 2 g (of which 16% saturated, 21% mono-unsaturated, 63% polyunsaturated), carbohydrate 64.5 g, ash 4 g, Ca 163 mg, Fe 3.5 mg, Mg 210 mg, P 626 mg, K 1368 mg, Na 5 mg, Zn 1 mg, Cu 0.3 mg, Mn 2.3 mg, vitamin A 3 µg RE (B_1 0.64 mg, B_2 0.15 mg, niacin 1.6 mg, B_6 0.63 mg, folate 104 µg, pantothenate 0.9 mg. A 15 g serving is a source of Mn, P.

lovage   Herb of the carrot family, *Ligusticum scoticum*, with a strong musky scent of celery. The stems can be candied like ANGELICA or used as a vegetable, and the leaves and stems are used in soup. The seeds can also be used as a seasoning, with a flavour like dill or fennel seed.

lovastatin   *See* STATINS.

love apple   Old name for TOMATO.

low birth weight   Infants born weighing significantly less than normal (2.5–4.5 kg) are considered to be premature; their chances of survival and normal development are considerably improved if they are fed special formula preparations to meet their needs, rather than being breast fed or fed normal infant formula.

low in   EU legislation states that for a food label or advertising to bear a claim that it is low in fat, saturates, cholesterol, sodium or alcohol, it must provide less than half of the amount of the specified nutrient of a reference product for which no claim is made. US legislation sets precise levels at which claims may be made.

Lowry reaction Sensitive technique for colorimetric determination of protein using the Folin–Cioucalteau tungstate, molybdate, phosphate reagent, which reacts with tyrosine in proteins. Sensitivity 1 ng/mL, maximum absorbance 660 nm.

lox American (originally Yiddish) name for smoked salmon; *see also* LAX.

lozenges Shapes stamped out of mixture of icing sugar, glucose syrup and GUM ARABIC or GELATINE with flavourings, then hardened at 32–43 °C.

LRNI Lower reference nutrient intake; *see* REFERENCE INTAKES.

LSM^{TM} A low-sodium milk containing 50 mg/L; ordinary milk contains 500 mg/L.

lucerne *See* ALFALFA.

luciferase An enzyme that catalyses an ATP-dependent oxidation of a bioluminescent compound (luciferins of various types), leading to emission of visible light. Widely used as a REPORTER GENE in genetic engineering, and for assay of ATP. Firefly luciferase is EC 1.13.12.7, bacterial luciferase is EC 1.14.14.3.

Luff–Schoorl method For determination of starch and sugars. Sugars are extracted using ethanol, then starch is hydrolysed using hydrochloric acid and the resultant glucose is extracted after neutralisation. Sugars are determined in the extracts after oxidation using copper reagent, linked to the reduction of potassium iodide to iodine, and titration of iodine with sodium thiosulphate.

luganeghe Italian; pork sausage that is not twisted into links.

lumichrome Product of ultraviolet irradiation of riboflavin (VITAMIN B$_2$) in neutral solution; some is formed *in vivo* on exposure to sunlight and is excreted in the urine. May also arise as a result of intestinal bacterial metabolism of riboflavin. Formed in milk on exposure to sunlight.

See also LUMIFLAVIN; SUNLIGHT FLAVOUR.

lumiflavin Product of ultraviolet irradiation of riboflavin (VITAMIN B$_2$) in alkaline solution; soluble in chloroform, and provides the basis of a fluorimetric assay for the vitamin.

See also LUMICHROME.

luminacoids Japanese term, introduced 2003, to include all OLIGOSACCHARIDES, POLYOLS, resistant STARCH, indigestible DEXTRINS, resistant proteins and other compounds of plant or animal origin that may undergo (bacterial) metabolism in the intestinal lumen; a broader definition than either DIETARY FIBRE or NON-STARCH POLYSACCHARIDE.

lumpfish Large sea fish, *Cylopterus lumpus*, the eggs of which are salted, pressed and coloured, as Danish or German CAVIARE.

luncheon meat Precooked, canned meat, usually pork.

lupeose *See* STACHYOSE.

lupins Legumes, *Lupinus* spp. The ordinary garden lupin contains toxic quinolizidine alkaloids and tastes bitter; varieties selected for animal feed and grain crop, low in alkaloids, are known as sweet lupins; rich in protein and fat.

lupulones Aromatic acids in HOPS, *see* HUMULONES.

lutein A hydroxylated CAROTENOID (a XANTHOPHYLL); not VITAMIN A active, but may be an important ANTIOXIDANT nutrient. Together with ZEAXANTHIN accumulates in the retina, and considered to be protective against damage by uv and blue light.

luteotrophin (luteotrophic hormone) *See* PROLACTIN.

luxus konsumption *See* DIET-INDUCED THERMOGENESIS.

Lycasin™ Hydrogenated glucose syrup, a bulk SWEETENER.

lychee (litchi) The fruit of *Litchi chinensis*, native of China; the size of a small plum, with a hard case and translucent white jelly-like sweet flesh surrounding the seed.

Composition/100 g: (edible portion 60%) water 81.8 g, 276 kJ (66 kcal), protein 0.8 g, fat 0.4 g, carbohydrate 16.5 g (15.2 g sugars), fibre 1.3 g, ash 0.4 g, Ca 5 mg, Fe 0.3 mg, Mg 10 mg, P 31 mg, K 171 mg, Na 1 mg, Zn 0.1 mg, Cu 0.1 mg, Mn 0.1 mg, Se 0.6 µg, Vitamin E 0.1 mg, K 0.4 mg, B_1 0.01 mg, B_2 0.06 mg, niacin 0.6 mg, B_6 0.1 mg, folate 14 µg, C 72 mg. A 50 g serving (5 fruits) is a rich source of vitamin C.

lycopene A CAROTENOID, not VITAMIN A active, found especially in TOMATOES. It does not have a characteristic ionone ring; both rings are open. Epidemiological evidence suggests that it may be associated with lower incidence of cardiovascular disease and cancer of the prostate and gastrointestinal tract. Sometimes used as a food colour (E-160d).

lye-peeling A method of removing skins from vegetables by immersion in hot caustic soda solution (lye) followed by tumbling in a wash to remove the skin and chemicals.

lymph The fluid between blood and the tissues; the medium in which oxygen and nutrients are conveyed from the blood to the tissues, and waste products back to the blood. Similar to BLOOD PLASMA in composition. Dietary fat is absorbed into the lacteals (lymphatic vessels of the intestinal villi) as chylomicrons which are formed in the intestinal mucosa, and enters the bloodstream at the thoracic duct. After a fatty meal, the lymph is rich in emulsified fat and is called chyle.

lymphatics Vessels through which the LYMPH flows, draining from the tissues and entering the bloodstream at the thoracic duct.

lymphocytes *See* LEUCOCYTES.

lymphokine *See* CYTOKINE.

lyophilic A solute that has a high affinity for the solvent medium. When the solvent is water the term hydrophilic is used.

lyophilisation *See* FREEZE DRYING.

lyophobic A solute that has little or no affinity for the solvent medium. When the solvent is water the term hydrophobic is used.

lysergic acid The toxin of ERGOT.

lysine An essential amino acid, abbr Lys (K), M_r 146.2, pK_a 2.16, 9.18, 10.79, CODONS AAPu. Of nutritional importance, since it is the limiting amino acid in many cereals.

lysinoalanine An amino acid formed when proteins are heated or treated with alkali by reaction between ε-amino group of lysine and dehydroalanine formed from cysteine or serine. Present in many foods at about 1000 ppm. Although high doses cause kidney tubule lesions (nephrocytomegaly) in rats, it is not considered hazardous to health.

lysolecithin LECITHIN from which the fatty acid at carbon-2 has been removed.

lysozyme An enzyme (EC 3.2.1.17) that hydrolyses high molecular weight carbohydrates of bacterial cell walls, and so lyses bacteria. Widely distributed (e.g. in tears); egg white is especially rich.

lyxoflavin An analogue of RIBOFLAVIN isolated from human heart muscle, containing the sugar lyxose; its function is unknown.

lyxulose *See* XYLULOSE.

M

MA Modified atmosphere. *See* PACKAGING, MODIFIED ATMOSPHERE.

maasa W. African; shallow fried cakes made from millet or sorghum dough that has been allowed to undergo lactic acid bacterial fermentation for a short time.

maatjes *See* MATJES HERRING.

macadamia nut Or Queensland nut, fruit of *Macadamia ternifolia.*

Composition/100 g: (edible portion 31%) water 1.4 g, 3006 kJ (718 kcal), protein 7.9 g, fat 75.8 g (of which 17% saturated, 81% mono-unsaturated, 2% polyunsaturated), carbohydrate 13.8 g (4.6 g sugars), fibre 8.6 g, ash 1.1 g, Ca 85 mg, Fe 3.7 mg, Mg 130 mg, P 188 mg, K 368 mg, Na 5 mg, Zn 1.3 mg, Cu 0.8 mg, Mn 4.1 mg, Se 3.6 µg, vitamin E 0.5 mg, B_1 1.2 mg, B_2 0.16 mg, niacin 2.5 mg, B_6 0.28 mg, folate 11 µg, pantothenate 0.8 mg, C 1 mg. A 10 g serving (6 nuts) is a source of Mn.

macaroni, maccaroncelli *See* PASTA.

macassar gum   *See* AGAR.

mace   *See* NUTMEG.

macedoine   Mixture of fruits or vegetables, diced, or cut into small even-shaped pieces.

macerases   A group of enzymes (usually extracted from the mould *Aspergillus*) used to break down PECTIN in fruits to facilitate maximum extraction of the juice.

mackerel   An oily FISH, *Scomber scombrus*.

Composition/100g: water 63.5g, 858kJ (205kcal), protein 18.6g, fat 13.9g (of which 27% saturated, 45% mono-unsaturated, 27% polyunsaturated), cholesterol 70mg, carbohydrate 0g, ash 1.4g, Ca 12mg, Fe 1.6mg, Mg 76mg, P 217mg, K 314mg, Na 90mg, Zn 0.6mg, Cu 0.1mg, Se 44.1µg, I 140µg, vitamin A 50µg RE (50µg retinol, E 1.5mg, K 5mg, B_1 0.18mg, B_2 0.31mg, niacin 9.1mg, B_6 0.4mg, folate 1µg, B_{12} 8.7µg, pantothenate 0.9mg. A 100g serving is a source of Fe, vitamin E, B_1, B_2, pantothenate, a good source of Mg, P, vitamin B_6, a rich source of I, Se, niacin, vitamin B_{12}.

macon   'BACON' made from mutton.

maconochie   A canned meat stew much used in the First World War; made by Maconochie Brothers.

macrobiotic diet   A system of eating associated with Zen Buddhism; consists of several stages finally reaching Diet 7 which is restricted to cereals. Cases of severe malnutrition have been reported on this diet. Based loosely on the Buddhist concept of *yin* and *yang* whereby foods (and indeed everything in life) are predominantly one or the other and must be balanced.

macrocytes   Large immature precursors of red BLOOD CELLS found in the circulation in pernicious anaemia (*see* ANAEMIA PERNICIOUS) and in VITAMIN B_{12} and FOLIC ACID deficiency, due to impairment of the normal maturation of red cells; hence macrocytic ANAEMIA.

macrogols   Polyethylene glycols used as osmotic LAXATIVES.

mad cow disease   Bovine spongiform encephalopathy, *see* BSE.

Madeira nuts   *See* WALNUTS.

Madeira wines   Fortified wines from the island of Madeira: sercial (dry); verdelho (semi-dry); bual (semi-sweet); malmsey (sweet).

madidi   *See* KENKEY.

MAFF   Former UK Ministry of Agriculture, Fisheries and Food, now replaced by DEFRA, the Department of the Environment, Food and Rural Affairs.

magma   Mixture of sugar syrup and sugar crystals produced during sugar refining.

magnesium   An essential mineral; present in all human tissues, especially bone. Involved in the metabolism of ATP. Present in chlorophyll and so in all green plant foods, and therefore generally plentiful in the diet. Deficiency in human beings leads to disturbances of muscle and nervous system; in cattle, grass tetany. Magnesium-deficient plants are yellow (chlorosed).

Magnesium salts (especially the sulphate, EPSOM SALTS) are used as osmotic LAXATIVES because they are poorly absorbed from the small intestine; magnesium hydroxide (milk of magnesia) and carbonate are used as ANTACIDS; magnesium trisilicate is used in the treatment of peptic ULCERS.

magnetic field system   For detection of magnetic metals in foods. The food is passed through a strong magnetic field; any particle of magnetic material is magnetised, and this generates a voltage in a detector coil. Can be used for foods in aluminium cans, since aluminium is non-magnetic.

See also BALANCED COIL SYSTEM.

magnum   Double size wine BOTTLE, 1.5 L.

maheu   African; sour non-alcoholic beverage made from maize or millet by lactic acid fermentation.

mahi-mahi   *See* DOLPHIN FISH.

mahleb   Spice prepared from black cherry kernels, Syrian in origin, widely used in Greek baked goods.

maidenhair tree   *See* GINGKO.

maids of honour   Small tartlets filled with almond-flavoured custard; said to have originated in the court of Henry VIII, where they were made by Anne Boleyn when she was lady-in-waiting to Catherine of Aragon.

Maillard reaction   Non-enzymic reaction between LYSINE in proteins and reducing sugars, leading to a brown colour. A similar reaction occurs in the GLYCATION of proteins in DIABETES mellitus.

The first step in the reaction is the formation of a Schiff base (aldimine) between the aldehyde group of the sugar and the ε-amino group of lysine, followed by isomerisation (Amadori rearrangement). May also occur with other amino acids at the amino terminal of a protein.

It takes place on heating or prolonged storage and is one of the deteriorative processes that take place in stored foods. It is accompanied by a loss in nutritional value, since the amino acid that reacts with the sugar is not available.

See also AVAILABILITY; AVAILABLE LYSINE.

maître d'hôtel   Simply prepared dishes garnished with butter creamed with parsley and lemon juice (maître d'hôtel butter); literally *in the style of the chief steward*. Used especially in the USA as a term for the head waiter.

maize Grain of *Zea mays*, also called Indian corn and (in USA) simply corn. Staple food in many countries, made into TORTILLAS in Latin America, POLENTA in Italy, and flaked as corn flakes breakfast cereal; various preparations in the southern states of the USA are known as hominy, samp and cerealine.

Two varieties of major commercial importance are flint corn (*Zea mays indurata*), which is very hard, and dent corn (*Z. mays dentata*); there is also sweet corn *Z. mays saccharata*, and a variety that expands on heating (*Zea mays everta; see* POPCORN).

The starch prepared from *Z. mays dentata* is termed cornflour; the ground maize is termed maize meal. There is a white variety; the usual yellow colour is partly due to cryptoxanthin (a vitamin A precursor). Because of its low content of the amino acid TRYPTOPHAN (and available NIACIN), diets based largely on maize are associated with the development of PELLAGRA.

Yellow sweet corn, composition/100g: (edible portion 36%) water 76g, 360kJ (86kcal), protein 3.2g, fat 1.2g (of which 18% saturated, 27% mono-unsaturated, 55% polyunsaturated), carbohydrate 19g (3.2g sugars), fibre 2.7g, ash 0.6g, Ca 2mg, Fe 0.5mg, Mg 37mg, P 89mg, K 270mg, Na 15mg, Zn 0.4mg, Cu 0.1mg, Mn 0.2mg, Se 0.6µg, vitamin A 10µg RE (961µg carotenoids), E 0.1mg, K 0.3mg, B_1 0.2mg, B_2 0.06mg, niacin 1.7mg, B_6 0.05mg, folate 46µg, pantothenate 0.8mg, C 7mg. A 90g serving (1 cob) is a source of Mg, vitamin B_1, pantothenate, a good source of folate.

maize, flaked Partly gelatinised maize used for animal feed. The grain is cracked to small pieces, moistened, cooked and flaked between rollers.

maize flour Highly refined and very finely ground maize meal from which all bran and germ have been removed.

Composition/100g: water 10.9g, 1511kJ (361kcal), protein 6.9g, fat 3.9g (of which 15% saturated, 30% mono-unsaturated, 55% polyunsaturated), carbohydrate 76.8g (0.6g sugars), fibre 13.4g, ash 1.5g, Ca 7mg, Fe 2.4mg, Mg 93mg, P 272mg, K 315mg, Na 5mg, Zn 1.7mg, Cu 0.2mg, Mn 0.5mg, Se 15.4µg, vitamin A 11µg RE (1515µg carotenoids), E 0.4mg, K 0.3mg, B_1 0.25mg, B_2 0.08mg, niacin 1.9mg, B_6 0.37mg, folate 25µg, pantothenate 0.7mg.

maize oil *See* CORN OIL.

maize, quality protein (QPM) A hybrid derived from the Opaque II strain, with a 10% higher yield than conventional maize, and 70–80% more TRYPTOPHAN and LYSINE.

maize rice Finely cut MAIZE with bran and germ partly removed, also called mealie rice.

maize starch, waxy   STARCH obtained from hybrids of MAIZE consisting wholly or largely of AMYLOPECTIN, compared with ordinary maize starch with 26% AMYLOSE and 74% amylopectin. The paste is semi-translucent, cohesive and does not form a gel.

malabsorption syndrome   Defect of absorption of one or more nutrients; signs include DIARRHOEA, STEATORRHOEA, abdominal distension, weight loss and specific signs of nutrient deficiency.

malacia   Abnormal softening of tissue or organ. *See* KERATOMALACIA; OSTEOMALACIA.

malai   Indian; cream prepared by boiling milk, leaving it to cool and then skimming off the clotted cream.

malic acid   Dicarboxylic acid (COOH—CHOH—CH$_2$—COOH); a metabolic intermediate occurring in many fruits, particularly in apples, tomatoes and plums. Used as a food additive to increase acidity (E-296).

mallorising   PASTEURISATION at high temperatures (up to 130 °C).

malmsey   *See* MADEIRA WINES.

malnutrition   Disturbance of form or function arising from deficiency or excess of one or more nutrients.

   See also CACHEXIA; OBESITY; PROTEIN–ENERGY MALNUTRITION; VITAMIN A TOXICITY; VITAMIN B$_6$ TOXICITY).

malolactic fermentation   The conversion of the malic acid in grape juice (and other fruit juices) into lactic acid, especially in red wines and CIDER as they mellow and become less acidic.

malpighia   *See* CHERRY, WEST INDIAN.

malt, malt extract   Mixture of starch breakdown products containing mainly MALTOSE (malt sugar), prepared from barley or wheat. The grain is allowed to sprout, when the enzyme diastase (AMYLASE) develops and HYDROLYSES the starch to maltose. The mixture is then extracted with hot water, and this malt extract contains a solution of starch breakdown products together with diastase. Malt extract may be the concentrated solution or evaporated to dryness.

maltase   Enzyme (EC 3.2.1.20) that hydrolyses MALTOSE.

malt flour   Germinated barley or wheat, in dried form. As well as dextrins, glucose, proteins and salts derived from the cereal, it is rich in diastase and is added to wheat flour of low DIASTATIC ACTIVITY for breadmaking; used as an ingredient of malt loaf.

Malthus, Thomas Robert   (1766–1835), author of an *Essay on the Principles of Population* (1798), postulating that any temporary or local improvement in living conditions will increase population faster than the food supply, and that disasters such as war and pestilence, which check population growth, are inescapable features of human society.

maltin, maltodextrin   *See* DEXTROSE EQUIVALENT VALUE.

maltitol   A SUGAR ALCOHOL produced by hydrogenation of maltose. Slowly hydrolysed in the digestive tract to GLUCOSE and SORBITOL and fairly completely utilised, providing 16 kJ (4 kcal)/g; sweeter than maltose, and 90% as sweet as sucrose (E-965).

maltobiose   *See* MALTOSE.

maltol   Also called laxarinic acid, palatone, veltol; chemically 3-hydroxy 2-methyl-γ-pyrone. Found in the bark of young larch trees, pine needles, chicory and roasted malt; synthesised for use as a fragrant, caramel-like flavour for addition to foods; imparts a 'freshly baked' flavour to bread and cakes.

maltonic acid   *See* GLUCONIC ACID.

maltose   Malt sugar, or maltobiose, a DISACCHARIDE, α-1,4-glucosyl-glucose. Hydrolysed by MALTASE. Does not occur in foods (unless specifically added as MALT) but formed during the acid or enzymic hydrolysis of starch. 33% as sweet as sucrose.

maltose figure   *See* DIASTATIC ACTIVITY.

maltose intolerance   *See* DISACCHARIDE INTOLERANCE.

malt sugar   *See* MALTOSE.

mamey   Fruit of the central American tree *Pouteria sapota*, sometimes known as SAPOTE.

Composition/100 g: (edible portion 60%) water 86 g, 213 kJ (51 kcal), protein 0.5 g, fat 0.5 g, carbohydrate 12.5 g, fibre 3 g, ash 0.3 g, Ca 11 mg, Fe 0.7 mg, Mg 16 mg, P 11 mg, K 47 mg, Na 15 mg, Zn 0.1 mg, Cu 0.1 mg, Se 0.6 µg, vitamin A 12 µg RE, B_1 0.02 mg, B_2 0.04 mg, niacin 0.4 mg, B_6 0.1 mg, folate 14 µg, pantothenate 0.1 mg, C 14 mg. A 200 g serving (quarter fruit) is a source of Cu, folate, a rich source of vitamin C.

manchego   Spanish sheep's milk hard cheese.

mandarin   Loose-skinned CITRUS fruit, *Citrus reticulata* or *C. nobilio*. Varieties include satsumas and tangerines (although all three names are used indiscriminately) with various hybrids including tangelo, tangor, temple, clementine.

manganese   An essential trace mineral which functions as the PROSTHETIC GROUP in a number of enzymes. Dietary deficiency has not been reported in humans; in experimental animals manganese deficiency leads to impaired synthesis of MUCOPOLYSACCHARIDES. Requirements are not known; a SAFE AND ADEQUATE INTAKE has been set at 1.8 (women) to 2.3 (men) mg/day.

mangelwurzel, mangoldwurzel   A root vegetable used as cattle feed, *Beta vulgaris rapa*; a cross between red and white BEETROOT.

mange tout   *See* PEA, MANGE TOUT.

mango   Fruit of *Mangifera indica*, originally of Indo-Burmese origin and now grown widely throughout the tropics; ovoid, with orange-coloured sweet aromatic flesh surrounding a central stone.

Composition/100 g: (edible portion 69%) water 81.7 g, 272 kJ (65 kcal), protein 0.5 g, fat 0.3 g, carbohydrate 17 g (14.8 g sugars), fibre 1.8 g, ash 0.5 g, Ca 10 mg, Fe 0.1 mg, Mg 9 mg, P 11 mg, K 156 mg, Na 2 mg, Cu 0.1 mg, Se 0.6 μg, vitamin A 38 μg RE (473 μg carotenoids), E 1.1 mg, K 4.2 mg, B_1 0.06 mg, B_2 0.06 mg, niacin 0.6 mg, B_6 0.13 mg, folate 14 μg, pantothenate 0.2 mg, C 28 mg. A 100 g serving (half fruit) is a source of vitamin E, a rich source of vitamin C.

mangosteen Fruit of *Garcinea mangostana*, the size of an orange with thick purple rind and sweet white pulp in segments.

manihot starch *See* CASSAVA.

manioc *See* CASSAVA.

manna Dried exudate from the manna-ash tamarisk tree (*Fraxinus ornus*). Abundant in Sicily and used as a mild laxative for children; it consists of 40–60% MANNITOL, 10–16% mannotetrose, 6–16% mannotriose, plus glucose, mucilage and fraxin. This is thought to be the food eaten by the Israelites in the wilderness. Manna sugar or mannite is MANNITOL.

manna bread A cake-like product made from crushed, sprouted wheat without yeast; said to be a recipe of the Essenes who lived by the Dead Sea at the beginning of the Christian era.

mannitol Mannite or manna sugar, a six-carbon SUGAR ALCOHOL found in beets, pumpkin, mushrooms, onions; 50–60% as sweet as sucrose. Extracted commercially from seaweed (*Laminaria* spp.) or by reduction of MANNOSE (E-421).

mannosans POLYSACCHARIDES containing MANNOSE.

mannose A six-carbon (hexose) sugar found in small amounts in legumes, MANNA and some gums. Also called seminose and carubinose.

mannotetrose *See* STACHYOSE.

manothermosonication Method of sterilisation using mild heat treatment combined with ultrasonication and moderately raised pressure.

Manucol™ Sodium ALGINATE.

MAP Modified atmosphere packaging, *see* PACKAGING, MODIFIED ATMOSPHERE.

MAP kinases Mitogen-activated PROTEIN KINASES – a family of enzymes that catalyse phosphorylation of target enzymes in response to hormones including INSULIN and insulin-like growth factor.

maple syrup Sap of the north American sugar maple tree, *Acer saccharum*. Evaporated either to syrup (63% sucrose, 1.5% invert sugar, *see* SUGAR, INVERT) or to dry sugar for use in confectionery.

maple syrup urine disease A rare GENETIC DISEASE affecting catabolism of the branched-chain amino acids LEUCINE, ISO-LEUCINE and VALINE, due to deficiency of branched-chain keto-acid dehydrogenase (EC 1.2.4.4), leading to accumulation of high concentrations of these amino acids and their keto-acids in plasma and urine. The keto-acids give the urine a characteristic smell like that of maple syrup. If untreated, leads to severe mental retardation and death in infancy.

marasmic kwashiorkor The most severe form of PROTEIN–ENERGY MALNUTRITION in children, with weight for height less than 60% of that expected and the oedema and other signs of kwashiorkor.

marasmus *See* PROTEIN–ENERGY MALNUTRITION.

marc (1) French; spirit distilled from the fermented residue of grape skins, stalks and seeds after the grapes have been pressed for wine making. The same as grappa (Italian), bagaciera (Portugal) and aguardiente (Spain). Often a harsh raw spirit, drunk young, although some are matured and smooth.

(2) Insoluble residue after extraction of soluble material from SUGAR BEET; mainly NON-STARCH POLYSACCHARIDES, used as livestock feed.

margarine (butterine, lardine, oleomargarine) Emulsion of about 80% vegetable, animal and/or marine fats and 20% water, originally made as a substitute for butter. Usually contains emulsifiers, antispattering agents, colours, vitamins A and D (sometimes E) and preservatives.

Ordinary margarines contain roughly equal proportions of saturated, mono-unsaturated and polyunsaturated fatty acids; special soft varieties are rich in polyunsaturated fatty acids. Low-fat spreads are made with 10–60% fat and correspondingly higher contents of air and water and less energy, and generally cannot legally be called margarine.

Kosher (and vegetarian) margarine is made only from vegetable oils, because ordinary margarine may include animal fats. It is fortified with carotene (which is derived from vegetable sources) as the source of vitamin A, instead of retinol (which may be obtained from non-kosher sources).

mariculture AQUACULTURE in saline environments.

marigold Pot or common marigold (*Calendula officinalis*); petals are used as flavouring and colouring, sometimes as a substitute for SAFFRON.

marinade Mixture of oil with wine, lemon juice or vinegar and herbs in which meat or fish is soaked before cooking, both to give flavour and to make it more tender. Hence to marinate.

marine biotoxins   Toxins in shellfish and marine fish, either produced naturally or accumulated by the fish from their diet (includes CIGUATERA and PARALYTIC SHELLFISH POISONING).

marine oils   *See* FISH OILS.

marjoram   Dried leaves of a number of aromatic plants of different species, used as seasoning. The most widely accepted marjoram herbs are the perennial bush *Origanum majorana* and the annual sweet marjoram *Majorana hortensis*. Spanish wild marjoram is *Thymus mastichina*.

marker gene   A readily detectable gene (e.g. conferring antibiotic or herbicide resistance) transferred into a TRANSGENIC organism together with the gene of interest, to permit ready identification of those cells in which the gene transfer has been achieved. Unlike a REPORTER GENE, it confers a survival advantage on the transfected cells when they are grown in the presence of the antibiotic or herbicide.

marmalade   Defined by EU Directive as JAM made from citrus peel; what was known as GINGER marmalade is now known as ginger preserve. The name comes from the Portuguese *marmalada*, the quince, which was used to make preserves. Used in French and German to mean jam or preserve in general.

marmite   (1) The original form of pressure cooker used by Papin in 1681; it was an iron pot with a sealing lid.

(2) Cookery term for a stock, or the pot in which stock is prepared.

Marmite™   YEAST EXTRACT flavoured with vegetable extract.

marron glacé   Chestnuts preserved in syrup; semi-crystallised.

marrow   (1) Bone marrow; tissue within internal cavities of bones. Red marrow is the site of formation of red BLOOD CELLS. In infants almost all of the marrow is red, and is gradually replaced by fat (yellow marrow) in the limb bones.

(2) Varieties of the gourd *Cucurbita pepo*.

Composition/100 g: (edible portion 87%) water 92.7 g, 88 kJ (21 kcal), protein 2.7 g, fat 0.4 g, carbohydrate 3.1 g, fibre 1.1 g, ash 1 g, Ca 21 mg, Fe 0.8 mg, Mg 33 mg, P 93 mg, K 459 mg, Na 3 mg, Zn 0.8 mg, Cu 0.1 mg, Mn 0.2 mg, Se 0.3 µg, vitamin B_1 0.04 mg, B_2 0.04 mg, niacin 0.7 mg, B_6 0.14 mg, folate 20 µg, pantothenate 0.4 mg, C 34 mg. A 100 g serving is a source of Mg, P, a rich source of vitamin C.

See also COURGETTE; PUMPKIN; SQUASH.

marshmallow   Soft sweetmeat made from an aerated mixture of gelatine or egg albumin with sugar or starch syrup. NOUGAT is harder, containing less water, and usually incorporates dried fruit and nuts. Originally, the root of the marshmallow plant (*Althaea* *officinalis*), which contains MUCILAGE as well as starch and sugar, was used.

marula   Fruit and nut from the southern African tree *Sclerocarya birrea* subsp. *caffra*.

Marumillon 50™   A mixture of the sweet glycosides extracted from stevia leaves.

See also STEVIOSIDE; REBAUDIOSIDE.

marzipan   *See* ALMOND PASTE.

MAS   Modified atmosphere storage. *See* PACKAGING, MODIFIED ATMOSPHERE.

mascarpone   Italian; soft cream CHEESE from the Lombardy region.

mashing   In the brewing of BEER, the process in which the malted barley is heated with water, to extract the soluble sugars and to continue enzymic reactions started during malting.

mash tun   Vessel used for MASHING.

maslin, mashum   (1) Old term, still used in Scotland, for mixed crop of beans and oats used as cattle food.

(2) In Yorkshire and N. England, a mixed crop of 2–3 parts of wheat and 1 part of rye, used for making bread.

(3) Also mesclin, miscellin; Medieval English; bread made from mixed wheat and rye.

Mason jar   Screw-topped glass jar for home bottling; patented 1858.

massecuite   The mixture of sugar crystals and syrup (mother liquor) obtained during the crystallisation stage of sugar refining.

mast   *See* MILK, FERMENTED.

mastic (mastic gum)   Resin from the evergreen shrub *Pistacia lenticus* and related species, with a flavour similar to liquorice, used in Greek and Balkan cookery.

mastication   Chewing, grinding and tearing food with the teeth while it becomes mixed with saliva.

matai   Chinese water chestnut, *see* CHESTNUT.

maté   Also yerba maté, or Paraguay or Brazilian tea. Infusion of the dried leaves of *Ilex paraguayensis*.

matjes herring   Dutch; young HERRING caught in spring, lightly salted and stored in barrels for a short time to allow fermentation to occur.

matoké   Steamed green BANANA or PLANTAIN.

matrix Gla protein   *See* OSTEOCALCIN.

matsutake   Edible wild fungus, *Tricholoma matsutake*, widely collected in Japan and exported canned or dried. *See* MUSHROOMS.

Matzka process   A low-temperature sterilisation process used for fruit juices by adding silver salts; in the presence of silver ions the pasteurisation temperature is only 8–11 °C. The KATADYN PROCESS employs silver ions alone.
See also OLIGODYNAMIC.

matzo, motza (plural matzoth)   Unleavened bread or Passover bread made as thin, flat, round or square water biscuits, and, according to the injunction in Exodus, eaten by Jews during the eight days of Passover in place of leavened bread.

maw   Fourth stomach of the ruminant.

mawseed   *See* POPPY SEED.

MaxEPA™   A standardised mixture of FISH OILS, rich in long-chain polyunsaturated FATTY ACIDS: eicosapentaenoic (EPA, C20:5 ω3) and docosohexaenoic (DHA, C22:6 ω3) acids.

mayonnaise   A SALAD DRESSING, reputedly invented by the duke of Richelieu in 1757, and originally named mahonnaise to celebrate the French victory at Mahon.

maysin   Coagulable globulin protein in maize.

mazindol   Anorectic (appetite suppressing, *see* APPETITE CONTROL) drug formerly used in the treatment of OBESITY.

mazun   *See* MILK, FERMENTED.

mazzard   *See* GEAN.

McGovern committee   USA; Senate Select Committee on Nutrition and Human Needs; published Dietary Goals for the United States, first draft 1977, final version 1980, based on the proposition that people should eat less of harmful foods rather than more of foods that are good for them. The basis of most current guidelines on healthy eating.

MCT   *See* MEDIUM CHAIN TRIGLYCERIDES.

mcv   *See* MEAN CELL VOLUME.

MDM   Mechanically deboned meat, *see* MEAT, MECHANICALLY RECOVERED.

mead   A traditional wine made by fermentation of honey, sometimes flavoured with herbs and spices. One of the most ancient of alcoholic drinks.

mealie(s)   *See* MAIZE.

mealie rice   *See* MAIZE RICE.

mean cell volume (mcv)   Average size of red BLOOD CELLS, determined using an electronic counter which sorts by size, or calculated from the HAEMATOCRIT and red cell count/L of blood. Low values occur with severe iron deficiency (microcytic ANAEMIA) and high values in FOLIC ACID and VITAMIN B$_{12}$ deficiency (megaloblastic anaemia).

meat   Generally refers to the muscle tissue of animal or bird, other parts being termed OFFAL or organ meat. Legally defined in UK as all that is found between the skin and bone of the animal.

meat bar Dehydrated cooked meat and fat; a modern form of PEMMICAN; 50% protein and 40% fat; provides 560 kcal (2350 kJ)/100 g.

meat conditioning After an animal has been slaughtered, muscle glycogen breaks down and is metabolised to lactic acid, which tends to improve the texture and keeping qualities of the meat. Meat that has been left until these changes have occurred is 'conditioned'. Electrical stimulation of muscles is sometimes used to hasten the development of RIGOR MORTIS, and shorten the time required for conditioning the meat.

See also MEAT, DFD.

meat, curing Pickling with the aid of sodium chloride (SALT), sodium nitrate (saltpetre) and sodium nitrite, which permits the growth of only salt-tolerant bacteria and inhibits the growth of *Clostridium botulinum*. The nitrite is the effective preserving agent and the nitrate is converted into nitrite during the pickling process. The red colour of cured meat is due to the formation of nitrosomyoglobin from MYOGLOBIN.

meat, DFD Dark, firm, dry; the condition of meat when the pH remains high through lack of GLYCOGEN (which would form LACTIC ACID). It poses a microbiological hazard.

See also MEAT CONDITIONING; RIGOR MORTIS.

meat extender Vegetable proteins added to meat products to replace part of the meat.

meat extract The water-soluble part of meat that is mainly responsible for its flavour. Commercially is made during the manufacture of CORNED BEEF; chopped meat is immersed in boiling water, when the water-soluble extractives are partially leached out and concentrated. Rich in the B vitamins (particularly vitamins B_1, B_{12} and niacin), meat bases and potassium, and a potent stimulator of gastric secretion.

meat factor Factor used to calculate the fat-free meat content of sausages and similar meat products, from a NITROGEN estimation.

meat, mechanically recovered Residual meat recovered from bones that have already been trimmed by knife. Also known as mechanically deboned meat and (in the USA) mechanically separated meat. It consists of meat and fat that were on the bone, comminuted by forcing through perforated filters (Paoli, Beehive, Bibun machines) or channels (Protecon machines), as well as bone fragments, depending on the pressure used in recovery.

meat, reformed Comminuted, flaked or ground meat that has been bound and shaped to resemble a cut of whole meat. In the UK even if it resembles a steak, it may not be so-called.

meat speciation   Identification of species of animal from which the meat originated.

meat sugar   Obsolete name for INOSITOL.

meat, water binding capacity (WBC)   The capacity of a piece of meat to retain added water during cutting, pressing or heating.
   See also MEAT, WATER HOLDING CAPACITY.

meat, water holding capacity (WHC)   The capacity of a piece of meat to retain its own water content during cutting, pressing or heating.
   See also MEAT, WATER BINDING CAPACITY.

medical foods   Legal definition (in the USA) of foods formulated for dietary treatment of a disease, to be administered enterally (i.e. by mouth or by naso-gastric tube, as opposed to PARENTERAL nutrition), under supervision of a physician; sometimes known as enteral foods.

medicinal paraffin   Liquid paraffin, a mineral oil of no nutritive value since it is not affected by digestive enzymes and passes through the intestine unchanged. Used as a LAXATIVE because of its lubricant properties. Formerly used to coat dried fruit.

medium chain triglycerides   TRIGLYCERIDES containing medium-chain (8–10 carbon) FATTY ACIDS used in treatment of MALABSORPTION; they are absorbed more rapidly than conventional fats, and the products of their digestion are transported to the liver, rather than in CHYLOMICRONS.

medlar   The fruit of *Mespilus germanica*. Can be eaten fresh from tree in Mediterranean areas but in colder climates, as the UK, does not become palatable until it is half rotten (bletted). Japanese medlar is the LOQUAT.

Meeh formula   *See* BODY SURFACE AREA.

megaloblast   Abnormal form of any of the cells that are precursors of red BLOOD CELLS; they occur in bone MARROW in ANAEMIA due to deficiency of FOLIC ACID or VITAMIN B_{12}.

megavitamin therapy   Treatment of diseases with very high doses of vitamins, several hundred-fold higher than REFERENCE INTAKES. Little or no evidence of efficacy; VITAMINS A, D, B_6 and NIACIN are known to be toxic at high levels of intake.

megrim   FLATFISH, the British smooth SOLE or scaldfish, *Psetta arnoglossa*.

mejing   *See* MONOSODIUM GLUTAMATE.

mekabu   Japanese; lobe leaf seaweed, normally dried.

melaena   Tarry black faeces due to partly digested blood as a result of bleeding into the gut.

melalgia, nutritional   *See* BURNING FOOT SYNDROME.

melampyrin   *See* DULCITOL.

melangeur Mixing vessel consisting of rollers riding on a rotating horizontal bed. Used to mix substances of pasty consistency (hence melangeuring).

melanin Brown pigments formed when phenolic compounds in cut fruit and vegetable are exposed to air and oxidise; also the pigments of skin and hair, formed from TYROSINE.

melano *See* KIWANO.

melanocortin Peptide HORMONE that regulates MELANIN synthesis in skin and hair, and also feeding behaviour through receptors in the hypothalamus. The agouti gene product antagonises melanocortin receptors, leading to OBESITY and INSULIN RESISTANCE in mutant mice (*see* AGOUTI MOUSE).

melba Peach poached in vanilla syrup, set in vanilla ice-cream with a purée of raspberries. Created by Escoffier, 1892, in honour of Dame Nellie Melba.

melegueta pepper *See* PEPPER, MELEGUETA.

melezitose Trisaccharide, glucosyl-glucosyl-fructose, hydrolysed to glucose plus the disaccharide turanose (α-1,3-glucosyl-fructose).

melibiose A DISACCHARIDE, α-1,6-galactosyl-glucose.

melissopalynology Analysis of pollens present in HONEY, in order to determine its botanical and geographical origin.

melitose, melitriose *See* RAFFINOSE.

mellorine US term for ICE CREAM made from non-butter fat.

melon GOURDS, sweet fruit of *Cucumis melo*.

Cantaloupe, composition/100 g: (edible portion 51%) water 90.2 g, 142 kJ (34 kcal), protein 0.8 g, fat 0.2 g, carbohydrate 8.2 g (7.9 g sugars), fibre 0.9 g, ash 0.6 g, Ca 9 mg, Fe 0.2 mg, Mg 12 mg, P 15 mg, K 267 mg, Na 16 mg, Zn 0.2 mg, Se 0.4 µg, vitamin A 169 µg RE (2063 µg carotenoids), E 0.1 mg, K 2.5 mg, B_1 0.04 mg, B_2 0.02 mg, niacin 0.7 mg, B_6 0.07 mg, folate 21 µg, pantothenate 0.1 mg, C 37 mg. A 230 g serving is a good source of folate, a rich source of vitamin A, C.

Honeydew, composition/100 g: (edible portion 46%) water 89.8 g, 151 kJ (36 kcal), protein 0.5 g, fat 0.1 g, carbohydrate 9.1 g (8.1 g sugars), fibre 0.8 g, ash 0.4 g, Ca 6 mg, Fe 0.2 mg, Mg 10 mg, P 11 mg, K 228 mg, Na 18 mg, Zn 0.1 mg, Se 0.7 µg, vitamin A 3 µg RE (57 µg carotenoids), K 2.9 mg, B_1 0.04 mg, B_2 0.01 mg, niacin 0.4 mg, B_6 0.09 mg, folate 19 µg, pantothenate 0.2 mg, C 18 mg. A 230 g serving is a good source of folate, a rich source of vitamin C.

melon, jelly (or horned) *See* KIWANO.

melting point The temperature at which a compound melts to a liquid. Often characteristic of a particular chemical and used as a means of identification, and as an index of purity, since impurities lower the melting point.

melts *See* SPLEEN.

membrane concentration Process of removing water, and some solutes, by use of a semipermeable membrane. It requires less heat than evaporation, so has less effect on flavour and texture.

membrane, semipermeable (selectively permeable) One that allows the passage of small molecules but not large ones; e.g. pig's bladder is permeable to water but not salt; collodion is permeable to salt but not protein molecules.

See also DIALYSIS; OSMOSIS; ULTRAFILTRATION.

menadione, menadiol Synthetic VITAMIN K analogue (vitamin K_3, sometimes known as menaquinone-0). Formerly used in prophylaxis of haemorrhagic disease of the newborn, but its use has declined since it was shown to support redox cycling reactions and may be associated with later development of cancers.

menaquinones Bacterial metabolites with VITAMIN K activity; vitamin K_2.

menarche The initiation of menstruation in adolescent girls, normally occurring between the ages of 11 and 15. The age at menarche has become younger in western countries, possibly associated with a better general standard of nutrition, and is later in less developed countries.

menhaden Oily FISH, *Brevoortia patronus, B. tyrannus*, from Gulf of Mexico and Atlantic seaboard of the USA, a rich source of FISH OILS. Menhaden oil is 33% saturated, 29% mono-unsaturated, 37% polyunsaturated, contains 521 mg cholesterol/100 g.

Menke's syndrome A GENETIC DISEASE involving failure of the intestinal copper transport mechanism, resulting in functional copper deficiency. Because of the effects on hair colour and structure, sometimes known as Menke's kinky or steely hair syndrome.

merguez North African; spiced sausage made from goat or mutton, flavoured with hrisa, a mixture of pepper and cumin.

mescal *See* TEQUILA.

mesocarp *See* ALBEDO.

meso-inositol *See* INOSITOL.

mesomorph Description given to a well-covered individual with well-developed muscles.

See also ECTOMORPH; ENDOMORPH.

mesophiles Pathogenic micro-organisms that grow best at temperatures between 25 and 40 °C; usually will not grow below 5 °C.

metabolic equivalent (MET)   Unit of measurement of heat production by the body; 1 MET = 50 kcal (210 kJ)/hour/m^2 body surface area.

metabolic rate   Rate of utilisation of ENERGY. *See* BASAL METABOLIC RATE.

metabolic syndrome   INSULIN RESISTANCE, HYPERTRIGLYCERIDAEMIA, low HDL, HYPERTENSION and HYPERGLYCAEMIA, associated with abdominal obesity, and sometimes also involving polycystic ovary syndrome and GOUT. Sometimes called 'syndrome X'. Mainly due to the metabolic effects of ADIPOSE TISSUE within the abdominal cavity (as opposed to subcutaneous adipose tissue). Commonly progresses to type II DIABETES mellitus when the capacity of the β-islet cells of the pancreas to secrete insulin in response to persistent hyperglycaemia is exhausted.

metabolic weight   ENERGY EXPENDITURE and BASAL METABOLIC RATE depend on the amount of metabolically active tissue in the body, not the total body weight; body weight to the power of 0.75 is often used to estimate metabolically active tissue.

metabolism   The processes of interconversion of chemical compounds in the body. Anabolism is the process of forming larger and more complex compounds, commonly linked to the utilisation of metabolic energy. Catabolism is the process of breaking down larger molecules to smaller ones, commonly oxidation reactions linked to release of energy.

metabolomics   Measurement of all the small molecules (metabolites) present in the organism, which represent interactions of the GENOME, transcriptome and proteome with the environment. *See also* PROTEOMICS; TRANSCRIPTOMICS.

metabonomics   Alternative term for METABOLOMICS.

metallisation   *See* METALLISED FILMS.

metallised films   For food packaging, manufactured by applying very thin layers of ALUMINIUM to a plastic film by vacuum deposition, to improve the barrier properties of the plastic. The thickness of the metal deposit is generally expressed as percentage light transmission through the film.

metalloproteins   Proteins containing a metal. For example, HAEMOGLOBIN, CYTOCHROMES, peroxidase, ferritin and siderophilin all contain IRON; many enzymes contain COPPER, MANGANESE or ZINC as a prosthetic group.

metallothionein   A small protein (M_r 6800, 61 amino acids) that binds ZINC, COPPER and CADMIUM. Important in both absorption and metabolism of essential metal ions, and also sequestration and excretion of metals such as cadmium. Plasma concentration may provide an index of zinc status.

metaphysis   Growing portion of a long BONE, between the EPI-PHYSIS and the shaft (DIAPHYSIS).

metaproteins   Products of the action of dilute acid or alkali on proteins; they are no longer soluble at their ISOELECTRIC points (*see* ISOELECTRIC FOCUSING) but will dissolve in weak acid or alkali.

metformin   *See* HYPOGLYCAEMIC AGENTS.

methaemoglobin   Oxidised HAEMOGLOBIN (unlike oxyhaemoglobin in which oxygen is reversibly bound without oxidising the iron); cannot transport oxygen. Present in small quantities in normal blood, increased after certain drugs and after smoking, and in babies after consumption of food or water containing moderately high levels of nitrates. Rarely occurs as a GENETIC DISEASE, methaemoglobinaemia.

methaglen (metheglin)   A traditional British wine made from honey (and thus a form of MEAD) to which herbs are added before fermentation. Originally for medicinal purposes.

methanogens   ARCHAEA found in RUMEN flora that produce methane (and hydrogen) as a metabolic end-product.

methanol (methyl alcohol, wood alcohol)   The first member of the alcohol series, chemically CH_3—OH. It is a highly toxic substance and leads to mental disturbance, blindness and death when consumed over a period. *See* ALCOHOL, DENATURED.

methionine   An essential amino acid, abbr Met (M), M_r 149.2, pK_a 2.13, 9.28, codon AUG. One of the three containing sulphur. Cystine and CYSTEINE (the other two sulphur amino acids) are not essential, but can only be made from methionine, and therefore the requirement for methionine is lower if there is an adequate intake of cyst(e)ine. Therefore the total sulphur amino acid content of foods is generally considered.

methionine load test   For VITAMIN B_6 status; measurement of urinary excretion of HOMOCYSTEINE after a test dose of 3 g of METHIONINE; the enzyme cystathionine synthetase (EC 4.2.1.22) is pyridoxal phosphate-dependent.

methionine sulphoximine   Formed by reaction between nitrogen trichloride (AGENE) and the amino acid METHIONINE when flour is treated with agene as a bleaching agent. Causes running fits in dogs, and although it has never been shown to be toxic to human beings, the use of agene as a FLOUR IMPROVER was abandoned in UK in 1955.

Methocel™   Methyl CELLULOSE.

méthode champenoise   Sparkling WINE made by a second fermentation in the bottle, as for CHAMPAGNE, but outside the Champagne region of north-eastern France.

Methofas™   Methyl hydroxypropyl CELLULOSE.

methotrexate   4-Amino-10-methyl folic acid, a FOLIC ACID antagonist used in cancer chemotherapy; inhibits dihydrofolate reductase (EC 1.5.1.3).

methylated spirits   *See* ALCOHOL, DENATURED.

methyl cellulose   *See* CELLULOSE.

methylene blue dye-reduction test   When the dye methylene blue is added to milk, any bacteria present take up oxygen and decolourise the dye. A similar test uses resazurin, which changes from blue-purple to pink. The speed of the change indicates the bacterial content. Pasteurised milk (*see* PASTEURISATION) must not reduce the dye in 30 min.

methylene tetrahydrofolate reductase   Enzyme (EC 1.7.99.5) involved in FOLIC ACID metabolism. A thermolabile variant occurs in 10–20% of the population leading to high blood levels of HOMOCYSTEINE, associated with ATHEROSCLEROSIS, THROMBOSIS and possibly NEURAL TUBE DEFECT.

methyl folate trap   Hypothesis to explain the occurrence of megaloblastic ANAEMIA and functional FOLIC ACID deficiency in VITAMIN B_{12} deficiency. Folic acid is transported between tissues as methyl folate, which can only be utilised by the vitamin B_{12}-dependent enzyme methionine synthetase (EC 2.1.1.13), so in vitamin B_{12} deficiency there is accumulation of folate as methyl folate, which cannot be utilised.

3-methylhistidine   Derivative of the amino acid HISTIDINE, found almost exclusively in the contractile proteins of muscle (myosin and actin). Useful as an index of lean meat content of foods, because it is not present in collagen or other added materials. Formed in protein after synthesis, and not reutilised when protein is catabolised. Urinary excretion has been proposed as an index of muscle protein turnover, but smaller pools of methyl histidine in non-muscle tissues turn over faster than muscle, and confound the interpretation of results.

methylisoborneol (MIB)   Microbial metabolite that can cause earthy or musty off-flavour in freshwater fish.

methylmalonic acid   Methylmalonyl CoA is an intermediate in the metabolism of VALINE, ISOLEUCINE and the side-chain of CHOLESTEROL, as well as (rare) odd-carbon FATTY ACIDS. It is normally metabolised by a VITAMIN B_{12}-dependent enzyme, methylmalonyl CoA mutase (EC 5.4.99.2); in deficiency, the activity of this enzyme is impaired and methylmalonic acid is excreted in the urine, especially after a test dose of valine or isoleucine. Methylmalonic aciduria also occurs as a GENETIC DISEASE due to deficiency of methylmalonyl CoA mutase.

N^1-methyl nicotinamide   Major urinary metabolite of NIACIN, and measured as an index of niacin status. Some methyl nicotinamide is oxidised to methyl pyridone carboxamide, and measurement of the ratio of the two metabolites is a more sensitive index of status.

methyl polysilicone (methyl silicone)   *See* DIMETHYLPOLYSILOXANE.

methyl pyridone carboxamide   *See* N^1-METHYL NICOTINAMIDE.

metmyoglobin   Brown oxidation product of MYOGLOBIN in meat when the iron has been oxidised to Fe^{3+}. Storage of pre-packed meat under low oxygen conditions slows the rate of oxidation.
 See also PACKAGING, MODIFIED ATMOSPHERE; NITROSOMYOGLOBIN.

metronidazole   Drug used to treat intestinal (and other) infections, including AMOEBIASIS and GIARDIASIS.

Meulengracht diet   Former treatment for peptic ULCER; sieved foods such as meat, chicken, vegetables, at two-hourly intervals. Richer in protein than the SIPPY DIET. The intention is to neutralise the acid in the stomach by the buffering effect of the protein.

meunière, à la   Fish dredged with flour, fried in butter and served with this butter and chopped parsley (literally *in the style of the miller's wife*).

micelle   Droplets of partially hydrolysed dietary lipid, emulsified by non-esterified FATTY ACIDS, mono-acylglycerol and BILE SALTS, small enough to be absorbed across the intestinal mucosa.

micro-aerophiles   Micro-organisms that grow best at oxygen concentrations well below atmospheric, but not ANAEROBIC (*see* AEROBIC). Lead to spoilage of foodstuffs unless all oxygen is excluded.

microbiological assay   Biological method of measuring compounds such as vitamins and amino acids, using micro-organisms. The principle is that the organism is inoculated into a medium containing all the growth factors needed except the one under examination; the rate of growth is then proportional to the amount of this nutrient added in the test substance.

microcapsules   *See* ENCAPSULATION.

microcytosis   Presence of abnormally small red BLOOD CELLS (microcytes) in the circulation; occurs in IRON deficiency ANAEMIA and other anaemias associated with impairment of HAEMOGLOBIN synthesis.

microencapsulation   *See* ENCAPSULATION.

microfiltration   Filtration under pressure through a membrane of small pore size (0.1–10μm; larger pores than for ULTRAFILTRATION). Used for clarification of beverages and to sterilise liquids by filtering out bacteria.

micronisation   Extremely rapid heating with infrared radiation. Suggested as an alternative to steam heating or toasting since the shorter heating time is less damaging to the foodstuff.

micronutrients   VITAMINS and MINERALS, which are needed in very small amounts (μg or mg per day), as distinct from fats, carbohydrates and proteins which are macronutrients, needed in considerably greater amounts.

micro-organisms   Bacteria, yeasts and moulds; can cause food spoilage, and disease (pathogens); used to process and preserve food by FERMENTATION and have been used as foodstuffs (single cell protein and mycoprotein).

See also FOOD POISONING.

microscope, atomic force   Microscope in which the surface of the specimen is scanned by a sharp probe that is repulsed away from the surface by atomic forces; measuring the deflection of the probe permits the production of a detailed topographical map of the sample at the molecular level.

microscope, confocal   Microscope in which a point light source (commonly from a laser) is focused on a small region of the sample, so that only the in-focus plane is illuminated, with the out of focus regions appearing as a black background.

microscope, electron   Microscope using a focused electron beam rather than light; permits resolution of the order of 0.2 nm, compared with light microscopy with a resolution of 0.25 μm. In scanning electron microscopy the electron beam is reflected from the surface of the sample; in transmission electron microscopy it is transmitted through the sample.

microvilli   Hair-like projections (~5 μm long) from the surface of epithelial cells, e.g. in the GASTROINTESTINAL TRACT. When microvilli form a dense covering on the surface of a cell, this is the brush border.

microwave cooking   Rapid heating by passing high-frequency electromagnetic waves (commonly 2450 MHz, sometimes 896 MHz in Europe and 915 MHz in the USA) from a magnetron through the food or liquid to be heated. The process is based on the electric dipole produced by the negatively charged oxygen atom and the positively charged hydrogen atoms in water. The application of a rapidly oscillating electric field causes the dipoles to reorient with each change in the field direction, dissipating energy as heat. The ratio of the capacitance of the food to the capacitance of air is the dielectric constant and depends on the number of dipoles, temperature and the changes induced by the electric fields.

middlings   *See* WHEATFEED.

mid-upper-arm circumference (MUAC)   A rapid way of assessing nutritional status, especially applicable to children.

See also ANTHROPOMETRY; QUAC STICK.

migaki-nishin   Japanese; mixture of dried fish fillets and ABALONE.

migration In food packaging, the release of compounds from the packaging material into the food; some diffusible compounds remaining from manufacture of plastics may present health hazards, or taint the food.

miki South-east Asian; noodles made from wheat flour, eggs and soda ash.

mikiyuk Alaskan Inuit; partially dried whale meat, allowed to undergo bacterial fermentation (*Micrococcus* and *Staphylococcus* spp. as well as lactic acid bacteria) for several months or years.

milchig Jewish term for dishes containing milk or milk products, which cannot be served with or after meat dishes.
See also FLEISHIG; PAREVE.

milfoil A common wild plant (*Achillea millefolium*, or yarrow) with finely divided leaves which can be used in salads or chopped to replace chervil or parsley as a garnish.

milk The secretion of the mammary gland of animals including cow, buffalo, goat, ass, mare, ewe, camel and human beings.

Cow's milk, composition/100 g: water 88 g, 251 kJ (60 kcal), protein 3.2 g, fat 3.3 g (of which 66% saturated, 28% mono-unsaturated, 7% polyunsaturated), cholesterol 10 mg, carbohydrate 4.5 g (5.3 g sugars) ash 0.7 g, Ca 113 mg, Mg 10 mg, P 91 mg, K 143 mg, Na 40 mg, Zn 0.4 mg, Se 3.7 µg, I 31 µg, vitamin A 28 µg RE (28 µg retinol, 5 µg carotenoids), E 0.1 mg, K 0.2 mg, B_1 0.04 mg, B_2 0.18 mg, niacin 0.1 mg, B_6 0.04 mg, folate 5 µg, B_{12} 0.4 µg, pantothenate 0.4 mg. A 585 ml serving (1 pint) is a source of Mg, Zn, vitamin B_1, B_6, folate, a good source of Se, vitamin A, a rich source of Ca, I, P, vitamin B_2, B_{12}, pantothenate.

Full cream milk is 3.9% fat, Channel Island 5.1%, semi-skimmed 1.6% and skimmed 0.1%.

Goat, composition/100 g: water 87 g, 289 kJ (69 kcal), protein 3.6 g, fat 4.1 g (of which 69% saturated, 28% mono-unsaturated, 3% polyunsaturated), cholesterol 11 mg, carbohydrate 4.4 g (4.4 g sugars) ash 0.8 g, Ca 134 mg, Fe 0.1 mg, Mg 14 mg, P 111 mg, K 204 mg, Na 50 mg, Zn 0.3 mg, Se 1.4 µg, I 31 µg, vitamin A 57 µg RE (56 µg retinol, 7 µg carotenoids), E 0.1 mg, K 0.3 mg, B_1 0.05 mg, B_2 0.14 mg, niacin 0.3 mg, B_6 0.05 mg, folate 1 µg, B_{12} 0.1 µg, pantothenate 0.3 mg, C 1 mg. A 585 ml serving (1 pint) is a source of Zn, vitamin B_6, a good source of Mg, vitamin B_1, pantothenate, a rich source of Ca, I, P, vitamin A, B_2, B_{12}.

Human, composition/100 g: water 87.5 g, 293 kJ (70 kcal), protein 1 g, fat 4.4 g (of which 48% saturated, 40% mono-unsaturated, 12% polyunsaturated), cholesterol 14 mg, carbohydrate 6.9 g (6.9 g sugars) ash 0.2 g, Ca 32 mg, Mg 3 mg, P 14 mg, K 51 mg, Na 17 mg, Zn 0.2 mg, Cu 0.1 mg, Se 1.8 μg, vitamin A 61 μg RE (60 μg retinol, 7 μg carotenoids), E 0.1 mg, K 0.3 mg, B_1 0.01 mg, B_2 0.04 mg, niacin 0.2 mg, B_6 0.01 mg, folate 5 μg, B_{12} 0.1 μg, pantothenate 0.2 mg, C 5 mg.

milk, accredited Term not used after October 1954; milk untreated by heat, from cows examined at specified intervals for freedom from disease.

milk, acidophilus Heat-treated milk inoculated with 1–2% *Lactobacillus acidophilus* or *Bifidobacterium bifidum* (*Lactobacillus bifidus*) which ferment milk slowly at 39 °C and form lactic and acetic acids, with small amounts of propionic and butyric acids, with final pH 3.9–4.4%; more than 10^6 live bacterial cells/mL. Claimed to enhance the growth of beneficial bacteria in the intestine.

Sweet acidophilus milk is made with a heavy inoculation of starter added to cold pasteurised milk to preserve the bacteria in the product.

See also PROBIOTICS.

milk, alcohol stability test For sourness of milk; milk that contains an acceptable level of lactic acid will not flocculate when shaken with double its volume of alcohol.

milk alkali syndrome Weakness and lethargy caused by prolonged adherence to a diet rich in milk, more than about 1 L daily, and alkalis.

milk baby Infant with iron deficiency ANAEMIA caused by excessive ingestion of milk and delayed or inadequate addition of iron-rich foods to the diet.

milk, citrated Milk to which sodium citrate has been added to combine with the calcium and inhibit the curdling of CASEINO-GEN which would normally occur in the stomach. Claimed, with little evidence, to be of value in feeding infants and invalids.

milk, clot on boiling test For sourness of milk, since milk that contains more than about 0.1% LACTIC ACID will not form a clot on boiling.

milk crumb In CHOCOLATE manufacture, a mix prepared from COCOA beans, milk and sugar. More expensive than using milk powder, but the product has a better texture, and a caramelised flavour from MAILLARD REACTION products.

milk, dye-reduction test *See* METHYLENE BLUE DYE-REDUCTION TEST.

milk, evaporated, condensed Full fat, skimmed or partly skimmed milk, sweetened or unsweetened, that has been concentrated by partial evaporation; fat and total solids for each type defined by law.

milk fat test   *See* GERBER TEST.

milk, feed flavours   Tainting of milk by volatile compounds in the animals' feedstuff; in severe cases the milk may need to be vacuum processed before it can be used.

milk, fermented   In various countries, milk is fermented with a mixture of bacteria (and sometimes yeasts) when the lactose is converted to lactic acid and in some cases to alcohol. The acidity (and alcohol) prevent the growth of potentially hazardous micro-organisms, and the fermentation thus acts to preserve the milk for a time.

Include busa (Turkestan), cieddu (Italy), dadhi (India), kefir (Balkans), kumiss (Steppes), laban zabadi (Egypt), mazun (Armenia), taette (N. Europe), skyr (Iceland), masl (Iran), crowdies (Scotland), kuban and YOGURT.

See also PROBIOTIC.

milk, filled   Milk from which the natural fat has been removed and replaced with fat from another source. The reason may be economic, if the butter-fat can be replaced by a cheaper one, or more recently, to replace a fat rich in saturated FATTY ACIDS with a more unsaturated vegetable oil.

milk, freezing-point test   A test for the adulteration of milk with water by measuring the freezing point; milk normally freezes between -0.53 and $-0.55\,°C$; if diluted with water it will freeze above $-0.53\,°C$. Also known as Hortvet test.

milk, homogenised   Mechanical treatment breaks up and redistributes the fat globules throughout the milk to prevent the cream rising to the surface.

milk, humanised   Cow's milk that has had its composition modified to resemble human milk, for infant feeding. The main change is a reduction in protein content, often achieved by dilution with carbohydrate and restoration of the fat content.

milk, irradiated   Milk that has been subjected to UV light, when the 7-dehydrocholesterol naturally present is partly converted into VITAMIN D.

milk, lactose-hydrolysed   Milk in which the LACTOSE has been hydrolysed to glucose and galactose by treatment with the enzyme LACTASE; intended for infants who are lactose intolerant. Lactose-free milk may also be prepared by physical removal of lactose by ULTRAFILTRATION.

See also DISACCHARIDE INTOLERANCE.

milk, long (ropy)   A Scandinavian soured milk which is viscous because of 'ropiness' caused by bacteria. *See* ROPE.

milk, malted A preparation of milk and the liquid separated from a mash of barley malt and wheat flour, evaporated to dryness.

Milkman's syndrome Form of OSTEOMALACIA with characteristic X-ray appearance of the bones; named after the American radiologist L. A. Milkman.

milk, methylene blue test *See* METHYLENE BLUE DYE-REDUCTION TEST.

milk of magnesia MAGNESIUM hydroxide solution used as an ANTACID and LAXATIVE.

milk, pasteurised *See* PASTEURISATION.

milk, protein Partially skimmed lactic acid milk plus milk curd (prepared from whole milk by RENNET precipitation); richer in protein and lower in fat than ordinary milk; supposed to be better tolerated in digestive disorders. Also known as albumin milk and eiweiss milch.

milk, ropy *See* MILK, LONG; ROPE.

milk stone Deposit of calcium and magnesium phosphates, protein, etc., produced when milk is heated to temperatures above 60 °C.

milk thistle An annual or biennial thistle, *Silybum marianum* (*Carduus marianus*) that has been used as a vegetable; the flower receptacle can be eaten like globe ARTICHOKE.

milk, toned Dried skim milk added to a high-fat milk such as buffalo milk, to reduce the fat content but maintain the total solids.

milk, tuberculin tested (TT) Applied to milk from a herd that has been attested free from tuberculosis.

milk, UHT (or long-life) Milk sterilised for a very short time (2 s) at ultra-high temperature (137 °C).

milk, witches' *See* WITCHES' MILK.

millerator Wheat-cleaning machine consisting of two sieves, the upper one retaining particles larger than wheat, the lower one rejecting particles smaller than wheat.

miller's offal *See* WHEATFEED.

millet Cereal of a number of species of Gramineae (grass family) smaller than wheat and rice and high in fibre content. Common millet (*Panicum* and *Setaria* spp.) also known as China, Italian, Indian, French hog, proso, panicled and broom corn millet, foxtail millet (*Setaria italica*); grows very rapidly, 2–2½ months from sowing to harvest.

Composition/100 g: water 8.7 g, 1582 kJ (378 kcal), protein 11 g, fat 4.2 g (of which 19% saturated, 22% mono-unsaturated, 58% polyunsaturated), carbohydrate 72.8 g, fibre 8.5 g, ash 3.3 g, Ca 8 mg, Fe 3 mg, Mg 114 mg, P 285 mg, K 195 mg, Na 5 mg, Zn

1.7 mg, Cu 0.8 mg, Mn 1.6 mg, Se 2.7 µg, vitamin E 0.1 mg, K 0.9 mg, B_1 0.42 mg, B_2 0.29 mg, niacin 4.7 mg, B_6 0.38 mg, folate 85 µg, pantothenate 0.8 mg. A 30 g serving is a source of Mg, folate, a good source of Cu, Mn.

Bulrush millet, pearl millet, bajoa or Kaffir manna corn is *Pennisetum typhoideum* or *P. americanum*. Other species are hungry rice (*Digitaria exilis*), jajeo millet (*Acroceras amplectens*), Kodo or haraka millet (*Paspalum scrobiculatum*), teff (*Eragrostis tefor, E. abyssinica*).

See also SORGHUM.

milling The term usually refers to the conversion of cereal grain into its derivative, e.g. wheat into flour, brown rice to white rice. Flour milling involves two types of rollers:

(1) break rolls are corrugated and exert shear pressure and forces which break up the wheat grain and permit sieving into fractions containing varying proportions of GERM, BRAN and ENDOSPERM;

(2) reducing rolls that are smooth and subdivide the endosperm to fine particles.

See also FLOUR, EXTRACTION RATE.

mills Various types of equipment used to reduce the size of fibrous foods to smaller pieces or to pulp and dry foods to powders. *See* BALL MILL; COMMINUTION; DISC MILL; HAMMER MILL; QUERNS; ROD MILL; ROLLER MILL.

milt (melt) Soft ROE (testes) of male fish. Also SPLEEN of animals.

miltone A toned milk (*see* MILK, TONED) developed in India in which peanut protein is added to buffalo or cow's milk to extend supplies.

mimetics *See* FAT REPLACERS.

Minafen™ Food low in PHENYLALANINE for treatment of PHENYLKETONURIA.

Minamata disease Poisoning by organic mercurial compounds, named after Minamata Bay in Japan, where fish contained high levels of organic mercurials during 1953–1956, as a result of mercury-rich industrial waste entering the river estuary.

minarine Name sometimes given to low-fat spreads with less than the statutory amount of fat in a MARGARINE.

mince (1) To chop or cut into small pieces with a knife or, more commonly, in a mincing machine or electric mixer.

(2) Meat which is finely divided by chopping or passing through a mincing machine; known as ground meat in the USA.

mincemeat A traditional product made from apple, sugar, vine fruits and citrus peel with suet, spices and acetic acid, coloured with caramel. Preserved by the sugar content and acid. Also called fruit mince. Originally a meat product; in the USA a spiced mixture of chopped meat, apples and raisins.

mineola A CITRUS fruit.

mineralocorticoids A general term for the STEROID hormones secreted by the adrenal cortex (*see* ADRENAL GLANDS) which control the excretion of salt and water (*see* WATER BALANCE).

mineral salts The inorganic salts, including sodium, potassium, calcium, chloride, phosphate, sulphate, etc. So-called because they are (or originally were) obtained by mining.

minerals, trace Those MINERAL SALTS present in the body, and required in the diet, in small amounts (parts per million): COPPER, CHROMIUM, IODINE, MANGANESE, SELENIUM; although required in larger amounts, ZINC and IRON are sometimes included with the trace minerals.

minerals, ultratrace Those MINERAL SALTS present in the body, and required in the diet, in extremely small amounts (parts per thousand million or less); known to be dietary essentials, although rarely if ever a cause for concern since the amounts required are small and they are widely distributed in foods and water, e.g. COBALT, MOLYBDENUM, SILICON, TIN, VANADIUM.

miners' cramp Cramp due to loss of SALT from the body caused by excessive sweating. Occurs in tropical climates and with severe exercise; mining often combines the two. Prevented by consuming salt, e.g., salt tablets in the tropics and for athletes.

minimum lethal dose (MLD) Smallest amount of a toxic compound that has been recorded as causing death.

See also LD$_{50}$; NO ADVERSE EFFECT LEVEL.

mint Aromatic herbs, *Mentha* spp., including spearmint, *M. spicata*; peppermint, *M. piperita*; garden mint is *M. spicata*. Oil of peppermint is distilled from stem and leaves of *M. piperita*, and used both pharmaceutically and as a flavour.

miracle berry The fruit of the West African bush *Richardella dulcifica* (*Synsepalum dulcificum*). It contains a taste-modifying glycoprotein (miraculin) that causes sour foods to taste sweet, hence the name.

miraculin The taste-modifying glycoprotein of the MIRACLE BERRY.

mirin Japanese; sweet alcoholic condiment made from rice fermented by addition of KOJI.

miscella The solution of oil in solvent obtained during solvent extraction of oilseeds.

miso Japanese sauce, prepared from autoclaved soya beans mixed with cooked rice and partly fermented with *Aspergillus oryzae* and *A. sojae* to form KOJI. Salt is added to stop further mould growth, bacterial fermentation continues with the addition of *Lactobacillus* (1–2 months).

Composition/100 g: water 43 g, 833 kJ (199 kcal), protein 11.7 g, fat 6 g (of which 20% saturated, 22% mono-unsaturated, 58% polyunsaturated), carbohydrate 26.5 g (6.2 g sugars), fibre 5.4 g, ash 12.8 g, Ca 57 mg, Fe 2.5 mg, Mg 48 mg, P 159 mg, K 210 mg, Na 3728 mg, Zn 2.6 mg, Cu 0.4 mg, Mn 0.9 mg, Se 7 µg, vitamin A 4 µg RE (52 µg carotenoids), K 30.1 mg, B_1 0.1 mg, B_2 0.23 mg, niacin 0.9 mg, B_6 0.2 mg, folate 19 µg, B_{12} 0.1 µg, pantothenate 0.3 mg.

mistelles French; partially fermented grape juice.

misua S.E. Asian; noodles made from wheat flour, eggs and soda ash.

mitochondrion (plural mitochondria) The subcellular organelles in all cells apart from red blood cells in which the major oxidative reactions of METABOLISM occur; linked to the formation of ATP from ADP.

mitogen Any compound that acts to stimulate cell division (mitosis).

mixed function oxidases A group of enzymes (EC 1.14.x.x) that catalyse oxidation of two substrates simultaneously, using molecular oxygen as the donor. Most hydroxylases and the CYTOCHROMES P_{450} are mixed-function oxidases.

mixiria Process of preserving meat and fish by roasting in their own fat and preserving in jars covered with a layer of fat.

mixograph Instrument for measuring the physical properties of a dough, similar in principle to the FARINOGRAPH.

MLD *See* MINIMUM LETHAL DOSE.

mocca Mixture of coffee and cocoa used in bakery and confectionery products.

mocha (1) Variety of arabica coffee.

(2) Flavoured with coffee.

(3) In the USA, a combination of coffee and chocolate flavouring.

See also MOCCA.

mock turtle soup Gelatinous soup made from calf's head, beef, bacon and veal; similar to turtle soup, but without the TURTLE; mock turtle is a calf's head dressed to resemble a turtle.

modified atmosphere *See* PACKAGING, MODIFIED ATMOSPHERE.

MODY Maturity onset DIABETES of the young. A rare type of diabetes mellitus due to genetic defects, sometimes of GLUCOKINASE (which is the pancreatic sensor for increased blood glucose).

mogroside Triterpenoid glycoside from the fruit of the Chinese plant *Momordica grosvenori* (known in Chinese as lo han kuo), 300 times as sweet as sucrose, and marketed as an intense SWEETENER.

moisture, bound   Water adsorbed onto solid foods and in solutions exhibits a vapour pressure less than that of free water at the same temperature, and it requires a higher temperature to dry the food or evaporate the solution.

moisture, free   Moisture in excess of the equilibrium moisture content at a given temperature and humidity, and so available to be removed.

molality   Concentration of a solution expressed as mol of solute per kg of solvent.

molarity   Concentration of a solution expressed as mol of solute per litre of solution.

molasses   The residue left after repeated crystallisation of sugar; it will not crystallise. Contains 67% sucrose, together with glucose and fructose and (if from beet) raffinose and small quantities of dextrans; 1100 kJ (260 kcal), >500 mg iron/100 g, with traces of other minerals.

mole   (1) Mexican; sauce made from sweet pepper, avocado, tomato and sesame, flavoured with aniseed, garlic, coriander, cinnamon, cloves, chilli and grated chocolate.

(2) Chemical term (abbreviated to mol), 1 mol of a compound is equivalent to its molecular mass in grams.

molecular sieve   Porous crystalline silicates that adsorb water and can be regenerated by heating; used, e.g., to remove water from alcohol or packaged foods.

molluscs   Marine bivalve shellfish with soft unsegmented body; most are enclosed in a hard shell and include ABALONE, CLAMS, COCKLES, MUSSELS, OYSTERS, SCALLOPS, WHELKS, WINKLES.

molybdenum   A dietary essential mineral, required for a number of enzymes in which it forms the functional part of the coenzyme MOLYBDOPTERIN. Deficiency is unknown; the reference intake is 45 µg and the upper tolerable intake 2 mg/day.

molybdopterin   A pterin derivative with MOLYBDENUM chelated by two sulphydryl groups; not a dietary essential but synthesised in the body. The coenzyme of molybdenum-dependent enzymes, including XANTHINE (EC 1.1.3.22), sulphite (EC 1.8.3.1), aldehyde (EC 1.2.3.1) and pyridoxal (EC 1.1.3.12) oxidases.

momoni   W African; various fish left to start fermenting in tropical heat for 6–10 hours, then salted for 1–2 days and sun-dried. Known in Ghana as stinking fish.

monellin   The active sweet principle, a protein, from the serendipity berry, *Dioscoreophyllum cumminsii*. 1500–2000 times as sweet as sucrose.

Monilia   Obsolete name for genus of fungi now known as CANDIDA.

318

moniliformin MYCOTOXIN formed by *Fusarium moniliforme, F. oxysporum, F. anthopilum* and *F. graminearum*, growing especially on maize. Toxic to experimental animals and associated with KESHAN DISEASE in areas of China where SELENIUM intake is extremely low.

monkey nut *See* PEANUT.

monkey orange Fruit of the southern African tree *Strychnos cocculoides.*

monkfish White fish, *Lophius piscatorius.*

Composition/100 g: water 83 g, 318 kJ (76 kcal), protein 14.5 g, fat 1.5 g (of which 27% saturated, 18% mono-unsaturated, 55% polyunsaturated), cholesterol 25 mg, carbohydrate 0 g, ash 1.2 g, Ca 8 mg, Fe 0.3 mg, Mg 21 mg, P 200 mg, K 400 mg, Na 18 mg, Zn 0.4 mg, Se 36.5 µg, vitamin A 12 µg retinol, B_1 0.03 mg, B_2 0.06 mg, niacin 2.1 mg, B_6 0.24 mg, folate 7 µg, B_{12} 0.9 µg, pantothenate 0.2 mg, C 1 mg. A 100 g serving is a source of niacin, vitamin B_6, a good source of P, a rich source of Se, vitamin B_{12}.

monoacylglycerol, monoglyceride *See* FAT, SUPERGLYCERINATED.

monoamine oxidase ENZYME (EC1.4.3.4) that oxidises AMINES; inhibitors are used clinically as antidepressants, and consumption of amine-rich foods such as cheese may cause a hypertensive crisis in people taking the drugs.

monocalcium phosphate *See* CALCIUM ACID PHOSPHATE.

monoethanolamine *See* ETHANOLAMINE.

monoglycerides *See* FAT, SUPERGLYCERINATED.

monokine *See* CYTOKINE.

monophagia Desire for one type of food.

monophenol oxidase *See* PHENOL OXIDASES.

monosaccharides Group name of the simplest sugars, including those composed of three carbon atoms (trioses), four (tetroses), five (pentoses), six (hexoses) and seven (heptoses). Formerly known as monoses or monosaccharoses. *See* CARBOHYDRATES.

monosaccharose **(monose)** Obsolete names for MONOSACCHARIDES.

monosodium glutamate (MSG) The sodium salt of GLUTAMIC ACID, used to enhance flavour of savoury dishes and often added to canned meat and soups. First isolated from seaweed by Tokyo chemist Kimunae Ikeda in 1908; he called it ajinomoto (aginomoto), meaning 'the essence of taste'.

See also FLAVOUR ENHANCER; UMAMI.

mono-unsaturates Commonly used term for mono-unsaturated FATTY ACIDS.

monstera Fruit of the Swiss cheese plant, *Monstera deliciosa,* also known as fruit salad fruit (Australia), and delicious fruit.

Monterey jack   American CHEDDAR-type cheese.

montmorillonite   *See* FULLER'S EARTH.

mooli   Long, white oriental variety of RADISH, *Raphanus sativa*.

Composition/100g: (edible portion 79%) water 95g, 75kJ (18kcal), protein 0.6g, fat 0.1g, carbohydrate 4.1g (2.5g sugars), fibre 1.6g, ash 0.6g, Ca 27mg, Fe 0.4mg, Mg 16mg, P 23mg, K 227mg, Na 21mg, Zn 0.2mg, Cu 0.1mg, Se 0.7µg, vitamin K 0.3mg, B$_1$ 0.02mg, B$_2$ 0.02mg, niacin 0.2mg, B$_6$ 0.05mg, folate 28µg, pantothenate 0.1mg, C 22mg.

moonshine   American term for illicit home-distilled spirit; Irish equivalent is poteen.

morbidity   The state of being diseased. Morbidity rate is the number of cases of a disease/million of the population.

See also INCIDENCE RATE; PREVALENCE RATE.

morel   Edible fungus *Morchella esculenta*, much prized for its delicate flavour; *see* MUSHROOMS.

Moreton Bay bug   Or Bay lobster. A variety of sand LOBSTER found in Australia.

moringa   Fruit of the kelor tree, *Moringa oleifera*; the leaves and seed pods are edible and are reported to taste like ASPARAGUS. The crushed seeds have antibacterial activity and can be used to purify drinking water. Ben oil, a fine oil used by watchmakers, is produced from the seeds. Also known as the horseradish tree, because its bulbous roots taste like horseradish.

moromi   East Asian; thick mash of cereal or cereal and soy bean left to undergo slow fermentation with bacteria, yeasts and moulds. A stage in the production of MISO, SOY SAUCE and SAKÉ.

morphine   *See* ANTIMOTILITY AGENTS.

mortality   The incidence of death in a population in a given period of time.

mortoban   *See* PHYLLO PASTRY.

moss, Irish   *See* CARRAGEENAN.

motilin   Peptide hormone secreted by the stomach and upper small intestine; increases intestinal motility.

mottled teeth   *See* FLUORIDE; FLUOROSIS.

motza   *See* MATZO.

mould bran   A fungal AMYLASE preparation produced by growing mould on moist wheat bran.

moulders   Machines that form dough or confectionery into different shapes.

mould inhibitors   *See* ANTIMYCOTICS.

moulds   FUNGI characterised by their branched filamentous structure (mycelium), including MUSHROOMS and smaller fungi. They can cause food spoilage very rapidly, e.g. white *Mucor*, grey-green *Penicillium*, black *Aspergillus*. Many also produce MYCOTOXINS.

Used for large-scale manufacture of citric acid (*Aspergillus niger*), ripening of cheeses (*Penicillium* spp.) and as source of enzymes for industrial use. A number of foods are fermented with moulds, e.g. IDLI, MISO and TEMPEH. The mycelium of *Fusarium* spp. is used as MYCOPROTEIN. Most of the ANTIBIOTICS are mould products.

mowrah fat (mowrah butter) *See* COCOA BUTTER EQUIVALENTS.

MPD Modified POLYDEXTROSE.

M_r Relative molecular mass, also known as molecular weight.

MRM *See* MEAT, MECHANICALLY RECOVERED.

mRNA Messenger RNA, synthesised in the nucleus as a copy of one strand of a region of DNA containing the information for the synthesis of one or more proteins.

> *See also* TRANSCRIPTION; TRANSLATION.

MRP Material resource planning.

MSG *See* MONOSODIUM GLUTAMATE.

MSM Mechanically separated meat, *see* MEAT, MECHANICALLY RECOVERED.

MUAC *See* MID-UPPER-ARM CIRCUMFERENCE.

mucilage Soluble but undigested polymers of the sugars arabinose and xylose found in some seeds and seaweeds; used as thickening and stabilising agents in food processing by virtue of their water-holding and viscous properties.

> *See also* GUM.

mucin A GLYCOPROTEIN, the main protein of MUCUS secreted by goblet cells of mucous epithelium as protection; it is resistant to hydrolysis by digestive enzymes. Especially rich in CYSTEINE and THREONINE; some 60% of the dietary requirement for threonine is accounted for by losses in intestinal mucus.

mucopolysaccharides GLYCOPROTEINS with a short polypeptide chain covalently linked to a long linear polysaccharide; commonly found in connective tissue.

mucoproteins GLYCOPROTEINS consisting of acidic MUCOPOLYSACCHARIDES covalently linked to specific proteins; sticky and slippery, found for example in saliva and mucous membrane secretions.

mucosa Moist tissue lining, e.g. the mouth (buccal mucosa), stomach (gastric mucosa), intestines and respiratory tract.

mucous colitis *See* IRRITABLE BOWEL SYNDROME.

mucus Viscous fluid secreted by mucous membranes, in the GASTRO-INTESTINAL TRACT. Acts both to lubricate the intestinal wall and also to prevent digestion of intestinal mucosal cells. Main constituent is MUCIN.

muesli Breakfast cereal; a mixture of raw cereal flakes (oats, wheat, rye, barley and millet) together with dried fruit, apple flakes, nuts, sugar, bran and wheatgerm. Originated in Switzerland in late 19th century.

mulberry Dark purple-red fruit of the tree *Morus nigra*, slightly sweet and acid, similar shape and size to a raspberry or loganberry. There is also a white mulberry, *M. alba*. Of little commercial importance as a fruit; the leaves of the mulberry are the only food plant of the silkworm.

Composition/100 g: water 87.7 g, 180 kJ (43 kcal), protein 1.4 g, fat 0.4 g, carbohydrate 9.8 g (8.1 g sugars), fibre 1.7 g, ash 0.7 g, Ca 39 mg, Fe 1.9 mg, Mg 18 mg, P 38 mg, K 194 mg, Na 10 mg, Zn 0.1 mg, Cu 0.1 mg, Se 0.6 µg, vitamin A 1 µg RE (157 µg carotenoids), E 0.9 mg, K 7.8 mg, B_1 0.03 mg, B_2 0.1 mg, niacin 0.6 mg, B_6 0.05 mg, folate 6 µg, C 36 mg. A 110 g serving is a source of Fe, a rich source of vitamin C.

mulled ale Beer that has been spiced and heated, traditionally by plunging a red-hot poker into the liquid.

mulled wine Wine mixed with fruit juice, sweetened and flavoured with spices (especially cinnamon, cloves and ginger), served hot.

mullet White FISH, Mugilidae and Mullidae families.

Composition/100 g: water 77 g, 490 kJ (117 kcal), protein 19.4 g, fat 3.8 g (of which 38% saturated, 38% mono-unsaturated, 24% polyunsaturated), cholesterol 49 mg, carbohydrate 0 g, ash 1.2 g, Ca 41 mg, Fe 1 mg, Mg 29 mg, P 221 mg, K 357 mg, Na 65 mg, Zn 0.5 mg, Cu 0.1 mg, Se 36.5 µg, I 190 µg, vitamin A 37 µg RE (37 µg retinol), E 1 mg, K 0.1 mg, B_1 0.09 mg, B_2 0.08 mg, niacin 5.2 mg, B_6 0.43 mg, folate 9 µg, B_{12} 0.2 µg, pantothenate 0.8 mg, C 1 mg. A 100 g serving is a source of pantothenate, a good source of P, niacin, vitamin B_6, B_{12}, a rich source of I, Se.

mulligatawny Anglo-Indian; CURRY-flavoured soup made with meat or chicken stock.

mulsum Roman; mixture of wine and honey, commonly drunk with the first course of a meal.

multiple effect The re-use of vapour from boiling liquor in one evaporator as the heating medium in another evaporator.

multiple sclerosis A slowly progressive disease involving nerve degeneration; it may take many years to develop to the stage of paralysis, and the disease is subject to random periods of spontaneous remission. There is some evidence that supplements of polyunsaturated FATTY ACIDS slow its progression.

munster Soft cheese made in wheel shapes with an orange-red rind. Originally French, now made in several countries.

muscatels Made by drying the large seed-containing grapes grown almost exclusively around Malaga (Spain). They are partially dried in the sun and drying is completed indoors; they are left on the stalk and pressed flat for sale. Muscatel is a sweet wine made from the grapes.

muscle The contractile unit of skeletal muscle is the cylindrical fibre, composed of many myofibrils. Chemically, muscle consists of four main proteins, actin, myosin, tropomyosin and troponin, as well as structural proteins such as COLLAGEN and ELASTIN. Contraction is achieved by formation of a complex between actin and myosin. The muscle fibre is surrounded by a thin membrane, the sarcolemma; within the muscle fibre, surrounding the myofibrils, is the sarcoplasm. Individual fibres are separated by a thin network of CONNECTIVE TISSUE, the endomysium, and the muscle as a whole is enclosed in the epimysium.

muscovado *See* SUGAR.

mushrooms The fruiting bodies of FUNGI (both mushrooms and toadstools). Altogether some 1100 species are sold, fresh or dried, in markets around the world; most of these are gathered wild rather than cultivated. 340 are poisonous to one degree or another (10 are fatal, 6 hallucinogenic); 250 have (potential) medicinal uses. The common cultivated mushroom, including flat, cup and button mushrooms is *Agaricus bisporus*, as is the chestnut or Paris mushroom.

Composition/100 g: (edible portion 97%) water 92.5 g, 92 kJ (22 kcal), protein 3.1 g, fat 0.3 g, carbohydrate 3.2 g (1.9 g sugars), fibre 1.2 g, ash 0.9 g, Ca 3 mg, Fe 0.5 mg, Mg 9 mg, P 85 mg, K 314 mg, Na 4 mg, Zn 0.5 mg, Cu 0.3 mg, Se 8.9 µg, vitamin K 0.1 mg, B_1 0.09 mg, B_2 0.42 mg, niacin 3.9 mg, B_6 0.12 mg, folate 16 µg, pantothenate 1.5 mg, C 2 mg. A 45 g serving is a source of Cu, vitamin B_2, pantothenate.

Other cultivated mushrooms include: shiitake or Black Forest mushroom; oyster mushroom; Chinese straw mushroom.

Some wild species are especially prized, including field mushroom; horse mushroom; parasol mushroom; beefsteak fungus; blewits; wood blewits; cèpe or boletus; chanterelle; matsutake; puffballs; morels; truffles, wood ears or Chinese black fungus; yellow mushroom.

mussels Marine bivalve MOLLUSCS, *Mytilus edulis*, *M. californianus*.

Composition/100 g: water 80.6 g, 360 kJ (86 kcal), protein 11.9 g, fat 2.2 g (of which 27% saturated, 33% mono-unsaturated, 40% polyunsaturated), cholesterol 28 mg, carbohydrate 3.7 g, ash 1.6 g, Ca 26 mg, Fe 4 mg, Mg 34 mg, P 197 mg, K 320 mg, Na

286 mg, Zn 1.6 mg, Cu 0.1 mg, Mn 3.4 mg, Se 44.8 μg, I 140 μg, vitamin A 48 μg retinol, E 0.6 mg, K 0.1 mg, B_1 0.16 mg, B_2 0.21 mg, niacin 1.6 mg, B_6 0.05 mg, folate 42 μg, B_{12} 12 μg, pantothenate 0.5 mg, C 8 mg. A 130 g serving is a source of Mg, Zn, vitamin B_1, B_2, niacin, C, a good source of folate, a rich source of Fe, I, Mn, P, Se, vitamin B_{12}.

Greenshell mussels (*Perna canaliculus*), so-called because of their emerald green shell markings, are native to New Zealand.

mustard Powdered seeds of black or brown mustard (*Brassica nigra* or *B. juncea*) or white or yellow (*Sinapsis alba*) or a mixture. English mustard contains not more than 10% wheat flour and turmeric (still referred to in parts of England as Durham mustard, after Mrs Clements of Durham). French mustard: Dijon made from dehusked seeds (and therefore light coloured) or black or brown seeds with salt, spices and white wine or unripe grape juice. Bordeaux (usually called French mustard) black and brown seeds mixed with sugar, vinegar and herbs. Meaux mustard is grainy and made with mixed seeds. American mustard is mild and sweet made with white seeds, sugar, vinegar and turmeric.

mustard and cress Salad herb mixture of leaves of mustard (*Brassica alba*) and garden cress (*Lepidium sativum*). Often mustard is replaced with rape (*Brassica napus* var. *oleifera*); a different strain from that used for RAPE seed oil, it has a larger leaf and grows faster than mustard.

mustard oil Oil from MUSTARD *Brassica juncea* (13% saturated, 64% mono-unsaturated, 23% polyunsaturated). Oil from varieties low in GLUCOSINOLATES and ERUCIC ACID is known as CANOLA.

mutachrome A yellow CAROTENOID pigment in orange peel which has vitamin A activity. Also known as citroxanthin.

mutagen Any compound that can modify DNA, causing a mutation in bacteria. Many mutagens are also CARCINOGENS, and early screening of compounds for safety involves testing for mutagenicity (the AMES TEST).

mutton Meat from fully grown sheep, *Ovis aries* (LAMB is from animals under 1 year old).

mwenge *See* ORUBISI.

mycelium Mass of fine branching threads that make up the feeding and growing (vegetative) part of a FUNGUS that produces a MUSHROOM or toadstool as a fruiting body.

mycoprotein Name given to mould MYCELIUM prepared as foodstuff. *Fusarium* and *Neurospora* spp. (grown on carbohydrate) have been used.

mycose *See* TREHALOSE.

mycotoxins Compounds produced by filamentous FUNGI (and so exclude MUSHROOM toxins) that may accumulate to harmful levels in foods without any adverse effect on the flavour or appearance of the food; many are acutely or chronically toxic or carcinogenic. The most important are: AFLATOXINS (produced by *Aspergillus* spp.), ochratoxins (*Aspergillus* and *Penicillium* spp.), monoliformin (*Fusarium* spp.), PATULIN (*Aspergillus* and *Penicillium* spp.) and ergot alkaloids formed by *Claviceps purpurea* growing on rye.

myenteron Muscle layers of the intestine, a layer of circular muscles inside a layer of longitudinal muscles, responsible for PERISTALSIS.

myocardial infarction Damage to heart muscle due to ISCHAEMIA (failure of the blood supply from the coronary arteries).

myofibril *See* MUSCLE.

myoglobin HAEM-containing oxygen binding protein in muscle. Responsible for the red colour of fresh meat, oxidised to brown METMYOGLOBIN as meat ages, or on cooking. When meat is cured (*see* MEAT, CURING) with nitrite, the myoglobin is converted to the bright red NITROSOMYOGLOBIN.

myo-inositol *See* INOSITOL.

myosin The major protein of MUSCLE, about 40% of the total. A globulin, insoluble in water but soluble in salt solution.

myristic acid A saturated FATTY ACID with 14 carbon atoms (C14:0).

myrosinase The enzyme (thioglycosidase, EC 3.2.3.1) in MUSTARD seed and HORSERADISH that hydrolyses myrosin or sinigrin to glucose and allyl isothiocyanate, the pungent principle.

Mysore flour A blend of 75% TAPIOCA and 25% PEANUT flour.

mysost *See* GJETOST.

myxoedema Severe hypothyroidism (underactivity of the thyroid gland, *see* THYROID HORMONES) in adults; the name is derived from puffiness of hands and face due to thickening of skin. Signs include coarsening of the skin, intolerance of cold, weight gain and dull mental apathy, as well as reduced BASAL METABOLIC RATE.

myxoxanthin CAROTENOID pigment in algae with VITAMIN A activity.

N

naartje Afrikaans; a small TANGERINE; *see* CITRUS fruit.

NAASO North American Association for the Study of Obesity, now called the Obesity Society; web site http://www.naaso.org/.

NAD, NADP Nicotinamide adenine dinucleotide and nicotinamide adenine dinucleotide phosphate, the coenzymes derived from NIACIN. Involved as hydrogen acceptors / donors in a wide variety of oxidation and reduction reactions.

NAEL *See* NO ADVERSE EFFECT LEVEL.

nalidixic acid Quinolone antibiotic used to treat intestinal (and urinary tract) infections.

nam pla Thai; salted paste made from shrimps and small fish.

nan Indian flat bread, an egg dough prepared with white flour and leavened with sodium bicarbonate, normally baked in a tandoor (*see* TANDOORI).

nanofiltration A membrane process to separate particles with molecular weights from 300–1000 Da, using lower pressures than reverse osmosis (*see* OSMOSIS, REVERSE).

naphthoquinone The chemical ring structure of VITAMIN K; the various chemical forms of vitamin K can be referred to as substituted naphthoquinones.

naringenin *See* NARINGIN.

naringin A GLYCOSIDE (trihydroxyflavonone rhamnoglucoside) found in grapefruit, especially in the immature fruit. Extremely bitter: dilutions of 1 part in 10000 parts of water can be detected. Sometimes found in canned grapefruit segments as tiny, white beads. Hydrolysed to the aglycone, naringenin, which is not bitter.

naseberry Alternative name for SAPODILLA.

nashi *See* PEAR, NASHI.

nasogastric tube Fine plastic tube inserted through the nose and thence into the stomach for ENTERAL NUTRITION.

nasturtium Both the leaves and seeds of *Tropaeolum officinalis* can be eaten; they have a hot flavour. The seeds can be pickled as a substitute for CAPERS, and the flowers can be used to decorate salads.

nata Filipino; thick gelatinous film grown on the surface of coconut, sugarcane or fruit juice by fermentation with the acetic acid bacterium *Acetobacter aceti*, which produces an extracellular cellulose polymer. Eaten as a dessert.

natamycin (or pimaricin) A polyene antifungal agent, from *Streptomyces natalensis*, used as a coating on the surface of cheeses to prevent the growth of mould or yeast.

national flour *See* FLOUR, WHEATMEAL.

natriuretic Any compound that promotes excretion of sodium salts in the urine; most DIURETICS are natriuretics.

natto Japanese; soya bean fermented using *Bacillus natto*.
Composition /100 g: water 55 g, 887 kJ (212 kcal), protein 17.7 g, fat 11 g (of which 16% saturated, 24% mono-unsaturated, 61% polyunsaturated), carbohydrate 14.4 g (3.6 g sugars), fibre 5.4 g, ash 1.9 g, Ca 217 mg, Fe 8.6 mg, Mg 115 mg, P 174 mg, K

729 mg, Na 7 mg, Zn 3 mg, Cu 0.7 mg, Mn 1.5 mg, Se 8.8 µg, vitamin K 23.1 mg, B_1 0.16 mg, B_2 0.19 mg, B_6 0.13 mg, folate 8 µg, pantothenate 0.2 mg, C 13 mg.

Natual™ Low CHOLESTEROL cheese, prepared by use of CYCLODEXTRIN.

natural foods A term widely used but with little meaning and sometimes misleading since all foods come from natural sources. No legal definition seems possible but guidelines suggest the term should be applied only to single foods that have been subjected only to mild processing, i.e. largely by physical methods such as heating, concentrating, freezing, etc., but not chemically or 'severely' processed.

natural water *See* WATER, MINERAL.

nature-identical Term applied to food additives, including vitamins, that are synthesised in the laboratory and are identical to those that occur in nature.

N balance (equilibrium) *See* NITROGEN BALANCE.

NCHS standards Tables of height and weight for age used as reference values for the assessment of growth and nutritional status of children, based on data collected by the US National Center for Health Statistics. The most comprehensive such set of data, and used in most countries of the world.

N conversion factor *See* NITROGEN CONVERSION FACTOR.

NDGA *See* NORDIHYDROGUAIARETIC ACID.

NDpCal *See* NET DIETARY PROTEIN–ENERGY RATIO.

neat's foot Ox or calf's foot used for making soups and jellies. Now called cow heels. Neat's foot oil is obtained from the knuckle bones of cattle; used in leather working and for canning sardines.

Necator Genus of HOOKWORMS that are parasitic in the small intestine; the human parasite is *N. americanus*.

necrosis Death of cells or tissues in an unprogrammed manner, in response to toxicity or ISCHAEMIA.

See also APOPTOSIS.

nectarine Smooth-skinned peach (*Prunus persica* var. *nectarina*). Composition /100 g: (edible portion 91%) water 87.6 g, 184 kJ (44 kcal), protein 1.1 g, fat 0.3 g, carbohydrate 10.6 g (7.9 g sugars), fibre 1.7 g, ash 0.5 g, Ca 6 mg, Fe 0.3 mg, Mg 9 mg, P 26 mg, K 201 mg, Zn 0.2 mg, Cu 0.1 mg, Mn 0.1 mg, vitamin A 17 µg RE (378 µg carotenoids), E 0.8 mg, K 2.2 mg, B_1 0.03 mg, B_2 0.03 mg, niacin 1.1 mg, B_6 0.03 mg, folate 5 µg, pantothenate 0.2 mg, C 5 mg. A 150 g serving (1 fruit) is a source of Cu, vitamin E, C.

Neeld–Pearson reaction *See* CARR–PRICE REACTION.

neep Scottish name for root vegetables; now used for TURNIP (and sometimes for SWEDE in England).

NEFA   Non-esterified FATTY ACIDS.

negus   Drink made from port or sherry with spices, sugar and hot water.

NEL   *See* NO EFFECT LEVEL.

nematode   Any one of a large group of unsegmented worms; most are free-living, but some, including HOOKWORMS and PINWORMS, are intestinal parasites.

neohesperidin dihydrochalcone (NEO-DHC)   A non-nutritive SWEETENER, 1000 times as sweet as sucrose; formed by hydrogenation of the naturally occurring FLAVONOID neohesperidin.

neomycin   Broad spectrum aminoglycoside ANTIBIOTIC isolated from *Streptomyces fradii* that is poorly absorbed from the GASTROINTESTINAL TRACT and is used to treat persistent intestinal bacterial infections.

neonate   Literally new-born, used to describe infants in the first four weeks of life.

neotame   Synthetic intense SWEETENER, 8000 times as sweet as sucrose, N-[N-(3,3-dimethylbutyl)-L-α-aspartyl]-L-phenylalanine 1-methyl ester. *See also* ASPARTAME.

nephrocalcinosis   Presence of calcium deposits in the kidneys; may result from VITAMIN D toxicity.

neroli oil   Prepared from blossoms of the bitter orange by steam distillation. Yellowish oil with intense odour of orange blossom.

net dietary protein calories   *See* NET DIETARY PROTEIN–ENERGY RATIO.

net dietary protein–energy ratio (NDpE)   A way of expressing the protein content of a diet or food taking into account both the amount of protein (relative to total energy intake) and the PROTEIN QUALITY. It is protein energy multiplied by net protein utilisation divided by total energy. If energy is expressed in kcal and the result expressed as a percentage, this is net dietary protein calories per cent, NDpCal%.

   See also NET PROTEIN VALUE.

net protein ratio (NPR), net protein utilisation (NPU)   Measures of PROTEIN QUALITY.

net protein value   A way of expressing the amount and quality of the protein in a food; the product of NET PROTEIN UTILISATION and protein content per cent.

   See also NET DIETARY PROTEIN–ENERGY RATIO; PROTEIN QUALITY.

neural tube defect   Congenital malformations of the spinal cord caused by failure of the closure of the neural tube in early embryonic development (before day 28 of gestation). Supplements of FOLIC ACID (400 µg/day) begun before conception reduce the risk significantly.

neuritis   Inflammatory disease of peripheral nerves.
See also NEUROPATHY.

neuropathy   Any disease of peripheral nerves, usually causing weakness and numbness.
See also NEURITIS.

neuropeptide Y   A peptide neurotransmitter involved in the control of appetite and feeding behaviour, especially in response to LEPTIN.

neutron activation analysis   The nuclei of a number of elements will capture a neutron on exposure to a neutron beam, leading to the formation of unstable (radioactive) ISOTOPES which can then be measured by the radiation emitted as they decay. Used for determination of whole body CALCIUM, chlorine and NITROGEN.

new cocoyam   *See* TANNIA.

New Zealand process   Drying process for meat. It is immersed in hot oil under vacuum when it dries to 3% moisture in about 4 h.

NFE   *See* NITROGEN-FREE EXTRACT.

NFLEA   US National Food Labelling and Education Act, 1993, the basis of NUTRITION LABELLING of foods and health claims that may be made.

nham   South-east Asian; semi-dry uncooked pork or beef sausage left to undergo lactic acid bacterial fermentation for 4–5 days.

niacin   (*see* p. 329) A VITAMIN; one of the B complex without a numerical designation. Sometimes (incorrectly) referred to as vitamin B_3, and formerly vitamin PP (pellagra preventative). Deficiency leads to PELLAGRA, photosensitive dermatitis resembling severe sunburn, a depressive psychosis and intestinal disorders; fatal if untreated.

Niacin is the GENERIC DESCRIPTOR for two compounds in foods that have the biological activity of the vitamin: nicotinic acid (pyridine carboxylic acid) and nicotinamide (the amide of nicotinic acid). In the USA niacin is sometimes used specifically to mean nicotinic acid, and niacinamide for nicotinamide.

The metabolic function of niacin is in the COENZYMES NAD (nicotinamide adenine dinucleotide) and NADP (nicotinamide adenine dinucleotide phosphate), which act as intermediate hydrogen carriers in a wide variety of oxidation and reduction reactions. In cereals niacin is largely present as NIACYTIN, which is not biologically available (*see* AVAILABILITY); therefore the preformed niacin content of cereals is generally ignored when calculating intakes.
See also NIACIN EQUIVALENTS.

nicotinic acid   nicotinamide

NIACIN

niacinamide   American name for nicotinamide, *see* NIACIN.

niacin equivalents   Nicotinamide can be formed in the body from the amino acid TRYPTOPHAN; on average 60 mg dietary tryptophan is equivalent to 1 mg preformed NIACIN. The total niacin content of foods is generally expressed as mg niacin equivalents; the sum of preformed niacin (excluding that in cereals, *see* NIACYTIN) plus one-sixtieth of the tryptophan.

niacinogens   Name given to protein–niacin complexes found in cereals; *see also* NIACYTIN.

niacin toxicity   High doses of nicotinic acid have been used to treat HYPERCHOLESTEROLAEMIA; they can cause an acute flushing reaction, with vasodilatation and severe itching (nicotinamide does not have this effect, but is not useful for treatment of hyper-cholesterolaemia). Intakes of niacin above 500 mg/day (the reference intake is 17 mg/day) can cause liver damage over a period of months; the risk is greater with sustained release preparations of niacin.

niacytin   The main form of NIACIN in cereals. Nicotinic acid ester-ified as nicotinoyl-glucose in oligosaccharides and non-starch polysaccharides; susceptible to alkaline hydrolysis and partially susceptible to acid hydrolysis in the stomach. However, because of variable availability, it is conventional to exclude the niacin content of cereals from calculations of intake.

   See also NIACINOGENS.

nib   *See* CHOCOLATE.

nibbler   Machine for COMMINUTION of dry foods using grating action rather than grinding as in MILLS.

niceritol   Penta-erythritol tetranicotinate, a derivative of NIACIN used as a hypolipidaemic agent.

nickel   A mineral (*see* MINERAL, ULTRATRACE) known to be essen-tial to experimental animals, although its function is not known. There is no information on requirements. Metallic nickel is used as a catalyst in the HYDROGENATION of fats.

nicotinamide (niacinamide)   One of the vitamers of NIACIN.

nicotinamide adenine dinucleotide (phosphate)   *See* NAD.

nicotinate, sodium   Sodium salt of nicotinic acid; has been used, among other purposes, to preserve the red colour in fresh and processed meats.

nicotinic acid   (*see* p. 329) One of the vitamers of NIACIN.

NIDDK   National Institute of Diabetes and Digestive and Kidney Diseases; web site http://www.niddk.nih.gov/.

nigella   Peppery seeds of the wild ONION, *Nigella sativa*.

Nigerian berry   *See* SERENDIPITY BERRY.

nigerseed   Or nug, *Guizotia abyssinica*; grown in India and Ethiopia as food crop.

night blindness   Nyctalopia. Inability to see in dim light as a result of VITAMIN A deficiency.
   See also DARK ADAPTATION; VISION.

nim leaf   Sweet nim, an aromatic Indian herb with an aroma resembling that of TRUFFLES.

ninhydrin test   For proteins and amino acids (actually for the amino group). Pink, purple or blue colour is developed on heating the amino acid or peptide with ninhydrin (triketohydrindene hydrate).

nip   The gap between rollers in a mill or a moulding/forming machine.

nisatidine   *See* HISTAMINE RECEPTOR ANTAGONISTS.

nisin   ANTIBIOTIC isolated from lactic *Streptococcus* group N; inhibits some but not all *Clostridia*; not used clinically. The only antibiotic permitted in the UK to preserve specified foods. It is naturally present in cheese, being produced by a number of strains of cheese starter organisms. Useful to prolong storage life of cheese, milk, cream, soups, canned fruits and vegetables, canned fish and milk puddings. It also lowers the resistance of many thermophilic bacteria (*see* THERMOPHILES) to heat and so permits a reduction in the time and/or temperature of heating when processing canned vegetables.

nitrates   The inorganic form of nitrogen used by plants; found in soils and included in inorganic fertiliser. Nitrate is a natural constituent of crops in amounts sometimes depending on the content in the soil. Also found in drinking water as a result of excessive use of fertilisers. Health problems can arise because within a day or two of harvesting some crop nitrates are converted into NITRITES which can react with the HAEMOGLOBIN (especially fetal haemoglobin) to form METHAEMOGLOBIN which cannot transport oxygen. An upper limit of 45–50 mg nitrate/L drinking water has been recommended for infants. Also used, together with nitrite, for curing meat (*see* MEAT, CURING).
   See also NITROSAMINES.

nitric oxide (NO)   Synthesised in most mammalian cells by the action of nitric oxide synthetase (EC 1.14.13.39) on ARGININE. It causes vasodilatation and inhibits platelet aggregation (and so has anticoagulant action), acting by cell surface receptors and intracellular guanylate cyclase (EC 4.6.1.2), leading to increased formation of cyclic GMP. Before it was identified, NO was known as the endothelium-derived relaxation factor.

nitrites   Found in many plant foods, since they are rapidly formed by the reduction of naturally occurring NITRATE. Nitrite is the essential agent in preserving meat by pickling, since it inhibits the growth of *Clostridia*; it also combines with the MYOGLOBIN of meat to form the characteristic red NITROSOMYOGLOBIN.

   See also NITROSAMINES.

nitrogen   A gas comprising about 80% of the atmosphere; in nutrition the term 'nitrogen' is used to refer to ammonium salts and nitrates utilised as plant fertilisers; proteins and amino acids as animal nutrients; and urea and ammonium salts as excretory products.

nitrogenase   The enzyme (EC 1.18.6.1 or 1.19.6.1) in nitrogen-fixing micro-organisms that catalyses the reduction of N_2 to ammonia. Irreversibly inactivated by oxygen.

   See also LEGHAEMOGLOBIN.

nitrogen balance (N balance)   The difference between the dietary intake of nitrogen (mainly protein) and its excretion (as urea and other waste products). Healthy adults excrete the same amount as is ingested, and so are in nitrogen equilibrium. During growth and tissue repair (convalescence) the body is in positive N balance, i.e. ingestion is greater than loss and there is an increase in the total body pool of nitrogen (protein). In fevers, fasting and wasting diseases (*see* CACHEXIA) the loss is greater than the intake and the individual is in negative balance; there is a net loss of nitrogen from the body.

nitrogen conversion factor   Factor by which total nitrogen content of a material (measured chemically, e.g. by the KJELDAHL DETERMINATION) is multiplied to determine the PROTEIN; depends on the amino acid composition of the proteins concerned. Wheat and most cereals 5.8, rice 5.95, soya 5.7, most legumes and nuts 5.3, milk 6.38, other foods 6.25. Errors arise if part of the nitrogen is non-protein nitrogen. In mixtures of proteins, as in dishes and diets, the factor of 6.25 is used. Crude protein is defined as N × 6.25.

nitrogen equilibrium   *See* NITROGEN BALANCE.

nitrogen-free extract (NFE)   In the analysis of foods and animal feedingstuffs, the fraction that contains the sugars and starches plus small amounts of other materials.

nitrogen, metabolic   Nitrogen in the faeces derived from internal or endogenous sources, as distinct from nitrogen-containing dietary sources (exogenous nitrogen). This nitrogen consists of unabsorbed digestive juices, mucus, shed intestinal mucosal cells and intestinal bacteria, and continues to be excreted on a protein-free diet.

nitrogen trichloride   *See* AGENE.

nitro-keg   BEER conditioned in kegs under nitrogen, to give a smoother, creamier beverage than traditional conditioning under carbon dioxide.

nitrosamines   *N*-Nitroso derivatives of AMINES. Found in trace amounts in mushrooms, fermented fish meal and smoked fish, and in pickled foods, where they are formed by reaction between NITRITE and amines. They cause cancer in experimental animals, but it is not known whether the small amounts in foods affect human beings. They are also found in human gastric juice, possibly as a result of reaction between dietary amines and nitrites or nitrates.

nitrosomyoglobin   The red colour of cured meat, formed by the reaction of NITRITE with MYOGLOBIN. Fades in light to yellow-brown metmyoglobin.

nitrous oxide N_2O, a gas used as a propellant in pressurised containers, e.g. to eject cream or salad dressing from containers.

nivalenol   Trichothecene MYCOTOXIN produced when cereals are infected with *Fusarium* spp.

nixtamal   The paste produced by steeping MAIZE in calcium hydroxide solution to make tortillas and tacos; the process is nixtamalisation.

N-lite^{TM} FAT REPLACER made from starch.

NMR   Nuclear magnetic resonance.

NO   *See* NITRIC OXIDE.

no adverse effect level (NAEL)   Highest dose or intake of a compound at which no adverse effect can be detected.
   See also LD_{50}; MINIMUM LETHAL DOSE.

noble rot   White grapes affected by the fungus *Botrytis cinerea*. It spoils the grapes if they are damaged by rain, but if they are ripe and healthy, and the weather is sunny, it causes them to shrivel and concentrates the sugar, so that top-quality sweet wines can be made.
   See also WINE CLASSIFICATION, GERMANY.

No Effect Level (NEL)   With respect to food additives, the maximum dose of an additive that has no detectable adverse effects.
   See also ACCEPTABLE DAILY INTAKE.

noggin Traditional measure of liquor = ¼ pint (140 mL); also known as a quartern.

N-oil™ FAT REPLACER made from starch.

nominal freezing time The time between the surface of the food reaching 0 °C and the thermal centre reaching 10 °C below the temperature of the first ice formation.

non-essential amino acids Those AMINO ACIDS that can be synthesised in the body and therefore are not dietary essentials.

non-esterified fatty acids (NEFA) *See* FATTY ACIDS, FREE.

non-hygroscopic foods Foods that have a constant water vapour pressure at different moisture contents, and so do not take up moisture from the atmosphere.

noni (Indian mulberry) Fruit of the south Pacific evergreen shrub *Morinda citrifolia*, with an unpleasant odour; the juice is claimed to have healing properties and to be beneficial in treatment of diabetes, heart disease and cancer.

non-Newtonian fluid *See* SHEAR RATE.

non-nutritive sweeteners *See* SWEETENERS, INTENSE.

non-saponified The water-insoluble material remaining in a fat or oil after SAPONIFICATION; mainly sterols, higher alcohols, hydrocarbons and pigments.

non-starch polysaccharides (NSP) (*see* p. 334) Those POLYSACCHARIDES (complex carbohydrates) found in foods other than STARCHES. They are the major part of dietary fibre (*see* FIBRE, DIETARY) and can be measured more precisely than total dietary fibre; include CELLULOSE, PECTINS, GLUCANS, GUMS, MUCILAGES, INULIN and CHITIN (and exclude LIGNIN). The NSP in wheat, maize and rice are mainly insoluble and have a laxative effect, while those in oats, barley, rye and beans are mainly soluble and have a blood cholesterol-lowering effect. In vegetables the proportions of soluble to insoluble are roughly equal but vary in fruits.

noodles PASTA made with flour from various grains (e.g. rice, wheat, buckwheat, mung bean starch) and water; may have egg added.

nopales Stems or pads of the PRICKLY PEAR cactus (*Opuntia* spp.).

Composition/100 g: (edible portion 96%) water 94.1 g, 67 kJ (16 kcal), protein 1.3 g, fat 0.1 g, carbohydrate 3.3 g (1.1 g sugars), fibre 2.2 g, ash 1.1 g, Ca 164 mg, Fe 0.6 mg, Mg 52 mg, P 16 mg, K 257 mg, Na 21 mg, Zn 0.3 mg, Cu 0.1 mg, Mn 0.5 mg, Se 0.7 µg, vitamin A 23 µg RE (298 µg carotenoids), K 5.3 mg, B_1 0.01 mg, B_2 0.04 mg, niacin 0.4 mg, B_6 0.07 mg, folate 3 µg, pantothenate 0.2 mg, C 9 mg.

334

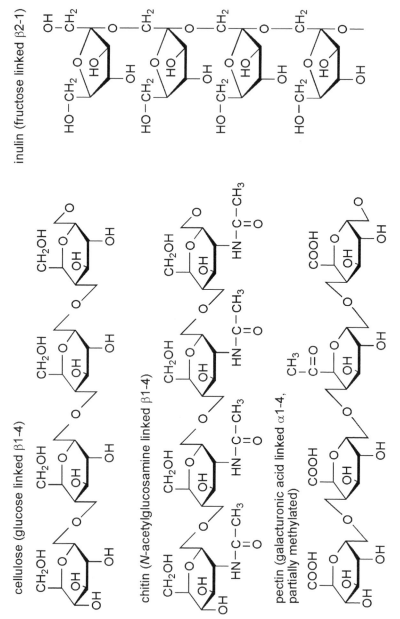

inulin (fructose linked β2-1)

cellulose (glucose linked β1-4)

chitin (N-acetylglucosamine linked β1-4)

pectin (galacturonic acid linked α1-4, partially methylated)

nor- Chemical prefix to the name of a compound indicating:

(1) One methyl (CH₃) group has been replaced by hydrogen (e.g. NORADRENALINE can be considered to be a demethylated derivative of adrenaline).

(2) A homologue of a compound containing one methylene (CH₂) group fewer than the parent compound.

(3) An ISOMER with an unbranched side-chain (e.g. norleucine, norvaline).

noradrenaline Hormone secreted by the adrenal medulla together with ADRENALINE; also a neurotransmitter. Physiological effects similar to those of adrenaline. Also known as norepinephrine.

norconidendrin *See* CONIDENDRIN.

nordihydroguaiaretic acid (NDGA) Extracted from the creosote bush, *Larrea divaricata* (*Covillea tridentata*); used as an antioxidant for fats.

norepinephrine *See* NORADRENALINE.

nori Edible seaweed, *Porphyra umbilicalis*.

norite Activated charcoal used to decolourise solutions.

norleucine 2-Aminohexanoic acid, a non-physiological AMINO ACID, an unbranched ISOMER of LEUCINE, commonly used as an internal standard in amino acid analysis.

northern blot *See* BLOTTING.

notatin *See* GLUCOSE OXIDASE.

nougat Sweetmeat made from a mixture of gelatine or egg albumin with sugar and starch syrup, and the whole thoroughly aerated. Originated in Montelimar in southern France.

Novadeloxᵀᴹ Benzoyl peroxide used for treating flour, *see* AGEING.

novain Obsolete name for CARNITINE.

novel foods Foods and food ingredients consisting of, or containing, chemical substances not hitherto used for human consumption to a significant extent in the locality in question (including micro-organisms, fungi or algae and substances isolated from them, and organisms obtained using genetic modification techniques). A food or ingredient to which has been applied a process not currently used for food manufacture or which has not been previously marketed and which gives rise to changes that affect its nutritional value or safety.

   See also SUBSTANTIAL EQUIVALENCE.

Noveloseᵀᴹ A preparation of resistant starch. *See* STARCH, RESISTANT.

NPR Net protein ratio, a measure of PROTEIN QUALITY.

NPU Net protein utilisation, a measure of PROTEIN QUALITY.

NPV Net protein value, a measure of PROTEIN QUALITY.

NSP *See* NON-STARCH POLYSACCHARIDES.

nubbing Term used in the canning industry for 'topping and tailing' of gooseberries.

nucellar layer Of wheat, the layer of cells that surrounds the endosperm and protects it from the entry of moisture.

nucleation The formation of a nucleus of water molecules that is required for ice crystal formation.

nucleic acids Polymers of PURINE and PYRIMIDINE sugar phosphates; two main classes: ribonucleic acid (RNA) and deoxyribonucleic acid (DNA). Collectively the purines and pyrimidines are called bases. DNA is a double-stranded polymer (the so-called 'double helix') containing the five-carbon sugar deoxyribose. RNA is a single-stranded polymer containing the sugar ribose.

Not nutritionally important, since dietary nucleic acids are hydrolysed to their bases, ribose and phosphate in the intestinal tract; purines and pyrimidines can readily be synthesised in the body, and are not dietary essentials.

nucleoproteins The complex of proteins and NUCLEIC ACIDS found in the cell nucleus.

nucleosides Compounds of PURINE or PYRIMIDINE bases with a sugar, most commonly ribose. For example, ADENINE plus ribose forms adenosine. With the addition of phosphate a NUCLEOTIDE is formed.

nucleotides Compounds of PURINE or PYRIMIDINE base with a sugar phosphate; the monomer units of DNA and RNA. Natural constituents of human milk, often used to supplement infant formulae.

nug *See* NIGERSEED.

nuoc mam Vietnamese, Cambodian; fermented fish sauce. The fish is digested by autolytic enzymes in the presence of salt added to inhibit bacterial growth.

nutmeg Dried ripe seed of *Myristica fragrans*; mace is the seed coat (arillus). Both mace and nutmeg are used as flavourings in meat products and bakery goods.

nutraceuticals Term for compounds in foods that are not nutrients but have (potential) beneficial effects.

See also FUNCTIONAL FOODS.

Nutrasweet™ *See* ASPARTAME.

nutricines Biologically active ingredients in animal feedstuff used to promote nutrition-based health.

nutrient density A way of expressing the nutrient content of a food or diet relative to the energy yield (i.e. per 1000 kcal or per MJ) rather than per unit weight.

nutrient enemata *See* RECTAL FEEDING.
   See also ENTERAL NUTRITION; PARENTERAL NUTRITION.

nutrients Essential dietary factors such as VITAMINS, MINERALS, AMINO ACIDS and FATTY ACIDS. Metabolic fuels (sources of energy) are not termed nutrients so that a commonly used phrase is 'energy and nutrients'.

nutrification The addition of nutrients to foods at such a level as to make a major contribution to the diet.

nutrigenetics The study of the effects of genotype on nutrient requirements and effects of diet on health.
   See also NUTRIGENOMICS.

nutrigenomics The study of how nutrients interact with the GENOME, and identification of nutrient-sensitive genes.
   See also NUTRIGENETICS.

nutrition The process by which living organisms take in and use food for the maintenance of life, growth, the functioning of organs and tissues and the production of energy; the branch of science that involves these processes.
   See also ENTERAL NUTRITION; PARENTERAL NUTRITION; RECTAL FEEDING.

nutritional claim Any representation that states, suggests or implies that a food has particular nutrition-related health properties. The extent of such claims on food labelling (*see* NUTRITIONAL LABELLING) and advertising are controlled by law in most countries.

nutritional disorder Any morbid process or functional abnormality of the body due to the consumption of a diet not conforming to physiological requirements, or to failure in absorption or utilisation of the food after ingestion.

nutritional genomics General term to include both NUTRIGENETICS and NUTRIGENOMICS.

nutritional labelling Any information appearing on labelling or packaging of foods relating to energy and nutrients in the food. Voluntary in the EU; if nutritional information is given, it must be in a standard format. The information must be given /100 g (or /100 mL), and may also, optionally, be given per serving of a stated size. In the USA nutritional labelling is obligatory, and information must be given in a standard format per SERVING (as defined by the Food and Drug Administration), and may optionally be given /100 g or /100 mL.

nutritional recommendations Recommendations comprising nutrient goals, food goals and dietary guidelines. In addition to REFERENCE INTAKES of nutrients, key recommendations in developed countries are reduction of total FAT intake to 30% of energy intake, with a more severe restriction of saturated fats (*see* FAT, SATURATED) (to 10% of energy intake); increase of CARBOHYDRATE intake to 55% of energy intake (with a reduction of sugars to 10% of energy intake); increased intake of NON-STARCH POLYSACCHARIDES and reduced intake of SALT.

nutritional status assessment   In adults, general adequacy of nutrition is assessed by measuring weight and height; the result is commonly expressed as the BODY MASS INDEX, the ratio of weight (kg)/height^2 (m). Body fat may also be estimated, by measuring SKINFOLD THICKNESS, and muscle diameter is also measured. For children, weight and height for age are compared with standard data for adequately nourished children. The increase in the circumference of the head and the development of bones may also be measured. Status with respect to individual vitamins and minerals is normally determined by laboratory tests, either measuring the blood and urine concentrations of the nutrients and their metabolites, or by testing for specific metabolic responses.

See also ANTHROPOMETRY; ENZYME ACTIVATION ASSAYS.

nutritionist   One who applies the science of nutrition to the promotion of health and control of disease; instructs auxiliary medical personnel; participates in surveys. Not legally defined in the UK, but there is a Register of Accredited Nutritionists maintained by the Nutrition Society.

See also DIETITIAN.

nutrition policy (or planning)   A set of concerted actions, based on a governmental mandate, intended to ensure good health of the population through informed access to safe, healthy and adequate food.

nutrition surveillance   Monitoring the state of health, nutrition, eating behaviour and nutrition knowledge of a given population for the purpose of planning and evaluating NUTRITION POLICY. Especially in developing countries, monitoring may include factors that may be potential causes of nutritional emergencies, in order to give early warning of such emergencies.

nutritive ratio   In animal feeding; a measure of the value of a feedstuff for growth (or milk production) compared with its fattening value. It is the sum of the digestible carbohydrate, protein and 2.3 × fat, divided by digestible protein. Ratio 4–5 for growth, 7–8 for fattening.

nutritive value index   In animal feeding; intake of digestible energy expressed as energy digestibility multiplied by voluntary intake of dry matter of a particular feed, divided by METABOLIC WEIGHT (weight$^{0.75}$), compared with standard feed.

nutro-biscuit   Indian; biscuit baked from a mixture of 60% wheat flour and 40% peanut flour; contains 16–17% protein.

nutro-macaroni   Indian; mixture of 80 parts WHEAT flour, 20 parts defatted PEANUT meal (19% protein).

nuts   Hard-shelled fruit of a wide variety of trees, e.g. ALMONDS, BRAZIL, CASHEW, PEANUT, WALNUT. All have high fat content, 45–60%; high protein content, 15–20%; 15–20% carbohydrate. The CHESTNUT is an exception, with 3% fat and 3% protein, being largely carbohydrate, 37%. A number of nuts are grown mainly for their oils; *see* OILSEED.

NVDP   Non-volatile decomposition products.

nyctalopia   *See* NIGHT BLINDNESS.

nystagmus   Rapid involuntary movement of the eyes, as when following a moving object; may also occur as a result of a congenital defect, and in the WERNICKE–KORSAKOFF SYNDROME due to VITAMIN B$_1$ deficiency.

O

Oatrim^{TM}   FAT REPLACER made from NON-STARCH POLYSACCHARIDE.

oats   Grain from *Avena* spp., especially *A. sativa, A. steritis* and *A. strigosa*. Oatmeal, ground oats; oatflour, ground and bran removed; groats, husked oats; Embden groats, crushed groats; Scotch oats, groats cut into granules of various sizes; Sussex ground oats, very finely ground oats; rolled oats, crushed by rollers and partially precooked.

Composition /100g: water 8g, 1628kJ (389kcal), protein 16.9g, fat 6.9g (of which 20% saturated, 37% mono-unsaturated, 42% polyunsaturated), carbohydrate 66.3g, fibre 10.6g, ash 1.7g, Ca 54mg, Fe 4.7mg, Mg 177mg, P 523mg, K 429mg, Na 2mg, Zn 4mg, Cu 0.6mg, Mn 4.9mg, vitamin E 1.1mg, B$_1$ 0.76mg, B$_2$ 0.14mg, niacin 1mg, B$_6$ 0.12mg, folate 56µg, pantothenate 1.3mg. A 30g serving is a source of Cu, Mg, P, vitamin B$_1$, a rich source of Mn.

obesity   Excessive accumulation of body fat. A BODY MASS INDEX (BMI) above 30kg/m^2 is considered to be obesity (and above 40 gross obesity). The desirable range of BMI for optimum life expectancy is 20–25; between 25 and 30 is considered to be OVERWEIGHT rather than obesity. People more than 50% above desirable WEIGHT are twice as likely to die prematurely as those within the desirable weight range.

obesity, dietary   Obesity in experimental animals induced by overfeeding, as opposed to pharmacological treatment or as a result of genetic defects.

***ob-ob* mouse**   A genetically obese mouse; the defective gene was cloned in 1994, and the gene product was identified as LEPTIN.

obstipation Extreme and persistent CONSTIPATION caused by obstruction of the intestinal tract.

oca Tuber of *Oxalis tuberosa*, formerly an important food of the Andean highlanders.

occlusal The biting surface of a premolar or molar tooth.

ochratoxins MYCOTOXINS formed by *Aspergillus* and *Penicillium* spp. growing on cereals. They have been associated with nephropathy in both animals and human beings, with evidence that they are carcinogenic and teratogenic. They can accumulate in relatively high concentrations in blood and tissues of monogastric animals but are cleaved by protozoan enzymes in RUMINANTS.

octave A cask for wine containing one-eighth of a PIPE, about 59 L (13 imperial gallons).

octopus Marine cephalopod (*Octopus* spp.) with beak-like mouth surrounded by eight tentacles bearing suckers.

Composition /100 g: water 80 g, 343 kJ (82 kcal), protein 14.9 g, fat 1 g, cholesterol 48 mg, carbohydrate 2.2 g, ash 1.6 g, Ca 53 mg, Fe 5.3 mg, Mg 30 mg, P 186 mg, K 350 mg, Na 230 mg, Zn 1.7 mg, Cu 0.4 mg, Se 44.8 µg, I 20 µg, vitamin A 45 µg RE (45 µg retinal), E 1.2 mg, K 0.1 mg, B_1 0.03 mg, B_2 0.04 mg, niacin 2.1 mg, B_6 0.36 mg, folate 16 µg, B_{12} 20 µg, pantothenate 0.5 mg, C 5 mg. An 85 g serving is a source of I, P, vitamin B_6, a good source of Cu, a rich source of Fe, Se, vitamin B_{12}.

odontoblasts Cells in teeth, lining the pulp and forming dentine.

odoratism Disease produced by feeding seeds of the sweet pea, *Lathyrus odoratus*, to rats. The toxin β-aminopropionitrile is present in both *L. odoratus* and the singletary pea (*L. pusillus*), but not the chickling pea, *L. sativa*, which causes LATHYRISM in human beings. The toxin inhibits lysyl oxidase (EC 1.4.3.13) which oxidises lysine to ALLYSINE for cross-linkage of COLLAGEN and ELASTIN, leading to loss of elasticity of elastin and potentially to rupture of the aorta.

ODS Office of Dietary Supplements of the US National Institutes of Health; web site http://dietary-supplements.info.nih.gov/.

oedema Excess fluid in the body; may be caused by cardiac, renal or hepatic failure and by starvation (famine oedema).

oenin An ANTHOCYANIDIN from the skin of purple grapes.

oesophagus The gullet, a muscular tube ~23 cm long, between the pharynx and stomach.

See GASTROINTESTINAL TRACT.

oestradiol, oestriol, oestrone *See* OESTROGENS.

oestrogens The female sex hormones; chemically they are STEROIDS, although non-steroidal compounds also have oestrogen activity, including the synthetic compounds stilboestrol and hexoestrol. These have been used for chemical caponisation (*see* CAPON) of cockerels and to increase the growth rate of cattle. Compounds with oestrogen activity are found in a variety of plants; collectively these are known as PHYTOESTROGENS.

offal Corruption of 'off-fall'.

(1) With reference to meat, the term includes all parts that are cut away when the carcass is dressed, including liver, kidneys, brain, spleen, pancreas, thymus, tripe and tongue. Known in the USA as organ meats or variety meat.

(2) With reference to wheat, offal is the bran discarded when milled to white flour. *See also* WHEATFEED.

ohelo Fruit of the Hawaiian shrub *Vaccinium reticulatum*, related to the CRANBERRY.

Composition /100g: water 92.3g, 117kJ (28kcal), protein 0.4g, fat 0.2g, carbohydrate 6.8g, ash 0.3g, Ca 7mg, Fe 0.1mg, Mg 6mg, P 10mg, K 38mg, Na 1mg, vitamin A 42µg RE, B_1 0.02mg, B_2 0.04mg, niacin 0.3mg, C 6mg.

ohmic heating Sterilisation by heat generated by passing an electric current through the food or mixture.

OHTC *See* OVERALL HEAT TRANSFER COEFFICIENT.

oilseed A wide variety of seeds are grown as a source of oils, e.g. cottonseed, sesame, groundnut, sunflower, soya, and nuts such as coconut, groundnut and palm. After extraction of the oil the residue is a valuable source of protein, especially for animal feedingstuffs, oilseed cake.

oils, essential *See* ESSENTIAL OILS.

oils, fixed The TRIACYLGLYCEROLS (triglycerides), the edible oils, as distinct from the volatile or ESSENTIAL OILS.

okra Also known as gumbo, bamya, bamies and ladies' fingers; the edible seed pods of *Hibiscus esculentus*. Small ridged mucilaginous pods resembling a small cucumber; used in soups and stews. Two varieties: oblong are gomba, round are bamya.

Composition /100g: (edible portion 86%) water 90.2g, 130kJ (31kcal), protein 2g, fat 0.1g, carbohydrate 7g (1.2g sugars), fibre 3.2g, ash 0.7g, Ca 81mg, Fe 0.8mg, Mg 57mg, P 63mg, K 303mg, Na 8mg, Zn 0.6mg, Cu 0.1mg, Mn 1mg, Se 0.7µg, vitamin A 19µg RE (741µg carotenoids), E 0.4mg, K 53mg, B_1 0.2mg, B_2 0.06mg, niacin 1mg, B_6 0.22mg, folate 88µg, pantothenate 0.2 mg, C 21mg. A 95g serving (8 pods) is a source of Mg, vitamin B_1, a rich source of Mn, folate, vitamin C.

olallie berry Cross between LOGANBERRY and YOUNGBERRY.

Olean^{TM} *See* OLESTRA.

oleandomycin Antibiotic sometimes used as an additive in chicken feed.

oleic acid   Mono-unsaturated FATTY ACID (C18:1 ω9); found to some extent in most fats; OLIVE and RAPESEED oils are especially rich sources.

oleomargarine   *See* MARGARINE.

oleo oil   *See* PREMIER JUS; TALLOW, RENDERED.

oleoresins   In the preparation of some spices such as pepper, ginger and capsicum, the aromatic material is extracted with solvents which are evaporated off, leaving behind thick oily products known as oleoresins.

   See also ESSENTIAL OILS.

oleostearin   *See* PREMIER JUS; TALLOW, RENDERED.

oleovitamin   Preparation of fish liver oil or vegetable oil containing one or more of the fat-soluble VITAMINS.

Olestra (Olean)™   A SUCROSE POLYESTER used as a FAT REPLACER; it has the cooking and organoleptic properties of triacylglycerol, but is not hydrolysed by LIPASE, and not absorbed from the intestinal tract.

olfaction   The sense or process of smelling. Sensory cells in the mucous membrane lining the nasal cavity communicate with the central nervous system via the olfactory (first cranial) nerve.

oligoallergenic diet   Comprising very few foods, or an elemental diet used to diagnose whether particular symptoms are the result of allergic response to food.

oligodipsia   Reduced sense of thirst.

oligodynamic   Sterilising effect of traces of certain metals. For example, SILVER at a concentration of 1 part in 5 million will kill *Escherichia coli* and staphylococci in 3 h.

oligopeptides   *See* PEPTIDES.

oligosaccharides   CARBOHYDRATES composed of 3–10 monosaccharide units (with more than 10 units they are termed POLYSACCHARIDES).

   See also PREBIOTICS.

olive   Fruit of the evergreen tree, *Olea europaea*; picked unripe when green or ripe when they have turned dark blue or purplish, and usually pickled in brine or used as a source of oil. Olives have been known since ancient times. The tree is extremely slow growing and continues to fruit for many years; there are claims that trees are still fruiting after 1000 years.

   Composition /100 g: water 75.3 g, 607 kJ (145 kcal), protein 1 g, fat 15.3 g (of which 14% saturated, 77% mono-unsaturated, 9% polyunsaturated), carbohydrate 3.8 g (0.5 g sugars), fibre 3.3 g, ash 4.5 g, Ca 52 mg, Fe 0.5 mg, Mg 11 mg, P 4 mg, K 42 mg, Na 1556 mg, Cu 0.1 mg, Se 0.9 µg, vitamin A 20 µg RE (750 µg carotenoids), E 3.8 mg, K 1.4 mg, B_1 0.02 mg, B_2 0.01 mg, niacin 0.2 mg, B_6 0.03 mg, folate 3 µg.

olive oil Pressed from ripe OLIVES, the fruit of *Olea europaea*. Virgin olive oil is not refined and the flavour varies with the locality where it is grown; extra virgin oil contains less than 1% acidity. Other types have been refined to varying extents. Used in cooking, as salad oil, for canning sardines and for margarine manufacture. 14% saturated, 76% mono-unsaturated, 10% polyunsaturated, contains 14 mg vitamin E, 60 mg vitamin K/100 g; also relatively rich in SQUALENE.

omasum *See* RUMINANTS.

omega fatty acids Polyunsaturated FATTY ACIDS (PUFA) are described by chain length, number of double bonds and (in biochemistry and nutrition) by the position of their first double bond counting from the terminal methyl group, labelled as omega (ω or n-). In systematic chemical nomenclature the position of a double bond is numbered from the carboxyl end (carbon-1), but what is important nutritionally is that human enzymes can desaturate fatty acids between an existing double bond and the carboxyl group, but not between an existing double bond and the methyl group.

There are three series of PUFA: $\omega 3$, $\omega 6$ and $\omega 9$, derived from linolenic, linoleic and oleic acids, respectively. The first two cannot be synthesised in the body and are the precursors of two families of EICOSANOIDS.

See also FATTY ACIDS, ESSENTIAL; Table 8.

omega-3 ($\omega 3$) marine triglycerides A mixture of triacylglycerols (triglycerides) rich in two long-chain polyunsaturated FATTY ACIDS, eicosapentaenoic acid (EPA, C20:5 $\omega 3$) and docosohexaenoic (DHA, C22:6 $\omega 3$).

omentum Double layer of PERITONEUM attached to the stomach and linking it to other abdominal organs. *See* GASTROINTESTINAL TRACT.

OMNI Organising Medical Networked Information; web site http://omni.ac.uk/.

omophagia Eating of raw or uncooked food.

oncogene Any gene associated with the development of cancer. Viral oncogenes are related to, and possibly derived from, normal mammalian genes (proto-oncogenes) that are involved in the regulation of cell proliferation and growth. Mutation to yield an active oncogene involves loss of the normal regulation of the expression of the proto-oncogene.

oncom Indonesian; fermented groundnut and soybean PRESS CAKE with cassava, fermented with moulds: *Neurospora sitophila* to produce a red product or *Rhizopus oligosporus* for a grey product.

onglet French; cut of beef corresponding to top of the skirt.

onion   Bulb of *Allium cepa*; many varieties with white, brown, red or purple skins.

Composition /100 g: (edible portion 90%) water 88.5 g, 176 kJ (42 kcal), protein 0.9 g, fat 0.1 g, carbohydrate 10.1 g (4.3 g sugars), fibre 1.4 g, ash 0.3 g, Ca 22 mg, Fe 0.2 mg, Mg 10 mg, P 27 mg, K 144 mg, Na 3 mg, Zn 0.2 mg, Mn 0.1 mg, Se 0.5 µg, 6 µg carotenoids, K 0.4 mg, B_1 0.05 mg, B_2 0.03 mg, niacin 0.1 mg, B_6 0.15 mg, folate 19 µg, pantothenate 0.1 mg, C 6 mg. A 160 g serving (1 medium) is a source of vitamin B_6, folate, C.

onion, Egyptian (tree onion)   *Allium cepa* proliform group. Type that produces clusters of aerial bulbs that develop shoots to form multi-tiered plant; the aerial bulbs are cropped.

onion, everlasting   *See* ONION, WELSH.

onion, green   *See* ONION, SPRING; ONION, WELSH.

onion, Japanese bunching   *Allium fistulosum*, similar to Welsh onion (*see* ONION, WELSH), but larger.

onion, perennial   *See* ONION, WELSH.

onion, spring   Young plants of *Allium cepa*, generally eaten whole (developing bulb and leaves) as a salad vegetable. Also known as salad onions or scallions.

Composition /100 g: (edible portion 96%) water 89.8 g, 134 kJ (32 kcal), protein 1.8 g, fat 0.2 g, carbohydrate 7.3 g (2.3 g sugars), fibre 2.6 g, ash 0.8 g, Ca 72 mg, Fe 1.5 mg, Mg 20 mg, P 37 mg, K 276 mg, Na 16 mg, Zn 0.4 mg, Cu 0.1 mg, Mn 0.2 mg, Se 0.6 µg, vitamin A 50 µg RE (1735 µg carotenoids), E 0.6 mg, K 207 mg, B_1 0.05 mg, B_2 0.08 mg, niacin 0.5 mg, B_6 0.06 mg, folate 64 µg, pantothenate 0.1 mg, C 19 mg.

onion, Welsh   The perennial onion, *Allium cepa perutile*. Leaves are cropped, leaving the plant to grow. Similar to, but smaller than, the Japanese bunching onion, *Allium fistulosum*. Also sometimes used as an alternative name for the LEEK.

Composition /100 g: (edible portion 65%) water 90.5 g, 142 kJ (34 kcal), protein 1.9 g, fat 0.4 g, carbohydrate 6.5 g, ash 0.7 g, Ca 18 mg, Fe 1.2 mg, Mg 23 mg, P 49 mg, K 212 mg, Na 17 mg, Zn 0.5 mg, Cu 0.1 mg, Mn 0.1 mg, Se 0.6 µg, vitamin A 58 µg RE, B_1 0.05 mg, B_2 0.09 mg, niacin 0.4 mg, B_6 0.07 mg, folate 16 µg, pantothenate 0.2 mg, C 27 mg.

opisthorchiasis   Infection with the FLUKE *Opisthorchis felineus*; a bile duct parasite of fish-eating mammals.

opsomania   Craving for special food.

OptaGrade™, OptaMax™   FAT REPLACERS made from starch.

optic   Dispenser attached to bottles of spirits, etc. in bars to ensure delivery of a precise volume.

optical activity (optical rotation)   The ability of some compounds to rotate the plane of polarised light because of the asymmetry of the molecule. If the plane of light is rotated to the right, the substance is dextrorotatory and is designated by the prefix (+); if laevorotatory, the prefix is (−). A mixture of the two forms is optically inactive and is termed racemic.

Sucrose is dextrorotatory but is hydrolysed to glucose (dextrorotatory) and fructose, which is more strongly laevorotatory, so hydrolysis changes optical activity from (+) to (−); hence, the mixture of glucose and fructose is termed invert sugar (*see* SUGAR, INVERT).

The obsolete notation for (+) was *d*- and for (−) was *l*-; this is quite separate from D- and L-, which are used to designate stereoisomerism, *see* D-, L- AND DL-.

opuntia *See* NOPALES; PRICKLY PEAR.

oral rehydration Administration of an isotonic solution of salt and glucose (or sucrose) to replace fluid and electrolytes lost in DIARRHOEA.

orange CITRUS fruit, from the subtropical tree *Citrus sinensis*.
Composition /100 g: (edible portion 73%) water 87 g, 197 kJ (47 kcal), protein 0.9 g, fat 0.1 g, carbohydrate 11.8 g (9.4 g sugars), fibre 2.4 g, ash 0.4 g, Ca 40 mg, Fe 0.1 mg, Mg 10 mg, P 14 mg, K 181 mg, Zn 0.1 mg, Se 0.5 µg, vitamin A 11 µg RE (327 µg carotenoids), E 0.2 mg, B_1 0.09 mg, B_2 0.04 mg, niacin 0.3 mg, B_6 0.06 mg, folate 30 µg, pantothenate 0.3 mg, C 53 mg. A 160 g serving (1 medium) is a good source of folate, a rich source of vitamin C.

orange, bitter The fruit of the subtropical tree *Citrus aurantium*; known as Seville orange in Spain, bigaradier in France, melangol in Italy and khush-khash in Israel. Used mainly as root stock, because of its resistance to the gummosis disease of citrus. The fruit is too acid to be edible; used in manufacture of MARMALADE; the peel oil is used in the LIQUEUR curaçao; the peel and flower oils (neroli oil) and the oils from the green twigs (petit-grain oils) are used in perfumery.

orange butter Chopped whole orange, cooked, sweetened and homogenised.

orange roughy A deep-water FISH (*Hoplostethus atlanticus*) that turns orange after being caught; mainly caught around New Zealand.

orcanella *See* ALKANNET.

oreganum Or Mexican sage; *see* MARJORAM.

orexigenic Stimulating appetite.

orexins Also called hypocretins, two small peptide HORMONES synthesised in the hypothalamus that stimulate appetite INCRETINS secreted by the hypothalamus.

organic (1) Chemically, the term means substances containing carbon in the molecule (with the exception of carbonates and cyanide). Substances of animal and vegetable origin are organic; MINERALS are inorganic.

(2) The term organic foods refers to 'organically grown foods', meaning plants grown without the use of (synthetic) pesticides, fungicides or inorganic fertilisers, prepared without the use of preservatives. Foodstuffs grown on land that has not been treated with chemical fertilisers, herbicides or pesticides for at least three years. Organic meat is from animals fed on organically grown crops without the use of growth promoters, with only a limited number of medicines to treat disease and commonly maintained under traditional, non-intensive, conditions.

organ meat *See* OFFAL (1).

organoleptic Sensory properties, i.e. those that can be detected by the sense organs. For foods used particularly of the combination of TASTE, texture and astringency (perceived in the mouth) and aroma (perceived in the nose).

orlistat Drug used in the treatment of OBESITY; it inhibits gastric and pancreatic LIPASES (EC 3.1.1.3) and prevents absorption of much of the dietary fat. Trade name Xenical.

ormer *See* ABALONE.

ornithine An amino acid that occurs as a metabolic intermediate (e.g. in the synthesis of UREA), but not involved in protein synthesis, and not of nutritional importance, M_r 132.2, pK_a 1.71, 8.69, 10.76.

orotic acid An intermediate in the biosynthesis of PYRIMIDINES; a growth factor for some micro-organisms and at one time called vitamin B_{13}. There is no evidence that it is a human dietary requirement.

orris root Peeled rhizomes of *Iris germanica* used as a flavouring in ice cream, confectionery and baked goods.

ortanique A Jamaican CITRUS fruit; cross between orange and tangerine.

orthophenylphenol (OPP) A compound used for the treatment of CITRUS fruit and NUTS after harvesting to prevent the growth of moulds (E-231). DIPHENYL (E-230) is also used.

ortolan Small wild song bird, *Emberisa hortulana*, sometimes caught in the wild and eaten in parts of Europe, where it is prized for its delicate flavour.

orubisi Tanzanian; traditional effervescent, opaque, slightly sour BEER produced by fermentation of bananas and sorghum. Also known as amarwa; Kenyan urwaga and Ugandan mwenge are similar.

oryzenin The major protein of RICE.

Oslo breakfast A breakfast requiring no preparation, introduced in Oslo, Norway, in 1929 for schoolchildren before classes started. It consisted of rye biscuit, brown bread, butter or vitaminised margarine, whey cheese and cod liver oil paste, 0.3 L milk, raw carrot, apple, half orange.

osmazome Obsolete name given to an aqueous extract of meat regarded as the 'pure essence of meat'.

osmolality Concentration of osmotically active particles per kg of solvent.

osmolarity Concentration of osmotically active particles per litre of solution.

osmole Unit of OSMOTIC PRESSURE. Equals molecular mass of a solute, in grams, multiplied by the number of ions when it dissociates in solution.

osmophiles Micro-organisms that can flourish under conditions of high OSMOTIC PRESSURE, e.g. in jams, honey, brine pickles; especially yeasts (also called xerophilic yeasts).

osmosis The passage of water through a semipermeable membrane, from a region of low concentration of solutes to one of higher concentration.

osmosis, reverse Or hyperfiltration, the passage of water from a more concentrated to a less concentrated solution through a SEMIPERMEABLE MEMBRANE by the application of pressure. Used for desalination of seawater, concentration of fruit juices and processing of whey. The membranes commonly used are cellulose acetate or polyamide with very small pores, 10^3–10^4 μm.

See also ULTRAFILTRATION; OSMOTIC PRESSURE.

osmotic dehydration Partial dehydration of fruit by use of a concentrated sugar solution to extract water.

osmotic pressure The pressure required to prevent the passage of water through a SEMIPERMEABLE MEMBRANE from a region of low concentration of solutes to one of higher concentration, by OSMOSIS.

Osmovac^{TM} **process** Two-stage drying of fruits. In the first stage, about half the moisture is removed by OSMOTIC DEHYDRATION, followed by vacuum drying.

ossein The organic matrix of the bone left behind when the mineral salts are removed by solution in dilute acid. Mainly COLLAGEN, and hydrolysed by boiling water to GELATINE.

osteoblasts Cells that are responsible for the formation of bone. Differentiation of osteoblast precursor cells is stimulated by VITAMIN D, after OSTEOCLASTS have been activated.

osteocalcin Calcium-binding protein in bone and cartilage that contains γ-CARBOXYGLUTAMATE (Gla) residues formed by a VITAMIN K-dependent reaction; synthesis regulated by VITAMIN D.

osteoclasts Cells that resorb calcified bone. Activated (*inter alia*) by VITAMIN D to maintain plasma concentration of calcium.

osteomalacia The adult equivalent of RICKETS; bone demineralisation due to deficiency of VITAMIN D and hence inadequate absorption of calcium and loss of calcium from the bones.

osteoporosis Degeneration of the bones with advancing age due to loss of bone mineral and protein; this is largely a result of loss of HORMONES with increasing age (oestrogens in women and testosterone in men). Although there is negative CALCIUM balance (net loss of calcium from the body) this is the result of osteoporosis, rather than the cause, although there is evidence that calcium and VITAMIN D supplements may slow progression. A high calcium intake in early life is beneficial, since this results in greater bone density at maturity, and regular exercise to stimulate bone metabolism is also important.

Ostermilk™ Dried milk for infant feeding. Ostermilk No. 1 is half-cream; No. 2 is full-cream.

ostrich Large flightless bird (*Struthio camelus*), up to 2.5 m tall, native of Africa, farmed in many regions.

Composition /100 g: water 71 g, 691 kJ (165 kcal), protein 20.2 g, fat 8.7 g (of which 38% saturated, 47% mono-unsaturated, 16% polyunsaturated), cholesterol 71 mg, carbohydrate 0 g, ash 0.7 g, Ca 7 mg, Fe 2.9 mg, Mg 20 mg, P 199 mg, K 291 mg, Na 72 mg, Zn 3.5 mg, Cu 0.1 mg, Se 33 µg, vitamin E 0.2 mg, B_1 0.18 mg, B_2 0.27 mg, niacin 4.4 mg, B_6 0.47 mg, folate 7 µg, B_{12} 4.6 µg, pantothenate 1.1 mg. A 100 g serving is a source of vitamin B_1, B_2, pantothenate, a good source of Fe, P, Zn, niacin, vitamin B_6, a rich source of Se, vitamin B_{12}.

ovalbumin The albumin of egg white; comprises 55% of the total solids.

Ovaltine™ A preparation of MALT EXTRACT, milk, eggs, cocoa and soya, with added thiamin, vitamin D and niacin, for consumption as a beverage when added to milk. Invented in 1863 by Swiss scientist George Wander, and originally called Ovomaltine.

oven spring The sudden increases in the volume of a dough during the first 10–12 min of baking, due to increased rate of fermentation and expansion of gases.

overall heat transfer coefficient (OHTC) The sum of the resistances to heat flow due to conduction and convection.

overrun In ice cream manufacture, the per centage increase in the volume of the mix caused by the beating-in of air. Optimum overrun, 70–100%. To prevent excessive aeration, US regulations state that ice cream must weigh 4.5 lb/gallon (0.48 kg/L).

overweight Excessive accumulation of body fat, but not so great as to be classified as OBESITY. Defined as BODY MASS INDEX 25–30 kg/m^2.

ovomucin A carbohydrate–protein complex in egg white, responsible for the firmness of egg white, 1–3% of the total solids.

ovomucoid A protein of egg white, 12% of the total solids. It inhibits the digestive enzyme TRYPSIN, but is inactivated by gastric PEPSIN.

oxalic acid A dicarboxylic acid, chemically COOH—COOH. Poisonous in large amounts; present especially in spinach, chocolate, rhubarb and nuts. The toxicity of rhubarb leaves is due to their high content of oxalic acid.

Reports that very high intakes of VITAMIN C (several grams per day) lead to formation of oxalic acid were based on detection of oxalic acid in urine, but this was almost certainly formed after collection; there is no known pathway for formation of oxalic acid from ascorbate.

Genetic diseases of GLYCINE and GLYOXYLATE metabolism lead to HYPEROXALURIA, as a result of reduction of glyoxylate to oxalate by lactate dehydrogenase (EC 1.1.1.27).

Oxfam Non-governmental organization concerned with famine relief and improvement of food resources in less developed countries. Originally founded by Gilbert Murray in 1942 as Oxford Committee for Famine Relief. Web site http://www.oxfam.org.uk/.

oxidases (oxygenases) Enzymes that oxidise substrates by reaction with oxygen to form water or hydrogen peroxide. They thus differ from dehydrogenases, which oxidise substrates by transfer of hydrogen to a COENZYME. Mixed function oxidases introduce oxygen into both the substrate and water.

oxidation The chemical process of removing electrons from an element or compound (e.g. the oxidation of iron compounds from ferrous, Fe^{2+} to ferric, Fe^{3+}), frequently together with the removal of hydrogen ions (H^+). The reverse process, the addition of electrons or hydrogen, is reduction. In biological oxidation and reduction reactions, CYTOCHROMES act to transfer electrons, while COENZYMES derived from the vitamins NIACIN and VITAMIN B_2 are hydrogen carriers, transferring both electrons and H^+ ions.

oxidative phosphorylation The formation of ATP from ADP and phosphate in the MITOCHONDRION, linked to the ELECTRON TRANSPORT CHAIN and the oxidation of metabolic fuels.

See also UNCOUPLING PROTEIN.

Oxo^{TM} A dried preparation of hydrolysed meat, meat extract, salt and cereal in cube form, used as a drink or gravy.

oxycalorimeter Instrument for measuring the oxygen consumed and carbon dioxide produced when a food is burned, as distinct from the CALORIMETER, which measures the heat produced.

oxycarotenoids *See* XANTHOPHYLLS.

oxygenases *See* OXIDASES.

oxygen scavengers Finely powdered iron or a mixture of glucose and GLUCOSE OXIDASE used to remove residual oxygen from packaged foods. Commonly included in the package as a sachet, but may also be an integral part of the packaging material (*see* BIOACTIVE POLYMERS).

oxyhaemoglobin Oxygenated HAEMOGLOBIN.

oxymyoglobin MYOGLOBIN is the muscle oxygen-binding protein; it takes up oxygen to form oxymyoglobin, which is bright red, while myoglobin itself is purplish-red. The surface of fresh meat that is exposed to oxygen is bright red from the oxymyoglobin, while the interior of the meat is darker in colour where the myoglobin is not oxygenated.

oxyntic cells *See* PARIETAL CELLS.

oxyntomodulin Peptide hormone released post-prandially from cells of the gastrointestinal mucosa in proportion to energy intake. It is derived from PROGLUCAGON, and inhibits food intake. Circulating levels are increased in ANOREXIA.

oxytetracycline *See* TETRACYCLINE.

oxythiamin Antimetabolite of thiamin, used in experimental studies of VITAMIN B_1 deficiency; it inhibits thiamin pyrophosphokinase (EC 2.7.6.2). Unlike PYRITHIAMIN it does not enter the central nervous system.

oxyuriasis Infestation of the large intestine with PINWORM.

oyster Marine bivalve MOLLUSC, *Ostreidae* and *Crassostrea* spp.

Composition /100 g: water 85.2 g, 285 kJ (68 kcal), protein 7.1 g, fat 2.5 g (of which 38% saturated, 14% mono-unsaturated, 48% polyunsaturated), cholesterol 53 mg, carbohydrate 3.9 g, ash 1.4 g, Ca 45 mg, Fe 6.7 mg, Mg 47 mg, P 135 mg, K 156 mg, Na 211 mg, Zn 90.8 mg, Cu 4.5 mg, Mn 0.4 mg, Se 63.7 µg, I 60 µg, vitamin A 30 µg RE (30 µg retinal), E 0.9 mg, K 0.1 mg, B_1 0.1 mg, B_2 0.09 mg, niacin 1.4 mg, B_6 0.06 mg, folate 10 µg, B_{12} 19.5 µg, pantothenate 0.2 mg, C 4 mg. An 85 g serving (6 oysters) is a source of Mg, Mn, P, a rich source of Cu, Fe, I, Se, Zn, vitamin B_{12}.

oyster crabs American; small young crabs found inside oysters, cooked and eaten whole, including the soft shell.

oyster mushroom *Pleurotus ostreatus*, *see* MUSHROOMS.

oyster plant (vegetable oyster) *See* SALSIFY.

ozone O_3, a powerful germicide, used to sterilise water and in antiseptic ice for preserving fish.

P

P. 4000   A class of synthetic SWEETENERS, chemically nitro-amino alkoxybenzenes (propoxyamino nitrobenzene is 4100 times as sweet as saccharin). They are not considered harmless and are not permitted in foods.

PA 3679   Designation of a putrefactive anaerobic bacterium widely used in investigations of heat sterilisation.

paak   South-east Asian; salty fish paste made by fermenting fish or shrimps with rice.

PABA   *See PARA-AMINO BENZOIC ACID.*

pacificarins   Compounds present in foods that resist micro-organisms; they may be of microbial origin or synthesised by the plant itself. Also known as phytoncides.

packaging, active   Packaging that changes the condition of the packed food to extend its shelf life or improve safety or sensory properties, while maintaining quality. May include OXYGEN SCAVENGERS, desiccants, antimicrobial compounds, etc.

   See also BIOACTIVE POLYMERS; PACKAGING, MODIFIED ATMOSPHERE.

packaging, green   Use of biodegradable materials to replace conventional plastics in food packaging.

   See also STARCH, THERMOPLASTIC.

packaging, intelligent   Packaging system that monitors the condition of packaged foods to give information about its quality during transport and storage. May include a variety of chemical, enzymic or immunological sensors to detect temperature, oxygen, products of spoilage and specific micro-organisms.

   See also TIME–TEMPERATURE INDICATOR.

packaging, modified atmosphere   Storage of fruits, vegetables and prepacked meat in a controlled atmosphere in which a proportion of the oxygen is replaced by carbon dioxide, sometimes with the addition of other gases such as argon and nitrous oxide. For some products a high oxygen atmosphere is used, to reduce enzymic BROWNING and anaerobic spoilage. In the passive process, the product is sealed in a selectively permeable polymer and allowed to undergo metabolism until the desired gas composition has been achieved; in the active process the package is evacuated, then flushed with the desired gas mixture before sealing.

packed cell volume (PCV)   *See* HAEMATOCRIT.

paddy   RICE in the husk after threshing; also known as rough rice.

pak choy   Chinese CABBAGE or Chinese leaves, *Brassica chinensis*.

PAL   *See* PHYSICAL ACTIVITY LEVEL.

Palatinat^{TM} *See* ISOMALT.

palatinose   Isomaltulose, a DISACCHARIDE, α-1,6-glucosyl-fructose.

palatone *See* MALTOL.

Palestine bee *See* BEE WINE.

Palestine soup English, 19th century, made from Jerusalem ARTI-CHOKES and named in the mistaken belief that the artichokes came from Jerusalem.

palmitic acid A saturated FATTY ACID with 16 carbon atoms (C16:0), widespread in fats and oils.

palmitoleic acid A mono-unsaturated fatty acid with 16 carbon atoms (C16:1 ω7), widespread in fats and oils.

palm kernel oil One of the major oils of commerce, widely used in cooking fats and margarines; oil extracted from the kernel of the nut of the oil palm, *Elaeis guineensis*. Pale in colour in contrast to red PALM OIL from the outer part of the nut; 86% saturated, 12% mono-unsaturated, 2% polyunsaturated, contains 3.8 mg vitamin E, 25 mg vitamin K/100 g.

palm oil From outer fibrous pulp of the fruit of the oil palm, *Elaeis guineensis*. Coloured red because of very high content of α- and β-carotene (30 mg of each /100 g); 52% saturated, 39% mono-unsaturated, 10% polyunsaturated, contains 16 mg vitamin E, 8 mg vitamin K /100 g.

palm, wild date *Phoenix sylvestris*, a relative of the true DATE palm, *P. dactylifera*, grown in India as a source of sugar, obtained from the sap.

palm wine Fermented sap from various palm trees, especially date and coconut palms.

palynology The study of pollens and spores.
See also MELISSOPALYNOLOGY.

PAM Passive atmosphere modification. *See* PACKAGING, MODIFIED ATMOSPHERE.

pan *See* BETEL.

panada Mixture of fat, flour and liquid (stock or milk) mixed to a thick paste; used to bind mixtures such as chopped meat, and also as the basis of soufflés and choux PASTRY.

panary fermentation Yeast fermentation of dough in breadmaking.

pancreas Abdominal gland with two functions: the endocrine pancreas (the islets of Langerhans) secretes the HORMONES INSULIN, GLUCAGON and GASTRIN; the exocrine pancreas (acinar cells) secretes the PANCREATIC JUICE. Known by the butcher as sweetbread or gut sweetbread, as distinct from chest sweetbread which is thymus.

pancreatic juice The alkaline digestive juice produced by the exocrine pancreas and secreted into the duodenum. It contains the inactive precursors of a number of PROTEIN digestive enzymes.

Trypsinogen is activated to trypsin (EC 3.4.21.4) by ENTEROPEP-
TIDASE (EC 3.4.21.9) in the intestinal lumen; in turn, trypsin
activates the other enzyme precursors: chymotrypsinogen to chymotrypsin (EC 3.4.21.1), pro-elastase to elastase (EC 3.4.21.36),
procarboxypeptidases to carboxypeptidases (EC 3.4.17.1 and 2).
Also contains LIPASE (EC 3.1.1.3), AMYLASE (EC 3.2.1.1) and
nucleases.

Secretion of alkaline pancreatic juice is stimulated by
SECRETIN; secretion of pancreatic juice rich in enzymes is stimulated by CHOLECYSTOKININ.

pancreatin Preparation made from the pancreas of animals containing the enzymes of PANCREATIC JUICE. Used to replace pancreatic enzymes in pancreatic insufficiency and CYSTIC FIBROSIS as
an aid to digestion.

pancreozymin Obsolete name for CHOLECYSTOKININ.

pandemain (paynemaine) Medieval English; fine white bread
made from sifted flour.

pandemic An EPIDEMIC that affects large numbers of people in
many different countries, or world-wide.

pan dowdy American; baked apple sponge pudding, served with
the apple side up.

pangamic acid N-Di-isopropyl glucuronate, claimed to be an
ANTIOXIDANT, and to speed recovery from fatigue. Sometimes
called vitamin B_{15}, but no evidence that it is a dietary essential,
nor that it has any metabolic function.

Paniplus[TM] A mixture of calcium peroxide and other salts added
to dough to permit use in high-speed manufacturing processes,
introduced in 1920.

panir Indian, Middle Eastern; soft mild-flavoured cheese. Milk is
left to ferment for 6–12 h, then heated to separate the curd.

panning In sugar confectionery (and pharmaceutical) manufacture, the application of many layers of coating to centres tumbling in a revolving pan. Coatings may be sugar syrup (hard
panning, each layer is dried with hot air) or glucose syrup (soft
panning, each layer is dried by the application of fine sugar.

panocha Candy made from brown sugar, milk, butter and nuts.

panthenol The alcohol of PANTOTHENIC ACID; biologically
active.

pantoprazole See PROTON PUMP.

pantothenic acid A vitamin with no numerical designation.
Chemically, the β-alanine derivative of pantoic acid. Required
for the synthesis of COENZYME A (and hence essential for the
metabolism of fats, carbohydrates and amino acids) and of acyl
carrier protein (and hence essential for the synthesis of fatty
acids).

Dietary deficiency is unknown; it is widely distributed in all living cells. Human requirements are not known with any certainty; the adequate intake for adults is 5 mg /day. Experimental deficiency signs in rats include greying of the hair (hence at one time known as the anti-grey hair factor; there is no evidence that it affects greying of human hair with age). Experimental deficiency in human beings leads to fatigue, headache, muscle weakness and gastrointestinal disturbances.

See also BURNING FOOT SYNDROME.

PANTOTHENIC ACID AND COENZYME A

papain   Proteolytic enzyme (*see* PROTEOLYSIS) (EC 3.4.22.2) from the juice of the PAWPAW used in tenderising meat; sometimes called vegetable pepsin. The enzyme is obtained as the dried latex on the skin of the fruit by scratching it while still on the tree, and collecting the flow. The rate of reaction is slow at room temperature, increasing to maximum activity at 80 °C and rapidly inactivated at higher temperatures; hence, it continues to tenderise the meat during the early stages of cooking.

papa seca   *See* CHUÑO.

papaw   Purple fruit of *Asiminia triloba*, related to the CUSTARD APPLE; distinct from the PAWPAW or papaya.

papaya   *See* PAWPAW.

papillote, en   Made or served in a paper case.

Papin's digester   Early version of the pressure cooker or AUTOCLAVE. Named after D. Papin, French physicist 1647–1712; originally invented for the purpose of softening bones for the preparation of GELATINE.

paprika   *See* PEPPER, SWEET.

PAR   *See* PHYSICAL ACTIVITY RATIO.

para-**amino benzoic acid (PABA)**   Essential growth factor for micro-organisms. It forms part of the molecule of FOLIC ACID and is therefore required for the synthesis of this vitamin. Mammals cannot synthesise folic acid, and PABA has no other known function; there is no evidence that it is a human dietary requirement. Sulphanilamides (sulpha drugs) are chemical analogues of PABA, and exert their antibacterial action by antagonising PABA utilisation.

parabens   Methyl, ethyl and propyl esters of *p*-hydroxybenzoic acid used together with their sodium salts as antimicrobials in food (E-214–219). Effective over a wide range of pH; more effective against moulds and yeast than against bacteria.

paracasein   Obsolete name for precipitated milk CASEIN.

paracrine   Production by a cell of locally acting HORMONE-like substances that act on nearby cells.
   See also AUTOCRINE; ENDOCRINE GLANDS.

paraffin, medicinal (liquid)   *See* MEDICINAL PARAFFIN.

Paraflow™   A plate heat exchanger used for pasteurising liquids.

parageusia   Abnormality of the sense of taste.
   See also DYSGEUSIA; GUSTIN; HYPOGEUSIA.

parakeratosis   Disease of swine characterised by cessation of growth, erythema, seborrhoea and hyperkeratosis of the skin; due to ZINC deficiency and possibly to changes in essential FATTY ACID metabolism.

paralactic acid   *See* SARCOLACTIC ACID.

paralytic shellfish poisoning   Caused by shellfish that have accumulated toxins from the dinoflagellate plankton, *Gonyaulax* spp.

parasol mushroom   *Macrolepiota procera*, *see* MUSHROOMS.

paratha   Indian; wholewheat unleavened bread.

parathormone   Commonly used as an abbreviation for the PARATHYROID HORMONE; correctly a trade name for a pharmaceutical preparation of the hormone.

parathyroid hormone   Hormone secreted by the four parathyroid glands (in the neck near the THYROID GLAND). The hormone is secreted in response to a fall in plasma calcium, and acts on the kidney to increase the formation of the active metabolite of VITAMIN D (calcitriol), leading to an increase in plasma calcium by increasing intestinal absorption and mobilising the mineral from bones. It also reduces urinary excretion of phosphate.

paratyphoid   *See* TYPHOID.

parboil   Partially cook. Of special interest in nutrition is the parboiling of brown rice, steaming rice in the husk before milling. The water-soluble vitamins diffuse from the husk into the grain;

when the rice is polished, it contains more of these vitamins than polished raw rice.

parchita *See* PASSION FRUIT.

parenteral nutrition Nutrition other than via the intestinal tract. Slow infusion of solution of nutrients into the veins through a catheter. This may be partial, to supplement food and nutrient intake, or total (TPN, total parenteral nutrition), providing the sole source of energy and nutrient intake for patients with major intestinal problems.

See also ENTERAL NUTRITION; RECTAL FEEDING.

pareve (parve) Jewish term for dishes containing neither milk nor meat. Jewish law prohibits mixing of milk and meat foods or the consumption of milk products for 3 h after a meat meal.

See also MILCHIG; FLEISHIG.

parevine USA; a frozen dessert resembling ice cream, but containing no dairy produce or meat products (such as gelatine), and hence PAREVE, to conform with Jewish dietary laws.

parietal cells Cells of the gastric mucosa that secrete gastric acid (see GASTRIC SECRETION) and INTRINSIC FACTOR. Also known as oxyntic cells.

See also ACHLORHYDRIA; ANAEMIA, PERNICIOUS; PROTON PUMP.

parillin Or smilacin; highly toxic glycoside of glucose, rhamnose and parigenin from SARSAPARILLA root.

parity The number of pregnancies that a woman has had that have resulted in the birth of an infant capable of survival.

See also PRIMIPARA.

parmesan cheese English and French name for the hard dry Italian CHEESE parmigiana. Made from semi-skimmed cow's milk cooked with RENNET, dried for at least six months. When 2 years old it is called vecchio, stravecchio is 3 years, stravecchione 4 years old.

Composition/100 g: water 29.2 g, 1641 kJ (392 kcal), protein 35.8 g, fat 25.8 g (of which 67% saturated, 31% mono-unsaturated, 2% polyunsaturated), carbohydrate 3.2 g (0.8 g sugars), ash 6 g, Ca 1184 mg, Fe 0.8 mg, Mg 44 mg, P 694 mg, K 92 mg, Na 1602 mg, Zn 2.8 mg, Se 22.5 μg, I 72 μg, vitamin A 108 μg RE (106 μg retinol, 28 μg carotenoids), E 0.2 mg, K 1.7 mg, B_1 0.04 mg, B_2 0.33 mg, niacin 0.3 mg, B_6 0.09 mg, folate 7 μg, B_{12} 1.2 μg, pantothenate 0.5 mg. A 20 g serving is a source of P, a good source of Ca, vitamin B_{12}.

PARNUTS EU term for foods prepared for particular nutritional purposes (intended for people with disturbed metabolism or in special physiological condition or young children). Also called dietetic foods.

paromomycin ANTIBIOTIC used to treat intestinal bacterial infections and amoebic DYSENTERY.

parosmia Any disorder of the sense of smell.

parotid glands Pair of SALIVARY GLANDS situated in front of the ears, with ducts that open in the cheek, opposite the second molar teeth.

parsley Leaves of the herb *Petroselinum crispum*, *P. hertense* or *P. sativum*.

Composition/100 g: (edible portion 95%) water 88 g, 151 kJ (36 kcal), protein 3 g, fat 0.8 g, carbohydrate 6.3 g (0.9 g sugars), fibre 3.3 g, ash 2.2 g, Ca 138 mg, Fe 6.2 mg, Mg 50 mg, P 58 mg, K 554 mg, Na 56 mg, Zn 1.1 mg, Cu 0.1 mg, Mn 0.2 mg, Se 0.1 µg, vitamin A 421 µg RE (10615 µg carotenoids), E 0.8 mg, K 1640 mg, B_1 0.09 mg, B_2 0.1 mg, niacin 1.3 mg, B_6 0.09 mg, folate 152 µg, pantothenate 0.4 mg, C 133 mg. A 5 g serving is a source of vitamin C.

parsley, Hamburg Root of *Petroselinum crispum* var. *tuberosum*, grown for its root (also called turnip-rooted parsley); similar in appearance to PARSNIP.

parsnip Root of *Pastinaca sativa*, eaten as a vegetable.

Composition/100 g: (edible portion 85%) water 80 g, 314 kJ (75 kcal), protein 1.2 g, fat 0.3 g, carbohydrate 18 g (4.8 g sugars), fibre 4.9 g, ash 1 g, Ca 36 mg, Fe 0.6 mg, Mg 29 mg, P 71 mg, K 375 mg, Na 10 mg, Zn 0.6 mg, Cu 0.1 mg, Mn 0.6 mg, Se 1.8 µg, E 1.5 mg, K 22.5 mg, B_1 0.09 mg, B_2 0.05 mg, niacin 0.7 mg, B_6 0.09 mg, folate 67 µg, pantothenate 0.6 mg, C 17 mg. A 65 g serving is a source of Mn, vitamin C, a good source of folate.

partial glyceride esters *See* ACETOGLYCERIDES.

partridge GAME bird, *Perdix perdix* and related species.

parts per million (ppm) Description of low concentrations meaning exactly what the term says = mg /kg.

pascal (Pa) SI unit of pressure = 1 newton/m^2.

Paselli Excel^{TM} FAT REPLACER made from starch.

passion fruit Also known as parchita, granadilla and water lemon; fruit of the tropical vine, *Passiflora* spp. Purple or greenish-yellow when ripe, watery pulp containing small seeds.

Composition/100 g: (edible portion 52%) water 73 g, 406 kJ (97 kcal), protein 2.2 g, fat 0.7 g, carbohydrate 23.4 g (11.2 g sugars), fibre 10.4 g, ash 0.8 g, Ca 12 mg, Fe 1.6 mg, Mg 29 mg, P 68 mg, K 348 mg, Na 28 mg, Zn 0.1 mg, Cu 0.1 mg, Se 0.6 µg, vitamin A 64 µg RE (784 µg carotenoids), K 0.7 mg, B_2 0.13 mg, niacin 1.5 mg, B_6 0.1 mg, folate 14 µg, C 30 mg.

pasta (Alimentary paste); dried dough, traditionally made with hard wheat (SEMOLINA) but soft wheat may be added, sometimes with egg and milk. Spinach, tomato or squid ink may be added to the dough to give a green, red or black colour. The dough is partly dried in hot air, then more slowly. Sold both completely dry, when it can be stored for a long period, and 'fresh', i.e. less dried and keeping for only a week or so.

Made in numerous shapes: spaghetti is a solid rod about 2 mm in diameter; vermicelli is about one-third this thickness, ravioli (envelopes stuffed with meat or cheese), fettucine and linguini (ribbons), and a range of twists, spirals and other shapes. Macaroni is tubular shaped, about 5 mm in diameter; at 10 mm it is known as zitoni, and at 15 mm fovantini or maccaroncelli. Cannelloni are tubes 1.5–2 cm wide and 10 cm long, stuffed with meat; penne are nib-shaped. Lasagna is sheets of pasta. Farfals are ground, granulated or shredded.

Composition/100 g: water 10.3 g, 1553 kJ (371 kcal), protein 12.8 g, fat 1.6 g (of which 20% saturated, 20% mono-unsaturated, 60% polyunsaturated), carbohydrate 74.7 g, fibre 2.4 g, ash 0.7 g, Ca 18 mg, Fe 1.3 mg, Mg 48 mg, P 150 mg, K 162 mg, Na 7 mg, Zn 1.2 mg, Cu 0.3 mg, Mn 0.7 mg, Se 62.2 µg, B_1 0.09 mg, B_2 0.06 mg, niacin 1.7 mg, B_6 0.11 mg, folate 18 µg, pantothenate 0.4 mg.

pasteurisation A means of prolonging the storage time of foods for a limited time, by killing the vegetative forms of many pathogenic organisms. These can be killed by mild heat treatment, whereas destruction of all bacteria and spores (sterilisation) requires higher temperatures for longer periods, often spoiling the product in the process.

In flash pasteurisation, the product is held at a higher temperature than for normal pasteurisation, but for a shorter time, so that there is less development of a cooked flavour.

Pasteurisation of milk destroys all pathogens, and although pasteurised milk will sour within a day or two, this is not a source of disease. It is achieved either by heating to 63–66 °C for 30 min (holder method), followed by immediate cooling, or (the high-temperature short-time process) heating to 71 °C for 15 s. The efficacy of pasteurisation is checked by either the METHYLENE BLUE DYE-REDUCTION TEST or the PHOSPHATASE TEST.

pasteuriser Equipment used to pasteurise liquids such as milk and fruit juices. The material is passed continuously over heated plates, or through pipes, where it is heated to the required temperature, maintained at that temperature for the required time, then immediately cooled.

pastillage Paste used on cakes, made from icing sugar, with gum tragacanth or gelatine and cornflour.

pastourma Greek and Turkish; black-rinded smoked bacon, highly flavoured with garlic.

pastrami Middle European (especially Rumanian-Jewish); smoked and seasoned beef (now also made from turkey). Known in Canada as smoked beef.

pastry Baked dough of flour, fat and water. Six basic types: shortcrust in which the fat is rubbed into the flour; suet crust in which chopped suet is mixed with the flour; puff and flaky, in which the fat is rolled into the dough; hotwater crust and choux, in which the fat is melted in hot water before being added to the flour (choux pastry also contains eggs and is whisked to a paste before cooking). PHYLLO PASTRY is made from flour and water only. Suet pastry is raised using baking powder or self-raising flour; puff and flaky and choux pastry are raised by the steam trapped between layers of dough.

pâte French for paste; used for pastry, dough or batter, also for PASTA.

pâté French for any savoury pie, now used almost exclusively to mean a savoury paste of liver, meat, fish or vegetables.

patent flour *See* FLOUR, EXTRACTION RATE.

pathogen Bacterium or other micro-organism that causes disease, as opposed to COMMENSAL or SYMBIOTIC organisms.

patty Small savoury pie, normally made with shortcrust pastry; also (in the USA) small cakes of minced meat or poultry, like croquettes but not dipped in breadcrumbs before cooking.

patulin Broad-spectrum ANTIBIOTIC, but also a carcinogenic and teratogenic MYCOTOXIN, produced by *Byssochlamys nivea*, *Penicillium* and *Aspergillus* spp.; *P. expansum* is the most important because it is a common cause of storage rot in fruit. Inactivated by alcoholic fermentation, pasteurisation or treatment with sulphur dioxide.

patum peperium *See* GENTLEMAN'S RELISH.

paua *See* ABALONE.

paunching Removing the entrails of rabbit, hare, etc.

paupiette Small thinly cut piece of meat wrapped round a filling of forcemeat and braised.

pavlova Australian; meringue cake topped with fruit and whipped cream; created in honour of the Russian ballerina Anna Pavlova on her visit to Australia in the 1920s.

pawpaw (papaya) Large green or yellow fruit of the tropical tree *Carica papaya*, widely grown in all tropical regions. The source of the proteolytic enzyme PAPAIN.

Composition/100g: (edible portion 67%) water 88.8g, 163kJ (39kcal), protein 0.6g, fat 0.1g, carbohydrate 9.8g (5.9g sugars), fibre 1.8g, ash 0.6g, Ca 24mg, Fe 0.1mg, Mg 10mg, P 5mg, K 257mg, Na 3mg, Zn 0.1mg, Se 0.6µg, vitamin A 55µg RE (1112µg carotenoids), E 0.7mg, K 2.6mg, B_1 0.03mg, B_2 0.03mg, niacin 0.3 mg, B_6 0.02 mg, folate 38 µg, pantothenate 0.2 mg, C 62 mg. A 110 g serving is a good source of folate, a rich source of vitamin C.

PBI   *See* IODINE, PROTEIN-BOUND.

PCM   Protein–calorie   malnutrition;   *see*   PROTEIN–ENERGY MALNUTRITION.

PCR   *See* POLYMERASE CHAIN REACTION.

PCV   Packed cell volume, *see* HAEMATOCRIT.

PDCAAS   Protein digestibility corrected amino acid score; a measure of PROTEIN QUALITY based on amino acid score, corrected for the digestibility of the protein.

peach   Fruit of the tree *Prunus persica.*

Composition/100 g: (edible portion 87%) water 88.9 g, 163 kJ (39 kcal), protein 0.9 g, fat 0.3 g, carbohydrate 9.5 g (8.4 g sugars), fibre 1.5 g, ash 0.4 g, Ca 6 mg, Fe 0.3 mg, Mg 9 mg, P 20 mg, K 190 mg, Zn 0.2 mg, Cu 0.1 mg, Mn 0.1 mg, Se 0.1 µg, vitamin A 16 µg RE (320 µg carotenoids), E 0.7 mg, K 2.6 mg, B_1 0.02 mg, B_2 0.03 mg, niacin 0.8 mg, B_6 0.03 mg, folate 4 µg, pantothenate 0.2 mg, C 7 mg. A 120 g serving (1 fruit) is a source of vitamin C.

pea, garden or green   Seed of the LEGUME *Pisum sativum.*

Composition/100 g: water 88.9 g, 176 kJ (42 kcal), protein 2.8 g, fat 0.2 g, carbohydrate 7.6 g (4 g sugars), fibre 2.6 g, ash 0.6 g, Ca 43 mg, Fe 2.1 mg, Mg 24 mg, P 53 mg, K 200 mg, Na 4 mg, Zn 0.3 mg, Cu 0.1 mg, Mn 0.2 mg, Se 0.7 µg, vitamin A 54 µg RE (1414 µg carotenoids), E 0.4 mg, K 25 mg, B_1 0.15 mg, B_2 0.08 mg, niacin 0.6 mg, B_6 0.16 mg, folate 42 µg, pantothenate 0.8 mg, C 60 mg. A 70 g serving is a source of folate, a rich source of vitamin C.

pea, mange tout   Immature pods and embryo seeds of the LEGUME *Pisum sativum* var. *macrocarpon* or *macrocarpum*, eaten whole. Also known as snap peas or sugar snap peas.

peanut   Fruit of *Arachis hypogaea*, also known as earthnut, groundnut, arachis nut, monkey nut; technically a LEGUME, not a nut. Peanut (arachis) oil is 18% saturated, 49% mono-unsaturated, 34% polyunsaturated, vitamin E 15.7 mg, K 0.7 mg.

Composition/100 g: water 6.5 g, 2373 kJ (567 kcal), protein 25.8 g, fat 49.2 g (of which 15% saturated, 52% mono-unsaturated, 33% polyunsaturated), carbohydrate 16.1 g (4 g sugars), fibre 8.5 g, ash 2.3 g, Ca 92 mg, Fe 4.6 mg, Mg 168 mg, P 376 mg, K 705 mg, Na 18 mg, Zn 3.3 mg, Cu 1.1 mg, Mn 1.9 mg, Se 7.2 µg, vitamin E 8.3 mg, B_1 0.64 mg, B_2 0.14 mg, niacin 12.1 mg, B_6 0.35 mg, folate 240 µg, pantothenate 1.8 mg. A 25 g serving is a source of Mg, P, vitamin B_1, niacin, a good source of Cu, Mn, vitamin E, a rich source of folate.

peanut butter   Ground, roasted peanuts; commonly prepared from a mixture of Spanish and Virginia peanuts, since the first alone is too oily and the second is too dry. Separation of the oil is prevented by partial HYDROGENATION of the oil and the addition of EMULSIFIERS.

pea, processed Garden PEAS (*Pisum sativum*) that have matured on the plant and subsequently been canned.

pear Fruit of many species of *Pyrus*; cultivated varieties all descended from *P. communis*. The UK National Fruit Collection has 495 varieties of dessert and cooking pears, and a further 20 varieties of PERRY pears.

Composition/100 g: (edible portion 92%) water 84 g, 243 kJ (58 kcal), protein 0.4 g, fat 0.1 g, carbohydrate 15.5 g (9.8 g sugars), fibre 3.1 g, ash 0.3 g, Ca 9 mg, Fe 0.2 mg, Mg 7 mg, P 11 mg, K 119 mg, Na 1 mg, Zn 0.1 mg, Cu 0.1 mg, Se 0.1 µg, vitamin A 1 µg RE (60 µg carotenoids), E 0.1 mg, K 4.5 mg, B_1 0.01 mg, B_2 0.03 mg, niacin 0.2 mg, B_6 0.03 mg, folate 7 µg, C 4 mg. A 150 g serving (1 large) is a source of Cu.

pearling In the milling of cereals such as rice, oats and barley, the tightly adhering husk is removed by an abrasion process known as pearling, as opposed to the break rolls that are used in MILLING other cereals.

pear, nashi (or Asian) Apple-shaped fruit of *Pyris pyrifolia* (sometimes known as apple pear because of its shape).

Composition/100 g: (edible portion 91%) water 88 g, 176 kJ (42 kcal), protein 0.5 g, fat 0.2 g, carbohydrate 10.6 g (7.1 g sugars), fibre 3.6 g, ash 0.4 g, Ca 4 mg, Mg 8 mg, P 11 mg, K 121 mg, Cu 0.1 mg, Mn 0.1 mg, Se 0.1 µg, 50 µg carotenoids, E 0.1 mg, K 4.5 mg, B_1 0.01 mg, B_2 0.01 mg, niacin 0.2 mg, B_6 0.02 mg, folate 8 µg, pantothenate 0.1 mg, C 4 mg.

pear, prickly *See* PRICKLY PEAR.

pease pudding English; dish prepared from dried peas, soaked, boiled, mashed and sieved, traditionally served with baked ham.

pecan nuts From the American tree *Carya illinoensis*, species of hickory nut.

Composition/100 g: (edible portion 53%) water 3.5 g, 2893 kJ (691 kcal), protein 9.2 g, fat 72 g (of which 9% saturated, 59% mono-unsaturated, 31% polyunsaturated), carbohydrate 13.9 g (4 g sugars), fibre 9.6 g, ash 1.5 g, Ca 70 mg, Fe 2.5 mg, Mg 121 mg, P 277 mg, K 410 mg, Zn 4.5 mg, Cu 1.2 mg, Mn 4.5 mg, Se 3.8 µg, vitamin A 3 µg RE (55 µg carotenoids), E 1.4 mg, K 3.5 mg, B_1 0.66 mg, B_2 0.13 mg, niacin 1.2 mg, B_6 0.21 mg, folate 22 µg, pantothenate 0.9 mg, C 1 mg. An 18 g serving (3 nuts) is a source of Cu, a rich source of Mn.

pecorino Italian hard sheep milk cheese with a grainy texture.

pectase An enzyme (EC 3.1.1.11) in the pith (albedo) of CITRUS fruits which demethylates PECTIN to form water-insoluble pectic acid. The intermediate compounds, with varying numbers of methoxyl groups, are pectinic acids. Also known as pectin esterase, pectin methyl esterase and pectin methoxylase. Unlike PECTINASE, present in both ripe and unripe fruit, and not associated with softening and ripening.

pectic acid   Demethylated PECTIN.

pectin   Plant tissues contain hemicelluloses (chemically polymers of galacturonic acid) known as protopectins, which cement the cell walls together. As fruit ripens, there is maximum protopectin present; thereafter it breaks down to pectin, pectinic acid and finally pectic acid and the fruit softens as the adhesive between the cells breaks down. High methoxypectins (with >50% esterification) form rigid gels at low pH; low methoxypectins (<50% esterification) form softer, spreadable gels, over a wide range of pH, in the presence of divalent cations.

Pectin is the setting agent in JAM; it forms a gel with sugar under acid conditions. Soft fruits, such as strawberry, raspberry and cherry, are low in pectin; plums, apples and oranges are rich. Apple pulp and orange pith are the commercial sources of pectin. Added to jams, confectionery, chocolate, ice cream as an emulsifier and stabiliser instead of agar; used in making jellies, and as antistaling agent in cakes. Included in NON-STARCH POLYSACCHARIDES.

pectin, amidated   The low-methoxyl PECTIN formed when pectin is de-esterified with ammonia, forming amides from methoxyl groups.

pectinase   Group of enzymes that hydrolyse PECTIN and pectic acid (demethylated pectin formed by the action of PECTASE). Important in the softening of fruit, by degradation of pectin during ripening, and used commercially to clarify fruit juices. Also known as pectolase, pectozyme.

Two endolyases hydrolyse methylated pectin to yield oligosaccharide fragments: pectin lyase (EC 4.2.2.10) is polymethoxygalacturonide lyase; pectate endolyase (EC 4.2.2.2) is poly α-D-glucuronide lyase. EC 3.2.1.15 is an endopolygalacturonidase, acting on pectic acid to produce oligosaccharides. EC 3.2.1.67 is an exopolygalacturonidase, removing galactonobiose units sequentially from the end of the pectic acid molecule.

pectinesterase   *See* PECTASE.

pectinic acid   Partially demethylated PECTIN.

pectins, low-methoxyl   Partially demethylated pectins that can form gels with little or no sugar and which are therefore used in low-calorie jams and jellies.

pectolase, pectozyme   *See* PECTINASE.

pedometer   Portable device that records number of paces walked, and therefore approximate distance travelled.

peeling   Five main techniques are used industrially to peel fruits and vegetables. Flash steam peeling using high-pressure steam to raise the surface temperature without cooking, followed by rapid release of pressure so that the surface layer flashes off. Knife peeling uses either stationary blades pressed against rotating food or rotating blades pressed against stationary food. In abrasion peeling the food is fed onto carborundum-coated rollers or into a rotating carborundum-coated drum. Caustic peeling (lye peeling) uses a solution of sodium hydroxide (known as lye) to soften the outer layer, followed by wet or dry tumbling to remove it. Flame peeling rotates the food through a furnace to burn off the outer layer.

Pekar test   A comparative test of flour colour.

pekmez   Turkish; thick jelly made by evaporating grape juice, the basis of Turkish delight and other sugar confectionery. Also general Balkan name for jam.

pekoe   *See* TEA.

pellagra   The disease due to deficiency of the vitamin NIACIN and the amino acid TRYPTOPHAN. Signs include a characteristic photosensitive dermatitis (especially on the face and back of hands), resembling severe sunburn; mental disturbances (a depressive psychosis sometimes called dementia); and digestive disorders (most commonly diarrhoea); fatal if untreated. Most commonly associated with a diet based on MAIZE or SORGHUM, which are poor sources of both tryptophan and niacin, with little meat or other vegetables.

PEM   *See* PROTEIN–ENERGY MALNUTRITION.

pemmican   Mixture of dried, powdered meat and fat, used as a concentrated food source, e.g. on expeditions.

penicillamine   Chelating agent used to enhance the excretion of COPPER in WILSON'S DISEASE.

penicillin   The first ANTIBIOTIC; found in the culture fluid of the MOULD *Penicillium notatum* in 1929. Active against a wide range of bacteria and of great value clinically. Not used as food preservative because of the danger that repeated small doses will increase the development of penicillin-resistant organisms.

Penicillium   A genus of MOULDS; apart from the production of PENICILLIN, several species are valuable in the ripening of CHEESES. *P. roquefortii* is responsible for the blue veining of Roquefort, Gorgonzola and other blue cheeses. Other species are responsible for spoilage, and may form MYCOTOXINS in foods (e.g. the unidentified nephrotoxin from *P. polonicum*).

pentagastrin   Synthetic peptide that has the same effect as the HORMONE GASTRIN on gastric acid secretion.

pentane   Hydrocarbon gas (C_5H_{12}) formed in small amounts by breakdown of oxidised linoleic acid, and exhaled on the breath; used as an index of oxygen RADICAL damage to tissue lipids, and indirectly as an index of ANTIOXIDANT status.

See also ETHANE; FATTY ACIDS.

pentosans   POLYSACCHARIDES of PENTOSES. Widely distributed in plants, e.g. fruit, wood, corncobs, oat hulls. Not digested, and hence a component of NON-STARCH POLYSACCHARIDES or dietary FIBRE.

pentose phosphate pathway   Or hexose monophosphate shunt, an alternative pathway of GLUCOSE METABOLISM.

See also FAVISM.

pentoses   MONOSACCHARIDE SUGARS with five carbon atoms.

pentosuria   The excretion of PENTOSE sugars in the urine. Idiopathic pentosuria is an inherited metabolic condition almost wholly restricted to Ashkenazi (N European) Jews, which has no adverse effects. Consumption of fruits rich in pentoses (e.g. pears) can also lead to (temporary) pentosuria.

penuche   Candy made from brown sugar and beaten until it is smooth and creamy.

P-enzyme   Potato PHOSPHORYLASE (EC 2.4.1.1), an enzyme that cleaves starch to yield glucose-1-phosphate; specific for α-1,4 links.

pepper, black, white   Fruit of the tropical climbing vine, *Piper nigrum*; the fruits are peppercorns. Black pepper is made from sun-dried unripe peppercorns when the red outer skin turns black. White pepper is made by soaking ripe berries and rubbing off outer skin. Usually ground as a condiment. Green peppercorns are dried or pickled unripe fruit. Pungency due to the alkaloids piperine, piperdine and chavicine.

pepper, chilli   Small red fruit of the bushy perennial plant *Capsicum frutescens*, various varieties known as red pepper, chilli (or chili), jalapeno. Usually sun-dried and therefore wrinkled. Very pungent, ingredient of CURRY powder, pickles and TABASCO sauce. Cayenne pepper is made from the powdered dried fruits. Unripe (green) chillis are also very pungent.

Composition/100 g: water 93 g, 88 kJ (21 kcal), protein 0.9 g, fat 0.1 g, carbohydrate 5.1 g (3.1 g sugars), fibre 1.3 g, ash 1.4 g, Ca 7 mg, Fe 0.5 mg, Mg 14 mg, P 17 mg, K 187 mg, Na 1173 mg, Zn 0.2 mg, Cu 0.1 mg, Mn 0.1 mg, Se 0.3 µg, vitamin A 36 µg RE (898 µg carotenoids), E 0.7 mg, K 8.7 mg, B_1 0.02 mg, B_2 0.05 mg, niacin 0.8 mg, B_6 0.15 mg, folate 10 µg, C 68 mg.

peppercorn   *See* PEPPER, BLACK.

pepper dulse Red aromatic seaweed (*Laurencia pinnatifida*), dried and used as a spice in Scotland.

peppergrass Peppery-tasting cress (*Lepidium sativum*), also known as pepperwort and (in USA) peppermint.

pepper, Jamaican *See* ALLSPICE.

pepper, Japan Black seeds of *Zanthoxylum piperitum* with a pungent peppery flavour.

pepper, melegueta (or Guinea) Seeds of the W. African tree *Amomum melegueta*, also known as grains of paradise.

peppermint A hybrid (*Mentha* × *piperita*) between *M. aquatica* and *M. spicata* (SPEARMINT). Not used for flavouring dishes but grown for the essential oil which is used in confectionery and medicinally.

pepper, sweet Fruit of *Capsicum annuum*; various varieties known as bell or bullnose pepper, capsicum, paprika, pimiento (distinct from pimento or ALLSPICE); may be red, yellow, purple or brown, very variable size and shape; some varieties can be spicy but mostly non-pungent.

Green, composition/100 g: (edible portion 82%) water 94 g, 84 kJ (20 kcal), protein 0.9 g, fat 0.2 g, carbohydrate 4.6 g (2.4 g sugars), fibre 1.7 g, ash 0.4 g, Ca 10 mg, Fe 0.3 mg, Mg 10 mg, P 20 mg, K 175 mg, Na 3 mg, Zn 0.1 mg, Cu 0.1 mg, Mn 0.1 mg, vitamin A 18 µg RE (577 µg carotenoids), E 0.4 mg, K 7.4 mg, B_1 0.06 mg, B_2 0.03 mg, niacin 0.5 mg, B_6 0.22 mg, folate 11 µg, pantothenate 0.1 mg, C 80 mg. An 80 g serving is a rich source of vitamin C.

Red, composition/100 g: (edible portion 82%) water 92 g, 109 kJ (26 kcal), protein 1 g, fat 0.3 g, carbohydrate 6 g (4.2 g sugars), fibre 2 g, ash 0.5 g, Ca 7 mg, Fe 0.4 mg, Mg 12 mg, P 26 mg, K 211 mg, Na 2 mg, Zn 0.3 mg, Mn 0.1 mg, Se 0.1 µg, vitamin A 157 µg RE (2493 µg carotenoids), E 1.6 mg, K 4.9 mg, B_1 0.05 mg, B_2 0.09 mg, niacin 1 mg, B_6 0.29 mg, folate 18 µg, pantothenate 0.3 mg, C 190 mg. An 80 g serving is a source of vitamin A, E, B_6, a rich source of vitamin C.

Pepsi-Cola™ A COLA DRINK. First made in 1896 in the USA by Caleb Bradham, druggist.

pepsin An enzyme (EC 3.4.23.1) in the GASTRIC JUICE; hydrolyses proteins to give smaller polypeptides, known as peptones; an endopeptidase. Active only at acid pH, 1.5–2.5. Secreted as the inactive precursor pepsinogen, which is activated by gastric acid. Vegetable pepsin is PAPAIN.

peptic ulcer *See* ULCER.

peptidases Enzymes that hydrolyse proteins, and which are therefore important in PROTEIN digestion. Endopeptidases cleave at specific points in the middle of protein molecules (between specific amino acids, depending on the enzyme); exopeptidases remove amino acids sequentially from either the amino terminal (aminopeptidases) or carboxy terminal (carboxypeptidases).

peptides Compounds formed when AMINO ACIDS are linked together through the —CO—NH— (peptide) linkage. Two amino acids so linked form a dipeptide, three a tripeptide, etc.; medium-length chains of amino acids (4–20) are known as oligopeptides, longer chains are polypeptides or proteins.

peptide YY HORMONE secreted by endocrine cells of the gastrointestinal tract, in proportion to the energy yield of a meal, that acts on the hypothalamus to signal satiety and decrease food intake. It also inhibits intestinal motility and gastric secretion.

peptidoglycans Conjugated proteins with complex chains of carbohydrate, found especially in bacterial cell walls. Especially rich in N-acetylglucosamine and N-acetylmuramic acid.

peptones Small polypeptides that are intermediate products in the hydrolysis of proteins. The term is often used for any partial hydrolysate of protein, e.g. bacteriological peptone, used as a growth medium for micro-organisms.

PER Protein efficiency ratio, a measure of PROTEIN QUALITY.

perch Freshwater FISH, *Perca fluviatilis*.
    Composition/100 g: water 79 g, 381 kJ (91 kcal), protein 19.4 g, fat 0.9 g, cholesterol 90 mg, carbohydrate 0 g, ash 1.2 g, Ca 80 mg, Fe 0.9 mg, Mg 30 mg, P 200 mg, K 269 mg, Na 62 mg, Zn 1.1 mg, Cu 0.2 mg, Mn 0.7 mg, Se 12.6 µg, vitamin A 9 µg RE (9 µg retinol, E 0.2 mg, K 0.1 mg, B_1 0.07 mg, B_2 0.1 mg, niacin 1.5 mg, B_6 0.12 mg, folate 5 µg, B_{12} 1.9 µg, pantothenate 0.8 mg, C 2 mg. A 100 g serving is a source of Cu, Se, pantothenate, a good source of P, a rich source of Mn, vitamin B_{12}.

percomorph oil Oil prepared from the liver of the percomorph, a member of the PERCH family; a rich source of VITAMIN D.

pericarp The fibrous layers next to the outer husk of cereal grains and outside the testa; of low digestibility and removed from grain during milling. The major constituent of BRAN.

perigo factor A postulated factor produced when bacterial growth medium is autoclaved with nitrite or meat is cured with nitrite: it is about 10 times more inhibitory to some bacteria than nitrite alone.

perilla Perrenial herb, *Perilla frutscens*, a member of the mint family; green-leafed and purple-leafed varieties (sometimes known as purple mint, Chinese basil or wild coleus). Also known as beefsteak plant, and shiso in Japan.

perillartine Non-nutritive SWEETENER derived from perillaldehyde, extracted from shiso (PERILLA) seed oil; 2000 times as sweet as sucrose.

perimysium *See* MUSCLE.

periodontal Relating to the tissues between the teeth; the periodontal membrane is the ligament around a tooth, attaching it to the bone.

peristalsis The wavelike rhythmic alternating contraction and relaxation of smooth muscle that forces food through the intestinal tract in peristaltic waves.

peritoneum Serous membrane of the abdominal cavity.

periwinkle *See* WINKLE.

perleche Dryness of the corners of the mouth; may be infected. Occurs in RIBOFLAVIN deficiency.

permeation In food packaging, the diffusion of molecules across the package wall, with adsorption from the external atmosphere and desorption into the internal atmosphere.

Permutit^{TM} An ION-EXCHANGE RESIN.

pernicious anaemia *See* ANAEMIA, PERNICIOUS.

peroxidase Enzyme (EC 1.11.1.17) that reduces HYDROGEN PEROXIDE (H_2O_2) to water, while oxidising another substrate. A relatively thermostable enzyme, frequently used as an index of the efficacy of BLANCHING of fruits and vegetables.

peroxide Any compound with the peroxy (—O—O—) group; atmospheric oxidation of unsaturated FATTY ACIDS produces peroxides. Also used to mean specifically HYDROGEN PEROXIDE (H_2O_2).

peroxide number Or peroxide value; a measure of the oxidative rancidity of fats by determination of the lipid peroxides present.

perry Fermented PEAR juice (in UK may include not more than 25% apple juice) analogous to CIDER from apples. Sparkling perry is sometimes known as champagne perry.

Persian apple *See* CITRON.

Persian berry Yellow colour obtained from the berries of the buckthorn, *Rhamnus* spp.; legally permitted in food in most countries. Contains the glucosides of rhamnetin and rhamnazin.

persimmon Fruit of *Diospyros virginiana* (American persimmon or Virginia date) and *D. kaki* (Japanese persimmon, date plum, kaki or sharon fruit). Kaki may be eaten raw or cooked; American persimmon develops a sour flavour if cooked.

American, composition/100 g: (edible portion 82%) water 64 g, 532 kJ (127 kcal), protein 0.8 g, fat 0.4 g, carbohydrate 33.5 g, ash 0.9 g, Ca 27 mg, Fe 2.5 mg, P 26 mg, K 310 mg, Na 1 mg, vitamin C 66 mg. A 25 g serving (1 fruit) is a good source of vitamin C.

Japanese, composition/100 g: (edible portion 84%) water 80 g, 293 kJ (70 kcal), protein 0.6 g, fat 0.2 g, carbohydrate 18.6 g (12.5 g sugars), fibre 3.6 g, ash 0.3 g, Ca 8 mg, Fe 0.2 mg, Mg 9 mg, P 17 mg, K 161 mg, Na 1 mg, Zn 0.1 mg, Cu 0.1 mg, Mn 0.4 mg, Se 0.6 µg, vitamin A 81 µg RE (2693 µg carotenoids), E 0.7 mg, K

2.6 mg, B$_1$ 0.03 mg, B$_2$ 0.02 mg, niacin 0.1 mg, B$_6$ 0.1 mg, folate 8 μg, C 8 mg. An 80 g serving (half fruit) is a source of Mn.

pervaporation Evaporation from a colloidal suspension (*see* COLLOID) by heating in a bag made from a semipermeable membrane. If there are crystalloids present, they pass through the membrane and are deposited on the outside of the bag.

pescetarian A partial VEGETARIAN who will eat fish but not meat.

PET Polyethylene terephthalate; clear plastic used in packaging, especially bottles for drinks; biodegradable within about 8 weeks when composted.

PETscan *See* POSITRON EMISSION TOMOGRAPHY SCANNING.

petechiae Small round, flat, dark red spots caused by bleeding into the skin or under mucous membrane; occur in VITAMIN C deficiency as a result of capillary fragility.

pétillant French; lightly sparkling wines.

petit-grain oils Prepared from twigs and leaves of the bitter ORANGE by steam distillation; similar to NEROLI OIL but less fragrant. Petit-grain Portugal prepared from leaves of sweet orange, mandarin petit-grain from TANGERINE leaves, and lemon petit-grain from LEMON leaves.

Petrifilm^{TM} **plates** Laminated plastic film containing dehydrated nutrients for bacterial culture, as an alternative to traditional agar plates.

Peyer's patches Oval masses of lymphoid tissue in the small intestinal mucous membrane, responsible for the production of lymphocytes (white BLOOD CELLS) and antibodies.

PGA Pteroylglutamic acid, *see* FOLIC ACID.

PGPR Polyglycerol polyricinoleate, used as an emulsifying agent in CHOCOLATE manufacture.

pH Potential hydrogen, measurement of acidity or alkalinity on a logarithmic scale. Defined as the negative logarithm of the hydrogen ion concentration. The scale runs from 0, which is very strongly acidic, to 14, which is very strongly alkaline. Pure water is pH 7, which is neutral; below 7 is acid, above is alkaline.

See also BUFFER.

phaeophytin Brownish-green derivative of CHLOROPHYLL, caused by the loss of MAGNESIUM in acid conditions. The formation of phaeophytin accounts for the colour change when green vegetables are cooked.

phage *See* BACTERIOPHAGE.

phagomania Morbid obsession with food; also known as sitomania.

phagophobia Fear of food; also known as sitophobia.

pharmafoods Alternative name for FUNCTIONAL FOODS.

phase inversion   CREAM is an emulsion of fat in water; BUTTER is an emulsion of water in fat. The change from cream to butter is termed phase inversion.

phase transition   Transition between solid and fluid states. Fluids (gases, liquids and particulate solids) flow under pressure; solids are deformed.

phase I metabolism   The first phase of metabolism of foreign compounds (xenobiotics), involving metabolic activation such as hydroxylation (catalysed by CYTOCHROMES P$_{450}$), deacylation, etc. Generally regarded as detoxication reactions, but may in fact convert inactive precursors into metabolically active compounds, and involved in activation of precursors to carcinogens.

phase II metabolism   The second phase of the metabolism of foreign compounds, in which the activated derivatives formed in PHASE I METABOLISM are conjugated with amino acids (e.g. glycine, alanine), GLUCURONIC ACID or GLUTATHIONE, to yield water-soluble derivatives that can be excreted in the urine or bile.

phaseolin   Globulin protein in kidney or haricot BEAN (*Phaseolus vulgaris*).

phaseolunatin   Cyanogenic (cyanide-forming) GLUCOSIDE found in certain LEGUMES (such as lima bean, chick pea, common vetch), which hydrolyses to glucose, acetone and hydrocyanic acid; not proven harmful when present in the diet.

phasin   Originally the LECTIN from the bean *Phaseolus vulgaris*, now used for non-toxic plant lectins in general.

PHB ester   *See* PARABENS.

pheasant   GAME bird, *Phasianus colchicus* and related species. Total weight 1.5 kg; traditionally sold as brace, i.e. cock and hen, although now commonly available as single birds; usually hung 3 days (up to 3 weeks in very cold weather) to develop flavour.

Composition/100 g: (edible portion 76%) water 72.8 g, 557 kJ (133 kcal), protein 23.6 g, fat 3.6 g (of which 40% saturated, 40% mono-unsaturated, 20% polyunsaturated), cholesterol 66 mg, carbohydrate 0 g, ash 1.4 g, Ca 13 mg, Fe 1.1 mg, Mg 20 mg, P 230 mg, K 262 mg, Na 37 mg, Zn 1 mg, Cu 0.1 mg, Se 16.2 µg, vitamin A 50 µg retinol, B$_1$ 0.08 mg, B$_2$ 0.15 mg, niacin 6.8 mg, B$_6$ 0.74 mg, folate 6 µg, B$_{12}$ 0.8 µg, pantothenate 1 mg, C 6 mg. A 100 g serving is a source of pantothenate, a good source of P, Se, a rich source of niacin, vitamin B$_6$, B$_{12}$.

phenetylurea   *See* DULCIN.

phenol oxidases   Group of enzymes that oxidise phenols to quinones, which then undergo non-enzymic polymerisation to red-brown pigments.

Tyrosinase (monophenol oxidase, EC 1.14.18.1) is a copper-dependent enzyme in mammalian tissues, responsible for formation of melanin.

Polyphenol oxidase (catechol oxidase, laccase EC 1.10.3.2) is a calcium-dependent enzyme responsible for browning of cut fruit and vegetables. It acts on catechols and other polyphenols, including FLAVONOIDS. Inhibited by chelating compounds such as EDTA, also by SULPHITES and CYSTEINE.

phenolphthalein *See* LAXATIVES.

phentermine An anorectic (appetite suppressant) drug formerly used in the treatment of obesity, especially in combination with FENFLURAMINE (fen-phen); withdrawn in 1995 in response to reports of heart valve damage.

phenylalanine An essential AMINO ACID; abbr Phe (F), M_r 165.2, pK_a 2.16, 9.18, codons UUPy. In addition to its role in protein synthesis, it is the metabolic precursor of the non-essential amino acid TYROSINE (and hence NORADRENALINE, ADRENALINE and the THYROID HORMONES). Tyrosine in the diet spares phenylalanine, so reducing the requirement.

*o***-phenylene diamine** Reagent used for determination of total VITAMIN C after oxidation to dehydroascorbic acid with iodine; forms a fluorescent quinoxaline derivative with dehydroascorbic acid.

phenylethylamine The AMINE formed by decarboxylation of the amino acid PHENYLALANINE.

phenylisothiocyanate *See* EDMAN REAGENT.

phenylketonuria A GENETIC DISEASE affecting the metabolism of PHENYLALANINE. Phenylalanine is normally metabolised to TYROSINE, catalysed by phenylalanine hydroxylase (EC 1.14.16.1). Impairment of this reaction leads to a considerable accumulation of phenylalanine in plasma and tissues (up to 100 times the normal concentration) and metabolism to phenylpyruvate, phenyllactate and phenylacetate, collectively known as phenylketones, which are excreted in the urine. The very high plasma concentration of phenylalanine causes disruption of brain development, and if untreated there is severe mental retardation.

Infants are screened for phenylketonuria shortly after birth (by measurement of plasma phenylalanine); treatment is by very strict limitation of phenylalanine intake, only providing sufficient to meet requirements for protein synthesis. Once brain development is complete (between the ages of 8 and 12 years), dietary restriction can be relaxed to a considerable extent, since high concentrations of phenylalanine seem to have little adverse effect on the developed brain. There may, however, be benefits

from continuing dietary restriction into adult life, and phenylke-
tonuric women require extremely careful dietary control through
pregnancy to avoid severe damage to the fetus's developing
brain.

phenylthiohydantoin Reacts with the amino group of AMINO
ACIDS; used in separation of amino acids by thin-layer CHRO-
MATOGRAPHY, and for detection in HIGH-PERFORMANCE LIQUID
CHROMATOGRAPHY.

pheophorbide Product of strong acid hydrolysis of CHLOROPHYLL;
both the chelated Mg^{2+} ion and the phytol side chain are lost.
See also CHLOROPHYLLIDE; PHEOPHYTIN.

pheophytin Brown pigment produced from CHLOROPHYLL by
removal of the Mg^{2+} ion in dilute acid.
See also CHLOROPHYLLIDE; PHEOPHORBIDE.

phitosite High-calorie food.

phlorizin (phloridzin) A glucoside from the roots and bark of
various *Rosaceae* spp. that inhibits the renal tubular reabsorption of glucose. Formerly used as an experimental model of DIA-
BETES mellitus, but it causes glucosuria and hence hypoglycaemia,
rather than the hyperglycaemia and subsequent glucosuria seen
in uncontrolled diabetes.

phosphatase test A test for the adequacy of PASTEURISATION of
milk. The enzyme phosphatase (EC 3.1.3.x), normally present in
milk, is denatured at a temperature slightly higher than that
required to destroy most pathogens; therefore the presence of
detectable phosphatase activity indicates inadequate pasteurisation. The test can detect 0.2% raw milk in pasteurised milk.

phosphate additives *See* POLYPHOSPHATES.

phosphates Salts of PHOSPHORIC ACID; the form in which the
element PHOSPHORUS is normally present in foods and body
tissues.
See also POLYPHOSPHATES.

phosphatides *See* PHOSPHOLIPIDS.

phosphatidic acid Glycerol esterified with two molecules of fatty
acid, with the third hydroxyl group esterified to phosphate;
chemically diacylglycerol phosphate; intermediates in the metabolism of PHOSPHOLIPIDS.

phosphatidylcholine A PHOSPHOLIPID containing CHOLINE; *see*
LECITHIN.

phosphatidylethanolamine A PHOSPHOLIPID containing
ETHANOLAMINE.

phosphatidylinositol A PHOSPHOLIPID containing INOSITOL.

phosphatidylserine A PHOSPHOLIPID containing SERINE.

phospholipids (phosphatides, phospholipins) Glycerol esterified
to two molecules of FATTY ACID, one of which is usually a polyun-

saturated fatty acid. The third hydroxyl group is esterified to phosphate and one of a number of water-soluble compounds, including SERINE (phosphatidylserine), ETHANOLAMINE (phosphatidylethanolamine), CHOLINE (phosphatidylcholine, also known as LECITHIN) and INOSITOL (phosphatidylinositol).

Cell membranes are a double layer of phospholipids with the fatty acid side-chains on the inside. The water-soluble compound esterified to the phosphate interacts with water. This is why phospholipids can be used to emulsify oils and fats in water and are commonly used in food manufacture as EMULSIFIERS. From the energy point of view they can be regarded as being equivalent to simple fats (TRIACYLGLYCEROLS); they also provide a source of choline and inositol, neither of which is a dietary essential.

phosphoproteins Proteins containing phosphate, other than as NUCLEIC ACIDS (nucleoproteins) or PHOSPHOLIPIDS (lipoproteins), e.g. CASEIN from milk, ovovitellin from egg yolk.

phosphoric acid May be one of three types, orthophosphoric acid (H_3PO_4), metaphosphoric acid (HPO_3) or pyrophosphoric acid ($H_4P_2O_7$). Orthophosphoric acid and its salts are E-338–341, used as ACIDITY REGULATORS and in acid-fruit-flavoured beverages such as lemonade.

phosphorus An essential element, occurring in tissues and foods as phosphate (salts of PHOSPHORIC ACID), PHOSPHOLIPIDS and phosphoproteins. In the body most (80%) is present in the skeleton and teeth as HYDROXYAPATITE; the remainder is in the phospholipids of cell membranes, in NUCLEIC ACIDS and in a variety of metabolic intermediates, including ATP.

The parathyroid glands (*see* PARATHYROID HORMONE) control the concentration of phosphate in the blood, mainly by modifying its excretion in the urine. Human dietary needs (about 1.3 g per day) are almost always met; deficiency rarely occurs in adults. The CALCIUM:phosphate ratio of infant foods is, however, important.

Phosphate deficiency is common in livestock and gives rise to OSTEOMALACIA (also known as sweeny or creeping sickness). Phosphate is also essential for plant growth, hence the use of inorganic phosphate or bone meal as fertiliser.

phosphorylase Enzyme (EC 2.4.1.1) responsible for the breakdown of glycogen and starch to glucose 1-phosphate. In vegetables associated with formation of sugars during ripening and on storage. Important in potatoes during storage because it remains active at low temperatures whereas enzymes of GLYCOLYSIS are cold labile, so that sugars accumulate rather than being utilised.

photon absorptiometry Technique for determination of BONE density, as an index of CALCIUM and VITAMIN D status.

photosynthesis Sequence of reactions, most commonly in plants, but also in some micro-organisms, that leads to synthesis of carbohydrates by reduction of carbon dioxide using light as the primary energy source. Considered in two separate reaction sequences: the light phase, in which light energy is captured by CAROTENOIDS, and transferred to CHLOROPHYLL, leading, via an electron transport chain, to the reduction of $NADP^+$ to NADPH and the synthesis of ATP from ADP and phosphate; the dark phase in which NADPH and ATP are used to reduce carbon dioxide to glucose.

There are two separate pathways for the dark phase reaction: the C3 pathway (Calvin cycle), in which phosphoglyceric acid is the first product of CO_2 fixation, and the C4 pathway (Hatch and Slack pathway), in which four-carbon dicarboxylic acids are the first products of CO_2 fixation. Both pathways may occur together in some plants; the C4 pathway is found especially in maize, sorghum, sugar cane and tropical grasses growing under high light intensity where water is scarce.

phrynoderma Blocked pores or 'toad-skin' (follicular hyperkeratosis of the skin) often encountered in malnourished people. Originally thought to be due to VITAMIN A deficiency but possibly due to other deficiencies, and also occurs mildly in adequately nourished people.

phthisis Obsolete name for any disease resulting in wasting of tissues; *see* CACHEXIA; PROTEIN–ENERGY MALNUTRITION.

phulka *See* CHAPPATI.

phycotoxins Marine biotoxins that accumulate in fish and shellfish from their diet (causing PARALYTIC SHELLFISH POISONING and CIGUATERA poisoning when the fish are eaten), as distinct from toxins naturally present (tetramine poisoning).

phyllo pastry (filo pastry) Plain paper-thin pastry made from flour and water, rolled into small balls then tossed in the air and stretched until it forms an extremely thin sheet. Multiple layers are used as the basis for Greek and Middle-Eastern pastry dishes. Known as mortoban in south-east Asia.

phylloquinone *See* VITAMIN K.

phylloxera An aphid which threatened to destroy the vineyards of Europe in the middle of the 19th century. They were saved by grafting susceptible varieties onto resistant American vine rootstock.

physalin A CAROTENOID, zeaxanthin dipalmitate, in the fruits of the CAPE GOOSEBERRY, *Physalis* spp.

Physalis *See* CAPE GOOSEBERRY.

physical activity level (PAL) Total ENERGY cost of physical activity throughout the day, expressed as a ratio of BASAL METABOLIC

RATE. Calculated from the PHYSICAL ACTIVITY RATIO for each activity, multiplied by the time spent in that activity. A desirable PAL for health is considered to be 1.7; the average in UK is 1.4.

physical activity ratio (PAR)   ENERGY cost of physical activity expressed as a ratio of BASAL METABOLIC RATE.

physin   Name given to a growth factor in liver, later identified as VITAMIN B$_{12}$.

physiological saline   A solution of sodium chloride that is isotonic with blood plasma, 0.15 mol/L (9 g/L).

phytase   Enzyme (inositol hexahydrate phosphohydrolase, EC 3.1.3.26) that hydrolyses PHYTATE to inositol mono- to tetrakis-phosphates (tetraphosphates), which do not chelate minerals, and free phosphate. Occurs in cereal grains, where it is activated by soaking or during germination and malting. Added to poultry feed to increase availability of PHOSPHATE; main commercial source is *Aspergillus* spp., but also expressed in genetically modified rapeseed, tobacco and tomato seeds.

phytic acid (phytate)   INOSITOL hexaphosphate, present in cereals, particularly in the bran, dried legumes and some nuts as both water-soluble salts (sodium and potassium) and insoluble salts of calcium and magnesium. Magnesium calcium phytate is phytin. Can bind calcium, iron and zinc to form insoluble complexes; it is not clear how far phytate reduces the availability of these minerals in the diet, especially since there is PHYTASE in yeast and legumes (and possibly in the human gut) which may liberate these minerals.

phytin   Magnesium calcium PHYTIC ACID, approximately 12% calcium, 1.5% magnesium and 22% phosphorus.

phytoagglutinins   *See* LECTINS.

phytoalexins   Compounds produced by plants under conditions of stress or in response to mechanical or fungal damage which may be toxic, or induce adverse reactions, when the plants are consumed.

phytochromes   Also known as florigens. Photosensitive polypeptides with a tetrapyrrole prosthetic group, responsible for day-length sensitivity in plants, and possibly also enhanced germination of seeds that have been vernalised (chilled to 4 °C). The protein undergoes a conformational change on exposure to red light (660 nm) and the reverse change on exposure to infrared (735 nm).

phytoestrogens   Polyphenols (*see* FLAVONOIDS) found in a variety of plant foods that have OESTROGEN activity.

phytohaemagglutinins   *See* LECTINS.

phytoncides   *See* PACIFICARINS.

phytoplankton   *See* PLANKTON.

phytosterol General name given to sterols occurring in plants, the chief of which is SITOSTEROL.

phytotoxin Any poisonous substance produced by a plant. *See also* ALKALOIDS.

phytylmenaquinone *See* VITAMIN K.

pica An unnatural desire for foods; alternative words, cissa, cittosis and allotriophagy. Also a perverted appetite (eating of earth, sand, clay, paper, etc.).

piccalilli Mixture of chopped, brine-preserved vegetables in mustard sauce.

pickling Also called BRINING. Vegetables immersed in 5–10% salt solution (brine) undergo lactic acid fermentation, while the salt prevents the growth of undesirable organisms. The sugars in the vegetables are converted to lactic acid; at 25 °C the process takes a few weeks, finishing at 1% acidity.

See also HALOPHILES; MEAT, CURING.

pidan *See* EGGS, CHINESE.

pigeon *Columba livia*; young about four weeks old is squab.

Composition/100 g: (edible portion 65%) water 72.8 g, 594 kJ (142 kcal), protein 17.5 g, fat 7.5 g (of which 32% saturated, 43% mono-unsaturated, 25% polyunsaturated), cholesterol 90 mg, carbohydrate 0 g, ash 1.2 g, Ca 13 mg, Fe 4.5 mg, Mg 25 mg, P 307 mg, K 237 mg, Na 51 mg, Zn 2.7 mg, Cu 0.6 mg, Se 13.5 µg, vitamin A 28 µg retinol, B_1 0.28 mg, B_2 0.28 mg, niacin 6.9 mg, B_6 0.53 mg, folate 7 µg, B_{12} 0.5 µg, pantothenate 0.8 mg, C 7 mg. A 100 g serving is a source of Se, Zn, vitamin B_2, pantothenate, C, a good source of vitamin B_1, B_6, a rich source of Cu, Fe, P, niacin, vitamin B_{12}.

pigeon pea Tropical LEGUME, *Cajanus cajan*, also known as red gram.

Composition/100 g: water 10.6 g, 1436 kJ (343 kcal), protein 21.7 g, fat 1.5 g (of which 27% saturated, 0% mono-unsaturated, 73% polyunsaturated), carbohydrate 62.8 g, fibre 15 g, ash 3.5 g, Ca 130 mg, Fe 5.2 mg, Mg 183 mg, P 367 mg, K 1392 mg, Na 17 mg, Zn 2.8 mg, Cu 1.1 mg, Mn 1.8 mg, Se 8.2 µg, vitamin A 1 µg RE, B_1 0.64 mg, B_2 0.19 mg, niacin 3 mg, B_6 0.28 mg, folate 456 µg, pantothenate 1.3 mg. An 85 g serving is a source of Ca, Zn, niacin, vitamin B_6, pantothenate, a rich source of Cu, Fe, Mg, Mn, P, vitamin B_1, folate.

pignoli (pignolias, pinoli) *See* PINENUTS.

pig nut *See* EARTH NUT.

pike Freshwater FISH, *Esox lucius*.

pilchard Oily FISH, *Sardina (Clupea) pilchardus*; young is the SARDINE.

piles *See* HAEMORRHOIDS.

pils Pale type of lager originally made in Czechoslovakia. *See* BEER.

pimaricin *See* NATAMYCIN.

pimento *See* ALLSPICE.

pimiento *See* PEPPER, SWEET.

Pimms™ A ready-mixed cocktail, based on spirits, flavoured with herbs and liqueurs, normally served as a long drink with ice and soda or lemonade, garnished with fruit, cucumber or mint. Originally there were four varieties: No. 1 based on gin, No. 2 whisky, No. 3 brandy, No. 4 rum; only No. 1, now based on vodka, survives.

pimpernel *See* BURNET.

pin and disc mill *See* DISC MILL.

pinang *See* BETEL.

pineapple Fruit of the tropical plant *Ananas sativus*, one of the bromeliad family. The fruit contains the proteolytic enzyme bromelain (EC 3.4.22.23), which has been used (like PAPAIN) to tenderise meat.

Composition/100 g: (edible portion 52%) water 87 g, 201 kJ (48 kcal), protein 0.5 g, fat 0.1 g, carbohydrate 12.6 g (9.3 g sugars), fibre 1.4 g, ash 0.2 g, Ca 13 mg, Fe 0.3 mg, Mg 12 mg, P 8 mg, K 115 mg, Na 1 mg, Zn 0.1 mg, Cu 0.1 mg, Mn 1.2 mg, Se 0.1 µg, vitamin A 3 µg RE (34 µg carotenoids), K 0.7 mg, B_1 0.08 mg, B_2 0.03 mg, niacin 0.5 mg, B_6 0.11 mg, folate 15 µg, pantothenate 0.2 mg, C 36 mg. An 80 g serving (1 slice) is a rich source of Mn, vitamin C.

pinenuts Or pine kernels, edible seeds of various species of pine cone, especially Mediterranean stone pine, *Pinus pinea*.

Composition/100 g: (edible portion 57%) water 5.9 g, 2633 kJ (629 kcal), protein 11.6 g, fat 61 g (of which 16% saturated, 39% mono-unsaturated, 44% polyunsaturated), carbohydrate 19.3 g, fibre 10.7 g, ash 2.3 g, Ca 8 mg, Fe 3.1 mg, Mg 234 mg, P 35 mg, K 628 mg, Na 72 mg, Zn 4.3 mg, Cu 1 mg, Mn 4.3 mg, vitamin A 1 µg RE, B_1 1.24 mg, B_2 0.22 mg, niacin 4.4 mg, B_6 0.11 mg, folate 58 µg, pantothenate 0.2 mg, C 2 mg.

pinking Of pickled onions, the development of pink discoloration, eventually darkening to brown, as a result of reaction between the onions and trace amounts of aldehydes in the acetic acid used in PICKLING.

pinnochio *See* PINENUTS.

pint, reputed 13 1/3 fluid oz = 285 mL; half a reputed quart.

pinworm Or threadworm; parasitic nematode worm (*Enterobius* and *Oxyuris* spp.) in upper part of large intestine.

pipe Cask for wine; the volume varies with the type of wine: port, 115 gallons (517 L); Tenerife, 100 gal (450 L); Marsala, 90 gal (418 L).

pipis Edible MOLLUSC, *Plebidonas deltoides*, widely distributed around Australian coastline.

piri-piri Small red peppers (*see* PEPPER, CHILLI), 1 cm long, extremely pungent. Also (Portuguese) sauce made from the peppers.

pirogi Russian; small baked pasties of yeast dough filled with chopped fish, meat, etc.

pistachio Fruit of *Pistacchio vera*; yellow-green coloured nut. May be roasted and salted or used as flavouring for ice-cream and (Indian) hot sweet milk beverage.

Composition/100 g: (edible portion 53%) water 4 g, 2332 kJ (557 kcal), protein 20.6 g, fat 44.4 g (of which 13% saturated, 55% mono-unsaturated, 32% polyunsaturated), carbohydrate 28 g (7.6 g sugars), fibre 10.3 g, ash 3 g, Ca 107 mg, Fe 4.2 mg, Mg 121 mg, P 490 mg, K 1025 mg, Na 1 mg, Zn 2.2 mg, Cu 1.3 mg, Mn 1.2 mg, Se 7 μg, vitamin A 28 μg RE (332 μg carotenoids), E 2.3 mg, B_1 0.87 mg, B_2 0.16 mg, niacin 1.3 mg, B_6 1.7 mg, folate 51 μg, pantothenate 0.5 mg, C 5 mg. A 25 g serving is a source of Mn, P, vitamin B_1, a good source of Cu, vitamin B_6.

pita (pitta) Middle Eastern; flat bread, made by sour dough process and baked at a high temperature for a short time, as an oval or circle, which can be opened up as an envelope. Also known as pocket, balady or burr bread.

pitanga Surinam cherry, *Eugenia uniflora* or *E. michelii*; small round fruit, deeply ribbed, cherry-like with single stone.

Composition/100 g: (edible portion 88%) water 91 g, 138 kJ (33 kcal), protein 0.8 g, fat 0.4 g, carbohydrate 7.5 g, ash 0.5 g, Ca 9 mg, Fe 0.2 mg, Mg 12 mg, P 11 mg, K 103 mg, Na 3 mg, vitamin A 75 μg RE, B_1 0.03 mg, B_2 0.04 mg, niacin 0.3 mg, C 26 mg.

pitaya (pitahaya) Fruit of various cacti, especially *Hylocereus* and *Selenicereus* spp.

pith *See* ALBEDO.

pits Stones from cherries, plums, peaches, apricots. Oil extracted from these pits is used in cosmetics and pharmaceuticals, for canning sardines and as table oil. The press cake left behind contains AMYGDALIN.

pitting (1) Removing the stones (pits) from cherries, olives, etc.

(2) Collapse of the structure of fruit tissue caused by low-temperature dehydration. *See also* CHILLING INJURY.

pivka Obsolete name for preprothrombin (protein induced by vitamin K absence), the undercarboxylated precursor of PRO-THROMBIN, released into the circulation in VITAMIN K deficiency. May be measured by immunoassay as a sensitive index of vitamin K status.

pizza Originally Italian; savoury tart on a base of yeast dough, traditionally cooked in a wood-burning oven. The topping varies with region and may contain tomatoes, cheese, salami or seafood.

placebo Inactive substance used as a control in trials of drugs, etc., in order to ensure that any response observed is due to the compound under test and not simply the result of an intervention.

plaice FLATFISH, *Pleuronectus platessa*.

plankton Microscopic organisms, both plants (phytoplankton) and animals (zooplankton), drifting in the sea, which are the basis of the marine food chain.

plansifter A nest of sieves mounted together so that material being sieved is divided into a number of fractions of different size. Widely used in flour milling.

plantago *See* PSYLLIUM.

plantain Or Adam's fig; variety of BANANA (*Musa* spp.) with higher starch and lower sugar content than dessert bananas, picked when flesh is too hard to be eaten raw and therefore cooked. Some varieties become sweet if left to ripen, others never develop a high sugar content.

Composition/100 g: (edible portion 65%) water 65 g, 511 kJ (122 kcal), protein 1.3 g, fat 0.4 g, carbohydrate 31.9 g (15 g sugars), fibre 2.3 g, ash 1.2 g, Ca 3 mg, Fe 0.6 mg, Mg 37 mg, P 34 mg, K 499 mg, Na 4 mg, Zn 0.1 mg, Cu 0.1 mg, Se 1.5 µg, vitamin A 56 µg RE (925 µg carotenoids), E 0.1 mg, K 0.7 mg, B_1 0.05 mg, B_2 0.05 mg, niacin 0.7 mg, B_6 0.3 mg, folate 22 µg, pantothenate 0.3 mg, C 18 mg. A 200 g serving is a source of Cu, vitamin A, a good source of Mg, folate, a rich source of vitamin B_6, C.

plaque (1) Dental plaque is a layer of bacteria in an organic matrix on the surface of teeth, especially around the neck of each tooth. May lead to development of gingivitis, PERIODONTAL disease and caries.

(2) Atherosclerotic plaque (*see* ATHEROSCLEROSIS) is the development of fatty streaks in the intima of blood vessels.

plasma, blood *See* BLOOD PLASMA.

plasmid Small circular region of extrachromosomal bacterial DNA, which has an origin of replication and is therefore maintained in a cell line. Especially amenable to the introduction of foreign genes, and widely used in genetic engineering. Between 5 and 90 kb in size.

plasminogen Inactive precursor of plasmin in the bloodstream; activation to plasmin is important in the lysis of blood clots.

plastic fluids Those that do not flow until a critical SHEAR STRESS is achieved, when the shear rate is either linear (Bingham-type) or non-linear (Casson-type).

plasticiser Chemical added to plastic films to make them more flexible.

plate count To estimate the number of bacteria in a sample, it is poured on to an AGAR plate, when each bacterial cell multiplies to produce a colony of bacteria which is visible to the naked eye. A count of the number of colonies gives the number of bacteria in the portion of the sample that was taken. Pasteurised milk contains about 100 000 bacteria/mL; good quality raw milk contains less than 500 000/mL.

PLC Programmable logic controllers; computer-based systems for controlling manufacturing processes.

plethysmography Technique for determination of body volume by immersion in water, for estimation of body fat (*see* BODY DENSITY).

Pliofilm^{TM} Rubber hydrochloride, the first transparent wrapping paper (1934) that could be heat sealed.

pluck Butchers' term for heart, liver and lungs of an animal.

plum Fruit of various *Prunus* spp. Common European plums are *P. domestica*; blackthorn or sloe is *P. spinosa*; bullace is *P. insititia*; damson is *P. damascena*; GREENGAGES are *P. italica*. The UK National Fruit Collection contains 336 varieties.

Composition/100 g: (edible portion 94%) water 87 g, 193 kJ (46 kcal), protein 0.7 g, fat 0.3 g, carbohydrate 11.4 g (9.9 g sugars), fibre 1.4 g, ash 0.4 g, Ca 6 mg, Fe 0.2 mg, Mg 7 mg, P 16 mg, K 157 mg, Zn 0.1 mg, Cu 0.1 mg, Mn 0.1 mg, vitamin A 17 μg RE (298 μg carotenoids), E 0.3 mg, K 6.4 mg, B_1 0.03 mg, B_2 0.03 mg, niacin 0.4 mg, B_6 0.03 mg, folate 5 μg, pantothenate 0.1 mg, C 10 mg. A 110 g serving (2 fruits) is a source of vitamin C.

plumcote American; cross between plum and apricot.

pneumatic conveying Transfer of material in powder form by means of air currents. Applied to flour, sugar, etc.

pneumatic dryers The material is dried almost instantaneously in a turbulent stream of hot air, which also acts as a conveyor system. Applicable to powdered, granular and flaky materials; used for starch, mashed potato, cereals, flour, powdered soups, etc.

poi Polynesian, Hawaiian; paste made from pounded TARO, often allowed to ferment, eaten with meat, fish and vegetables.

Composition/100 g: water 71.6 g, 469 kJ (112 kcal), protein 0.4 g, fat 0.1 g, carbohydrate 27.2 g (0.4 g sugars), fibre 0.4 g, ash 0.6 g, Ca 16 mg, Fe 0.9 mg, Mg 24 mg, P 39 mg, K 183 mg, Na 12 mg, Zn 0.2 mg, Cu 0.2 mg, Mn 0.4 mg, Se 0.7 μg, vitamin A 3 μg RE (48 μg carotenoids), E 2.3 mg, K 1 mg, B_1 0.13 mg, B_2 0.04 mg, niacin 1.1 mg, B_6 0.27 mg, folate 21 μg, pantothenate 0.3 mg, C 4 mg.

polarimeter, polariscope Instrument used to determine the degree of rotation of POLARISED LIGHT, as a means of measuring concentrations of OPTICALLY ACTIVE compounds.

polarised light Ordinary light vibrates in many planes; after passing through a crystal of quartz or a polarising filter, it vibrates in only one plane, i.e. it is polarised.

Polenske number Measure of the water-soluble fatty acids in a lipid that are not steam volatile.

> See also KIRSCHNER NUMBER; REICHERT–MEISSL NUMBER; STEAM DISTILLATION.

polenta Traditional Italian porridge made from maize meal, often with cheese added. May be further cooked by baking or frying. Also Italian name for coarsely ground maize meal (called hominy grits in USA).

policosanols Long-chain (C24–30) aliphatic alcohols from hydrolysis of sugar cane wax, that lower LDL cholesterol, increase HDL, prevent platelet aggregation and may inhibit foam cell formation from macrophages. Trade name Ateromixol.

pollack (pollock) White FISH, *Pollachius virens*, also known as coalfish.

pollards *See* WHEATFEED.

polony Italian smoked pork and veal sausage, ready to slice and eat; also known as bologna.

polydextrose, modified A randomly bonded GLUCOSE polymer prepared by heating glucose and SORBITOL with citric acid. It is more resistant to enzymic digestion than normal POLYSACCHARIDES and 60% is excreted undigested, so providing only about 4 kJ (1 kcal)/g; hence termed 'non-sweetening sucrose replacement', or BULKING AGENT.

polydipsia Abnormally intense thirst; a typical symptom of DIABETES mellitus and insipidus.

polygalacturonase *See* PECTINASE.

polyglucose *See* POLYDEXTROSE.

polymerase chain reaction (PCR) An *in vitro* method for rapid amplification of specific DNA sequences. Starting from minute amounts of DNA, repetitive cycles of template denaturation, primer annealing and the extension of the annealed primers by DNA polymerase result in the exponential accumulation of the DNA; 10^6-fold in 20 cycles, each of which takes 4 min.

The basis of DNA fingerprinting techniques, and widely used for rapid identification of potentially pathogenic organisms in foods.

polymer in oil An index of degradation of oil used in frying by the formation of viscous polymers of lipids due to heating and oxidation.

polymorphism (1) The ability to crystallise in two or more different forms. For example, depending on the conditions under which it is solidified, the fat tristearin can form three kinds of crystal, each with a different melting point: 54, 65, 71 °C.

(2) Genetic polymorphism is the relatively widespread occurrence in the population of one or more variants of a gene.

polymyxins Antibiotics isolated from *Bacillus polymyxin* (*B. aerosporin*); polymyxin A is aerosporin. They are polypeptides, active against coliform bacteria; apart from clinical use, they are of value in controlling infection in brewing.

polyneuritis Any disease involving inflammation of all of the peripheral nerves.

See also POLYNEUROPATHY.

polyneuropathy Any disease involving all of the peripheral nerves; symptoms first affect the extremities (fingers and toes), then ascend towards the trunk. Occurs in BERIBERI due to VITAMIN B$_1$ deficiency.

See also POLYNEURITIS.

polyols *See* SUGAR ALCOHOLS.

polyoxyethylene *See* CRUMB SOFTENERS.

polypeptides *See* PEPTIDES.

polyphagia Excessive or continuous eating.

polyphenol oxidase *See* PHENOL OXIDASES.

polyphosphates Complex PHOSPHATES added to foods as EMULSIFIERS, BUFFERS, SEQUESTRANTS, to prevent discoloration of sausages, aid mixing of the fat, speed penetration of the brine in curing, hold water in meat and fish products. E-450a, b, c and E-541, 544, 545.

polysaccharides Complex CARBOHYDRATES formed by the condensation of large numbers of MONOSACCHARIDE units, e.g. STARCH, GLYCOGEN, CELLULOSE, DEXTRINS, INULIN. Formerly called polysaccharoses. Collectively, polysaccharides other than starch and dextrins are known as NON-STARCH POLYSACCHARIDES, a major component of DIETARY FIBRE.

polysome An array of several RIBOSOMES along a molecule of mRNA, engaged in the process of TRANSLATION.

polysorbates *See* CRUMB SOFTENERS.

polyunsaturates *See* FATTY ACIDS, POLYUNSATURATED.

polyuria Production of a large volume of dilute urine; may be due simply to high fluid intake, or to kidney disease or DIABETES mellitus or insipidus.

pomace Residue of fruit pulp after expressing juice; also applied to fish from which oil has been expressed.

pombé African BEER brewed from millet.

POMC *See* PRO-OPIOMELANOCORTIN.

pomegranate The fruit of the subtropical tree *Punica granatum*. Juice contained in a pulpy sac surrounding each of a mass of seeds; outer skin contains tannin and is therefore bitter. Sweet juice used to prepare grenadine SYRUP for alcoholic and fruit drinks.

Composition/100 g: (edible portion 56%) water 81 g, 285 kJ (68 kcal), protein 0.9 g, fat 0.3 g, carbohydrate 17.2 g (16.6 g sugars), fibre 0.6 g, ash 0.6 g, Ca 3 mg, Fe 0.3 mg, Mg 3 mg, P 8 mg, K 259 mg, Na 3 mg, Zn 0.1 mg, Cu 0.1 mg, Se 0.6 µg, vitamin A 5 µg RE (90 µg carotenoids), E 0.6 mg, K 4.6 mg, B_1 0.03 mg, B_2 0.03 mg, niacin 0.3 mg, B_6 0.1 mg, folate 6 µg, pantothenate 0.6 mg, C 6 mg. A 150 g serving (1 fruit) is a source of Cu, pantothenate, vitamin C.

pomelo (pomeloe, pummelo) A CITRUS fruit, fruit of *Citrus grandis*, from which the GRAPEFRUIT is descended; also called shaddock, after Captain Shaddock, who introduced it into Barbados in the 16th century.

Composition/100 g: (edible portion 56%) water 89 g, 159 kJ (38 kcal), protein 0.8 g, fat 0 g, carbohydrate 9.6 g, fibre 1 g, ash 0.5 g, Ca 4 mg, Fe 0.1 mg, Mg 6 mg, P 17 mg, K 216 mg, Na 1 mg, Zn 0.1 mg, 10 µg carotenoids, B_1 0.03 mg, B_2 0.03 mg, niacin 0.2 mg, B_6 0.04 mg, C 61 mg. A 150 g serving (quarter fruit) is a rich source of vitamin C.

pomes Botanical name for fruits such as apple or pear, formed by the enlargement of the receptacle which becomes fleshy and surrounds the carpels.

pomfret *See* PONTEFRACT CAKES.

pompano Oily FISH, *Trachinotus carolinus*, related to MACKEREL.

ponceau (ponceau 4R) Strawberry red colour, E-124.

ponderal index An index of fatness, used as a measure of OBESITY: height divided by cube root of weight. Confusingly, the index is higher for thin people, and lower for fat people.

See also BODY MASS INDEX.

ponderocrescive Foods stimulating weight gain.

pondoperditive Foods stimulating weight loss.

pone bread Colloquial name for corn bread in the southern states of the USA. (Corn pone are small corn cakes, a specialty of Alabama.)

Pontefract cakes A round, flat sweetmeat made from LIQUORICE originally in Pontefract in England, also called pomfret.

poonac The residue of COCONUT after the extraction of the oil.

popcorn Variety of MAIZE (parch maize, *Zea mays everta*) that expands on heating; also the name of the fluffy white mass so formed.

pope's eye The small circle of fat in the centre of a leg of pork or mutton.

poppadom Indian; thin roasted or fried crisps made from lentil flour; may be spiced.

poppy seed Seeds of the opium poppy, *Papaver somniferum*, used mixed with honey in cakes, and as a flavouring on the crust of bread and rolls. Also called maw seed.

Composition/100 g: water 6.8 g, 2231 kJ (533 kcal), protein 18 g, fat 44.7 g (of which 12% saturated, 15% mono-unsaturated, 73% polyunsaturated), carbohydrate 23.7 g (13.7 g sugars), fibre 10 g, ash 6.8 g, Ca 1448 mg, Fe 9.4 mg, Mg 331 mg, P 849 mg, K 700 mg, Na 21 mg, Zn 10.2 mg, Cu 1.6 mg, Mn 6.8 mg, Se 1.6 μg, vitamin E 1.1 mg, B_1 0.85 mg, B_2 0.17 mg, niacin 1 mg, B_6 0.44 mg, folate 58 μg, C 3 mg.

Population Reference Intake, PRI *See* REFERENCE INTAKES.

porgy American term for various food and game fish of the sea bream family, including *Pagrus* (red porgy) and *Senostomus* spp. *See also* SCUP.

pork Meat from the pig (swine, hog), *Suidae* spp. eaten fresh, as opposed to bacon and ham, which are cured.

Composition/100 g (depending on joint): (edible portion 78–83%) water 63–67 g, 830–1030 kJ (200–245 kcal), protein 17–20 g, fat 12–19 g (of which 38% saturated, 50% mono-unsaturated, 12% polyunsaturated), cholesterol 73 mg, ash 1 g, Ca 5–18 mg, Fe 0.9 mg, Mg 20 mg, P 200 mg, K 315–360 mg, Na 50 mg, Zn 1.7–1.9 mg, Cu 0.1 mg, Se 29–33 μg, vitamin A 2 μg retinol, B_1 0.7–0.9 mg, B_2 0.2 mg, niacin 4.6 mg, B_6 0.4–0.5 mg, folate 1–7 μg, B_{12} 0.5–0.6 μg, pantothenate 0.7 mg, C 1 mg. A 150 g serving is a source of Cu, Zn, vitamin B_2, pantothenate, a rich source of P, Se, vitamin B_1, niacin, B_6, B_{12}.

porphyra Red seaweed used to make LAVER bread.

porphyrin One of a number of pigments consisting of a substituted tetrapyrrole ring and a chelated metal ion, including HAEM and CHLOROPHYLL.

porridge Oatmeal (*see* OATS) cooked in water or milk as a breakfast dish; originally Scottish. Also similar thick soups made with other cereals.

port Fortified wines from the upper Douro valley of north-east Portugal. Mostly aged in wood and bottled when ready for drinking; vintage port is aged in wood for 2 years, then in the bottle for at least 10; late bottled vintage is aged less than 6 years. Crusted port is blended from quality vintages, bottled young and develops a sediment (crust) in the bottle. Ruby port is young, old tawny is aged for 10 or more years; fine old tawny is a blend of young and old wines. Tawny port is aged in wood, vintage in the bottle. White port is made from white grapes; generally served chilled as an apéritif.

porter *See* BEER.

positron emission tomography scanning Radiographic technique that utilises positrons emitted by the decay of ^{15}O after a dose of H_2^{15}O.

Poskitt index Index of fatness in children; per cent of expected weight for age.

posset (1) Drink made from hot milk curdled with ale or wine, sometimes thickened with breadcrumbs and spiced. Formerly used as remedy for colds; popular in late Middle Ages.

(2) Small amount of milk regurgitated by babies after feeding.

post-cibal Occurring after eating.

post-mature Baby born after 42 weeks of gestation.

See also PREMATURE.

post-partum Relating to the first few days after birth.

postprandial After a meal.

potassium An essential mineral, widespread in nature; the human body contains about 125 g. Mostly present inside the cells. Reference intake for adults 3.5 g/day; abundant in fruit and vegetables. Important in plant fertilisers.

potassium nitrate *See* NITRATE.

potassium sorbate Potassium salt of SORBIC ACID (E-202).

potato Or Irish potato; the 'ordinary' potato, tuber of *Solanum tuberosum*.

Composition/100 g: water 79 g, 322 kJ (77 kcal), protein 2 g, fat 0.1 g, carbohydrate 17.5 g (0.8 g sugars), fibre 2.2 g, ash 1.1 g, Ca 12 mg, Fe 0.8 mg, Mg 23 mg, P 57 mg, K 421 mg, Na 6 mg, Zn 0.3 mg, Cu 0.1 mg, Mn 0.2 mg, Se 0.3 µg, 9 µg carotenoids, K 1.9 mg, B_1 0.08 mg, B_2 0.03 mg, niacin 1.1 mg, B_6 0.29 mg, folate 16 µg, pantothenate 0.3 mg, C 20 mg. A 180 g serving is a source of Cu, Mg, Mn, P, niacin, folate, a good source of vitamin B_6, a rich source of vitamin C.

potato, air Tubers of *Dioscorea bulbifera*, the aerial YAM.

potato crisps Flavoured thin slices of potato, deep fried and eaten cold, sometimes as an accompaniment to meals, more commonly as a snack. Called chips in USA.

potato, fairy *See* EARTH NUT.

potato flour Dried potato tuber.

potato starch Or farina, prepared from POTATO tuber and widely used as a stabilising agent when gelatinised by heat.

potato, sweet Tubers of the herbaceous climbing plant *Ipomoea batatas*, known in Britain before the Irish POTATO. The flesh may be white, yellow or pink (if carotene is present); the leaves are also edible.

Composition/100 g: (edible portion 72%) water 77 g, 360 kJ (86 kcal), protein 1.6 g, fat 0.1 g, carbohydrate 20.1 g (4.2 g sugars), fibre 3 g, ash 1 g, Ca 30 mg, Fe 0.6 mg, Mg 25 mg, P 47 mg, K 337 mg, Na 55 mg, Zn 0.3 mg, Cu 0.2 mg, Mn 0.3 mg, Se 0.6 µg, vitamin A 709 µg RE (8516 µg carotenoids), E 0.3 mg, K 1.8 mg, B_1 0.08 mg, B_2 0.06 mg, niacin 0.6 mg, B_6 0.21 mg, folate 11 µg, pantothenate 0.8 mg, C 2 mg. A 65 g serving is a rich source of vitamin A.

potato, tule *See* ARROWHEAD.

poteen Irish name for illicit home-distilled spirit; American equivalent is moonshine.

pot liquor Liquid left in the pan after cooking vegetables.

pot pie American; meat or poultry pie baked in an uncovered vessel with a crust of pastry or biscuit dough.

pottage A thick soup of stewed vegetables (sometimes with meat); literally 'what is put in a pot'.

pottle Traditional English wine measure; $\frac{1}{2}$ gallon (= 2.25 L).

poularde A neutered hen bird.

poultry General term for farmyard birds (as opposed to wild GAME birds) kept for eggs and/or meat; CHICKEN, DUCK, GOOSE, GUINEA FOWL, PIGEON and TURKEY.

poultry, New York dressed Poultry that has been slaughtered and plucked but not eviscerated.

pound cake American name for Madeira cake; rich cake containing a pound, or equal quantities, of each of the major ingredients, flour, sugar and butter (and eggs).

poussin Young CHICKEN, 4–6 weeks old.

powdor fort, powdor douce Medieval English; mixed spices. Powdor fort was hot, containing ginger, pepper and mace, powdor douce was milder, containing ginger, cinnamon, nutmeg and cloves.

pozol Latin American; balls of fermented maize dough mixed with water and eaten as a porridge; various bacteria and yeasts are involved in the fermentation. Chorote is similar, but ground cocoa beans are mixed with the dough.

PPAR receptor Peroxisome proliferation activation receptor, a steroid hormone-like nuclear receptor protein that binds long-chain polyunsaturated fatty acids or EICOSANOID derivatives (prostaglandins and leukotrienes). Also activated by FIBRIC ACID derivatives used as hypolipidaemic agents, and THIAZOLINDINE-DIONE hypoglycaemic agents. May act to modulate gene expression alone or as a heterodimer with the RETINOID X receptor.

PP factor or vitamin *See* NIACIN.

ppm Parts per million (= mg/kg).

PPP Product processing packaging.

prahoc   Cambodian; fermented fish paste prepared by pressing fish under banana leaves before salting and sun-drying.

prairie chicken   American GAME bird, *Tympanuchus cupido* and *T. pallidicinctus*.

prairie oyster   Traditional cure for a hangover; a raw egg with WORCESTERSHIRE SAUCE and brandy; the egg is swirled with the liquid but the yolk remains intact.

pravastatin   *See* STATINS.

prawns   Shellfish of various tribes of suborder Macrura; *Palaemonida* spp., *Penaeida* spp. and *Pandalida* spp. In UK smaller fish are known as SHRIMP and larger as prawns; in USA all are called shrimp. The deep-water prawn is *Pandalus borealis*; common pink shrimp is *Pandalus montagui*; brown shrimp is *Crangon* spp.

Composition/100 g: water 76 g, 444 kJ (106 kcal), protein 20.3 g, fat 1.7 g (of which 23% saturated, 23% mono-unsaturated, 54% polyunsaturated), cholesterol 152 mg, carbohydrate 0.9 g, ash 1.2 g, Ca 52 mg, Fe 2.4 mg, Mg 37 mg, P 205 mg, K 185 mg, Na 148 mg, Zn 1.1 mg, Cu 0.3 mg, Mn 0.1 mg, Se 38 μg, I 100 μg, vitamin A 54 μg retinol, E 1.1 mg, B_1 0.03 mg, B_2 0.03 mg, niacin 2.6 mg, B_6 0.1 mg, folate 3 μg, B_{12} 1.2 μg, pantothenate 0.3 mg, C 2 mg. A 50 g serving is a source of Cu, P, a good source of Se, a rich source of I, vitamin B_{12}.

See also DUBLIN BAY PRAWN; LOBSTER; SCAMPI.

PRE   Protein retention efficiency, a measure of PROTEIN QUALITY.

pre-albumin   *See* TRANSTHYRETIN.

Pream^{TM} Non-dairy CREAMER.

prebiotics   Non-digestible OLIGOSACCHARIDES that support the growth of colonies of certain bacteria in the colon. They include derivatives of FRUCTOSE and GALACTOSE, and lead to the growth of bifidobacteria, so changing and possibly improving the colonic flora. PROBIOTICS and prebiotics are sometimes termed synbiotics. They are considered to play a role as FUNCTIONAL FOODS.

precipitator, electrostatic   A device for removing powder particles from an air stream by passing it between two electrodes, so that particles become charged and can be removed at an earthed electrode.

precision   Of an assay; the degree of reproducibility of a result, determined by calculation of the variance between replicate analyses.

See also ACCURACY.

preforms   Small dense pellets made in an extruder from pre-gelatinised cereal dough, which are suitable for extended storage until they are converted to used to make snack foods by frying, toasting or puffing. (Also known as 'half products'.)

pregnancy, nutritional needs Pregnant women have slightly increased energy and protein requirements compared with their needs before pregnancy, although there are metabolic adaptations in early pregnancy which result in laying down increased reserves for the great stress of the last trimester, and high requirements for iron and calcium. These increased needs are reflected in the increased REFERENCE INTAKES for pregnancy (*see* Tables 3–6 of the Appendix).

premature Usually a PRETERM birth, but also used when the infant weighs less than 2.5 kg when born at term, as a result of intrauterine undernutrition.

premier jus Best-quality SUET prepared from fat surrounding ox and sheep kidneys. The fat is chilled, shredded and heated at moderate temperature. When pressed, premier jus separates into a liquid fraction (oleo oil or liquid oleo) and a solid fraction (oleostearin or solid tallow).

preservation Protection of food from deterioration by microorganisms, enzymes and oxidation, by cooling, destroying the micro-organisms and enzymes by heat treatment or IRRADIATION, reducing their activity through dehydration or the addition of chemical PRESERVATIVES, and by smoking, SALTING and PICKLING.

preservation index In pickling, the acetic acid content expressed as a percentage of total volatile constituents.

preservatives Substances capable of retarding or arresting the deterioration of food; examples are SULPHUR DIOXIDE, BENZOIC ACID, specified ANTIBIOTICS, SALT, acids and essential oils. *See* Table 7 of the Appendix.

press cake Solid residue remaining after extraction of liquid component from foods; especially residue from oilseeds. Used as animal feed and in a number of fermented foods, including BONGKREK, DAGÉ and ONCOM.

pressure, absolute Total pressure above zero (a perfect vacuum), as opposed to pressure expressed above atmospheric pressure (measured using a pressure gauge) or below atmospheric (measured using a vacuum gauge).

pressure cooking *See* AUTOCLAVE; PAPIN'S DIGESTER.

preterm Birth before 37 weeks of gestation.
See also POST-MATURE; PREMATURE.

pretzels German; hard brittle biscuits in the shape of a knot, made from flour, water, shortening, yeast and salt. Also called bretzels.

prevalence rate Measure of morbidity based on current sickness in a population at a particular time (point prevalence) or over a stated period of time (period prevalence).
See also INCIDENCE RATE.

PRI Population reference intake of nutrients; *see* REFERENCE INTAKES.

prickly ash Bark and berries of *Zanthoxylum americanum* and *Z. clava-herculis*, used as a food flavour, reputed to be a circulatory stimulant, and antirheumatic. Also known as toothache bark.

prickly pear Fruit of the cactus *Opuntia* spp., also called Indian fig, barberry fig, tuna or sabra fruit, an important part of the diet in certain areas of Mexico. The stems or pads are NOPALES.

Composition/100 g: (edible portion 75%) water 88 g, 172 kJ (41 kcal), protein 0.7 g, fat 0.5 g, carbohydrate 9.6 g, fibre 3.6 g, ash 1.6 g, Ca 56 mg, Fe 0.3 mg, Mg 85 mg, P 24 mg, K 220 mg, Na 5 mg, Zn 0.1 mg, Cu 0.1 mg, Se 0.6 µg, vitamin A 2 µg RE (28 µg carotenoids), B_1 0.01 mg, B_2 0.06 mg, niacin 0.5 mg, B_6 0.06 mg, folate 6 µg, C 14 mg. A 100 g serving (1 fruit) is a good source of Mg, vitamin C.

primigravida Woman experiencing her first pregnancy.

primipara Woman who has given birth to one infant capable of survival.

See also PARITY.

principal component analysis Mathematical technique for condensing a METABOLOMIC spectrum to a single point on a graph, permitting rapid comparison between different species, experimental and control groups, etc.

prions Small, glycosylated proteins (M_r 27 000–30 000) in the brain cell membranes; to a considerable extent they are species-specific. A modified prion, designated PrPsc, resistant to digestion, heat and chemical agents, is the cause of SPONGIFORM ENCEPHALOPATHIES.

Pritikin programme Low-fat, low-cholesterol diet combined with exercise, to prevent heart disease, developed by Nathan Pritikin, 1979.

probiotics Preparations of microbial culture added to food or animal feed, claimed to be beneficial to health by restoring balance to the intestinal flora. Organisms commonly involved include *Bifidobacterium* spp., *Enterococcus faecium*, *Lactobacillus* spp., *Saccharomyces bulardii*.

See also BACTERIOCINS; MILK, ACIDOPHILUS; PREBIOTICS.

probucol Drug used in treatment of primary hypercholesterolaemia; acts by inhibiting synthesis of CHOLESTEROL and increasing catabolism of low-density lipoprotein (*see* LIPOPROTEINS, PLASMA).

procarcinogen A compound that is not itself carcinogenic, but undergoes metabolic activation in the body to yield a CARCINOGEN, commonly as a result of PHASE I METABOLISM.

processing Any and all processes to which food is subjected after harvesting, for the purposes of improving its appearance, texture, palatability, nutritive value, keeping properties and ease of preparation, and for eliminating micro-organisms, toxins and other undesirable constituents.

processing aids Compounds used in manufacturing to enhance the appeal or utility of a food or component; clarifying and clouding agents, catalysts, flocculants, filtration aids, crystallisation inhibitors.

proctitis Inflammation of the rectum.

proctocolitis Inflammation of the colon and rectum.

pro-enzyme *See* ZYMOGEN.

proglucagon Precursor of the peptide HORMONE GLUCAGON, synthesised in pancreatic α-islet cells and endocrine cells of the gastrointestinal tract; post-synthetic modification leads to formation of glucagon, OXYNTOMODULIN and GLP-1.

progoitrins Substances found in plant foods which are precursors of GOITROGENS.

programming The idea that nutritional and environmental factors *in utero* or during early post-natal life can modify gene expression and hence programme metabolism permanently. *See also* EPIGENETICS.

pro-insulin The inactive precursor of INSULIN, in which the A- and B-chains are joined by the C-PEPTIDE; the form in which insulin is stored in pancreatic β-islet cells before release. A small proportion of insulin secretion is pro-insulin. A rare variant of insulin-dependent DIABETES mellitus is due to genetic lack of the pro-insulin converting enzyme (CARBOXYPEPTIDASE E), so that only pro-insulin is secreted.

prolactin Hormone secreted by the anterior pituitary that stimulates milk secretion after childbirth. Also known as lactogenic or luteotrophic hormone, and luteotrophin.

prolamins The major storage proteins of the ENDOSPERM of cereals, including gliadin (WHEAT), zein (MAIZE), hordein (BARLEY) and avenin (OATS). Characterised by solubility in 70% alcohol, but not water or absolute alcohol; especially rich in PROLINE and GLUTAMINE, low in LYSINE.

proline A non-essential amino acid, abbr Pro (P), M_r 115.1, pK_a 1.95, 10.64, CODONS CCNu.

Promega™ Mixture of long-chain marine FATTY ACIDS: eicosapentaenoic (EPA, C20:5 ω3) and docosohexaenoic (DHA, C22:6 ω3) acids.

promoter A compound that is not itself carcinogenic, but enhances the activity of a CARCINOGEN if given subsequently. *See also* COCARCINOGEN.

Pronutro™ Protein-rich baby food (22% protein) developed in South Africa; made from maize, skim-milk powder, groundnut flour, soya flour and fish protein concentrate with added vitamins.

proof spirit An old method of describing the ALCOHOL content of SPIRITS; originally defined as a solution of alcohol of such strength that it will ignite when mixed with gunpowder. Proof spirit contains 57.07% alcohol by volume or 49.24% by weight in Great Britain. In the USA it contains 50% alcohol by volume. Pure (absolute) alcohol is 175.25° proof UK or 200° proof USA. Spirits were described as under or over proof; a drink 30° over proof contains as much alcohol as 130 volumes of proof spirit; 30° under proof means that 100 volumes contains as much alcohol as 70 volumes of proof spirit. Nowadays alcohol content is usually measured as per cent alcohol by volume.

pro-opiomelanocortin (POMC) Peptide HORMONE precursor that is normally modified by CARBOXYPEPTIDASE E. POMC neurons in the central nervous system mediate feeding behaviour and insulin levels, and peptides derived from POMC are ligands for the hypothalamic MELANOCORTIN receptor, which inhibits feeding behaviour. *See also* AGOUTI MOUSE; FAT MOUSE.

propantheline *See* ATROPINE.

propellant Gas used to expel a product from a container.

propionates Salts of propionic acid, CH_3CH_2COOH, a normal metabolic intermediate. The free acid and salts are used as mould inhibitors, e.g. on cheese surfaces; to inhibit ROPE in bread and baked goods (E-280–283).

propolis Waxy substance produced by bees, used to seal the hive; has antioxidant and antibacterial activities, and sold as a nutritional supplement, with little evidence of efficacy.

propyl gallate An ANTIOXIDANT, E-310.

Prosparol™ An emulsion containing 50% vegetable fat, 1.7 MJ (405 kcal)/100 g; used as a concentrated source of energy.

prostaglandins Locally acting HORMONES (PARACRINE agents) synthesised from long-chain polyunsaturated fatty acids; *see* EICOSANOIDS.

prosthetic group Non-protein part of an ENZYME molecule, unlike a coenzyme, covalently bound to the protein; either an organic compound or a metal ion. Essential for catalytic activity. The enzyme protein without its prosthetic group is the apo-enzyme and is catalytically inactive. With the prosthetic group, it is known as the holo-enzyme.

See also COENZYME; ENZYME ACTIVATION ASSAYS.

protamines Small water-soluble proteins found especially in sperm, rich in basic AMINO ACIDS, especially ARGININE, and not coagulated by heat. So basic that they form salts with mineral acids, e.g. salmine from salmon, sturine from sturgeon, clupeine from herring, scombrine from mackerel.

proteans Slightly altered proteins that have become insoluble, probably an early stage of denaturation.

proteases Alternative name for PROTEINASES.

Protecon[TM] A bone press for preparation of mechanically recovered meat (*see* MEAT, MECHANICALLY RECOVERED).

protein All living tissues contain proteins; they are polymers of AMINO ACIDS, joined by peptide bonds (*see* PEPTIDES). 21 amino acids are incorporated into proteins during synthesis, and others are formed by post-synthetic modification. Any one protein may contain several hundred or thousand amino acids. The sequence of the amino acids in a protein determines its overall structure and function: many proteins are ENZYMES; others are structural (e.g. COLLAGEN in connective tissue and KERATIN in hair and nails); many HORMONES are polypeptides. Proteins are constituents of all living cells and are dietary essentials. Chemically distinguished from fats and carbohydrates by containing nitrogen.

proteinases Enzymes that hydrolyse proteins, also known as peptidases.

See also CHILLPROOFING; ENDOPEPTIDASES; EXOPEPTIDASES; TENDERISERS.

protein calorie malnutrition *See* PROTEIN–ENERGY MALNUTRITION.

protein calories per cent *See* PROTEIN–ENERGY RATIO.

protein, conjugated Proteins that include a non-protein PROSTHETIC GROUP, e.g. HAEMOGLOBIN and CYTOCHROMES contain HAEM; many oxidative enzymes contain a prosthetic group derived from VITAMIN B_2; glycoproteins proteins are conjugated with carbohydrates; other proteins are conjugated with fatty acids.

protein conversion factor *See* NITROGEN CONVERSION FACTOR.

protein, crude Total NITROGEN multiplied by 6.25.

See also KJELDAHL DETERMINATION; NITROGEN CONVERSION FACTORS.

protein efficiency ratio (PER) A measure of PROTEIN QUALITY.

protein–energy malnutrition (PEM) A spectrum of disorders, especially in children, due to inadequate feeding. Marasmus is severe wasting and also occurs in adults; the result of a food intake inadequate to meet energy expenditure. Emaciation, similar to that seen in marasmus, occurs in patients with advanced cancer and AIDS; in this case it is known as CACHEXIA.

Kwashiorkor affects only young children and includes severe oedema, fatty infiltration of the liver and a sooty dermatitis; it is likely that deficiency of ANTIOXIDANT nutrients and the stress of infection may be involved. The name kwashiorkor is derived from the Ga language of Ghana to describe the illness of the first child when it is weaned (on to an inadequate diet) on the arrival of the second child.

See also GOMEZ CLASSIFICATION; MARASMIC KWASHIORKOR; WATER-LOW CLASSIFICATION; WELLCOME CLASSIFICATION.

protein–energy ratio The protein content of a food or diet expressed as the proportion of the total energy provided by protein (17 kJ, 4 kcal/g). The average requirement for protein is about 7% of total energy intake; western diets provide about 14%.

protein equivalent A measure of the digestible nitrogen of an animal feedingstuff in terms of protein. It is measured by direct feeding or calculated from the digestible pure protein plus half the digestible non-protein nitrogen.

protein, first class An obsolete system of classifying proteins into first and second class, to indicate their relative nutritional value or PROTEIN QUALITY. Generally, but not invariably, animal proteins were considered 'first class' and plant proteins 'second class', but this classification has no validity in the diet as a whole.

protein hydrolysate Mixture of AMINO ACIDS and POLYPEPTIDES prepared by hydrolysis of PROTEINS with acid, alkali or PROTEASES, used in ENTERAL and PARENTERAL nutrition and in supplements.

protein intolerance An adverse reaction to one or more specific proteins in foods, commonly the result of an ALLERGY. General protein intolerance may be due to a variety of GENETIC DISEASES affecting amino acid metabolism. Treatment is normally by severe restriction of protein intake.

See also ADVERSE REACTIONS TO FOODS; AMINO ACID DISORDERS; HYPERAMMONAEMIA.

protein kinases Enzymes that catalyse phosphorylation of target enzymes in cells in response to the action of HORMONES and neurotransmitters. Protein kinase A is activated by 5′-AMP, protein kinase B by the activated insulin receptor substrate, protein kinase C by cyclic AMP; MAP KINASES are activated by a variety of mitogenic hormones.

protein quality A measure of the usefulness of a protein food for maintenance and repair of tissue, growth and formation of new tissues and, in animals, production of meat, eggs, wool and milk. It is important only if the total intake of protein barely meets the requirement. Furthermore, the quality of individual proteins is relatively unimportant in mixed diets, because of COMPLEMENTA-TION between different proteins. Two types of measurement are used to estimate protein quality: biological assays and chemical analysis.

Biological value (BV) is the proportion of absorbed protein retained in the body (i.e. taking no account of digestibility). A protein that is completely usable (e.g. egg and human milk) has a BV = 0.9–1; meat and fish have BV = 0.75–0.8; wheat protein 0.5; gelatine 0.

Net protein utilisation (NPU) is the proportion of dietary protein that is retained in the body under specified experimental conditions (i.e. it takes account of digestibility; NPU = BV × digestibility). By convention NPU is measured at 10% dietary protein (NPU_{10}) at which level the protein synthetic mechanism of the animal can utilise all of the protein so long as the balance of ESSENTIAL AMINO ACIDS is correct. When fed at 4% dietary protein, the result is NPU standardised. If the food or diet is fed as it is normally eaten, the result is NPU operative (NPU_{op}).

Protein efficiency ratio (PER) is the gain in weight of growing animals per gram of protein eaten.

Net protein retention (NPR) is the weight gain of animals fed the test protein, minus the weight loss of a group fed a protein-free diet, divided by the amount of protein consumed.

Protein retention efficiency (PRE) is the NPR converted into a percentage scale by multiplying by 16; it then becomes numerically the same as net protein utilisation.

Relative protein value (RPV) is the ability of a test protein, fed at various levels of intake, to support NITROGEN BALANCE, relative to a standard protein.

Chemical score is based on chemical analysis of the protein; it is the amount of the limiting AMINO ACID compared with the amount of the same amino acid in egg protein.

Amino acid score (protein score) is similar to chemical score, but uses an amino acid mixture as the standard.

Protein digestibility corrected amino acid score (PDCAAS) is the amino acid score × digestibility

Essential amino acid index is the sum of all the essential amino acids compared with those in egg protein or the amino acid target mixture.

protein rating Used in Canadian food regulations to assess the overall PROTEIN QUALITY of a food. It is protein efficiency ratio × per cent protein content of food × the amount of food that is reasonably consumed. Foods with a rating above 40 may be designated excellent dietary sources; foods with rating below 20 are considered to be insignificant sources; 20–40 may be described as good sources.

protein, reference A theoretical concept of the perfect protein which is used with 100% efficiency at whatever level it is fed in the diet. The nearest approach to this theoretical protein are egg and human milk proteins, which are used with 90–100% efficiency (BV = 0.9–1.0) when fed at low levels in the diet (4%), but not when fed at high levels (10–15%).

protein retention efficiency (PRE) A measure of PROTEIN QUALITY.

protein score A measure of PROTEIN QUALITY based on chemical analysis.

protein, second class *See* PROTEIN, FIRST CLASS.

protein turnover *See* HALF-LIFE (1).

proteoglycans *See* GLYCOPROTEINS.

proteolysis The hydrolysis of proteins to their constituent AMINO ACIDS, catalysed by alkali, acid or enzymes.

proteomics Identification of all the proteins present in a cell, tissue or organism. The proteome cannot be predicted from the TRANSCRIPTOME, because of post-translational modifications such as glycosylation, esterification and phosphorylation that are involved in the synthesis of many proteins.

proteoses Partial degradation products of proteins; soluble in water. The stages of breakdown are protein → proteoses → peptones → polypeptides → oligopeptides → amino acids.

Proteus Genus of flagellate and highly motile rod-like GRAM-negative bacteria, common in intestinal flora. Some species are pathogenic.

prothrombin Protein in plasma involved in coagulation of BLOOD. Prothrombin time is an index of the coagulability of blood (and hence of VITAMIN K nutritional status) based on the time taken for a citrated sample of blood to clot when calcium ions and thromboplastin are added.

protoalkaloids Amines synthesised by decarboxylation of AMINO ACIDS.
See also ALKALOIDS.

protogen *See* LIPOIC ACID.

proton pump Enzyme (H^+/K^+ ATPase, EC 3.6.1.36) in parietal (oxyntic) cells of gastric mucosa that causes secretion of gastric acid; acts by exchanging H^+ and K^+ across the cell membrane. Irreversible inhibitors (e.g. lansoprazole, pantoprazole and omeprazole) are used in the treatment of gastric ULCERS and HIATUS HERNIA.

protopectin *See* PECTIN.

protoporphyrin The iron-free precursor of HAEM. Normally present in red blood cells in low concentrations, an increased concentration is an early index of IRON deficiency. Also increased by LEAD toxicity.
See also PORPHYRIN.

proving The stage in breadmaking when the dough is left to rise.

provitamin   A substance that is converted into a vitamin, such as 7-dehydrocholesterol, which is converted into VITAMIN D, or those CAROTENES that can be converted to VITAMIN A.

provolone   Smoked drawn curd cheese, originally made from buffalo milk, now mainly cow milk.

proximate analysis   Analysis of foods and feedingstuffs for NITRO-GEN (for protein), ether extract (for fat), crude FIBRE and ASH (mineral salts) together with soluble carbohydrate calculated by subtracting these values from the total (*see* CARBOHYDRATE BY DIF-FERENCE). Also known as Weende analysis, after the Weende Experimental Station in Germany, which in 1865 outlined the methods of analysis to be used.

Prozac   *See* FLUOXETINE.

prunin   *See* NARINGIN.

Prunus   Genus of plants including PLUMS, PEACHES, NECTARINES, CHERRIES and ALMONDS.

Pruteen^{TM}   Microbial protein produced by growing *Methylophilus methylotrophus*, on methanol; 70% protein in dry weight.

pseudoalkaloids   Pharmacologically active compounds in plants, unlike ALKALOIDS and PROTOALKALOIDS, not derived from amino acids; two major groups: (i) STEROID and TERPENE derivatives and (ii) purines (e.g. CAFFEINE).

pseudoglobulin   Water-soluble GLOBULIN which is not precipitated from salt solutions by dialysis against distilled water. Pseudoglobulins occur in blood plasma, in animal tissues, and in milk.
> *See also* EUGLOBULIN.

pseudokeratins   *See* KERATIN.

pseudoplastic   Material whose VISCOSITY decreases with increasing SHEAR RATE.
> *See also* DILATANT; RHEOPECTIC; THIXOTROPIC.

PSL   Practical storage life.

PSP   *See* PARALYTIC SHELLFISH POISONING.

P:S ratio   The ratio between polyunsaturated and saturated FATTY ACIDS. In western diets the ratio is about 0.6; it is suggested that increasing to near 1.0 will reduce the risk of atherosclerosis and coronary heart disease.

PSW   Pulsed shock waves, a technology proposed for preservation of foods by inactivation of ENZYMES without heating, through generating shock waves by powerful electric discharge in liquids.

psychrometer   *See* HYGROMETER.

psychrometry   Study of the interrelationships of temperature and humidity relevant to drying with hot air.

psychrophiles (psychrophilic organisms)   Bacteria and fungi that tolerate low temperatures. Their preferred temperature range is

15–20 °C, but they will grow in cold stores at or below 0 °C; the temperature must be reduced to about −10 °C before growth stops, but the organisms are not killed and will regrow when the temperature rises.

Bacteria of the genera *Achromobacter, Flavobacterium, Pseudomonas* and *Micrococcus; Torulopsis* yeasts; and moulds of the genera *Penicillium, Cladosporium, Mucor* and *Thamnidium* are psychrophiles.

psyllium   Also known as plantago or flea seed, *Plantago psyllium.* Small, dark reddish-brown seeds which form a mucilaginous mass with water; used as a bulk-forming LAXATIVE.

pteroylglutamic acid (pteroylglutamate), pteroylpolyglutamic acid (pteroylpolyglutamate)   *See* FOLIC ACID.

PTFE   Polytetrafluoroethylene, a polymer resistant to heat and many chemicals, and with low coefficient of friction, used to make non-stick coatings for cooking utensils.

ptomaines   Obsolete name for amines formed by decarboxylation of amino acids during putrefaction of proteins; putrescine from ARGININE, cadaverine from LYSINE, muscarine in MUSHROOMS (also neurine formed by dehydration of CHOLINE). They have an unpleasant smell and were formerly thought to cause food poisoning, but are in fact harmless, albeit sometimes the products of pathogenic bacteria.

ptyalin   Obsolete name for salivary AMYLASE.

ptyalism   Or sialorrhoea, excessive flow of SALIVA.

puberty, delayed   The normal onset of puberty in boys is between the ages of 12 and 15; a number of factors may delay this, especially deficiency of ZINC. Severely zinc-deficient boys of 20 are still prepubertal.

PUFA   Polyunsaturated fatty acids.

puffballs   Edible wild fungi; mosaic puffball *Calvatia* (*Lycoperdon*) *caelata*, giant puffball *C. gigantea* (may grow to 30 cm in diameter), normally eaten while still relatively small and fleshy, much prized for their delicate flavour. *See* MUSHROOMS.

puffer fish   *See* TETRODONTIN POISONING.

puffing gun   For manufacture of puffed cereals by EXPLOSION PUFFING. A chamber (the gun) is charged with the grain material, subjected to high-pressure steam, then the pressure is released very rapidly. The shot of grain is propelled into an expansion vessel, when it expands to 3–10 times its original volume.

pullulanase   *See* DEBRANCHING ENZYMES.

pulque   Sourish beer produced in central and south America by the rapid natural fermentation of aquamiel, the sweet mucilaginous sap of the agave (American aloe or century plant, *Agave americana*). Contains 6% alcohol by volume.

puls (pulmentus)   Roman; barley or wheat that has been roasted, pounded and boiled to make a gruel; probably a precursor of POLENTA.

Pulse™   Capsules of fish oil rich in ω3 polyunsaturated fatty acids.

pulsed light   Technique for sterilisation of packaging, food surfaces and water by exposure to very short bursts (typically 100–300 μs) of very high-intensity broad spectrum light, about 25% of which is UV.

pulses   Name given to the dried seeds (matured on the plant) of LEGUMES such as PEAS, BEANS and LENTILS. In the fresh, wet form they contain about 90% water, but the dried form contains about 10% water and can be stored.

pumpernickel   Dense sour-flavoured black bread made from rye, originally German; in USA name for any rye bread.

pumpkin   A GOURD, fruit of *Cucurbita pepo*.

Composition/100 g: water 79 g, 377 kJ (90 kcal), protein 16.1 g, fat 1.4 g (of which 40% saturated, 30% mono-unsaturated, 30% polyunsaturated), cholesterol 50 mg, carbohydrate 2 g, ash 1.3 g, Ca 10 mg, Fe 3.5 mg, Mg 250 mg, P 272 mg, K 382 mg, Na 70 mg, Zn 1 mg, Cu 0.4 mg, Se 27.4 μg, vitamin A 30 μg retinol, E 5 mg, K 0.1 mg, B_1 0.01 mg, B_2 0.12 mg, niacin 1.4 mg, B_6 0.13 mg, folate 6 μg, B_{12} 0.5 μg.

Seeds, composition/100 g: (edible portion 74%) water 6.9 g, 2265 kJ (541 kcal), protein 24.5 g, fat 45.8 g (of which 20% saturated, 33% mono-unsaturated, 48% polyunsaturated), carbohydrate 17.8 g (1 g sugars), fibre 3.9 g, ash 4.9 g, Ca 43 mg, Fe 15 mg, Mg 535 mg, P 1174 mg, K 807 mg, Na 18 mg, Zn 7.5 mg, Cu 1.4 mg, Mn 3 mg, Se 5.6 μg, vitamin A 19 μg RE (228 μg carotenoids), K 51.4 mg, B_1 0.21 mg, B_2 0.32 mg, niacin 1.7 mg, B_6 0.22 mg, folate 58 μg, pantothenate 0.3 mg, C 2 mg. A 15 g serving is a source of Cu, Fe, Mn, a good source of Mg, P.

PureBright™   *See* PULSED LIGHT.

purgative   *See* LAXATIVES.

puri (poori)   Indian; unleavened wholewheat bread prepared from a butter-rich dough, shaped into small pancakes and deep fried in hot oil.

purines   (*see* p. 398) Nitrogenous bases that occur in NUCLEIC ACIDS (adenine and guanine) and their precursors and metabolites; inosine, caffeine and theobromine are also purines. They are not dietary essentials; both dietary and endogenously formed purines are excreted as URIC ACID.

purl   Old English winter drink; warmed ale with bitters and brandy or milk, sugar and spirit.

puto   South-east Asian; steamed bread made from rice that has been allowed to undergo a lactic acid fermentation.

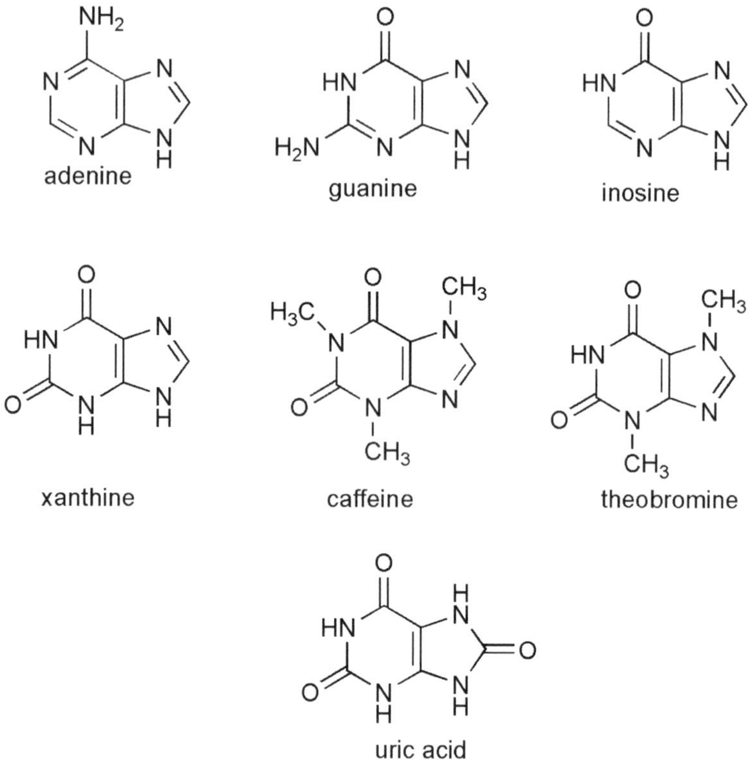

398

adenine

guanine

inosine

xanthine

caffeine

theobromine

uric acid

PURINES

Leuconostoc mesenteroides and yeasts produce carbon dioxide as a raising agent.

putromaine Any toxin produced by the decay of food within the body.

pyloric stenosis Narrowing of the PYLORUS, leading to repeated vomiting and sometimes visible distension of the stomach.

pylorus Lower end of the STOMACH, where it enters the duodenum, via the pyloric SPHINCTER.

pyorrhea Obsolete name for PERIODONTAL disease.

pyrazines Derivatives of six-membered heterocyclic aromatic compounds with two N atoms in the ring; they impart nutty, roasted, 'green' and fruity flavours to foods.

pyridine nucleotides Obsolete name for the COENZYMES NAD and NADP.

pyridorin Term used for pyridoxamine (*see* VITAMIN B_6) when used to inhibit the Amadori reaction (the rearrangement of the initial product of protein GLYCATION to the advanced glycation end-product); potentially useful in preventing the adverse effects of poor glycaemic control in DIABETES mellitus.

pyridoxal, pyridoxamine, pyridoxine *See* VITAMIN B$_6$.

4-pyridoxic acid The main urinary metabolite of VITAMIN B$_6$.

pyridoxyllysine A SCHIFF BASE formed by condensation between pyridoxal and the ε-amino group of LYSINE in proteins. Renders both the VITAMIN B$_6$ and the lysine unavailable, and also has antivitamin B$_6$ antimetabolic activity.

pyrimidines Nitrogenous bases that occur in NUCLEIC ACIDS, cytosine, thymine and uracil.

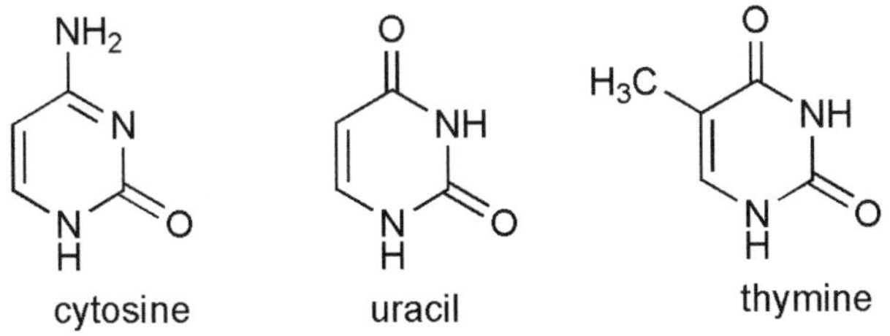

cytosine   uracil   thymine

PYRIMIDINES

pyrithiamin Antimetabolite of thiamin, used in experimental studies of VITAMIN B$_1$ deficiency; it inhibits thiamin pyrophosphokinase (EC 2.7.6.2) and competes for uptake across the blood–brain barrier, accumulating in the central nervous system. *See also* OXYTHIAMIN.

pyrocarbonate *See* DIETHYL PYROCARBONATE.

pyrosis Alternative name for heartburn (USA). *See* INDIGESTION.

pyrroles Derivatives of five-membered heterocyclic compounds (C$_4$H$_4$NH) that impart a 'burnt' flavour to foods; mainly formed by the MAILLARD REACTION.

pyruvic acid An intermediate in the metabolism of carbohydrates, formed by the anaerobic GLYCOLYSIS of GLUCOSE. It may then either be converted to acetyl CoA, and oxidised through the CITRIC ACID cycle or be reduced to lactic acid. The oxidation to acetyl CoA is THIAMIN dependent, and blood concentrations of pyruvate and lactate rise in thiamin deficiency.

Q

QPM Quality protein MAIZE.

QUAC stick Quaker arm circumference measuring stick. A stick used to measure height which also shows the 80th and 85th

centiles of expected MID-UPPER ARM CIRCUMFERENCE. Developed by a Quaker Service Team in Nigeria in the 1960s as a rapid and simple tool for assessment of nutritional status.
See also ANTHROPOMETRY.

quahog   American bivalve mollusc, *Venus mercenaria*.

quail   Formerly a GAME bird, now so endangered in the wild that shooting is prohibited, but farmed to some extent. Two main species, *Bonasa umbellus* and *Colinus virginianus*; Californian quail is *Lophortyx californica*. The small EGGS are prized as a delicacy.

Composition/100 g: (edible portion 76%) water 70 g, 561 kJ (134 kcal), protein 21.8 g, fat 4.5 g (of which 34% saturated, 34% mono-unsaturated, 32% polyunsaturated), cholesterol 70 mg, carbohydrate 0 g, ash 1.3 g, Ca 13 mg, Fe 4.5 mg, Mg 25 mg, P 307 mg, K 237 mg, Na 51 mg, Zn 2.7 mg, Cu 0.6 mg, Se 17.4 µg, vitamin A 17 µg retinol, B_1 0.28 mg, B_2 0.28 mg, niacin 8.2 mg, B_6 0.53 mg, folate 7 µg, B_{12} 0.5 µg, pantothenate 0.8 mg, C 7 mg. A 100 g serving is a source of Zn, vitamin B_2, pantothenate, C, a good source of Se, vitamin B_1, B_6, a rich source of Cu, Fe, P, niacin, vitamin B_{12}.

quality assurance   The planned actions necessary to provide adequate confidence that a product will satisfy requirements for quality.

quality control   The operational techniques and activities that are used to fulfil requirements for quality.

quality management   That aspect of management that determines and implements the QUALITY POLICY.

quality policy   The overall quality intentions and direction of an organisation, formally expressed by management.

quality system   The organisational structure, responsibilities, procedures and resources for implementing QUALITY MANAGEMENT.

quamash   Or camash; starchy roots of *Camassia quamash*, formerly the staple food of west coast native Americans.

quantitative ingredients declaration (QUID)   Obligatory on food labels in the EU since February 2000; previous legislation only required declaration of ingredients in descending order of quantity, not specific declaration of the amount of each ingredient present.

quark (quarg)   Originally German; unripened soft CHEESE, known in France as fromage frais.

quart   Imperial measure of volume, equal to $\frac{1}{4}$ Imperial gallon or 2 pints (i.e. 1.1 L). Reputed quart is the traditional 'bottle' of wine or spirits; approximately $\frac{2}{3}$ Imperial quart, or $26\frac{2}{3}$ fluid ounces (730 mL). Reputed pint is $13\frac{1}{3}$ fluid ounces.

quartern   *See* NOGGIN.

quebracho   Or aspidosperma; obtained from the bark of *Aspidosperma quebrachoblanco*; used as source of tannins and alkaloids.

queen substance   *See* ROYAL JELLY.

quercitin   A flavone (*see* FLAVONOIDS), found in onion skins, tea, hops and horse chestnuts. Not known to be a dietary essential or to have any function in the body.

quercitol   *See* ACORN SUGAR.

querns   Pair of grinding stones used for pulverising grain (from about 4000–2000 BC). The lower stone was slightly hollowed and the upper stone was rolled by hand on the lower one.

Quetelet's index   *See* BODY MASS INDEX.

quick breads   Baked goods such as biscuits, muffins, popovers, griddles, cakes, waffles and dumplings, in which no yeast is used. The raising is carried out quickly with baking powder or other chemical agents.

quick freezing   Rapid freezing of food by exposure to a blast of air at a very low temperature. Unlike slow freezing, very small crystals of ice are formed, which do not rupture the cells of the food and so the structure is relatively undamaged. A quick-frozen food is commonly defined as one that has been cooled from a temperature of $0\,°C$ to $-5\,°$ or lower, in a period of not more than 2 h and then cooled to $-18\,°C$.

QUID   *See* QUANTITATIVE INGREDIENTS DECLARATION.

quillaja (quillaia)   Or soapbark; the dried bark of the shrub *Quillaja saponaria*, which contains SAPONINS and TANNINS. Used to produce foam in soft drinks, shampoos and fire extinguishers.

quince   Pear-shaped fruit of *Cydonia oblongata*, with flesh similar to that of the apple; sour but strong aromatic flavour when cooked; rich in pectin and used chiefly in jams and jellies.

Composition/100 g: (edible portion 61%) water 84 g, 239 kJ (57 kcal), protein 0.4 g, fat 0.1 g, carbohydrate 15.3 g, fibre 1.9 g, ash 0.4 g, Ca 11 mg, Fe 0.7 mg, Mg 8 mg, P 17 mg, K 197 mg, Na 4 mg, Cu 0.1 mg, Se 0.6 µg, vitamin A 2 µg RE, B_1 0.02 mg, B_2 0.03 mg, niacin 0.2 mg, B_6 0.04 mg, folate 3 µg, pantothenate 0.1 mg, C 15 mg. A 90 g serving (1 fruit) is a good source of vitamin C.

Japanese quince is fruit of the ornamental shrub *Chaenomeles lagenaria*, hard, sour and aromatic, used in preserves and jellies.

quinine   Bitter ALKALOID extracted from bark of the cinchona tree (*Cinchona officinalis*), formerly used to treat or prevent malaria and in apéritif wines, BITTERS and TONIC WATER.

quinoa   Glutinous   seeds   of   the   south   American   plant *Chenopodium album*, used in Chile and Peru to make bread.

Composition/100 g: water 9.3 g, 1566 kJ (374 kcal), protein 13.1 g, fat 5.8 g (of which 14% saturated, 34% mono-unsaturated,

52% polyunsaturated), carbohydrate 68.9 g, fibre 5.9 g, ash 2.9 g, Ca 60 mg, Fe 9.3 mg, Mg 210 mg, P 410 mg, K 740 mg, Na 21 mg, Zn 3.3 mg, Cu 0.8 mg, Mn 2.3 mg, vitamin B_1 0.2 mg, B_2 0.4 mg, niacin 2.9 mg, B_6 0.22 mg, folate 49 µg, pantothenate 1 mg. A 30 g serving is a source of Fe, P, a good source of Cu, Mg, a rich source of Mn.

quintal   100 kg (220 lb).

Quorn™   MYCOPROTEIN from the mould *Fusarium graminearum*.

R

***R*- and *S*-**   Systematic chemical nomenclature for assigning conformation of four different groups around an asymmetric carbon atom, in which the two ISOMERS are *R*- (for *rectus*, right) and *S*- (for *sinistra*, left). It is based on a hierarchy of substituent groups, and does not give the same conformation for all the naturally occurring amino acids, unlike the DL-system. It is little used in biochemistry and nutrition, apart from naming the isomers of VITAMIN E.

See also D-, L- AND DL-; OPTICAL ACTIVITY.

rabbit   (1) *Lepus cuniculus*; both wild and farmed rabbits are eaten.

Composition/100 g: water 73 g, 569 kJ (136 kcal), protein 20 g, fat 5.6 g (of which 40% saturated, 35% mono-unsaturated, 26% polyunsaturated), cholesterol 57 mg, carbohydrate 0 g, ash 0.7 g, Ca 13 mg, Fe 1.6 mg, Mg 19 mg, P 213 mg, K 330 mg, Na 41 mg, Zn 1.6 mg, Cu 0.1 mg, Se 23.7 µg, vitamin B_1 0.1 mg, B_2 0.15 mg, niacin 7.3 mg, B_6 0.5 mg, folate 8 µg, B_{12} 7.2 µg, pantothenate 0.8 mg. A 210 g serving (half rabbit) is a source of Cu, Mg, vitamin B_1, B_2, a good source of Fe, Zn, pantothenate, a rich source of P, Se, niacin, VITAMIN B_6, B_{12}.

(2) Original form of rarebit, *see* WELSH RAREBIT.

racemic   The mixture of the D- and L-isomers of a compound, commonly shown as DL-.

rad   A non-SI unit of the energy absorbed from ionising radiation; the absorption of 100 ergs per gram of substance. Now superseded by the GRAY.

radappertisation   Sterilisation of food by high-dose IRRADIATION for destruction of (virtually) all organisms.

See also RADICIDATION; STERILE.

radiation sterilization   *See* IRRADIATION.

radical (free radical)   A highly reactive molecular species with an unpaired electron.

radicchio   Red variety of CHICORY.

Composition/100 g: (edible portion 91%) water 93 g, 96 kJ

(23 kcal), protein 1.4 g, fat 0.3 g, carbohydrate 4.5 g (0.6 g sugars), fibre 0.9 g, ash 0.7 g, Ca 19 mg, Fe 0.6 mg, Mg 13 mg, P 40 mg, K 302 mg, Na 22 mg, Zn 0.6 mg, Cu 0.3 mg, Mn 0.1 mg, Se 0.9 μg, vitamin A 1 μg RE (8848 μg carotenoids), E 2.3 mg, K 255.2 mg, B_1 0.02 mg, B_2 0.03 mg, niacin 0.3 mg, B_6 0.06 mg, folate 60 μg, pantothenate 0.3 mg, C 8 mg.

radicidation Low-level IRRADIATION treatment to kill non-spore-forming pathogens and prevent food poisoning; less severe treatment than RADAPPERTISATION.

radioallergosorbent tests (RAST) Tests for food allergy. *See* ADVERSE REACTIONS TO FOODS.

radio frequency heating *See* MICROWAVE COOKING.

radioimmunoassay (RIA) Sensitive and specific analytical technique for determination of analytes present at very low concentrations in biological samples. Based on competition between unlabelled and labelled analyte for a limited number of binding sites on an ANTIBODY; after calibration, measurement of either the bound or unbound labelled analyte permits determination of the amount present in the sample. Bound and free analyte may be separated by a variety of techniques, including ultrafiltration, solvent extraction, equilibrium dialysis, adsorption onto charcoal and binding of the antiserum to a solid phase.

Also known as saturation analysis or radio-ligand binding assay, especially when a binding protein or plasma transport protein is used rather than an antibody.

See also ELISA; FLUORESCENCE IMMUNOASSAY.

radio-ligand binding assay *See* RADIOIMMUNOASSAY.

radiolysis Chemical changes caused by IRRADIATION, producing compounds that have antibacterial activity.

radish The root of *Raphanus* spp.

Composition/100 g: (edible portion 90%) water 95 g, 67 kJ (16 kcal), protein 0.7 g, fat 0.1 g, carbohydrate 3.4 g (2.1 g sugars), fibre 1.6 g, ash 0.6 g, Ca 25 mg, Fe 0.3 mg, Mg 10 mg, P 20 mg, K 233 mg, Na 39 mg, Zn 0.3 mg, Cu 0.1 mg, Mn 0.1 mg, Se 0.6 μg, 14 μg carotenoids, vitamin K 1.3 mg, B_1 0.01 mg, B_2 0.04 mg, niacin 0.3 mg, B_6 0.07 mg, folate 25 μg, pantothenate 0.2 mg, C 15 mg.

radurisation PASTEURISATION of food by low-dose IRRADIATION to destroy a sufficient number of yeasts, moulds and non-spore-forming bacteria to prolong shelf-life.

raffinade Best-quality refined sugar.

raffinose Trisaccharide, galactosyl-glucosyl-fructose, found in cotton seed, sugar-beet molasses and Australian manna; also known as gossypose, melitose or melitriose. 23% of the sweetness of sucrose. Not digested.

Raftiline™ FAT REPLACER made from NON-STARCH POLYSACCHARIDE.

Raftilose™ Fructo-oligosaccharide derived from INULIN, a PREBIOTIC.

ragi Dried balls of STARTER containing moulds, yeast and bacteria on cereal or starch, used as a starter inoculation for production of LAO-CHAO, SAKÉ, tape, and other fermented foods.

raisin Dried seedless GRAPES of several kinds. Valencia raisins from Spanish grapes; Thompson seedless raisins produced mainly in California from the sultanina grape (the skins are coarser than the sultana).

Composition/100 g: water 15.4 g, 1252 kJ (299 kcal), protein 3.1 g, fat 0.5 g, carbohydrate 79.2 g (59.2 g sugars), fibre 3.7 g, ash 1.9 g, Ca 50 mg, Fe 1.9 mg, Mg 32 mg, P 101 mg, K 749 mg, Na 11 mg, Zn 0.2 mg, Cu 0.3 mg, Mn 0.3 mg, Se 0.6 µg, vitamin E 0.1 mg, K 3.5 mg, B_1 0.11 mg, B_2 0.13 mg, niacin 0.8 mg, B_6 0.17 mg, folate 5 µg, pantothenate 0.1 mg, C 2 mg.

raisin oil Extracted from the seeds of muscat GRAPES, which are removed before drying them to yield RAISINS. The oil is used primarily to coat the raisins to prevent them sticking together, to render them soft and pliable and less subject to insect infestation.

raising powder *See* BAKING POWDER.

rambutan Fruit of *Nephelium lappaceum*; covered with yellowish-red soft spines with large seed surrounded by white juicy flesh, similar to LYCHEE, and sometimes called hairy lychee. The name means *hairy man of the jungle* in Bahasa-Malay, reflecting the appearance of the fruit.

ramekin (1) Porcelain or earthenware mould in which a mixture is baked and then brought to the table, or the savoury served in a ramekin dish. Paper soufflé cases are called ramekin cases.

(2) Formerly the name given to toasted cheese; now tarts filled with cream cheese.

rancidity The development of unpleasant flavours in oils and fats as a result of LIPASE action or oxidation.

See also ACID NUMBER.

rancimat Apparatus for determining oxidative stability of fats by dissolving the gases produced by oxidation in distilled water and measuring electrical conductivity.

See also ACTIVE OXYGEN METHOD.

randomisation of fats *See* INTERESTERIFICATION.

ranitidine *See* HISTAMINE RECEPTOR ANTAGONISTS.

Rankine scale *See* TEMPERATURE, ABSOLUTE.

rapeseed *Brassica napus* and *B. rapa*, also known as cole, coleseed or colza. Grown for its seed, as source of oil for both industrial and food use. Varieties low in erucic acid are termed '0' or single low (also called canbra oil); varieties low in glucosinolates and erucic acid yield CANOLA oil.

rarebit   *See* WELSH RAREBIT.

rasgulla   Indian; dessert of small balls of milk curd, ground almond and semolina, boiled in syrup.

rasher   Slice of BACON or HAM.

raspberry   Fruit of *Rubus idaeus*. Black raspberry is *Rubus occidentalis*, native of eastern USA.

Composition/100g: (edible portion 96%) water 85.8g, 218kJ (52kcal), protein 1.2g, fat 0.6g, carbohydrate 11.9g (4.4g sugars), fibre 6.5g, ash 0.5g, Ca 25mg, Fe 0.7mg, Mg 22mg, P 29mg, K 151mg, Na 1mg, Zn 0.4mg, Cu 0.1mg, Mn 0.7mg, Se 0.2µg, vitamin A 2µg RE (164µg carotenoids), E 0.9mg, K 7.8mg, B_1 0.03mg, B_2 0.04mg, niacin 0.6mg, B_6 0.05mg, folate 21µg, pantothenate 0.3mg, C 26mg. A 110g serving is a source of folate, a rich source of Mn, vitamin C.

RAST   Radio-allergosorbent tests for food allergy; *see* ADVERSE REACTIONS TO FOODS.

rastrello   Sharp-edged spoon used to cut out the pulp from halved citrus fruit.

ratafia   (1) Flavouring essence made from bitter almonds.

(2) Small macaroon-like biscuits flavoured with almonds.

(3) Almond-flavoured liqueur.

rat line test   Obsolete biological assay for VITAMIN D. Rats were maintained on a rachitogenic (rickets-inducing) diet, then given the test substance or standard vitamin D for 7–10 days. At postmortem examination the long bones were stained with silver nitrate; in newly calcified regions silver phosphate is precipitated, and on exposure to light gives a stain that can be quantified.

ravioli   Square envelope of PASTA stuffed with minced meat or cheese.

raw sugar   Brown unrefined sugar, 96–98% pure, as imported for refining. Contaminated with mould spores, bacteria, cane fibre and dirt.

ray   Cartilaginous FISH, *Raja* spp.

RBP   *See* RETINOL BINDING PROTEIN.

RDA   Recommended daily (or dietary) allowance (or amount) of nutrients; *see* REFERENCE INTAKES.

RE   Retinol equivalents, *see* VITAMIN B.

reactive oxygen species (ROS)   A variety of compounds derived from oxygen, including superoxide, hydroxyl and perhydroxyl RADICALS, hydrogen peroxide and singlet oxygen.

rebaudioside   Very sweet substance extracted from the leaves of *Stevia rebaudiana* (same source as STEVIOSIDE); 400 times as sweet as sucrose.

recombinant DNA   Product of ligating (joining) two separate pieces of DNA, produced using the same RESTRICTION ENZYME, so as to permit introduction of foreign DNA into a host genome or PLASMID.

recommended daily amount (or allowance), RDA   *See* REFERENCE INTAKES.

recrystallisation   Changes in shape, size or orientation of ice crystals in frozen foods that cause a loss of quality.

rectal feeding   Also known as nutrient enemata. The colon can absorb 1–2 L of solution per day; maximum daily amount of glucose that can be given is 75 g (equivalent to 1260 kJ, 300 kcal), and 1 g of nitrogen, in the form of hydrolysed protein (equivalent to 6 g of protein).

red blood cells   *See* BLOOD CELLS.

red colours   AMARANTH (E-123), CARMOISINE (E-122), COCHINEAL (E-120), ERYTHROSINE (E-127), PONCEAU 4R (E-124), red 2G (E-128).

red cooking   Chinese method of cooking; meat or poultry is first stir fried, then simmered in broth or water.

redcurrants   Fruit of *Ribes sativum* (same species as whitecurrants); the UK National Fruit Collection contains 78 varieties.

Composition/100 g: (edible portion 98%) water 84 g, 234 kJ (56 kcal), protein 1.4 g, fat 0.2 g, carbohydrate 13.8 g (7.4 g sugars), fibre 4.3 g, ash 0.7 g, Ca 33 mg, Fe 1 mg, Mg 13 mg, P 44 mg, K 275 mg, Na 1 mg, Zn 0.2 mg, Cu 0.1 mg, Mn 0.2 mg, Se 0.6 µg, vitamin A 2 µg RE (72 µg carotenoids), E 0.1 mg, K 11 mg, B_1 0.04 mg, B_2 0.05 mg, niacin 0.1 mg, B_6 0.07 mg, folate 8 µg, pantothenate 0.1 mg, C 41 mg. A 110 g serving a rich source of vitamin C.

red fish   *See* ROSEFISH.

red herring   HERRING that has been well salted and smoked for about 10 days. Also called Yarmouth bloater. Bloaters are salted less and smoked for a shorter time; KIPPERS lightly salted and smoked overnight.

redox potential   Oxidation/reduction potential, the potential of an electrode in a 1 mol /L solution of each of the oxidant and reductant, relative to a hydrogen electrode.

red pepper   *See* PEPPER, SWEET.

red tide   Sudden, unexplained increase in numbers of toxic dinoflagellate organisms in the sea which cause fish and shellfish feeding on them to become seasonally toxic.

reduced   EU and US legislation state that for a food label or advertising to bear a claim that it contains a reduced amount of fat, saturates, cholesterol, sodium or alcohol it must contain 25% less of the specified nutrient than a reference product for which no claim is made. A food may not claim to have a reduced content of a nutrient if it is already classified as LOW IN or FREE FROM that nutrient.

reducing sugars SUGARS that are chemically reducing agents, including GLUCOSE, FRUCTOSE, LACTOSE, many PENTOSES, but not SUCROSE.

reduction *See* OXIDATION.

reduction rolls *See* MILLING.

reference intakes (of nutrients) Amounts of nutrients greater than the requirements of almost all members of the population, determined on the basis of the average requirement plus twice the standard deviation, to allow for individual variation in requirements, and thus covering the theoretical needs of 97.5% of the population. Reference intakes for energy are based on the average requirement, without the allowance for individual variation. Used for planning institutional catering, assessing the adequacy of diets of groups of people, but not strictly applicable to individuals. Tables of reference intakes published by different national and international authorities differ because of differences in the interpretation of the available data.

Variously called in different countries and by different expert committees: RDA, the recommended daily (or dietary) amount (or allowance); RDI, recommended daily (or dietary) intake; RNI, reference nutrient intake; PRI, population reference intake; safe allowances. *See* Tables 3-6.

Levels of intake below that at which health and metabolic integrity are likely to be maintained are generally taken as the average requirement minus twice the standard deviation. Variously known as minimum safe intake (MSI), lower reference nutrient intake (LRNI) or lowest threshold intake.

reference man, woman An arbitrary physiological standard; defined as a person aged 25, weighing 65 kg, living in a temperate zone of a mean annual temperature of 10 °C. Reference man performs medium work, with an average daily energy requirement of 13.5 MJ (3200 kcal). Reference woman is engaged in general household duties or light industry, with an average daily requirement of 9.7 MJ (2300 kcal).

reference nutrient intake, RNI *See* REFERENCE INTAKES.

reference protein *See* PROTEIN, REFERENCE.

refractive index Measure of the bending or refraction of a beam of light on entering a denser medium (the ratio between the sine of the angle of incidence of the ray of light and the sine of the angle of refraction). It is constant for pure substances under standard conditions. Used as a measure of sugar or total solids in solution, purity of oils, etc.

refractometer Instrument to measure the REFRACTIVE INDEX. The Abbé refractometer consists of two prisms between which the substance under examination (jam, fruit juice, sugar syrup, etc.) is spread, and light is reflected through the solution. The immersion refractometer dips into the solution.

refried beans *See* FRIJOLES.

refrigerants Cooling agents in refrigerators and freezers; originally ammonia or carbon dioxide were used, subsequently replaced by chlorofluorocarbons (CFCs), freons and arctons. Because of the persistence of CFCs in the upper atmosphere, where they destroy the protective ozone layer, manufacture of fully halogenated chlorofluorocarbons (CFCs) ceased in most countries in 1995, and they are being replaced by hydrofluorocarbons (HFCs) and hydrochlorofluorocarbons (HCFCs), sometimes collectively known as hydrofluoroalkanes (HFAs), although production of these compounds is to be phased out by 2015–2020.

See also HEAT PUMP.

refrigeration, mechanical Equipment that evaporates and compresses a refrigerant in a continuous cycle, using the cooled air, cooled liquid or cooled surfaces to freeze foods.

regional enteritis *See* CROHN'S DISEASE.

Rehfuss tube A small diameter tube with a slotted metal tip for removing samples of food from the stomach after a test meal.

See also RYLE TUBE.

Reichert–Meissl number Measure of the steam-volatile fatty acids in a lipid.

See also KIRSCHNER NUMBER; POLENSKE NUMBER; STEAM DISTILLATION.

relative dose response test For vitamin A status. The increase in circulating RETINOL BINDING PROTEIN after an oral dose of vitamin A; greater in vitamin A deficient subjects because in the absence of vitamin A reserves in the liver there is accumulation of the apo-protein.

relative humidity *See* HUMIDITY.

relative protein value A measure of PROTEIN QUALITY.

release agents Compounds used to lubricate surfaces that come into contact with food to prevent ingredients and finished products from sticking to them, e.g. fatty acid amides, microcrystalline waxes, petrolatums, starch, methyl cellulose.

relish Culinary term for any spicy or piquant preparation used to enhance flavour of plain food.

remove Obsolete term for the main course of dinner.

Remyline™ FAT REPLACER made from starch.

renal threshold Concentration of a compound in the blood above which it is not reabsorbed in the kidney, and so is excreted in the urine.

rendering Liberation of fat from ADIPOSE TISSUE. Dry rendering, heating the fat dry; wet rendering may use steam or hot water, either in open vessels or sealed under a pressure of 280–490 kPa (40–70 psi).

renin Proteolytic enzyme (angiotensin-forming enzyme, angiotensinogenase, EC 3.4.23.15) secreted by the kidney; specific for the leucine–leucine bond in angiotensinogen, yielding ANGIOTENSIN I. This is then cleaved to yield active angiotensin II by the angiotensin converting enzyme (ACE, EC 3.4.15.1), a peptidase in the blood vessels of the lungs and other tissues.

rennet Extract of calf stomach; contains the enzyme CHYMOSIN (rennin) which clots milk. Used in cheese-making and for JUNKET.

rennet, fungal A mixture of proteolytic enzymes from *Mucor pusillus*, *M. michei* and *Endothia parasitica*, used as substitutes for RENNET.

rennet, vegetable The name given to proteolytic enzymes derived from plants, such as BROMELAIN (from the pineapple) and FICIN (from the fig), as well as biosynthetic CHYMOSIN. Used for the preparation of vegetarian cheeses.

rennin *See* CHYMOSIN.

rentschlerising Sterilising by treatment with ultraviolet light, named after Dr H.C. Rentschler, who developed the lamp.

reovirus One of a small group of RNA-containing viruses that infect the intestinal and respiratory tracts without causing specific or serious disease.

See also ECHOVIRUS; ENTEROVIRUS.

REPFED Ready to eat products for extended durability, or refrigerated pasteurised foods for extended durability.

reporter gene A readily detectable gene (e.g. that for β-glucuronidase, firefly LUCIFERASE or GREEN FLUORESCENT PROTEIN) transferred into a TRANSGENIC organism together with the gene of interest, to permit ready identification of those cells in which the gene transfer has been achieved. Unlike a MARKER GENE, it does not confer a survival advantage on the transfected cells under laboratory conditions, but leads to the expression of a readily measured protein.

repression Inhibition of gene expression leading to a decrease in the rate of synthesis of a protein.

See also INDUCTION.

resazurin test *See* METHYLENE BLUE DYE-REDUCTION TEST.

resins, ion-exchange *See* ION-EXCHANGE RESINS.

resistant starch *See* STARCH, RESISTANT.

resistin Small protein secreted by ADIPOSE TISSUE that antagonises INSULIN action in the liver and acts on adipose tissue to inhibit differentiation of pre-ADIPOCYTES. Expression is low in DIABETES mellitus and during food deprivation, increased on refeeding, administration of INSULIN and in OBESITY. Also known as adipocyte secreted factor.

respiratory quotient (RQ) Ratio of the volume of carbon dioxide produced when a substance is oxidised to the volume of oxygen used. The oxidation of carbohydrate results in an RQ of 1.0; of fat, 0.7; and of protein, 0.8.

respirometer *See* SPIROMETER.

restoration The addition of nutrients to replace those lost in processing, as in milling of cereals.

   See also FORTIFICATION.

restriction enzymes (restriction endonucleases) Endonucleases (EC 3.2.21.3–5) that hydrolyse DNA at specific sequences (commonly palindromic sequences of 4–5 nucleotides). Some leave flush ends, others a region of single-stranded DNA (a 'sticky end') that can be annealed with a different fragment of DNA produced using the same enzyme, the basis of genetic engineering and the introduction of DNA from one species into the genome of another. Also used to split genomic DNA into fragments that can be sequenced. More than 160 restriction sites have been identified for different enzymes.

reticulocyte Immature precursor of the red blood cell (normocyte or erythrocyte) in which the remains of the nucleus are visible as a reticulum. Normally <1% of total red blood cells, but increased on remission of ANAEMIA, when there is a high rate of red cell production.

reticulum *See* RUMINANT.

retinal (retinaldehyde), retinene, retinoic acid, retinal *See* VITAMIN A.

retinoid Collective term for compounds chemically related to, or derived from, VITAMIN A. Synthetic retinoids have some of the biological activities of the vitamin, but have lower toxicity, and are used for treatment of serious skin disorders and some cancers.

retinoid receptors Two families of RETINOID binding proteins in cell nuclei that bind to retinoid response elements on DNA, and modulate gene expression in response to retinoids. The RAR (retinoic acid receptor) family bind all-*trans* (and 9-*cis*) retinoic acid, the RXR (originally 'unknown retinoid' receptor) family bind 9-*cis* retinoic acid. Retinoid receptors also interact with calcitriol (VITAMIN D) and THYROID HORMONE and other nuclear-acting hormone receptors.

retinol binding protein (1) Plasma protein (RBP) required for transport of retinol; synthesis falls in protein–energy malnutrition and ZINC deficiency, leading to functional VITAMIN A deficiency despite adequate liver reserves. Because apo-retinol binding protein does not occur in plasma, measurement of RBP provides a sensitive index of vitamin A status.

See also RELATIVE DOSE RESPONSE TEST; TRANSTHYRETIN.

(2) Cellular retinol (and retinoic acid) binding proteins (CRBP and CRABP) are essential for uptake of retinol and retinoic acid into cells, before onward metabolism and binding to RETINOID RECEPTORS.

retinol equivalents *See* VITAMIN A.

retort In food technology, an AUTOCLAVE.

retort pouches Laminated plastic or plastic and metal film packaging for AMBIENT-STABLE FOODS that are cooked in the factory and then reheated in the pouch at home.

retrogradation Cooked starch has an amorphous structure; the STALING of bread and other starchy foods is due to crystallisation of the starch, so that crumb loses its softness, a process that can be delayed by addition of emulsifiers (CRUMB SOFTENERS) such as polyoxyethylene and fatty acid monoglycerides. A number of modified starches (*see* STARCH, MODIFIED) are used to slow the process of retrogradation.

retroretinol Isomer of retinol (*see* VITAMIN A); one of the physiologically active RETINOIDS.

retrovirus RNA-containing virus that can incorporate its genetic material into the DNA of a host cell by making a DNA copy of the RNA using REVERSE TRANSCRIPTASE.

reverse osmosis *See* OSMOSIS, REVERSE.

reverse transcriptase Enzyme (EC 2.7.7.49) encoded by RNA viruses that catalyses the synthesis of DNA from an RNA template (the reverse of the process that occurs in TRANSCRIPTION). This permits incorporation of a copy of the virus genome into the host DNA. Reverse transcriptase is widely used in molecular biology and biotechnology to insert novel genes derived from mRNA into PLASMIDS.

Reynolds number (Re) Used to categorise fluid flow = (diameter of pipe × average velocity × fluid density)/fluid VISCOSITY. A value <2100 is streamline or laminar flow, >4000 is turbulent.

RF heating *See* MICROWAVE COOKING.

rhamnose A methylated PENTOSE; 33% as sweet as sucrose; widely distributed in plant foods.

rheology The science of the deformation and flow of materials.

rheopectic (rheopexic) A fluid whose structure builds up with continued SHEAR STRESS, so that VISCOSITY increases, as is the case with whipping cream.

See also DILATANT; PSEUDOPLASTIC; THIXOTROPIC.

rhizome Botanical term for swollen stem that produces roots and leafy shoots.

rhizopterin Obsolete name for FOLIC ACID.

rhodopsin The pigment in the cone cells of the retina of the eye, also known as visual purple, consisting of the protein opsin and retinaldehyde, which is responsible for the visual process. In rod cells of the retina the equivalent protein is iodopsin.

See also VITAMIN A; DARK ADAPTATION; VISION.

Rhodotorula Yeasts that may cause red, pink or yellow discoloration in foods.

rhubarb Leaf-stalks of the perennial plant, *Rheum rhaponticum*. Has a high content of OXALIC ACID (the leaves contain even more, and are toxic).

Composition/100g: (edible portion 75%) water 94g, 88kJ (21kcal), protein 0.9g, fat 0.2g, carbohydrate 4.5g (1.1g sugars), fibre 1.8g, ash 0.8g, Ca 86mg, Fe 0.2mg, Mg 12mg, P 14mg, K 288mg, Na 4mg, Zn 0.1mg, Mn 0.2mg, Se 1.1µg, vitamin A 5µg RE (231µg carotenoids), E 0.4mg, K 41mg, B_1 0.02mg, B_2 0.03mg, niacin 0.3mg, B_6 0.02mg, folate 7µg, pantothenate 0.1mg, C 8mg. A 140g serving is a source of Ca, Mn, vitamin C.

RIA *See* RADIOIMMUNOASSAY.

Ribena^{TM} A BLACKCURRANT juice cordial.

riboflavin *See* VITAMIN B_2.

ribonucleic acid (RNA) *See* NUCLEIC ACIDS.

ribose A pentose (five-carbon) sugar that occurs as an intermediate in the metabolism of glucose; especially important in the NUCLEIC ACIDS and various COENZYMES: occurs widely in foods.

ribosomes Intracellular organelles consisting of proteins and RNA that catalyse the synthesis of proteins (TRANSLATION). Ribosomes bind to, and travel along, mRNA, binding aminoacyl tRNA to each CODON in turn, and catalysing the synthesis of peptide bonds. A series of ribosomes translating the same strand of mRNA is known as a polysome. Proteins destined for export from the cell are synthesised by ribosomes attached to the rough endoplasmic reticulum of the cell.

Ribotide^{TM} A mixture of the PURINE derivatives, disodium inosinate and guanylate, used as a FLAVOUR enhancer for savoury dishes.

ribotyping Method for identification of bacteria using DNA probes to identify their ribosomal RNA.

ribozyme An RNA molecule that can catalyse a chemical reaction, an enzyme composed solely of RNA, with no protein.

rice Grain of *Oryza sativa*; the major food in many countries. Rice when threshed is known as paddy, and is covered with a fibrous husk making up nearly 40% of the grain. When the husk has been removed, brown rice is left. When the outer bran layers up to the endosperm and germ are removed, the ordinary white rice of commerce or polished rice is obtained (usually polished with glucose and talc).

Composition/100g: water 11.6g, 1528kJ (365kcal), protein 7.1g, fat 0.7g, carbohydrate 79.9g (0.1g sugars), fibre 1.3g, ash 0.6g, Ca 28mg, Fe 4.3mg, Mg 25mg, P 115mg, K 115mg, Na 5mg, Zn 1.1mg, Cu 0.2mg, Mn 1.1mg, Se 15.1µg, vitamin E 0.1mg, K 0.1mg, B_1 0.58mg, B_2 0.05mg, niacin 4.2mg, B_6 0.16mg, folate 231µg, pantothenate 1mg. A 30g serving is a source of Mn, vitamin B_1, a rich source of folate.

rice, American *See* BULGUR.

rice cones Granular rice particles the size of sand grains; the rice equivalent of SEMOLINA.

rice, fermented South American; whole rice is moistened and left to ferment for 10–15 days, then dried and milled. Bacterial and fungal fermentation reduces the time required for cooking – there is some loss of protein, but synthesis of VITAMIN B_2. Also known as arroz fermentado, arroz Amarillo or sierra rice.

rice, glutinous For most dishes, separate rice grains that do not stick together in a glutinous mass are preferred. Glutinous rice is rich in soluble starch, dextrin and maltose and on boiling the grains adhere in a sticky mass; used for sweetmeats and cakes.

rice, golden Variety of rice genetically engineered to contain large amounts of CAROTENE.

rice grass *See* INDIAN RICE GRASS.

rice, hungry W African variety of MILLET, *Digitaria exilis*.

rice, maize or mealie *See* MAIZE RICE.

rice paper Smooth edible white 'paper' made from the pith of the Taiwanese shrub *Tetrapanax papyriferus* and the Indo-Pacific shrub *Scaevola sericea*.

rice, red W. African species, *Oryza glaberrima*, with red bran layer.

rice, synthetic *See* TAPIOCA-MACARONI.

rice, unpolished American term; rice that has been undermilled in that the husk, germ and bran layers have been only partially removed.

rice vinegar Japanese; VINEGAR prepared from SAKÉ.

rice, wild Also known as zizanie, Tuscarora rice, Indian rice and American wild rice (American rice is BULGUR); *Zizania aquatica*, native to eastern N. America, grows 4 m (12 feet) high; long, thin, greenish grain; little is grown and difficult to harvest, so is a gourmet food. Higher in protein content than ordinary rice.

Composition/100 g: water 7.8 g, 1494 kJ (357 kcal), protein 14.7 g, fat 1.1 g (of which 18% saturated, 18% mono-unsaturated, 64% polyunsaturated), carbohydrate 74.9 g (2.5 g sugars), fibre 6.2 g, ash 1.5 g, Ca 21 mg, Fe 2 mg, Mg 177 mg, P 433 mg, K 427 mg, Na 7 mg, Zn 6 mg, Cu 0.5 mg, Mn 1.3 mg, Se 2.8 µg, vitamin A 1 µg RE (231 µg carotenoids), E 0.8 mg, K 1.9 mg, B_1 0.12 mg, B_2 0.26 mg, niacin 6.7 mg, B_6 0.39 mg, folate 95 µg, pantothenate 1.1 mg. A 30 g serving is a source of Cu, Mg, Mn, P, Zn, niacin, folate.

rice wine *See* SAKÉ.

ricin A LECTIN in the castor oil bean.

ricing Culinary term: cutting into small pieces about the size of rice grains.

rickets Malformation and undermineralisation of the bones in growing children due to deficiency of VITAMIN D, leading to poor absorption of calcium. In adults the equivalent is OSTEOMALACIA. In early (subclinical) rickets there is a marked elevation of plasma ALKALINE PHOSPHATASE.

Refractory or vitamin D-resistant rickets does not respond to normal amounts of vitamin D but requires massive doses. Usually a result of a congenital defect in the metabolism of vitamin D or cellular vitamin D receptors; may also be due to strontium poisoning.

ricotta Italian soft WHEY cheese; American ricotta is made from a mixture of whey and skimmed milk.

Composition/100 g: water 71.7 g, 728 kJ (174 kcal), protein 11.3 g, fat 13 g (of which 67% saturated, 29% mono-unsaturated, 3% polyunsaturated), cholesterol 51 mg, carbohydrate 3 g (0.3 g sugars), ash 1 g, Ca 207 mg, Fe 0.4 mg, Mg 11 mg, P 158 mg, K 105 mg, Na 84 mg, Zn 1.2 mg, Se 14.5 µg, vitamin A 120 µg RE (117 µg retinol, 33 µg carotenoids), E 0.1 mg, K 1.1 mg, B_1 0.01 mg, B_2 0.19 mg, niacin 0.1 mg, B_6 0.04 mg, folate 12 µg, B_{12} 0.3 µg, pantothenate 0.2 mg. A 110 g serving is a source of vitamin A, B_2, a good source of Ca, P, Se, a rich source of vitamin B_{12}.

riffle flumes Washing equipment consisting of stepped channels along which the product being washed is carried in a flow of water; stones and grit are retained on the steps.

rigor mortis Stiffening of muscle that occurs after death. As the flow of blood ceases, anaerobic metabolism leads to the formation of lactic acid and the soft, pliable muscle becomes stiff and rigid. If meat is hung in a cool place for a few days ('conditioned'), the meat softens again. Fish similarly undergo rigor mortis usually of shorter duration than in mammals.

See also MEAT CONDITIONING; MEAT, DFD.

rijstaffel Dutch, Indonesian; meal consisting of a variety of different dishes (20 or more) served at the same time.

risk factor A factor that can be measured to indicate the statistical or epidemiological probability of an adverse condition, effect or disease. Does not imply that it is a causative factor, nor that reversing the risk factor will reduce the hazard.

Rittinger's law Equation to calculate the energy cost of reducing particle size, based on the difference in surface area.
See also BOND'S LAW; COMMINUTION; KICK'S LAW.

RNA Ribonucleic acid, see NUCLEIC ACIDS.

RNAi (RNA interference) A technique for silencing the expression of specific genes by use of double-stranded RNA; it serves as an antiviral defence mechanism and may play a role in the formation and maintenance of heterochromatin during cell division.

RNI Reference nutrient intake, see REFERENCE INTAKES.

rocambole Mild variety of GARLIC, *Allium scordoprasum*, also called sand leek.

rock eel, rock salmon Alternative names for DOGFISH.

rocket Cruciferous plant, *Eruca sativa*, with small spear-shaped leaves and peppery taste, eaten raw in salads or cooked. Also called arugula, rucola, Italian cress.
    Composition/100g: (edible portion 60%) water 91.7g, 105kJ (25kcal), protein 2.6g, fat 0.7g, carbohydrate 3.7g (2g sugars), fibre 1.6g, ash 1.4g, Ca 160mg, Fe 1.5mg, Mg 47mg, P 52mg, K 369mg, Na 27mg, Zn 0.5mg, Cu 0.1mg, Mn 0.3mg, Se 0.3µg, vitamin A 119µg RE (4979µg carotenoids), E 0.4mg, K 108mg, B_1 0.04mg, B_2 0.09mg, niacin 0.3mg, B_6 0.07mg, folate 97µg, pantothenate 0.4mg, C 15mg.

rock fish Saltwater FISH, *Sebastodes* spp., with a flavour resembling crab.

rock lobster New Zealand salt-water CRAYFISH (*Jasus edwardsii*).

rocou See ANNATTO.

rod mill Variant of BALL MILL, using cylindrical steel rods instead of balls, to prevent balls sticking in foods.

roe Hard roe is the eggs of the female fish. Soft roe is from the male fish, also known as milt or melt. Hard roe of sturgeon and lumpfish are used to make CAVIARE and mock caviare.

Rohalase™ Bacterial and fungal AMYLASES used in brewing.

roller dryer The material to be dried is spread over the surface of internally heated rollers and drying is complete within a few seconds. The rollers rotate against a knife that scrapes off the dried film as soon as it forms. There is little damage to nutrients by this method; for example, roller-dried milk is not scorched, but there is more loss of vitamins B_1 and C than in spray drying.

roller mill Pairs of horizontal cylindrical rollers, separated by only a small gap and revolving at different speeds. The material is thus ground and crushed in one operation. Used in flour milling.

rollmop Filleted uncooked HERRING pickled in spiced vinegar.

roll-on closure (RO) Aluminium or lacquered tinplate cap for sealing on to narrow-necked bottles with a threaded neck. The unthreaded cap is moulded on to the neck of the bottle and forms an airtight seal.

romaine French and American name for cos LETTUCE.

rooibos tea Fermented leaves of the S African bush *Aspalathus linearis*. Contains a unique polyphenol, aspalathin, which becomes red during preparation and produces a reddish herbal tea; free from CAFFEINE and THEAFLAVIN.

root beer American; non-alcoholic carbonated beverage flavoured with extract of SASSAFRAS root and oil of wintergreen.

rope Spore-forming bacteria (*Bacillus mesentericus* and *B. subtilis*) occur on wheat and hence in flour. The spores can survive baking and are present in the bread. Under the right conditions of warmth and moisture the spores germinate and the mass of bacteria convert the bread into sticky, yellowish patches that can be pulled out into rope-like threads, hence the term ropy bread. The bacterial growth is inhibited by acid substances. Can also occur in milk, called long milk in Scandinavia.

roquefort Green-blue marbled French CHEESE made in Roquefort-sur-Soulzon from ewe's milk; ripened in limestone caves where the mould, *Penicillium roquefortii* is present and inoculates the cheese.

ROS *See* REACTIVE OXYGEN SPECIES.

rosefish (red fish) Saltwater FISH with red flesh, *Sebastes marinus*, sometimes called ocean perch.

Rose-Gottlieb test Gravimetric method for determination of fat in milk, by extraction with diethyl ether and petroleum ether from an ammoniacal alcoholic solution of the sample.

rosella Caribbean plant (*Hibiscus sabdariffa*) grown for its fleshy red sepals, used to make drinks, jams and jelly. Also known as sorrel, flor de Jamaica.

rosemary A bushy shrub, *Rosmarinus officinalis*, cultivated commercially for its essential oil, used in medicine and perfumery. The leaves are used to flavour soups, sauces and meat.

rose water Fragrant water made by distillation or extraction of the ESSENTIAL OILS of rose petals. Used in confectionery (especially TURKISH DELIGHT) and baking.

rotary louvre dryer Hot air passes through a moving bed of the solid inside a rotating drum.

Roth–Benedict spirometer *See* SPIROMETER.

Rothera's test For KETONES in urine; reaction with ammonium hydroxide, ammonium sulphate and sodium nitroprusside to give a purple colour in the presence of ketones.

roti *See* CHAPPATI.

rôtisserie Method of cooking which developed from the traditional rotating spit above an open fire; the food is rotated while roasting, so bastes itself.

roughage *See* FIBRE, DIETARY; NON-STARCH POLYSACCHARIDES.

round worm *See* NEMATODE.

roux The foundation of most sauces; prepared by cooking together equal amounts of fat and plain flour, for a short time for white sauces, and longer for blond or brown sauces. The sauce is then prepared by stirring in milk or stock.

Rovimix™ Stabilised preparations of vitamins, as beadlets coated with a gelatine–starch mixture, used to enrich foods.

royal jelly The food on which bee larvae are fed and which causes them to develop into queen bees. Although it is a rich source of PANTOTHENIC ACID and other vitamins, in the amounts consumed it would make a negligible contribution to human nutrition. 2% of its dry weight is hydroxydecenoic acid, which is believed to be the active queen substance. Claimed, without foundation, to have rejuvenating properties for human beings.

RPV Relative protein value, a measure of PROTEIN QUALITY.

RQ *See* RESPIRATORY QUOTIENT.

RTE Ready to eat.

rubble reel Machine for cleaning materials such as wheat. The material is fed into a long inclined reel made of perforated metal that rotates inside a frame. The perforations become larger nearer the bottom, so that there is a graded sieving of the material as it passes down the reel.

Rubner factors *See* ENERGY CONVERSION FACTORS.

rum Spirit distilled from fermented sugar cane juice or molasses; may be colourless and light tasting or dark and with a strong flavour. Traditionally rum is darker and more strongly flavoured the further south in the Caribbean it is made. There are three main categories: Cuban, Jamaican and Dutch East Indies; and several types: aguardiente (Spain, Portugal and S America), Bacardi (trade name, originally from Cuba), cachaca (Brazil), cane spirit (S Africa), Demerara rum (Guyana), 35–60% alcohol by volume, 1.0–1.8 MJ (250–420 kcal) per 100 mL.

rumen *See* RUMINANTS.

ruminants Animals such as the cow, sheep and goat, which possess four stomachs, as distinct from monogastric animals, such as human, pig, dog and rat. The four are: the rumen, or first stomach, where bacterial fermentation produces volatile fatty acids, and whence the food is returned to the mouth for further mastication (chewing the cud); the reticulum, where further bacterial fermentation produces volatile fatty acids; the omasum; and the abomasum or true stomach. The bacterial fermentation allows ruminants to obtain nourishment from grass and hay which cannot be digested by monogastric animals.

rumpbone   Cut of meat: (USA) = aitchbone, (UK) = loin or haunch.

rush nut   *See* TIGER NUT.

rusk   (1) Sweetened biscuit or piece of bread or cake crisped in the oven, especially as food for young children when teething.

(2) Cereal added to SAUSAGES and HAMBURGERS.

rutabaga   American name for SWEDE.

rutin   The disaccharide derivative of QUERCITIN, containing GLUCOSE and RHAMNOSE. Found in grains, tomato stalk and elderflower. Not known to be a dietary essential or to have any function in the body.

See also FLAVONOIDS.

rye   Grain of *Secale cereale*, the predominant cereal in some parts of Europe; very hardy and withstands adverse conditions better than wheat. Rye flour is dark and the dough lacks elasticity; rye bread is usually made with sour dough or leaven rather than yeast.

Composition/100 g: water 10.9 g, 1402 kJ (335 kcal), protein 14.8 g, fat 2.5 g (of which 18% saturated, 18% mono-unsaturated, 65% polyunsaturated), carbohydrate 69.8 g (1 g sugars), fibre 14.6 g, ash 2 g, Ca 33 mg, Fe 2.7 mg, Mg 121 mg, P 374 mg, K 264 mg, Na 6 mg, Zn 3.7 mg, Cu 0.4 mg, Mn 2.7 mg, Se 35.3 µg, vitamin A 1 µg RE (217 µg carotenoids), E 1.3 mg, K 5.9 mg, B_1 0.32 mg, B_2 0.25 mg, niacin 4.3 mg, B_6 0.29 mg, folate 60 µg, pantothenate 1.5 mg.

Ryle tube   A narrow rubber tube with a blind end containing a lead weight, with holes above this level, for removing samples of the contents from the stomach at intervals after a test meal.

See also REHFUSS TUBE.

Ryvita™   A rye CRISPBREAD.

S

S- and R-   *See* R- AND S-.

saccharases   Enzymes (including INVERTASE) that HYDROLYSE sugars to their constituent MONOSACCHARIDES.

saccharic acid   The dicarboxylic acid derived from glucose.

saccharimeter POLARIMETER used to determine the purity of sugar; graduated on the International Sugar Scale, degrees sugar (distinct from SACCHAROMETER).

saccharin Sulphobenzimide, a synthetic SWEETENER, 550 times as sweet as sucrose. Soluble saccharin is the sodium salt.

saccharometer Floating device used to determine the specific gravity of sugar solutions (distinct from SACCHARIMETER).

Saccharomyces bulardii *See* PROBIOTICS.

saccharose *See* SUCROSE.

sachertorte Austrian; chocolate sponge cake with rich chocolate icing and whipped cream.

sack Old name for various white wines from Spain and the Canaries, e.g. sherry.

safe allowances, level of intake *See* REFERENCE INTAKES.

safe and adequate intake Where there is inadequate scientific evidence to establish requirements and REFERENCE INTAKES for a nutrient for which deficiency is rarely seen, if ever, the observed levels of intake are assumed to be greater than requirements, and thus provide an estimate of intakes that are safe and (more than) adequate to meet needs.

safflower Oil extracted from the seeds of *Carthamus tinctoria*. Mexican saffron is a substitute for SAFFRON made from the stigmata.

Linoleic safflower oil is 7% saturated, 15% mono-unsaturated, 78% polyunsaturated; oleic safflower oil is 7% saturated, 78% mono-unsaturated, 15% polyunsaturated; both contain 34.1 mg vitamin E, and 7.1 mg vitamin K/100 g.

saffron Deep orange-red powder from the powdered stigmata of the saffron crocus, *Crocus sativus*; 1g requires stigmata of 1500 flowers and yields about 50 mg of extract. Used as natural dyestuff (permitted food colour, with no E-number) and spice. Very soluble in water. Indian saffron is TURMERIC; Mexican saffron is SAFFLOWER.

sage Leaf of the Dalmatian sage, *Salvia officinalis*; fragrant and spicy, used to flavour meat and fish dishes and in poultry stuffing. Other sages (Greek, Spanish, English) differ in flavour from the Dalmatian variety.

sago Starchy grains prepared from the pith of the swamp sago (*Metroxylon sagu*) and the sugar palm (*Arenga pinnuta*); almost pure starch.

saithe A white FISH, *Polachius virens*, also known as coley and coal fish.

saké Japanese fermented beverage made from rice; although commonly called rice wine, it is technically a beer, since it is made from a cereal, although it does not contain gas. The fungus *Aspergillus oryzae* (Koji) is used as a source of AMYLASE, then yeast is added; the final product contains 14–20% alcohol.

salad dressing Emulsions of oil and vinegar, which may or not contain other flavourings. French dressing (vinaigrette) is a temporary EMULSION of oil and vinegar; heavy French dressing is stabilised with PECTIN or vegetable GUM.

Mayonnaise is a stable emulsion of vinegar in oil, made with egg. Salad cream was originally developed as a commercial substitute for mayonnaise (mid-19th century); an emulsion made from vegetable oil, vinegar, salt, spices, emulsified with egg yolk and thickened. Legally, in the UK, must contain not less than 25% by weight of vegetable oil and not less than 1.35% egg yolk solids. Mayonnaise usually contains more oil, less carbohydrate and water.

By US regulations salad dressing contains 30% vegetable oil and 4% egg yolk; mayonnaise contains 65% oil plus egg yolk.

Red mayonnaise is prepared by adding beetroot juice and the coral (eggs) of lobster to mayonnaise; an accompaniment to lobster and other seafood dishes. Russian dressing is in fact American; made from mayonnaise with pimento, chilli sauce, green pepper and celery, or sometimes by mixing mayonnaise with tomato ketchup. Thousand Island dressing is made from equal parts of mayonnaise and Russian dressing, with whipped cream.

salamander Traditional round metal cooking implement, heated in the fire until red hot and held over the surface of pastry and other foods to brown it.

salami Type of SAUSAGE speckled with pieces of fat, flavoured with garlic; originally Italian.

salatrims Family of triacylglycerols prepared from hydrogenated SOY or CANOLA oil and short-chain triacylglycerols by INTER-ESTERIFICATION; only partially absorbed. The name derives from short and long-chain acid triacylglycerol molecules.

salep, salepi Turkish, Greek; beverage prepared from orchid tubers. Milky white in appearance, with only a slight flavour.

sal fat Vegetable butter prepared from seeds of the Indian sal tree (*Shorea robusta*).

See also COCOA BUTTER EQUIVALENTS

saline *See* PHYSIOLOGICAL SALINE.

salinometer (salimeter, salometer) Hydrometer to measure concentration of salt solutions by density.

Salisbury steak American; similar to HAMBURGER, minced beef mixed with bread, eggs, milk and seasoning, shaped into cakes and fried.

saliva Secretion of the salivary glands in the mouth: 1–1.5 L secreted daily. A dilute solution of the protein MUCIN (which lubricates food) and the enzyme AMYLASE, with small quantities of urea, and mineral salts.

salivary glands Three pairs of glands in the mouth, which secrete SALIVA: parotid, submandibular and submaxillary glands.

Sally Lunn A sweet, spongy, yeast cake, named after a girl who sold her tea cakes in Bath in the 18th century. In southern USA a variety of yeast and soda breads.

salmagundi (salamagundi) Old English dish consisting of diced fresh and salt meats mixed with hard-boiled eggs, pickled vegetables and spices, arranged on a bed of salad.

salmine *See* PROTAMINES.

salmon Fish of a number of species including Atlantic salmon (*Salmo salar*), and chinook, chum, coho (or silver), pink (or humpback), sockeye (or red) which are *Oncorhynchus* spp., and in UK must be described as red or pink salmon. Although wild salmon are caught on a large scale, much is farmed in deep inlets of the sea.

Composition/100 g: water 69 g, 766 kJ (183 kcal), protein 19.9 g, fat 10.9 g (of which 22% saturated, 39% mono-unsaturated, 39% polyunsaturated), cholesterol 59 mg, carbohydrate 0 g, ash 1 g, Ca 12 mg, Fe 0.4 mg, Mg 28 mg, P 233 mg, K 362 mg, Na 59 mg, Zn 0.4 mg, Se 36.5 μg, vitamin A 15 μg RE (15 μg retinal), B_1 0.34 mg, B_2 0.12 mg, niacin 7.5 mg, B_6 0.64 mg, folate 26 μg, B_{12} 2.8 μg, pantothenate 1.4 mg, C 4 mg. A 100 g serving is a source of folate, a good source of P, vitamin B_1, pantothenate, a rich source of Se, niacin, VITAMIN B_6, B_{12}.

salmon berry Fruit of American wild raspberry, *Ribes spectabilis*.

***Salmonella* spp.** Bacteria (Enterobacteriaceae) that are a common cause of food poisoning. Found in eggs from infected hens, sausages, etc.; can survive in brine and at refrigerator temperatures; destroyed by adequate heating. Most species invade intestinal epithelial cells. Infective dose 10^3–10^6 organisms, onset 6–72 h, duration 2–7 days, TX 4.1.2.2.

Salmonella enterica serovars Typhi and *Paratyphi* (formerly *S. typhi* and *S. paratyphi*) cause systemic infection: infective dose 1–10^2 organisms, onset 10–21 days, duration weeks.

There was a large increase in salmonellosis in Britain in the 1980s when *S. enteritidis* became endemic in poultry, levelling off in 1990–1995. *Subsequently* there was an increase (also in USA) in *S. typhimurium* DT with a relatively high mortality. Found in cereals, beef, pork and chicken.

salmon, rock Alternative name for DOGFISH.

salometer *See* SALINOMETER.

salsify (oyster plant, vegetable oyster) Long, white, tapering root of the biennial plant *Tragopogon porrifolius*.

Composition/100g: (edible portion 87%) water 77g, 343kJ (82kcal), protein 3.3g, fat 0.2g, carbohydrate 18.6g, fibre 3.3g, ash 0.9g, Ca 60mg, Fe 0.7mg, Mg 23mg, P 75mg, K 380mg, Na 20mg, Zn 0.4mg, Cu 0.1mg, Mn 0.3mg, Se 0.8µg, vitamin B_1 0.08mg, B_2 0.22mg, niacin 0.5mg, B_6 0.28mg, folate 26µg, pantothenate 0.4mg, C 8mg.

Black salsify is very similar; hardy perennial, *Scorzonera hispanica* (sometimes used roasted as coffee substitute).

salt Usually refers to sodium chloride, common salt or table salt (chemically any product of reaction between an acid and an alkali is a salt). The main sources are either mining in areas where there are rich deposits of crystalline salt, or evaporation of seawater in shallow pans (known as sea salt).

See also BUFFERS; SODIUM.

salt-free diets Diets low in SODIUM, for the treatment of HYPERTENSION and other conditions. Most of the sodium of the diet is consumed as sodium chloride or SALT, and hence such diets are referred to as salt-restricted or low-salt diets, or sometimes 'salt-free', to emphasise that no salt is added to foods in preparation or at the table. Since foods naturally contain sodium chloride, a truly salt-free diet is not possible. It is the sodium and not the chloride that is important.

See also HYPERTENSION; SALT, LIGHT.

salting Method of preserving meat, fish and some vegetables using salt and saltpetre.

salt, light (lite) Mixtures of sodium chloride with potassium and ammonium chlorides together with citrates, formates, phosphates, glutamates, as well as herbs and spices and/or other substances to reduce the intake of SODIUM and improve the palatability of SALT-FREE DIETS.

saltpetre (Bengal saltpetre) Potassium NITRATE.

salts, Indian Ancient Greek and Roman name for sugar.

sambal goring *See* TRASSI.

SAMI Socially acceptable monitoring instrument. A small heart-rate-counting apparatus used to estimate ENERGY EXPENDITURE of human subjects.

samna Clarified butter fat, *see* BUTTER; GHEE.

samosa Indian; deep-fried stuffed pancakes, rolled into a cone or folded into an envelope.

samp Coarsely cut portions of MAIZE with bran and germ partly removed.

See also HOMINY.

samphire (1) Rock samphire, St Peter's herb, succulent plant of cliffs and salt marshes (*Crithmum maritimum*); grows on coastal rocks, fleshy aromatic leaves may be eaten raw, boiled or pickled.

(2) Marsh samphire (glasswort, sea asparagus), *Salicornia* spp., grows in salt marshes, salty, eaten cooked as a vegetable.

samso Danish hard CHEESE.

Sanatogen™ A preparation of casein and sodium glycerophosphate for consumption as a beverage when added to milk.

sanding In sugar confectionery, coating with sugar crystals, used mainly on jellies.

sand leek *See* ROCAMBOLE.

sandwich Two slices of bread enclosing a filling (meat, cheese, fish, etc.). Invention attributed to the fourth Earl of Sandwich (1718–1792), who spent long periods at the gaming table and carried a portable meal of beef sandwiched with bread. Decker sandwiches consist of several layers of bread, each separated by filling; Neapolitan sandwiches are decker sandwiches made with alternating slices of white and brown bread. Open sandwiches (SMØRREBRØD) consist of a single slice of bread, biscuit or small roll.

Sanecta™ *See* ASPARTAME.

Sanka™ Decaffeinated instant coffee. *See* CAFFEINE; COFFEE.

sapodilla Fruit of the sapodilla tree (*Achras sapota*); size of a small apple, rough-grained, yellow to greyish pulp. Chicle, the basis of CHEWING GUM, is made from the latex of the tree.

Composition/100 g: (edible portion 80%) water 78 g, 347 kJ (83 kcal), protein 0.4 g, fat 1.1 g, carbohydrate 20 g, fibre 5.3 g, ash 0.5 g, Ca 21 mg, Fe 0.8 mg, Mg 12 mg, P 12 mg, K 193 mg, Na 12 mg, Zn 0.1 mg, Cu 0.1 mg, Se 0.6 µg, vitamin A 3 µg RE, B_2 0.02 mg, niacin 0.2 mg, B_6 0.04 mg, folate 14 µg, pantothenate 0.3 mg, C 15 mg. An 85 g serving (half fruit) is a good source of vitamin C.

saponification Alkaline hydrolysis of FATTY ACID esters (including TRIACYLGLYCEROLS) prior to analysis. The saponification value of a fat or oil is the amount of potassium hydroxide required to hydrolyse (saponify) 1 g of the fat.

saponins Group of substances that occur in plants and can produce a soapy lather with water. Extracted commercially from soapwort (*Saponaria officinalis*) or soapbark (*Quillaja saponaria*) and used as foam producer in beverages and fire extinguishers, as detergents and for emulsifying oils. Bitter in flavour.

See also QUILLAJA.

sapote Fruit of the central American sub-tropical evergreen tree *Casimiroa edulis.*

Composition/100 g: (edible portion 71%) water 62.4 g, 561 kJ (134 kcal), protein 2.1 g, fat 0.6 g, carbohydrate 33.8 g, fibre 2.6 g, ash 1.1 g, Ca 39 mg, Fe 1 mg, Mg 30 mg, P 28 mg, K 344 mg, Na 10 mg, vitamin A 21 µg RE, B_1 0.01 mg, B_2 0.02 mg, niacin 1.8 mg, C 20 mg. A 110 g serving (half fruit) is a source of Mg, niacin, a rich source of vitamin C.

See also MAMEY.

sapsago   Swiss cheese made from soured skimmed milk and whole milk; clover is added to the curd, giving it a green colour.

saracen corn   *See* BUCKWHEAT.

saran   Generic name for thermoplastic materials made from polymers of vinylidene chloride and vinyl chloride. They are clear transparent films (cling film) used for wrapping food; resistant to oils and chemicals; can be heat-shrunk onto the product.

sarcolactic acid   Obsolete name for (+)lactic acid (which rotates the plane of polarised light to the right), found in muscle, as distinct from the optically inactive LACTIC ACID (a mixture of (+) and (−) isomers) found in sour milk. Also known as paralactic acid.

See also MEAT CONDITIONING; MEAT, DFD; RIGOR MORTIS.

sarcolemma   *See* MUSCLE.

sarcomere   The basic contractile unit of striated MUSCLE.

sarcosine   *N*-Methylglycine, an intermediate in the metabolism of CHOLINE. Found in relatively large amounts in starfish and sea urchins, used as an intermediate in the synthesis of antienzyme agents in toothpaste.

sardell   *See* ANCHOVY.

sardine   Young PILCHARD *Sardina* (*Clupea*) *pilchardus*; commonly canned in oil, brine or tomato paste. Norwegian canned sardines are salted and smoked before canning; French are salted and steamed.

Saridele   Protein-rich baby food (26–30% protein) developed in Indonesia; extract of soya bean with sugar, calcium carbonate, vitamins B_1, B_{12} and C.

sarsaparilla   (1) Flavour prepared from oil of SASSAFRAS and oil of wintergreen or oil of sweet birch.

(2) Roots of a south American plant (*Smilax officinalis*). Both used to flavour the beverage called sarsaparilla.

sassafras   American tree (*Sassafras albidum*) with aromatic bark and leaves. The root is used to make ROOT BEER and the young leaves are powdered to make filé powder, an essential flavouring of GUMBO. Sassafras oil from the root bark is used medicinally and as a flavour in beverages, but banned in some countries because of its toxicity.

satiety   The sensation of fullness after a meal.

satsuma   *See* CITRUS.

saturates   Commonly used term for saturated FATTY ACIDS.

saturation analysis   *See* RADIOIMMUNOASSAY.

saturation humidity   *See* HUMIDITY.

saturation temperature   *See* DEW POINT.

sauerkraut   German, Dutch, Alsatian; prepared by lactic fermentation of shredded cabbage. In the presence of 2–3% salt, acid-forming bacteria thrive and convert sugars in the cabbage into acetic and lactic acids, which then act as preservatives.

sauermilchkase   German cheeses made from low-fat milk using a lactic acid starter and no RENNET.

sauerteig   *See* BREAD.

sausage   Chopped meat, commonly beef or pork, seasoned with salt and spices, mixed with cereal (usually wheat rusk prepared from crumbed unleavened biscuits) and packed into casings (*see* SAUSAGE CASINGS). In UK pork sausages must be at least 65% meat and beef sausages 50% meat.

Six main types: fresh, smoked, cooked, smoked and cooked, semi-dry and dry. Frankfurters, Bologna, Polish and Berliner sausages are made from cured meat and are smoked and cooked. Thuringer, soft salami, mortadella and soft cervelat are semi-dry sausages. Pepperoni, chorizos, dry salami, dry cervelat are slowly dried to a hard texture.

sausage casings   Natural casings are made from hog intestines for fresh frying sausages, and from sheep intestines for chipolatas and frankfurters, now mainly replaced by artificial casings made from CELLULOSE, polyvinyl dichloride or COLLAGEN. Skinless sausages are prepared in cellulose casing, which is then peeled off.

sausage factor   *See* MEAT FACTOR.

sausages, emulsion   Also known as bratwurst. Sausages made from a meat mixture that is finely chopped with added water and salt. Much of the fat is liberated but remains emulsified by the lean meat mixture, giving a homogeneous paste (known in German as *brat*) that gels to a firm sliceable mass on heating.

savarin   *See* BABA.

saveloy   Highly seasoned smoked SAUSAGE; the addition of saltpetre gives rise to the bright red colour. Originally a sausage made from pig brains.

savory   Herb with strongly flavoured leaves used as seasoning in sauces, soups, salad dishes. Summer savory is an annual, *Satureja hortensis*; winter savory is a perennial, *S. montana*.

savoy   Variety of CABBAGE (*Brassica oleracea* var. *capitata*) with crimped leaves.

saw palmetto   North American palm (*Serenoa repens, S. serrulata*); the berries were eaten by native Americans, and there is some evidence that the oil (which contains STEROLS) may have beneficial effects in treatment of benign prostate enlargement.

Saxin™ *See* SACCHARIN.

sbrinz Swiss hard cheese similar to PARMESAN.

SCADA Supervisory control and data acquisition; software to display data from monitoring of manufacturing processes as real-time graphics, developed in the 1980s. Now superseded by open database connectivity (ODBC) and object linking exchange (OLE) software.

scald (1) Pouring boiling water over a food to clean it, loosen hairs (e.g. on a joint of pork) or remove the skin of fruit and tomatoes.

See also BLANCHING.

(2) Heating milk almost to boiling point, to retard souring or to make clotted CREAM.

(3) Defect occurring in stored apples; the formation of brown patches under the skin, with browning and softening of the tissue underneath. Due to accumulation of gases given off during ripening.

scaldfish *See* MEGRIM.

scallion Small ONION which has not developed a bulb, widely used in Chinese cooking; also used for shallots and spring onion (especially in USA).

scallops Marine bivalve MOLLUSCS, species of the Pectinidae family; Queen scallop is *Chamys opercularis.*

Composition/100 g: water 79 g, 368 kJ (88 kcal), protein 16.8 g, fat 0.8 g, cholesterol 33 mg, carbohydrate 2.4 g, ash 1.5 g, Ca 24 mg, Fe 0.3 mg, Mg 56 mg, P 219 mg, K 322 mg, Na 161 mg, Zn 0.9 mg, Cu 0.1 mg, Mn 0.1 mg, Se 22.2 µg, I 20 µg, vitamin A 15 µg retinol, K 0.1 mg, B_1 0.01 mg, B_2 0.06 mg, niacin 1.1 mg, B_6 0.15 mg, folate 16 µg, B_{12} 1.5 µg, pantothenate 0.1 mg, C 3 mg. A 60 g serving is a source of Mg, P, Se, a rich source of vitamin B_{12}.

scampi Shellfish, Norway lobster or Dublin Bay prawn, *Nephrops norvegicus. See* LOBSTER.

scapula The shoulder blade, a triangular BONE.

Scenedesmus See ALGAE.

Schiff base An aldimine linkage formed by condensation between an aldehyde and an amino group.

See also MAILLARD REACTION; PYRIDOXYLLYSINE.

Schilling test For VITAMIN B_{12} absorption; an oral dose of [57]Co-labelled vitamin B_{12} is given 1 h after a large (1000 µg) parenteral dose of non-radioactive vitamin, and radioactivity in urine is determined over the next 24 hours.

See also ANAEMIA, PERNICIOUS; INTRINSIC FACTOR.

schnitzel Austrian, German; cutlet or escalope of veal or pork.

Schoenheimer–Sperry reaction A modification of the LIEBER-MANN–BURCHARD reaction for CHOLESTEROL.

scifers Cornish name for Welsh onion (*see* ONION, WELSH).

scintillation counter Instrument for measurement of radioactivity by emission of light from a solid or liquid scintillator that emits a photon after absorbing a β-particle or γ-ray.

sclerosis Hardening of tissue due to scarring, inflammation or ageing.

See also ARTERIOSCLEROSIS; ATHEROSCLEROSIS.

scolex Head of a TAPEWORM, with hooks or suckers to permit attachment to the intestinal wall.

scombroid poisoning Apparently caused by bacterial spoilage of fish including many of the Scombridae (TUNA, bonito, MACKEREL) but also non-scombroid fish and other foods. Symptoms (including skin rash, nausea, tingling) resemble HISTAMINE poisoning and were previously thought to be due to bacterial formation of histamine, now doubted.

scone A variety of tea cake originally made from white flour or barley meal and sour milk or buttermilk in Scone, Scotland; baked on a griddle and cut in quarters. Drop scone is a small pancake made by dropping batter onto a griddle.

scorbutic *See* SCURVY.

scorzonera *See* SALSIFY.

Scotch egg Hard-boiled egg cased in seasoned sausage meat and breadcrumbs, fried and served cold.

scotopic Conditions of poor illumination; hence scotopic VISION is vision in dim light (*see* DARK ADAPTATION).

SCP *See* SINGLE CELL PROTEIN.

scrapple USA; meat dish prepared from pork carcass trimmings, maize meal, flour, salt and spices, cooked to a thick consistency.

scratchings, pork Small pieces of crisply cooked pork skin.

screening (1) Sorting of foods or food particles by size using sieves (known as screens).

(2) Comparison of measurements made on individuals or population groups using predetermined risk levels or cut-off points of reference ranges.

scrod Young COD or HADDOCK.

scrumpy Rough, unsweetened CIDER.

scup American term for various food and game fish of the sea bream family, especially *Senostomus* spp.

See also PORGY.

scurvy Deficiency of VITAMIN C, fatal if untreated. Nowadays extremely rare, but in the past a major problem in winter, when there were few sources of the vitamin available. It was especially a problem of long sea voyages during the 16th and 17th centuries;

when fresh supplies of fruit and vegetables were not available the majority of the crew often succumbed to scurvy.

scurvy, alpine *See* PELLAGRA.

scurvy grass A herb, *Cochlearia officinalis*, recommended as far back as the late 16th century as a remedy for scurvy.

scutellum Area surrounding the embryo of the cereal grain; scutellum plus embryo is the germ; rich in vitamins.

scybalum Lump or mass of hard FAECES.

SDA Specific dynamic action, *see* DIET-INDUCED THERMOGENESIS.

SDS (1) Sucrose distearate, a SUCROSE ester.

(2) The detergent sodium dodecyl sulphate.

SDS–PAGE Polyacrylamide gel ELECTROPHORESIS of proteins in the presence of the detergent sodium dodecyl sulphate to cause denaturation and a uniform charge, so that proteins are separated on the basis of their molecular weight.

SE *See* STARCH EQUIVALENT.

sea kale Coastal plant, *Crambe maritime*; the tender shoots are eaten like ASPARAGUS. Sea kale beet is SWISS CHARD.

sea slug *See* BÊCHE-DE-MER.

seasoning Normally used to mean salt and pepper, but may include any herbs, spices and condiments added to a savoury dish.

sea truffle SHELLFISH, a bivalve MOLLUSC, *Venus verrucosa*.

seaweed Marine algae of interest as food; include BADDERLOCKS, CARAGEENAN, DULSE, FINGERWARE, IRISH MOSS, KELP, LAVER, NORI, SUGARWARE and WAKAME, which are eaten as local delicacies and serve as a mineral supplement in animal feed.

See also AGAR; ALGAE; ALGINATES.

second messenger Small molecule released inside a cell in response to binding of a hormone or neurotransmitter to a receptor on the cell surface, which directly or indirectly activates or inhibits target enzymes.

secretin Peptide hormone secreted by the S-cells of the duodenum in response to acid food entering from the stomach. Stimulates secretion of alkaline PANCREATIC JUICE containing only low levels of enzyme, and also secretion of bile; decreases gastric secretion and GASTRIN release.

sedoheptulose (sedoheptose) A seven-carbon sugar, a metabolic intermediate.

Seitz filter A filter disc with pores so fine that they will not permit passage of bacteria, permitting sterilisation of liquids by filtration.

sekt German, central European; sparkling WINE, usually dry, made by tank fermentation, not the MÉTHODE CHAMPENOISE.

selenium A dietary essential mineral, found as SELENOCYSTEINE in the active sites of GLUTATHIONE PEROXIDASE (EC 1.11.1.9) and thyroxine deiodinase (EC 3.8.1.4). Through its role in glutathione peroxidase it acts as an ANTIOXIDANT, and to some extent can compensate for VITAMIN E deficiency. Similarly, vitamin E can compensate for selenium deficiency to some extent.

Requirements are of the order of 50 μg/day; in parts of New Zealand, Finland and China soils are especially poor in selenium and deficiency occurs. In China, selenium deficiency is associated with KESHAN DISEASE and KASHIN–BECK SYNDROME.

Selenium is toxic in excess; mild selenium intoxication results in production of foul-smelling hydrogen selenide, which is excreted on the breath and through the skin. Intakes above 200 μg/day are considered hazardous.

See also THYROID HORMONES.

Selenium-ACE™   Yeast-based product providing SELENIUM and VITAMINS A, C and E.

selenocysteine   The selenium analogue of the AMINO ACID CYSTEINE. Incorporated during ribosomal protein synthesis, and formed as a result of the action of selenocysteine synthetase (EC 2.9.1.1) on serine bound to tRNA. The codon for selenocysteine is UGA, one of the stop CODONS, read in a context-sensitive manner in an untranslated stem-loop sequence of the mRNA.

seltzer   Effervescent mineral water, originally from Niederselters, Germany.

See also SODA WATER.

seminose   *See* MANNOSE.

semipermeable membrane   A membrane with pores that permit the passage of small molecules, but not larger molecules such as proteins. Used in DIALYSIS and ULTRAFILTRATION.

semolina   The inner, granular, starchy endosperm of hard or durum wheat (not yet ground into flour); used to make PASTA and a milk pudding.

Composition/100 g: water 12.7 g, 1507 kJ (360 kcal), protein 12.7 g, fat 1 g, carbohydrate 72.8 g, fibre 3.9 g, ash 0.8 g, Ca 17 mg, Fe 1.2 mg, Mg 47 mg, P 136 mg, K 186 mg, Na 1 mg, Zn 1 mg, Cu 0.2 mg, Mn 0.6 mg, vitamin B_1 0.28 mg, B_2 0.08 mg, niacin 3.3 mg, B_6 0.1 mg, folate 72 μg, pantothenate 0.6 mg.

senna   Dried fruits of *Cassia* spp., used as an irritant LAXATIVE.

sensitivity   Of an assay; the smallest amount that can be determined with acceptable PRECISION.

sensory properties   *See* ORGANOLEPTIC.

sequestrants   Compounds that form soluble complexes with polyvalent metal ions, preventing them from undergoing reactions, and so improving the quality and stability of the product.

sequestrene, sequestrol *See* EDTA.

sercial *See* MADEIRA WINES.

sereh powder *See* LEMON GRASS.

serendipity berry Or Nigerian berry, fruit of the W. African plant *Dioscoreophyllum cumminsii*. It has an extremely sweet taste due to the protein monellin.

serine A non-essential amino acid; abbr Ser (S), M_r 105.1, pK_a 2.19, 9.21, CODONS UCNu, AGPy.

serotonin *See* 5-HYDROXYTRYPTAMINE.

serum Clear liquid left after protein has been coagulated; the serum from milk, occasionally referred to as lactoserum, is whey. Blood serum is the result of BLOOD CLOTTING; the fibrinogen in BLOOD PLASMA is converted to insoluble fibrin, which forms the clot. The clear liquid that is exuded is the serum.

serving US food labelling legislation (introduced in 1994) requires that nutrients be shown per standard serving of the food. The US Food and Drug Administration has defined serving or portion sizes, based on surveys of amounts customarily eaten, so that definitions of portions are not left to the manufacturer.

sesame A tropical and subtropical plant, *Sesamum indicum*. Known as sim-sim in E. Africa, benniseed in W. Africa, gingelly and til in Asia. Seeds are small and, in most varieties, white; used whole in sweetmeats, in stews and to decorate cakes and bread, and for extraction of the oil, which is used as a seasoning.

Composition /100 g: water 4.7 g, 2399 kJ (573 kcal), protein 17.7 g, fat 49.7 g (of which 15% saturated, 39% mono-unsaturated, 46% polyunsaturated), carbohydrate 23.5 g (0.3 g sugars), fibre 11.8 g, ash 4.4 g, Ca 975 mg, Fe 14.6 mg, Mg 351 mg, P 629 mg, K 468 mg, Na 11 mg, Zn 7.8 mg, Cu 4.1 mg, Mn 2.5 mg, Se 5.7 µg, 5 µg carotenoids, E 0.3 mg, B_1 0.79 mg, B_2 0.25 mg, niacin 4.5 mg, B_6 0.79 mg, folate 97 µg, pantothenate 0.1 mg. A 5 g serving is a source of Cu.

Sesame oil is 15% saturated, 42% mono-unsaturated, 44% polyunsaturated, contains 1.4 mg vitamin E, and 13.6 mg vitamin K/100 g.

See also TAHINI.

setback (of starch) *See* RETROGRADATION.

seto fuumi Japanese seasoning consisting of dried seaweed, tuna, sesame seed and MONOSODIUM GLUTAMATE.

sfumatrice Machine for obtaining the oil from the peel of citrus fruit by folding, when the natural turgor of the oil sacs forces out the oil.

shad Oily FISH, *Alosa* spp. (American shad is *A. sapidissima*), related to HERRING, that spawn in fresh water. The ROE is especially prized.

shaddock   *See* POMELO.

shallot   Bulb of the plant *Allium escalonium* (*A. cepa aggregatum*) related to the ONION, with similar flavour but less pungent; each plant has a cluster of small bulbs rather than the single large bulb of the onion.

sharon fruit   *See* PERSIMMON.

Sharples centrifuge   Continuous high-speed centrifuge (15–30 000 rpm), consisting of a vertical cylinder. Used to separate liquids of different densities or to clarify by sedimenting solids.

sharps   *See* WHEATFEED.

shashlik   *See* KEBAB.

shea butter   Vegetable butter from the nuts of the shea tree (*Butyrospermum parkii*) which grows wild in W. and central Africa. 49% saturated, 46% mono-unsaturated, 5% polyunsaturated, and contains 10% non-saponifiable lipids.

   See also COCOA BUTTER EQUIVALENTS

shearling   15–18-month-old sheep. *See* LAMB.

shear rate   The velocity gradient in a liquid subjected to a shear stress. For Newtonian fluids there is a linear relationship between shear stress and shear rate; non-Newtonian fluids (which include many emulsions, suspensions and concentrated solutions of starches, gums and proteins) show a non-linear relationship.

   See also DILATANT; PLASTIC FLUIDS; PSEUDOPLASTIC; RHEOPECTIC; THIXOTROPIC.

shear stress (or shearing force)   The force that moves a liquid.

   See also SHEAR RATE; VISCOSITY.

shellfish   A wide range of marine molluscs (ABALONE, CLAM, COCKLE, MUSSEL, SCALLOP, OYSTER, WHELK, WINKLE) and crustacea (order Decapoda: CRAB, CRAYFISH, LOBSTER, PRAWN, SHRIMP).

shellfish poisoning   Paralysis caused by eating shellfish contaminated with toxic organisms (dinoflagellates) that contain saxitoxin and related toxins. *See also* RED TIDE.

sherbet   (1) Arabic name for water-ice (sugar, water and flavouring), also known by French name, sorbet, and the Italian name, granita. Used to be served between courses during a meal to refresh the palate.

   (2) Originally a Middle Eastern drink made from fruit juice, often chilled with snow. Modern version is made with bicarbonate of soda and tartaric acid (to fizz) with sugar and flavours. Sherbet powder is the same mixture in dry form.

   (3) In the USA a frozen dessert containing 1–2% milk fat, 2–5% dairy solids; as opposed to sorbet, which contains no dairy solids.)

sherry   Fortified wines (around 15% ALCOHOL by volume) from the south-west of Spain, around Jerez and Cadiz. Matured by the solera process, rather than by discrete vintages; each year 30% of the wine in the oldest barrel is drawn off for bottling and replaced with wine from the next oldest; this in turn is replaced from the next barrel, and so on. In order of increasing sweetness, sherries are: fino (very dry); manzanilla; amontillado; oloroso (may be medium-dry or sweetened and more highly fortified); amoroso or cream.

Dry sherry contains 1–2% sugar and 100 mL supplies 500 kJ (120 kcal); medium sherry 3–4% sugar, 530 kJ (125 kcal); sweet sherry 7% sugar, supplies 590 kJ (140 kcal).

Sherry-type wines are also produced in other countries, including South Africa, Cyprus and the UK (made from imported grape juice) and may legally be described as sherry as long as the country of origin is clearly shown.

Shigella spp. Food-poisoning organisms that invade intestinal epithelial cells and cause DYSENTERY. Infective dose 10^2–10^5 organisms; onset 1–7 days; duration weeks; TX 4.1.4.1.

shiitake Or Black Forest mushroom, *Lentinula (Lentinus) edodes*. *See* MUSHROOMS.

shir To bake food (usually eggs) in a small shallow container or ramekin dish.

shirataki Chinese, Japanese; noodles made from tubers of the devil's tongue plant *Amorphallus rivieri*.

shortening Soft fats that produce a crisp, flaky effect in baked products. LARD possesses the correct properties to a greater extent than any other single fat. Shortenings compounded from mixtures of fats or prepared by hydrogenation are still called lard compounds or lard substitutes. Unlike oils, shortenings are plastic and disperse as a film through the batter and prevent the formation of a hard, tough mass.

showarma *See* KEBAB.

shrimp Small shellfish, species of the Paleamonidea and Pandalidae (PRAWNS), *Crangon crangon* (brown shrimp) and *Pandalus montagui* (pink shrimp). In the UK smaller fish are known as SHRIMP and larger as prawns; in the USA all are called shrimp. Three species are farmed commercially: the black tiger or giant tiger shrimp (*Penaeus monodon*), the Chinese white (*P. chinensis*) and the eastern Pacific white shrimp (*P. vannamet*).

Composition/100 g: water 76 g, 444 kJ (106 kcal), protein 20.3 g, fat 1.7 g (of which 23% saturated, 23% mono-unsaturated, 54% polyunsaturated), cholesterol 152 mg, carbohydrate 0.9 g, ash 1.2 g, Ca 52 mg, Fe 2.4 mg, Mg 37 mg, P 205 mg, K 185 mg, Na 148 mg, Zn 1.1 mg, Cu 0.3 mg, Mn 0.1 mg, Se 38 µg, I 100 µg, vitamin A 54 µg retinol, E 1.1 mg, B_1 0.03 mg, B_2 0.03 mg, niacin

2.6 mg, B_6 0.1 mg, folate 3 µg, B_{12} 1.2 µg, pantothenate 0.3 mg, C 2 mg. A 50 g serving is a source of Cu, P, a good source of Se, a rich source of I, vitamin B_{12}.

sialic acids N-Acetyl-neuraminic acid (amino sugar) derivatives; constituents of gangliosides, glycoproteins and bacterial cell walls.

sialogogue   Substance that stimulates the flow of saliva.

sialorrhoea   Or ptyalism, excessive flow of SALIVA.

sidemeats   *See* OFFAL.

sideroblast   Red BLOOD CELL precursor in which IRON-containing granules are visible. May be present in normal individuals, absent in iron deficiency ANAEMIA. Sideroblastic anaemia is characterised by the presence of abnormal ringed sideroblasts in the blood.

sideropenia   IRON deficiency.

siderophilin   *See* IRON TRANSPORT.

siderosis   Accumulation of the iron–protein complex, haemosiderin, in liver, spleen and bone marrow in cases of excessive red cell destruction and in diets exceptionally rich in IRON.
   See also HAEMOCHROMATOSIS.

sierra rice   *See* RICE, FERMENTED.

sigmoidoscope   Instrument that is inserted through the anus to view the interior of the rectum and sigmoid colon.

sign   Indication of a disorder that is observed by a physician but is not apparent to the patient.
   See also SYMPTOM.

sild   Traditional UK name applied to a mixture of young HERRING and young SPRAT when canned, since they are caught together and cannot be separated on a commercial scale. When fresh or frozen the mixture is termed WHITEBAIT.

silica gel   Sodium silicate, used as a drying agent in packaging. It can be regenerated by heating to drive off adsorbed water.

silicones   Organic compounds of silicon; in the food field they are used as antifoaming agents, as semipermanent glazes on baking tins and other metal containers, and on non-stick wrapping paper.

silver   Not of interest in foods apart from its use in covering 'nonpareils', the silver beads used to decorate confectionery. Present in traces in all plant and animal tissues but not known to be a dietary essential, and has no known function, nor is enough ever absorbed to cause toxicity.
   See also OLIGODYNAMIC.

silver beet   *See* SWISS CHARD.

simethicone   *See* DIMETHICONE.

simnel cake   Fruit cake with a layer of almond paste on top and sometimes another baked in the middle. Originally baked for Mothering Sunday, now normally eaten at Easter.

Simplesse^{TM}   FAT REPLACER made from protein.

simvastatin   *See* STATINS.

single cell oil   Fats produced by fungi or bacteria growing on a non-fat substrate.

single cell protein   Collective term used for biomass of bacteria, algae and yeast, and also (incorrectly) moulds, of potential use as animal or human food.

   See also MYCOPROTEIN.

sinharanut   *See* CHESTNUT.

sinkability   The ability of powder particles to sink quickly into a liquid for reconstituting a dried material.

sippy diet   Former treatment for peptic ulcer; hourly feeds of small quantities, 150 mL of milk, cream or other milky food. Lower in protein than the MEULENGRACHT DIET.

sitapophasis   Refusal to eat as expression of mental disorder.

sitology   Science of food (from the Greek *sitos*, food).

sitomania   Mania for eating, morbid obsession with food; also known as phagomania.

sitophobia   Fear of food; also known as phagophobia.

sitosterol   The main STEROL found in vegetable oils; reduces the absorption of CHOLESTEROL from the intestinal tract and therefore used in prevention and treatment of HYPERLIPIDAEMIA.

skate   Cartilaginous FISH, *Raja undutata*.

skinfold thickness   Index of subcutaneous fat and hence body fat content. Measured at four sites: biceps (midpoint of front upper arm), triceps (midpoint of back upper arm), subscapular (directly below point of shoulder blade at angle of 45°), supra-iliac (directly above iliac crest in mid-axillary line). Rapid surveys often involve only biceps. Precision callipers for measurement of skinfold thickness exert a pressure of 10g/mm^2, with a skin contact (pinch) area of $20–40 \text{mm}^2$ and require regular recalibration.

   See also ANTHROPOMETRY.

skipjack reaction   *See* SCOMBROID POISONING.

skyr   *See* MILK, FERMENTED.

Slendid^{TM}   FAT REPLACER made from NON-STARCH POLYSACCHARIDE.

Slimsweet^{TM}   A bulk SWEETENER, 15-times sweeter than sucrose, derived from natural sources, and believed to be mainly TAGATOSE.

sling   Drink made from gin and fruit juice.

Slite^{TM}   A preparation of 82% SUCROSE with intense SWEETENERS and bulking agents. The mixture has twice the sweetness of sucrose, and is stable to cooking.

slivovitz (sliwowitz) E European (originally Yugoslavia); distilled spirit made from fermented plums; similar to German quetsch and French mirabelle. Some of the stones are included with the fruit and produce a characteristic bitter flavour from the hydrocyanic acid (0.008% cyanide is present in the finished brandy).

sloe Wild PLUM, fruit of the blackthorn (*Prunus spinosa*) with a sour and astringent flavour; almost only use is for the preparation of sloe gin, a liqueur made by steeping wild sloes in gin or neutral spirit. Known in France as prunelle.

sloke *See* LAVER.

slot Shetland; dumplings made from pounded cod ROE and flour.

slow virus Obsolete term for infective agents with some properties resembling viruses, but not containing any nucleic acid. Now known as PRIONS.

SMA™ (Scientific Milk Adaptation) A milk preparation for infant feeding modified to resemble the composition of human milk; *see* MILK, HUMANISED.

smallage Wild CELERY, *Apium graveolens*.

smell *See* ORGANOLEPTIC.

smelt Small oily FISH, *Osmerus* spp.

smetana Thin soured cream, originally Russian.

smilacin *See* PARILLIN.

smoke point The temperature at which the decomposition products of frying oils become visible as bluish smoke. The temperature varies with different fats, ranging between 160 and 260 °C.

 See also FIRE POINT; FLASH POINT.

smoked beef *See* PASTRAMI.

smoke, liquid Either condensate from wood smoke or an aqueous extract of smoke, applied to the surface of foods as an alternative to traditional SMOKING.

smoking The process of flavouring and preserving meat or fish by drying slowly in the smoke from a wood fire; the type of wood used affects the flavour of the final smoked product.

smörgåsbord Scandinavian; buffet table laden with delicacies as a traditional gesture of hospitality, a traditional way of serving meals.

smørrebrød Scandinavian; open SANDWICHES, often on rye bread, with a variety of toppings and garnishes. Literally *smeared bread*.

SMS Sucrose monostearate. *See* SUCROSE ESTERS.

smut Group of fungi that attack wheat; includes loose or common smut (*Ustilago tritici*) and stinking smut or bunt (*Tilletia tritici*).

snail The small snail eaten in Europe is *Helix pomatia*; giant African snail (which weighs several hundred grams) is *Achatima fulica*.

H. pomatia composition/100 g: water 79 g, 377 kJ (90 kcal), protein 16.1 g, fat 1.4 g (of which 40% saturated, 30% mono-unsaturated, 30% polyunsaturated), cholesterol 50 mg, carbohydrate 2 g, ash 1.3 g, Ca 10 mg, Fe 3.5 mg, Mg 250 mg, P 272 mg, K 382 mg, Na 70 mg, Zn 1 mg, Cu 0.4 mg, Se 27.4 µg, vitamin A 30 µg retinol, E 5 mg, K 0.1 mg, B_1 0.01 mg, B_2 0.12 mg, niacin 1.4 mg, B_6 0.13 mg, folate 6 µg, B_{12} 0.5 µg.

snap pea, snow pea   *See* PEA, MANGE TOUT.

SNF   *See* SOLIDS-NOT-FAT.

SNP   (pronounced snip) Single nucleotide POLYMORPHISM.

snubbing   Topping and tailing of GOOSEBERRIES.

SO_2   *See* SULPHUR DIOXIDE.

soapbark   *See* QUILLAJA.

soapstock   In the refining of crude edible oils the free fatty acids are removed by agitation with alkali. The fatty acids settle to the bottom as alkali soaps and are known as soapstock or 'foots'.

soba   Japanese; noodles made from golden BUCKWHEAT.

SOD   *See* SUPEROXIDE DISMUTASE.

soda bread   Irish; made from flour and whey, or buttermilk, using sodium bicarbonate and acid in place of yeast.

soda water   Artificially carbonated water, also known as club soda; if sodium bicarbonate is also added, the product is seltzer water.

sodium   A dietary essential mineral; requirements are almost invariably satisfied by the normal diet. The body contains about 100 g of sodium and the average diet contains 3–6 g, equivalent to 7.5–15 g of sodium chloride (salt); the requirement is less than 0.5 g sodium/day. The intake varies enormously among different individuals and excretion varies accordingly.

Excessive intake of sodium is associated with high blood pressure, hence often treated with low-salt diets. Sodium controls the retention of fluid in the body, and reduced retention, aided by low-sodium diets, is required in cardiac insufficiency accompanied by OEDEMA, in certain kidney diseases, toxaemia of pregnancy and HYPERTENSION.

See also SALT-FREE DIETS; SALT, LIGHT; SODIUM : POTASSIUM RATIO; WATER BALANCE.

sodium bicarbonate   Sodium hydrogen carbonate, $NaHCO_3$, also known as baking soda or bicarbonate of soda; liberates carbon dioxide when in contact with acid (*see* BAKING POWDER). Used as a raising agent in baking flour confectionery.

sodium:potassium ratio In the body, the ratio of sodium (in the extracellular fluid) to potassium (in the intracellular fluid) is about 2:3. The ratio in unprocessed food, no salt added, is much lower, and when salt is added during processing it is much higher.

Fruits and vegetables are relatively low in sodium and rich in potassium; animal foods are rich in sodium.

sodom apple Tropical plant, *Calotropis procera*; fruit is inedible, but the leaves are used in W. Africa as a source of proteolytic milk-clotting enzymes as an alternative to RENNET in CHEESE production.

soft swell *See* SWELLS.

sol Colloidal suspension (*see* COLLOID) consisting of a solid dispersed in a liquid. In lyophobic sols there is little interaction between the dispersed particles and the dispersing medium; in lyophilic sols there is affinity between the dispersed and dispersant phases.

Solanaceae Family of plants including AUBERGINE (*Solanum melongena*), CAPE GOOSEBERRY (*Physalis peruviana*), POTATO (*Solanum tuberosum*), TOMATO (*Lycopersicon esculentum*).

solanine Heat-stable toxic GLYCOSIDE of the ALKALOID solanidine, found in small amounts in potatoes, and larger and sometimes toxic amounts in sprouted potatoes and potato skin when they become green through exposure to light. Causes gastrointestinal disturbances and neurological disorders; the upper acceptable limit is 20 mg solanine per 100 g fresh weight of potato.

sole FLATFISH, *Solea* spp.; Dover sole is *S. solea*.

solera *See* SHERRY.

solids-not-fat (SNF) Refers to the solids of milk excluding the fat, i.e. protein, lactose and salts. Used as an index of milk quality, determined by measuring the specific gravity using the LACTOMETER.

somatomedins Circulating growth factors, synthesised in the liver, with broad anabolic properties. Their structure resembles that of PRO-INSULIN, and they are sometimes known as insulin-like growth factors. Synthesis is much impaired in children with protein–energy malnutrition, and responds rapidly to nutritional rehabilitation.

somatostatin Peptide hormone secreted throughout gut; decreases gastric secretion and GASTRIN release, pancreatic secretion of bicarbonate and enzymes, expression and release of gut peptides, gastric emptying, intestinal motility, gall bladder contractility, absorption of glucose, triacylglycerols, amino acids, intestinal ion secretion, splanchnic blood flow.

somatotrophin A peptide HORMONE (growth hormone) secreted by the pituitary gland that promotes growth of bone and soft tissues. It also reduces the utilisation of GLUCOSE, and increases breakdown of fats to fatty acids; because of this it has been promoted as an aid to weight reduction, but with little evidence of efficacy.

somatotrophin, bovine (BST) A peptide hormone produced by cows in the anterior pituitary gland. High-yielding dairy cows have higher circulating levels and injection of BST increases the yield of milk by minimising the rate of yield decline after peak lactation. Approved for use in the USA in 1993, prohibited in the EU.

Differs in amino acid sequence from human SOMATOTROPHIN by about 35% and has negligible activity in human beings.

somen Thin fine white noodles made from wheat.

Somogyi–Nelson reagent Cupric tartrate/arsenomolybdate reagent for the detection and semiquantitative determination of glucose and other reducing sugars.

See also BENEDICT'S REAGENT, FEHLING'S REAGENT.

sorbestrin SORBITOL ester of fatty acids, developed as a FAT REPLACER because it is only partially absorbed from foods.

sorbet A water-ice containing sugar, water and flavouring (commonly fruit juice or pulp). Also known as SHERBET or granita.

sorbic acid Hexadienoic acid, $CH_3CH{=}CH{-}CH{=}CH{-}COOH$, used together with its sodium, potassium and calcium salts to inhibit growth of fungi in wine, cheese, soft drinks, low-sugar jams, flour, confectionery, etc. (E-200–203).

Sorbistat^{TM} SORBIC ACID and its potassium salt (Sorbistat K).

sorbitan esters Fatty acid esters of SORBITOL (mainly the mono-stearate) used as an emulsifying agent.

sorbitol Also known as glycitol, glucitol. A six-carbon SUGAR ALCOHOL found in plums, apricots, cherries and apples; manufactured by reduction of glucose; 50–60% as sweet as sucrose. Although it is metabolised, with the same energy yield as other carbohydrates, 16 kJ (4 kcal)/g, it is only slowly absorbed from the intestine and has an effective energy yield of 10 kJ (2.4 kcal)/g. Used in baked products, jam and confectionery suitable for diabetics (E-420).

sorcerers' milk *See* WITCHES' MILK.

sorghum *Sorghum vulgare, S. bicolor;* cereals that thrive in semi-arid regions, staple food in tropical Africa, central and N. India and China. Sorghum produced in the USA and Australia is used for animal feed. Also known as kaffir corn (in S. Africa), guinea corn (in W. Africa), jowar (in India), Indian millet and millo maize.

The white grain variety is eaten as meal; red grained has a bitter taste and is used for BEER; sorghum syrup is obtained from the crushed stems of the sweet sorghum.

Composition/100 g: water 9.2 g, 1419 kJ (339 kcal), protein 11.3 g, fat 3.3 g (of which 17% saturated, 34% mono-unsaturated, 48% polyunsaturated), carbohydrate 74.6 g, ash 1.6 g, Ca 28 mg,

Fe 4.4 mg, P 287 mg, K 350 mg, Na 6 mg, B_1 0.24 mg, B_2 0.14 mg, niacin 2.9 mg.

sorption The process by which foods gain (adsorption) or lose (desorption) moisture.

sorption isotherm The curve produced from different values of relative humidity plotted against equilibrium moisture content.

sorrel A common wild plant (*Rumex acetosa*); the leaves have a strong acid flavour, and are cooked together with spinach or cabbage; used to make soup and used in salads.

   See also ROSELLA.

sorting Separation of foods into categories on the basis of a measurable physical property (e.g. size or colour). Part of the process of GRADING.

soul food Afro-Caribbean term for food with traditional or cultural links, having emotional significance.

source In this book, foods are listed as sources of nutrients. A rich source of a nutrient means that 30% or more, a good source 20–30% and a source 10–20%, of the EU labelling recommended daily amount (*see* Table 2 of the Appendix) of the nutrient is supplied in the stated portion.

soursop *See* CUSTARD APPLE.

sous vide French-originated term for cooking in special pouches under vacuum, when the food has a shelf-life of weeks; claimed also to retain flavour and nutrients. Derived from the French *cuisine en papillote sous vide*, cooking in sealed container (originally a parchment paper case).

Southern blot *See* BLOTTING.

sowans (or virpa) Shetland; thick beverage made from oat and wheat meal, stepped in water for several days until sour, then strained.

Soxhlet method For determination of extractable lipids. The sample is extracted by constant perfusion with a stream of freshly distilled solvent.

soya (soy) A BEAN (*Glycine max*) important as a source of both oil and protein. The protein is of higher biological value than many other vegetable proteins, and is of great value for animal and human food. When raw it contains a TRYPSIN INHIBITOR, which is destroyed by heat. Native of China, where it has been cultivated for 5000 years; grows 60–100 cm high with 2–3 beans per pod.

   Composition/100 g: (edible portion 53%) water 67.5 g, 615 kJ (147 kcal), protein 12.9 g, fat 6.8 g (of which 15% saturated, 25% mono-unsaturated, 60% polyunsaturated), carbohydrate 11.1 g, fibre 4.2 g, ash 1.7 g, Ca 197 mg, Fe 3.5 mg, Mg 65 mg, P 194 mg, K 620 mg, Na 15 mg, Zn 1 mg, Cu 0.1 mg, Mn 0.5 mg, Se 1.5 µg, vitamin B_1 0.44 mg, B_2 0.17 mg, niacin 1.6 mg, B_6 0.06 mg, folate 165 µg, pantothenate 0.1 mg, C 29 mg.

Soybean oil is 15% saturated, 24% mono-unsaturated, 61% polyunsaturated, contains 9.2 mg vitamin E, 198 mg vitamin K/100 g.

soya flour   Dehulled, ground SOYA bean. The unheated material is a rich source of AMYLASE and PROTEINASE and is useful as a baking aid.

Composition/100 g: water 7.3 g, 1381 kJ (330 kcal), protein 47 g, fat 1.2 g (of which 13% saturated, 25% mono-unsaturated, 63% polyunsaturated), carbohydrate 38.4 g (20 g sugars), fibre 17.5 g, ash 6.2 g, Ca 241 mg, Fe 9.2 mg, Mg 290 mg, P 674 mg, K 2384 mg, Na 20 mg, Zn 2.5 mg, Cu 4.1 mg, Mn 3 mg, Se 1.7 µg, vitamin A 2 µg RE (24 µg carotenoids), E 0.2 mg, K 4.1 mg, B_1 0.7 mg, B_2 0.25 mg, niacin 2.6 mg, B_6 0.57 mg, folate 305 µg, pantothenate 2 mg.

soybean curd   *See* TOFU.

Soyolk™   Full fat SOYA FLOUR.

soy sauce   A condiment prepared from fermented SOYA bean, commonly used in China and Japan. Traditionally the bean, often mixed with wheat, is fermented with *Aspergillus oryzae* over a period of 1–3 years. The modern process is carried out at a high temperature or in an autoclave for a short time.

spaghetti   *See* PASTA.

spaghetti squash   A GOURD, also called cucuzzi, calabash, suzza melon; often classed as summer squash but not a true SQUASH. Only after cooking does the flesh resemble spaghetti in appearance.

Composition/100 g: (edible portion 71%) water 92 g, 130 kJ (31 kcal), protein 0.6 g, fat 0.6 g, carbohydrate 6.9 g, ash 0.3 g, Ca 23 mg, Fe 0.3 mg, Mg 12 mg, P 12 mg, K 108 mg, Na 17 mg, Zn 0.2 mg, Mn 0.1 mg, Se 0.3 µg, vitamin A 3 µg RE, B_1 0.04 mg, B_2 0.02 mg, niacin 0.9 mg, B_6 0.1 mg, folate 12 µg, pantothenate 0.4 mg, C 2 mg.

Spam™   Canned pork luncheon meat; a contraction of 'spiced ham'.

Spanish toxic oil syndrome   Widespread disease in Spain, 1981–1982, with 450 deaths and many people chronically disabled, because of consumption of an oil containing aniline-denatured industrial rape seed oil, sold as olive oil. The precise cause is unknown.

Spans™   Non-ionic surface active agents derived from fatty acids and hexahydric alcohols. Oil soluble, in contrast to TWEENS which are water-soluble or disperse well in water. Used in bread, cakes and biscuits as crumb softeners (antistaling agents), to improve dough, and as emulsifiers.

sparging Spraying fine droplets of aqueous alkali onto oil heated to 75–95 °C to remove free fatty acids as soaps that are water-soluble.

  See also ACID NUMBER; RANCIDITY.

spastic colon *See* IRRITABLE BOWEL SYNDROME.

spatchcock Small birds split down the back and flattened before grilling. Spitchcock is eel treated similarly.

SPE *See* SUCROSE POLYESTERS.

spearmint The common garden (culinary) mint; hybrid of *Mentha spicata*, *M. suaveolens* (apple mint) and *M. villosa* (*M. alopecuroides*, Bowles' mint).

specific dynamic action *See* DIET-INDUCED THERMOGENESIS.

specific electrical resistance Electrical resistance of $1\,cm^3$ of a product, placed between two $1\,cm^2$ electrodes that are located $1\,cm$ apart.

specific gravity Of a liquid, its mass divided by the mass of the same volume of water at the same temperature, or its DENSITY divided by the density of water at the same temperature.

specificity (1) Of an assay; the extent to which what is measured is due to the analyte under investigation, rather than other compounds that may also react.

  (2) In relation to enzymes, the ability of an enzyme to catalyse only a limited range of reactions, or, in some cases, a single reaction, and to show considerable specificity for the substrates undergoing reaction.

spectrograph Instrument that produces a photographic record of wavelength and intensity of light or other electromagnetic radiation.

spectrometer Instrument for measuring wavelength and intensity of light or other electromagnetic radiation.

spectrophotofluorimeter (spectrophotofluorometer) Instrument for measuring wavelength and intensity of light emitted by a solute at right angles to the beam of exciting light of a specific wavelength.

  See also FLUORIMETRY.

spectrophotometer Instrument that measures the amount of light absorbed at any particular wavelength, which is directly related to the concentration of the material in the solution. Used extensively to measure substances that have specific absorption in the visible, infrared or ultraviolet range, or can react to form coloured derivatives.

spelt Coarse type of WHEAT, mainly used as cattle feed.

spent wash Liquor remaining in the WHISKY still after distilling the spirit. A source of (unidentified) growth factors detected by chick growth. When dried is known as distillers' dried solubles.

spermyse Medieval English; soft cheese made and eaten in summer. Also called green cheese.

spherocyte Abnormal red BLOOD CELL that is spherical rather than disc shaped. Characteristic of some types of haemolytic ANAEMIA.

sphincter A ring of concentric muscle that surrounds an orifice and can close it partially or completely on contraction.

sphingolipids Class of phosphatides in which the 18-carbon dihydroxyalcohol sphingosine serves a similar function to GLYCEROL in PHOSPHOLIPIDS. Important in cell membranes, especially in nerve tissue. The major sphingolipid is sphingomyelin.

sphingomyelin *See* SPHINGOLIPIDS.

sphygmomanometer Instrument for measuring arterial BLOOD PRESSURE.

spices Distinguished from HERBS in that part, instead of the whole, of the aromatic plant is used: root, stem or seeds. Originally used to mask putrefactive flavours. Some have a preservative effect because of their essential oils, e.g. cloves, cinnamon and mustard.

spina bifida Congenital NEURAL TUBE DEFECT due to developmental anomaly in early embryonic development. Supplements of FOLIC ACID (400 μg/day) begun before conception reduce the risk.

spinach Leaves of *Spinacia oleracea*.

Composition /100 g: (edible portion 72%) water 91.4 g, 96 kJ (23 kcal), protein 2.9 g, fat 0.4 g, carbohydrate 3.6 g (0.4 g sugars), fibre 2.2 g, ash 1.7 g, Ca 99 mg, Fe 2.7 mg, Mg 79 mg, P 49 mg, K 558 mg, Na 79 mg, Zn 0.5 mg, Cu 0.1 mg, Mn 0.9 mg, Se 1 μg, vitamin A 469 μg RE (17 824 μg carotenoids), E 2 mg, K 482.9 mg, B_1 0.08 mg, B_2 0.19 mg, niacin 0.7 mg, B_6 0.19 mg, folate 194 μg, pantothenate 0.1 mg, C 28 mg. An 85 g serving is a source of Fe, vitamin E, a good source of Mg, a rich source of Mn, vitamin A, folate, C.

spinach beet *See* SWISS CHARD.

spinach, Chinese Leaves of *Amaranthus gangeticus*, also known as bhaji and callaloo.

spinach, Philippine Variety of purslane (*Talinum triangulare*) cultivated in the USA and cooked in the same way as SPINACH.

Spinkganz German; goose breast, dry-brined and smoked.

spiny lobster SHELLFISH, family Palinuridae, *see* LOBSTER.

spirits Beverages of high ALCOHOL content made by distillation of fermented liquors, including BRANDY, GIN, RUM, VODKA, WHISKY; usually 40% alcohol by volume (equivalent to 31.7 g per 100 mL). Silent spirit is highly purified alcohol, or neutral spirit, distilled from any fermented material.

spirometer Or respirometer; apparatus used to measure the amount of oxygen consumed (and in some instances carbon dioxide produced) from which to calculate the energy expended (indirect calorimetry).

spirulina Blue-green alga which can fix atmospheric nitrogen; eaten for centuries round Lake Chad in Africa and in Mexico. Many health claims are made, but are negated by the small amounts eaten.

Composition /100g: water 91g, 109kJ (26kcal), protein 5.9g, fat 0.4g, carbohydrate 2.4g, ash 0.6g, Ca 12mg, Fe 2.8mg, Mg 19mg, P 11mg, K 127mg, Na 98mg, Zn 0.2mg, Cu 0.6mg, Mn 0.2mg, Se 0.7μg, vitamin A 3μg RE, B_1 0.22mg, B_2 0.34mg, niacin 1.2mg, B_6 0.03mg, folate 9μg, pantothenate 0.3mg, C 1mg.

splanchnic Relating to the viscera.

spleen Abdominal organ whose main function is destruction of aged red blood cells and recycling the iron. As a food it is called melts.

Composition /100g: water 78g, 423kJ (101kcal), protein 17.2g, fat 3.1g (of which 50% saturated, 40% mono-unsaturated, 10% polyunsaturated), cholesterol 250mg, carbohydrate 0g, ash 1.3g, Ca 9mg, Fe 41.9mg, Mg 21mg, P 280mg, K 358mg, Na 84mg, Zn 2.8mg, Cu 0.1mg, Mn 0.1mg, Se 32.4μg, vitamin B_1 0.05mg, B_2 0.35mg, niacin 7.9mg, B_6 0.11mg, folate 4μg, B_{12} 5.3μg, C 23mg. A 100g serving is a source of Zn, a good source of vitamin B_2, a rich source of Fe, P, Se, niacin, vitamin B_{12}, C.

SPME Solid phase microextraction, a rapid technique for extracting volatile flavour components using fibres of polar or non-polar polymers, prior to chromatographic separation and identification.

spongiform encephalopathy Progressive degenerative neurological diseases including scrapie (in sheep), bovine spongiform encephalopathy (BSE, in cattle) and Creutzfeldt–Jakob disease (in human beings). Believed to be caused by PRIONS. BSE is believed to originate from infected meat and bone meal in cattle feed concentrates, and early onset Creutzfeldt–Jakob disease (new variant or nvCJD) has been linked to consumption of beef from animals affected by BSE.

A ban on specified bovine offal in food and feedstuffs, a ban on sale of meat from cattle more than 30 months old (reducing to 24 months in 2005) and a policy of slaughtering affected animals have resulted in a dramatic fall in the number of confirmed cases of BSE. The important unknown factor is the incubation period in human beings.

spores Bacterial spores are a resting state, resistant to heat, which can germinate to produce bacteria under suitable conditions. Spore formation only occurs in some species, when the organism encounters adverse conditions (e.g. dryness, lack of nutrients).

Spore-forming species, especially of *Bacillus* and *Clostridium*, are a health hazard because the spores are resistant to most sterilisation techniques.

sports drinks Solutions of glucose plus electrolytes to mimic those lost in sweat; generally isotonic with blood plasma to avoid potential problems of water intoxication. Sometimes known as 'bottled sweat'.

sprat Small oily FISH, *Sprattus* (*Clupea*) *sprattus,* fresh or frozen; young are canned as brisling.

See also HERRING; WHITEBAIT.

spray dryer Equipment in which the material to be dried is sprayed as a fine mist into a hot-air chamber and falls to the bottom as dry powder. Heating is very brief, so nutritional and functional damage are minimal. Dried powder consists of light, hollow particles.

spread, fat A general term for fats that are spread on bread (yellow fats), including BUTTER, MARGARINE and low-fat spreads that cannot legally be called margarine. Reduced fat spreads contain not more than 60% fat, and low-fat spreads not more than 40%, compared with 80% fat in butter and margarine. Very low-fat spreads contain less than 20% fat.

springers *See* SWELLS.

spring greens Young leafy CABBAGE eaten before the heart has formed, or leaf sprouts formed after cutting off the head.

See also COLLARD.

spring rolls Chinese (and general south-east Asian); pancakes filled with quick fried vegetables and meat; may be served as soft pancakes prepared at the table or rolled and deep fried. Also known as pancake rolls and Imperial rolls; loempia in Indonesian, and nem in Vietnamese, cuisine.

sprouts (1) *See* BRUSSELS SPROUTS (2) *See* BEAN SPROUTS.

spruce beer Western Canada; branches, bark and cones of black spruce (*Picea mariana*) boiled for several hours, then put in a cask with molasses, hops and yeast, and allowed to ferment.

sprue, tropical Name given (by Dutch in Java) to a tropical disease characterised by atrophy of the intestinal VILLI, with fatty diarrhoea and sore mouth, and signs of undernutrition due to poor absorption of nutrients. Both an unidentified infectious agent and FOLIC ACID deficiency have been suggested as causes.

spurtle Scottish; wooden stick traditionally used to stir porridge. Also known as theevil.

squab Young PIGEON; also general name for pigeon in the USA; squab pie is W. of England dish made from meat, apples and onions.

squalene Acyclic intermediate (triterpene hydrocarbon) in the synthesis of CHOLESTEROL. Acts as a feedback inhibitor and repressor of the rate-limiting enzyme of cholesterol synthesis (HMG COA reductase, EC 1.1.1.34), so may have a hypocholesterolaemic action. Found in small amounts in fish liver oils and in relatively large amounts in OLIVE OIL, but only small amounts in most other plant oils.

squash (1) Varieties of the GOURD *Cucurbita pepo*. Grouped with courgettes, squashes and pumpkins.

Butternut squash, composition /100 g: (edible portion 84%) water 86.4 g, 188 kJ (45 kcal), protein 1 g, fat 0.1 g, carbohydrate 11.7 g (2.2 g sugars), fibre 2 g, ash 0.8 g, Ca 48 mg, Fe 0.7 mg, Mg 34 mg, P 33 mg, K 352 mg, Na 4 mg, Zn 0.2 mg, Cu 0.1 mg, Mn 0.2 mg, Se 0.5 µg, vitamin A 532 µg RE (8531 µg carotenoids), E 1.4 mg, K 1.1 mg, B_1 0.1 mg, B_2 0.02 mg, niacin 1.2 mg, B_6 0.15 mg, folate 27 µg, pantothenate 0.4 mg, C 21 mg. A 100 g serving is a source of Mg, vitamin E, folate, a rich source of vitamin A, C.

Summer squash, composition /100 g: (edible portion 95%) water 95 g, 67 kJ (16 kcal), protein 1.2 g, fat 0.2 g, carbohydrate 3.3 g (2.2 g sugars), fibre 1.1 g, ash 0.6 g, Ca 15 mg, Fe 0.3 mg, Mg 17 mg, P 38 mg, K 262 mg, Na 2 mg, Zn 0.3 mg, Cu 0.1 mg, Mn 0.2 mg, Se 0.2 µg, vitamin A 10 µg RE (2245 µg carotenoids), E 0.1 mg, K 3 mg, B_1 0.05 mg, B_2 0.14 mg, niacin 0.5 mg, B_6 0.22 mg, folate 29 µg, pantothenate 0.2 mg, C 17 mg. A 100 g serving is a source of vitamin B_6, folate, a good source of vitamin C.

Winter squash, composition /100 g: (edible portion 71%) water 90 g, 142 kJ (34 kcal), protein 0.9 g, fat 0.1 g, carbohydrate 8.6 g (2.2 g sugars), fibre 1.5 g, ash 0.6 g, Ca 28 mg, Fe 0.6 mg, Mg 14 mg, P 23 mg, K 350 mg, Na 4 mg, Zn 0.2 mg, Cu 0.1 mg, Mn 0.2 mg, Se 0.4 µg, vitamin A 68 µg RE (858 µg carotenoids), E 0.1 mg, K 1.1 mg, B_1 0.03 mg, B_2 0.06 mg, niacin 0.5 mg, B_6 0.16 mg, folate 24 µg, pantothenate 0.2 mg, C 12 mg. A 100 g serving is a source of folate, a good source of vitamin C.

(2) Fruit squash is a concentrated sweetened fruit juice preparation which is diluted before drinking.

squid (or calamar) Marine cephalopod with elongated body and eight arms, *Loligo* and *Illex* spp.

Composition /100 g: water 79 g, 385 kJ (92 kcal), protein 15.6 g, fat 1.4 g (of which 40% saturated, 10% mono-unsaturated, 50% polyunsaturated), cholesterol 233 mg, carbohydrate 3.1 g, ash 1.4 g, Ca 32 mg, Fe 0.7 mg, Mg 33 mg, P 221 mg, K 246 mg, Na 44 mg, Zn 1.5 mg, Cu 1.9 mg, Se 44.8 µg, I 20 µg, vitamin A 10 µg retinol, E 1.2 mg, B_1 0.02 mg, B_2 0.41 mg, niacin 2.2 mg, B_6 0.06 mg, folate 5 µg, B_{12} 1.3 µg, pantothenate 0.5 mg, C 5 mg. An 85 g serving is a source of I, a good source of P, vitamin B_2, a rich source of Cu, Se, vitamin B_{12}.

squirrel cage disintegrator Machine for shredding food, consisting of two concentric cages fitted with knife blades along their length, which rotate in opposite directions, subjecting the food to cutting and shearing forces.

SRD State registered DIETITIAN; legal qualification to practise as a dietitian in the UK.

stabilizers Substances that stabilise emulsions of fat and water, e.g. GUMS, AGAR, egg albumin, CELLULOSE derivatives, LECITHIN (E-322) for crumb softening in bread and confectionery, glyceryl monostearate (E-471) and polyoxyethylene stearate (E-430–436) for crumb softening. The legally permitted list also includes superglycerinated fats (*see* FAT, SUPERGLYCINERATED), propylene glycol alginate and stearate (E-570), methyl-, methylethyl- and sodium carboxymethyl-celluloses (E-466), stearyl tartrate (E-483), sorbitan esters of fatty acids (E-491–495). Bread may contain only superglycerinated fats and stearyl tartrate. *See* Table 7 of the Appendix.

See also EMULSIFIERS.

stachyose Tetrasaccharide, galactosyl-galactosyl-glucosyl-fructose; not hydrolysed in the small intestine, and a substrate for bacterial fermentation in the colon. Present in SOYA beans and some other LEGUMES; gives rise to the flatulence commonly associated with eating beans. Also known as mannotetrose or lupeose.

stachys *See* ARTICHOKE, CHINESE.

stackburn The deterioration in colour and quality of canned foods that have not been sufficiently cooled after canning, then stored in stacks which cool slowly.

stadiometer Portable device for measuring height, with a vertical measuring board and a horizontal headboard.

stagnant loop syndrome *See* BLIND LOOP SYNDROME.

staling The crystalline structure of STARCH is lost during baking. Subsequently it recrystallises (undergoes RETROGRADATION) and in bread the crumb loses its softness. Staling can be delayed by emulsifiers (CRUMB SOFTENERS) such as polyoxyethylene and monoglyceride derivatives of fatty acids. Retrogradation of starch also takes place in dehydrated potatoes.

stanols Analogues of CHOLESTEROL that inhibit the absorption of cholesterol from the intestinal tract; trade name Benecol.

St Anthony's Fire *See* ERGOT.

Staphylococcus aureus Food poisoning organism that produces ENTEROTOXINS (TX 1.2.3.1–7) in the food. Onset of symptoms 1–6 h, duration 8–24 h.

starch A POLYSACCHARIDE, a polymer of GLUCOSE units; the form in which carbohydrate is stored in the plant (GLYCOGEN is sometimes referred to as animal starch.) Starch is broken down by acid or enzymic hydrolysis (AMYLASE), ultimately yielding glucose; it is the principal carbohydrate of the diet and, hence, the major source of energy for human beings and animals.

Starches from different sources (e.g. potato, maize, cereal, arrowroot, sago) have different structures, and contain different proportions of two major forms: AMYLOSE, which is a linear polymer and AMYLOPECTIN, which has a branched structure. The mixture of dietary starches consists of about 25% amylose and 75% amylopectin.

α1-6 link forms branch point in amylopectin

STARCH

starch, A and B Refers to larger granules of wheat starch, A 25–35 μm, and smaller particles, B 2–8 μm.

starch, animal *See* GLYCOGEN.

starch, arum From root of the arum lily (*Arum maculatum* and other spp.); similar to SAGO and ARROWROOT.

starch blockers Compounds that inhibit amylase action and so reduce the digestion of STARCH. Used as a slimming aid, with little evidence of efficacy.

starch, cold water swellable Starch that has been heated in a small amount of water so that it forms granules that will swell in cold water to form a gel, for use in instant desserts and other products.

starch, derivatised *See* STARCH, MODIFIED.

starch, enzyme-resistant *See* STARCH, RESISTANT.

starch equivalent A measure of the energy value of animal feedingstuffs; the amount of pure starch that would be equivalent to 100 g of the ration as a source of energy.

starch, inhibited *See* STARCH, MODIFIED.

starch, modified Starch altered by physical or chemical treatment to give special properties of value in food processing, e.g. change in gel strength, flow properties, colour, clarity, stability of the paste.

Acid-modified starch (thin boiling starch): acid treatment reduces the viscosity of the paste (used in sugar confectionery, e.g. gum drops, jelly beans).

Cross-linked starch: chains are cross-linked by phosphate or adipic diesters, to strengthen the granule and so control texture and provide heat, acid, and shear tolerance.

Derivatised starch (or stabilised starch): chemical derivatives such as ethers and esters show properties such as reduced gelatinisation in hot water and greater stability to acids and alkalis (inhibited starch); useful where food has to withstand heat treatment, as in canning or in acid foods. Further degrees of treatment can result in starch being unaffected by boiling water and losing its gel-forming properties.

Oxidised starch: peroxide, permanganate, chlorine, etc., alter the viscosity, clarity and stability of the paste (major use is outside the food industry).

See also STARCH, PREGELATINISED.

starch, oxidized   *See* STARCH, MODIFIED.

starch, pregelatinised   Raw starch does not form a paste with cold water and therefore requires cooking if it is to be used as a thickening agent. Pregelatinised starch, mostly maize starch, has been cooked and dried. Used in instant puddings, pie fillings, soup mixes, salad dressings, sugar confectionery, as binder in meat products.

starch, resistant   Starch that escapes digestion in the small intestine but can be fermented in the colon. Depending on the analytical method, resistant starch may be included with dietary FIBRE. Chemically it is a glucan formed when starch is heated (apparently formed after gelatinisation by spontaneous self-association of hydrated amylose).

starch, stabilized   *See* STARCH, MODIFIED.

starch, thermoplastic (or destructurised)   A homogeneous thermoplastic material made from native starch by swelling in a solvent (plasticiser) followed by heating and an extrusion process; used to make biodegradable packaging films and foam trays (to replace polystyrene foam).

starch, thin boiling   *See* STARCH, MODIFIED.

starch, waxy   Starch containing a high percentage of AMYLOPECTIN; they form soft pastes rather than rigid gels when gelatinised (*see* GELATINISATION).

See also MAIZE STARCH, WAXY.

star fruit   *See* CARAMBOLA.

starter   Culture of bacteria used to inoculate or start growth in a fermentation, e.g. milk for cheese production, or butter to develop the flavour.

Sta-Slim™   FAT REPLACER made from starch.

statins   A family of related compounds (lovastatin, pravastatin, simvastatin) used to treat hypercholesterolaemia. They act by inhibiting hydroxymethylglutaryl CoA reductase (HMG COA REDUCTASE, EC 1.1.1.34), the first and rate-limiting enzyme of CHOLESTEROL synthesis.

steam baking   An even temperature is maintained in the oven by means of closed pipes through which steam circulates. It is sometimes erroneously assumed that the bread is baked in steam.

steam distillation   Process for removal of volatile components by passing steam through the heated mixture, followed by condensation of the steam and volatiles. May be used either to purify a volatile compound such as an ESSENTIAL OIL or to remove undesirable flavours from oils and fats.

steam economy   In evaporation of liquids, the amount of steam required to evaporate 1 kg of water.

steapsin   Obsolete name for LIPASE.

stearic acid   Saturated FATTY ACID with 18 carbon atoms (C18:0); present in most animal and vegetable fats.

stearyl citrate   Ester of stearyl alcohol and citric acid, used to CHELATE metal ions that might otherwise cause RANCIDITY in oils.

steatohepatitis   Fatty infiltration of the liver.

steatopygia   Accumulation of large amounts of fat on the buttocks.

steatorrhoea   Faeces containing a large amount of fat (>5 g/day), and generally foul smelling. Characteristic of COELIAC DISEASE, and may also be due to fat malabsorption as a result of lack of BILE or intestinal LIPASE. Treatment by feeding low-fat diet.

steatosis   Fatty infiltration of the liver; occurs in PROTEIN–ENERGY MALNUTRITION and alcoholism.

steely hair syndrome   *See* MENKES SYNDROME.

steep   The process of leaving a food to stand in water, either to soften it or to extract its flavour and colour. Also the preparation of fruit liqueurs by steeping fruit in SPIRIT.

Stellar™   FAT REPLACER made from starch.

stenosis   Abnormal narrowing of blood vessels or heart valves.

stercobilin   One of the brown pigments of the faeces; formed from the BILE pigments, which, in turn, are formed as breakdown products of HAEMOGLOBIN.

stercolith   Stone formed of dried compressed FAECES.

sterculia   A bulk-forming LAXATIVE. *See* KARAYA GUM.

stereoisomerism   *See* ISOMERS.

sterigmatocystin   A MYCOTOXIN.

sterile   Free from all micro-organisms, bacteria, moulds and yeasts. When foods are sterilised, as in canning, they are preserved indefinitely, since they are protected from recontamination in the can, and also from chemical and enzymic deterioration.

sterilisation, cold   Applied to preservation with SULPHUR DIOXIDE or by IRRADIATION, high pressure, ULTRASONICATION or ELECTROPORATION.

sterilisation, radiation   *See* IRRADIATION.

sterility, commercial   In heat sterilisation, used to indicate that substantially all micro-organisms and spores which, if present, would be capable of growing in the food under defined storage conditions, have been inactivated.

steroids   Chemically, compounds that contain the cyclopenteno-phenanthrene ring system. All the biologically important steroids are derived metabolically from CHOLESTEROL; they include VITAMIN D (chemically a secosteroid rather than a steroid), and HORMONES including the sex hormones (androgens, oestrogens and progesterone) and the hormones of the adrenal cortex.

   See also PHYTOSTEROLS; SITOSTEROL; STANOLS.

stevia leaves   Leaves of the Paraguayan shrub, *Stevia rebaudiana*, the source of STEVIOSIDE and REBAUDIOSIDE, also known as yerba dulce.

stevioside   Naturally occurring GLUCOSIDE of steviol, a STEROID derivative, which is 300 times as sweet as sucrose. Isolated from leaves of the Paraguayan shrub, yerba dulce (*Stevia rebaudiana*), the same source as REBAUDIOSIDE.

Stevix^{TM}   Mixture of the sweet GLYCOSIDES extracted from STEVIA LEAVES.

stickwater   The aqueous fraction from pressing cooked fish in the manufacture of FISH MEAL. Contains amino acids, vitamins and minerals, and is either added to animal feed or mixed back with the fish meal and dried. Also known as fish solubles.

stilboestrol (stilbestrol)   Dihydroxystilbene, a synthetic compound with potent oestrogenic activity; the first non-steroidal oestrogen synthesised (1938). Formerly widely used both clinically and for chemical caponisation of cockerels (*see* CAPON) and to stimulate the growth of cattle.

Stilton   Semi-hard, creamy white or blue-veined English CHEESE made only in a very restricted area of the Vale of Belvoir in Leicestershire, UK, but named after the village of Stilton, Huntingdonshire. Matured 3–4 months; for production of blue Stilton the cheese is pricked with stainless steel wires during ripening to encourage growth of the mould *Penicillium roquefortii*.

stiparogenic   Foods that tend to cause constipation.

stiparolytic   Foods that tend to prevent or relieve constipation.

stirabout   Irish name for PORRIDGE.

stir frying   Chinese method of cooking; sliced vegetables and meat fried for a short time in a small amount of oil, normally in a WOK, over high heat with constant stirring.

St John's bread   *See* CAROB.

stobb   Strawberry stalk.

stocker cattle   Weaned calves grazed on grass, small grain pastures, grain stubble or legume pastures.

stockfish   Unsalted fish that has been dried naturally in air and sunshine; mostly prepared in Norway. Contains 12–15% water; 4.5 kg of fresh fish yield 1 kg stockfish.

   See also KLIPFISH.

Stoke's law   Equation to predict the stability of an EMULSION as the rate of separation of the phases, based on the diameter of droplets in the dispersed phase, the density of the two phases and the viscosity of the continuous phase.

Stomacher^{TM} Paddle-action blender used to prepare food samples for microbiological testing.

stomatitis   Inflammation of the mucous membrane of the mouth.

stondyng   Medieval English; thick POTTAGE such as FRUMENTY.

stork process   The process of ultra-high temperature sterilisation of milk followed by sterilisation again inside the bottle.

stout   *See* BEER.

strain   Horticultural term for seed-raised plants exhibiting certain characteristics, which are not stable or predictable enough when propagated to be a CULTIVAR.

strawberry   Fruit of *Fragaria* spp., a perennial herb of American origin, introduced into UK around 1600.

   Composition /100 g: (edible portion 94%) water 90.9 g, 134 kJ (32 kcal), protein 0.7 g, fat 0.3 g, carbohydrate 7.7 g (4.7 g sugars), fibre 2 g, ash 0.4 g, Ca 16 mg, Fe 0.4 mg, Mg 13 mg, P 24 mg, K 153 mg, Na 1 mg, Zn 0.1 mg, Mn 0.4 mg, Se 0.4 µg, vitamin A 1 µg RE (33 µg carotenoids), E 0.3 mg, K 2.2 mg, B_1 0.02 mg, B_2 0.02 mg, niacin 0.4 mg, B_6 0.05 mg, folate 24 µg, pantothenate 0.1 mg, C 59 mg. A 100 g serving is a source of Mn, folate, a rich source of vitamin C.

   Alpine strawberry is *Fragaria vesca semperflorens*, a variety of the European wild strawberry.

strawberry tomato   *See* CAPE GOOSEBERRY.

straw mushroom   *Volvariella volvacea, see* MUSHROOMS.

straw potatoes   Very thin strips of potato, deep fried. Also known as pommes allumettes.

Strecker degradation   A non-enzymic BROWNING REACTION between free amino acids and di- or tri-carbonyl compounds to form pyrazine derivatives. Will lead to loss of amino acids, and may be aesthetically damaging to food, but also exploited to yield desirable flavours in chocolate, honey and a variety of cooked and baked products.

See also MAILLARD REACTION.

streptavidin Protein from *Streptomyces* spp. that is similar to AVIDIN, and binds BIOTIN with high affinity.

streptozotocin ANTIBIOTIC isolated from *Streptomyces achromogenes* culture broth; specifically cytotoxic to the β-cells of the pancreatic islets, and used to induce experimental insulin-dependent DIABETES mellitus.

See also ALLOXAN.

streusel Also known as chocolate vermicelli or chocolate strands, made by extruding a chocolate paste through a perforated die plate and setting the strands as they emerge.

stroke Also known as cerebrovascular accident (CVA); damage to brain tissue by hypoxia due to blockage of a blood vessel as a result of thrombosis, atherosclerosis or haemorrhage. The severity and nature of the effects of the stroke depend on the region of the brain affected and the extent of damage. HYPERTENSION and HYPERCHOLESTEROLAEMIA are major risk factors.

Strongyloides Genus of small nematode worms that infest the small intestine.

struvite Small crystals of magnesium ammonium phosphate that occasionally form in canned fish, resembling broken glass.

STS Sorbitan tristearate, used as an emulsifying agent in CHOCOLATE manufacture.

Stubbs and More factor For calculating the amount of fat-free meat in a product from total NITROGEN content.

See also KJELDAHL DETERMINATION; NITROGEN CONVERSION FACTOR.

stunting Reduction in the linear growth of children, leading to lower height for age than would be expected, and generally resulting in life-long short stature. A common effect of PROTEIN–ENERGY MALNUTRITION, and associated especially with inadequate protein intake.

See also ANTHROPOMETRY; HARVARD STANDARDS; NCHS STANDARDS; NUTRITIONAL STATUS ASSESSMENT; TANNER STANDARDS; WATERLOW CLASSIFICATION.

sturgeon White FISH, *Acipenser* spp. The ROE is the source of CAVIAR.

sublimation A change in state of directly from solid to vapour without melting.

submaxillary gland One of the SALIVARY GLANDS.

submucosa Layer of loose (areolar) connective tissue underlying a mucous membrane.

substantial equivalence   Term used to denote oil, starch, etc., from a genetically modified crop, that does not contain protein or DNA, and cannot be distinguished from the same product from the unmodified crop.

substrate   The compound on which an ENZYME acts, or the medium on which MICRO-ORGANISMS grow.

subtilin   ANTIBIOTIC isolated from a strain of *Bacillus subtilis* grown on a medium containing asparagine. Used as a food preservative (not permitted in the UK), as it reduces the thermal resistance of bacterial SPORES and so permits a reduction in the processing time.

Sucaryl^{TM}   Sodium or calcium salt of cyclohexyl sulphamate (*see* CYCLAMATE).

succory   *See* CHICORY.

succotash   American; sweetcorn (MAIZE) kernels cooked with green or lima (butter) beans.

succus   Any juice or secretion of animal or plant origin. Succus entericus is the INTESTINAL JUICE.

suchar   Activated CHARCOAL, used to decolourise solutions.

sucking pig   Piglet aged 4–5 weeks, usually stuffed and roasted whole.

sucralfate   Complex of aluminium hydroxide and sulphated sucrose used to form a protective coat over the gastric or duodenal mucosa in treatment of peptic ULCERS.

Sucralose^{TM}   Chlorinated sucrose (trichlorogalactosucrose); 2000 times as sweet as sucrose, stable to heat and acid.

sucrase (sucrase-isomaltase)   *See* INVERTASE.

sucrol   *See* DULCIN.

Sucron^{TM}   Mixture of SACCHARIN and SUCROSE, four times as sweet as sucrose alone.

sucrose   Cane or beet SUGAR. A DISACCHARIDE, glucosyl-fructose.

sucrose distearate   *See* SUCROSE ESTERS.

sucrose esters   Di- and trilaurates and mono- and distearates of sucrose. Used as emulsifiers, wetting agents and surface active agents, e.g. for washing fruits and vegetables, as antispattering agents, antifoam agents and antistaling or crumb-softening agents (E-473).

  See also SUCROSE POLYESTERS.

sucrose intolerance   *See* DISACCHARIDE INTOLERANCE.

sucrose monostearate   *See* SUCROSE ESTERS.

sucrose polyesters (SPE)   Mixtures of hexa- hepta- and octa-esters of sucrose and common FATTY ACIDS (C-12 to C-20 and above). Can replace fats and oils in foods and food preparation (trade names OLESTRA, Olean) but pass through the gastroin-

testinal tract without being absorbed, hence known as fat substitutes or FAT REPLACERS.

Sudan gum *See* GUM ARABIC.

suet Solid white fat around the kidneys of oxen and sheep, used
in baking and frying. 58.3% saturated, 39% mono-unsaturated,
2.5% polyunsaturated, cholesterol 82 mg/100 g.

suet crust *See* PASTRY.

sufu Chinese cheese, made by inoculating soybean curd (TOFU)
with the mould *Actinomucor elegans*; stored after adding salt and
alcohol.

sugar Table sugar or SUCROSE, which is extracted from the SUGAR
BEET or SUGAR CANE, concentrated and refined. MOLASSES is the
residue left after the first stage of crystallisation and is bitter and
black. The residue from the second stage is TREACLE, less bitter
and viscous than molasses. The first crude crystals are muscovado or Barbados sugar, brown and sticky. The next stage is light
brown, demerara sugar. Refined white sugar is essentially 100%
pure sucrose; officially described in EU as semi-white, white and
extra-white. Yields 16 kJ (3.9 kcal) /g. Soft sugars are fine grained
and moister, white or brown (excluding large-grained demerara
sugar).

See also SUGARS.

sugar alcohols Also called polyols, chemical derivatives of SUGARS
that differ from the parent compound in having an alcohol group
(CH₂OH) instead of the aldehyde group (CHO); thus MANNITOL
from MANNOSE, XYLITOL from XYLOSE, LACTITOL from LACTULOSE
(also SORBITOL, ISOMALT and hydrogenated glucose SYRUP).
Several occur naturally in fruits, vegetables and cereals. They
range in sweetness from equal to sucrose to less than half. They
provide bulk in foods such as confectionery (in contrast to
intense sweeteners, *see* SWEETENERS, INTENSE), and so are called
bulk sweeteners.

They are slowly and incompletely metabolised so that they
are tolerated by diabetics and provide less energy than
sucrose: they are less CARIOGENIC than sucrose, especially
hydrogenated glucose syrup, isomalt, sorbitol and xylitol.
The energy yields differ, but the EU has adopted a value of
10 kJ (2.4 kcal)/g for all polyols (compared with 16 for
carbohydrates).

Considered safe and have no specified ADI, meaning that they
can be used in foods in any required amount; however a fairly
large amount, more than 20–50 g per day, varying with the rest
of the diet and the individual, can cause gastrointestinal discomfort and osmotic DIARRHOEA. For labelling purposes they are
included with carbohydrates not sugars; they do not ferment and

so do not damage teeth, and are used in manufacture of TOOTH-FRIENDLY SWEETS.

sugar beet *Beta vulgaris* subsp. *cicla*, biennial plant related to the garden BEETROOT but with white, conical roots; the most important source of SUGAR (SUCROSE) in temperate countries; contains 15–20% sucrose.

sugar, blood *See* GLUCOSE.

sugar, bottlers' *See* SUGAR, CANNERS'.

sugar cane The tropical grass, *Saccharum officinarum*; the juice of the stems contains about 15% SUCROSE and provides about 70% of the world's sugar production.

sugar, canners' Sugar with a higher standard of microbiological quality control than highly refined table sugar because some bacterial spores can survive the high temperatures of canning and even small numbers can damage canned food. Similarly bottlers' sugar must be virtually free from yeasts, moulds and certain bacteria.

sugar, caster Ordinary SUGAR (sucrose) crystallised in small crystals.

sugar confectionery A range of sugar-based products, including boiled sweets (hard glasses), fatty emulsions (toffees and caramels), soft crystalline products (fudges), fully crystalline products (fondants) and gels (gums, pastilles and jellies).

sugar doctor To prevent the crystallisation or 'graining' of SUGAR in sugar confectionery, a substance called the sugar doctor or candy doctor is added. This may be a weak acid, such as cream of tartar, which 'inverts' (HYDROLYSES) part of the sugar during the boiling, or invert sugar or starch syrup (*see* SUGAR, INVERT).

sugar esters *See* SUCROSE ESTERS.

sugar, icing Powdered SUGAR.

sugaring A type of deterioration of dried fruit on storage, most frequently on prunes and figs. A sugary substance appears on the surface or under the skin, consisting of glucose and fructose, with traces of citric and malic acids, lysine, asparagine and aspartic acid. When occurring under the skin of prunes, it is called 'red sugar'.

sugar, invert The mixture of glucose and fructose produced by hydrolysis of SUCROSE, 1.3 times sweeter than sucrose. So-called because the OPTICAL ACTIVITY is reversed in the process. It is important in the manufacture of sugar confectionery, and especially boiled sweets, since the presence of 10–15% invert sugar prevents the crystallisation of sucrose.

sugar, London demerara White sugar coloured with molasses to resemble partly refined sugar.

sugar maple   N. American tree; *Acer saccharum*. *See* MAPLE SYRUP.

sugar palm   *Arenga saccharifera*; grows wild in Malaysia and Indonesia; sugar (sucrose) is obtained from the sap.

sugar pea   *See* PEA, MANGE-TOUT.

sugars   The simplest CARBOHYDRATES; monosaccharides may contain three (triose), four (tetrose), five (pentose), six (hexose) or seven (heptose) carbon atoms, with hydrogen and oxygen. Di- and tri-saccharides consist of two or three monosaccharide units respectively.

sugar tolerance   *See* GLUCOSE TOLERANCE.

sugar, turbinado   Washed raw sugar, with a thin film of molasses.

sugarware   Edible seaweed, *Laminaria saccharina*.

sulphaguanidine (sulfaguanidine)   Poorly absorbed antibacterial agent (a sulphonamide) used in treatment of persistent bacterial DIARRHOEA and gastrointestinal infection.

sulphasalazine (sulfasalazine)   A sulphonamide drug (salicyl-azosulphapyridine) used in treatment of inflammatory bowel disease. Inhibits absorption of FOLIC ACID.

sulphites (sulfites)   Salts of sulphurous acid (H_2SO_3) used as sources of SULPHUR DIOXIDE (E-221–227).

sulphonamides (sulfonamides)   Family of drugs derived from sulphanilamide that prevent the growth of bacteria (i.e. bacteriostatic, not bactericidal), acting as antagonists of PARA-AMINOBENZOIC ACID.

sulphonylureas   *See* HYPOGLYCAEMIC AGENTS.

sulphoraphane (sulforafane)   Isothiocyanate derivative in *Brassica* spp. that induces PHASE II METABOLISM of XENOBIOTICS, and hence has a potentially anticarcinogenic action.

sulphur (sulfur)   An element that is part of the amino acids cysteine and methionine and therefore present in all proteins. It is also part of the molecules of vitamin B_1 and biotin and occurs in foods and in the body as sulphates. Apart from these amino acids and vitamins, there appears to be no requirement for sulphur in any other form and no deficiency has ever been observed, although it is essential for plants. Not only was the old-fashioned remedy of sulphur and molasses (brimstone and treacle) quite unnecessary, but elemental sulphur is not used by the body.

sulphur dioxide (SO_2)   Preservative used in gaseous form or as salts (SULPHITES) for fruit drinks, wine, comminuted meat, as a processing aid to control physical properties of flour; also prevents enzymic and non-enzymic browning (*see* BROWNING REACTIONS) by inhibition of PHENOL OXIDASES. Protects vitamin C but destroys vitamin B_1. Prepared by ancient Egyptians and Romans by burning sulphur and used to disinfect wine (E-220).

sulphuring (sulfuring) Preservation by treatment with SULPHUR DIOXIDE or SULPHITES; also used for treatment of vegetables prior to dehydration to prevent BROWNING REACTIONS.

sultanas Made by drying the golden sultana grapes grown in Turkey, Greece, Australia and S. Africa; the bunches are dipped in alkali, washed, sulphured and dried. Sultanas of the European type produced in the USA are termed seedless raisins.

See also CURRANTS, DRIED; RAISIN.

summer pudding Cold sweet of stewed fruit cased in bread or sponge cake.

sum-sum See SESAME.

Sunett^{TM} See ACESULPHAME K.

sunflower Annual plant, *Helianthus annuus*. Seeds used for oil; 11% saturated, 20% mono-unsaturated, 69% polyunsaturated, contains 41.1 mg vitamin E, 5.4 mg vitamin K/100 g.

Seeds, composition/100 g: (edible portion 54%) water 5.4 g, 2386 kJ (570 kcal), protein 22.8 g, fat 49.6 g (of which 11% saturated, 20% mono-unsaturated, 69% polyunsaturated), carbohydrate 18.8 g (2.6 g sugars), fibre 10.5 g, ash 3.5 g, Ca 116 mg, Fe 6.8 mg, Mg 354 mg, P 705 mg, K 689 mg, Na 3 mg, Zn 5.1 mg, Cu 1.8 mg, Mn 2 mg, Se 59.5 µg, vitamin A 3 µg RE (30 µg carotenoids), E 34.5 mg, K 2.7 mg, B_1 2.29 mg, B_2 0.25 mg, niacin 4.5 mg, B_6 0.77 mg, folate 227 µg, pantothenate 6.7 mg, C 1 mg. A 15 g serving is a source of Mg, Mn, P, Se, folate, pantothenate, a good source of Cu, vitamin B_1, a rich source of vitamin E.

sunlight flavour Name given to unpleasant flavours developing in foods after exposure to sunlight. In milk it is said to be due to the oxidation of METHIONINE in the presence of riboflavin (vitamin B_2). At the same time riboflavin undergoes photolysis to metabolically inactive lumichrome, so a significant loss of the vitamin can occur when milk is exposed to sunlight. In beer due to a change in the bitter principles from the hops.

superchill Cool to –1 to –4°C (chill temperature is usually 2°C).

supercooled liquid One that remains a liquid below its normal freezing point.

supercooling A phenomenon in which a liquid does become solid even though the temperature is below its freezing point.

supercritical fluid extraction Technique for extraction especially of non-polar compounds, e.g. decaffeination of coffee. A gas (commonly carbon dioxide) is compressed to above its critical pressure, but above its critical temperature, to yield a supercritical fluid with physical properties intermediate between those of a dense gas and a liquid with low viscosity and surface tension, high solvating properties and a high diffusion constant of solutes.

superoxide dismutase (SOD) COPPER- and ZINC-containing enzyme (EC 1.15.1.1), important as a scavenger of the superoxide radical. Activity in red BLOOD CELLS may provide an index of copper status.

supplementation *See* FORTIFICATION.

suprarenal glands *See* ADRENAL GLANDS.

surface area *See* BODY SURFACE AREA.

surface film *See* BOUNDARY FILM.

surface finishing agents Glazes, polishes, waxes and protective coatings on the surface of foods to increase palatability, enhance appearance or prevent discoloration.

surface heat transfer coefficient A measure of the resistance to heat flow caused by a boundary film of liquid.

surfactants (surface active agents) Compounds (other than EMULSIFIERS) that are both hydrophobic and hydrophilic, so act to emulsify lipids and water, e.g. soaps and detergents. Used to modify the surface properties of liquids, include solubilisers, dispersants, detergents, wetting agents, foaming and ANTIFOAMING AGENTS and compounds that enhance reconstitution of dried foods.

surimi Traditional Japanese, now widely used in food manufacture; minced non-oily FISH that has been washed with water to remove soluble proteins and odorants, leaving the myofibrillar proteins that give an elastic and chewy texture. When prepared with cryoprotectants (SUCROSE and SORBITOL), it has a better stability to freeze DENATURATION than minced fish, and is used to manufacture SEAFOOD analogues such as 'crab sticks'. The main commercial sources are Alaska pollock and southern blue whiting.

Composition /100 g: water 76 g, 414 kJ (99 kcal), protein 15.2 g, fat 0.9 g, cholesterol 30 mg, carbohydrate 6.8 g, ash 0.7 g, Ca 9 mg, Fe 0.3 mg, Mg 43 mg, P 282 mg, K 112 mg, Na 143 mg, Zn 0.3 mg, Se 28.1 µg, vitamin A 20 µg retinol, E 0.6 mg, K 0.1 mg, B_1 0.02 mg, B_2 0.02 mg, niacin 0.2 mg, B_6 0.03 mg, folate 2 µg, B_{12} 1.6 µg, pantothenate 0.1 mg.

See also KAMABOKO.

surveillance Continuous monitoring of (the nutritional status of) selected population groups. Differs from surveys in that data are collected and analysed over a prolonged period of time, hence longitudinal rather than cross-sectional data.

susceptor Packaging material used to achieve a localised high temperature in MICROWAVE COOKING, commonly a metallised plastic film (usually powdered ALUMINIUM). It concentrates the energy on the outside of the food to brown and crisp it.

sushi Japanese; thinly sliced raw fish.

suspensoids *See* COLLOID.

süssreserve Unfermented grape juice added to wines after fermentation to increase sweetness, especially in Germany, England and New Zealand.

Sustagen™ A powdered food concentrate, a mixture of whole and skim milk, casein, maltose, dextrins and glucose.

Svedberg Unit of the rate of sedimentation of biological particles and proteins in centrifugation.

swainsonine *See* LOCOWEED.

sweating Process of leaving sun dried fruit in wooden boxes (sweat boxes) to allow equilibration between drier and moister pieces, resulting in a more uniform product.

swede Root of *Brassica rutabaga* or Swedish turnip; called rutabaga in the USA.

Composition /100 g: (edible portion 85%) water 90 g, 151 kJ (36 kcal), protein 1.2 g, fat 0.2 g, carbohydrate 8.1 g (5.6 g sugars), fibre 2.5 g, ash 0.8 g, Ca 47 mg, Fe 0.5 mg, Mg 23 mg, P 58 mg, K 337 mg, Na 20 mg, Zn 0.3 mg, Mn 0.2 mg, Se 0.7 µg, 1 µg carotenoids, E 0.3 mg, K 0.3 mg, B$_1$ 0.09 mg, B$_2$ 0.04 mg, niacin 0.7 mg, B$_6$ 0.1 mg, folate 21 µg, pantothenate 0.2 mg, C 25 mg. A 60 g serving is a good source of vitamin C.

sweeney OSTEOMALACIA in livestock due to PHOSPHATE deficiency.

sweetbread Butchers' term for PANCREAS (gut sweetbread) or THYMUS (chest sweetbread).

sweet cecily *See* CHERVIL (3).

sweet clover disease Haemorrhagic disease of cattle caused by eating hay made from spoiled sweet clover (*Melilotus officinalis*), which contains dicoumarol, an antimetabolite of VITAMIN K.

sweetcorn *See* MAIZE.

sweeteners Four groups of compounds are used to sweeten foods:

(1) The SUGARS, of which the commonest is SUCROSE. FRUCTOSE has 173% of the sweetness of sucrose; GLUCOSE, 74%; MALTOSE, 33% and LACTOSE, 16%. HONEY is a mixture of glucose and fructose. *See also* SYRUP.

(2) Bulk sweeteners (*see* SWEETENERS, BULK), including SUGAR ALCOHOLS.

(3) Synthetic non-nutritive sweeteners which are many times sweeter than sucrose (*see* SWEETENERS, INTENSE).

(4) Various other chemicals such as GLYCEROL and GLYCINE (70% as sweet as sucrose), and certain PEPTIDES.

sweeteners, artificial *See* SWEETENERS, INTENSE.

sweeteners, bulk Used to replace sucrose and glucose syrups; unlike intense sweeteners (*see* SWEETENERS, INTENSE) they provide bulk in the food. Include SUGAR ALCOHOLS and hydro-genated glucose syrup (*see* SYRUP, HYDROGENATED).

sweeteners, intense (non-nutritive) Chemical substances that have no calorific value but are intensely sweet and so are useful as a replacement for sucrose in foods intended for diabetics and those on slimming regimes. Unlike bulk sweeteners (*see* SWEETENERS, BULK) do not replace the volume of sucrose.

See also ACESULPHAME, ASPARTAME, CYCLAMATE, MIRACLE BERRY, MONELLIN, NEOHESPERIDIN DIHYDROCHALCONE, SACCHARIN, STEVIO-SIDE, THAUMATIN.

Sweetex™ *See* SACCHARIN.

sweetness One of the five basic senses of TASTE.

Sweet'N Low™ A SWEETENER containing SACCHARIN.

sweet sop *See* CUSTARD APPLE.

swells Infected cans of food swollen at the ends by gases pro-duced by fermentation. A 'hard swell' has permanently extended ends. If the ends can be moved under pressure, but not forced back to the original position, they are 'soft swells'. 'Springers' can be forced back, but the opposite end bulges. A 'flipper' is a can of normal appearance in which the end flips out when the can is struck. Hydrogen swells are harmless, and due to acid fruits attacking the can.

Swift test Method for determining the emulsifying capacity of a protein or a meat suspension by measuring the volume of oil that can be emulsified, under specified conditions.

See also ACTIVE OXYGEN METHOD.

Swiss chard The spinach-like leaves and broad mid-rib of *Beta vulgaris* var. *cicla*, also known as leaf beet, leaf chard, sea kale beet, silver beet, white leaf beet, spinach beet.

Composition/100g: (edible portion 92%) water 93g, 80kJ (19kcal), protein 1.8g, fat 0.2g, carbohydrate 3.7g (1.1g sugars), fibre 1.6g, ash 1.6g, Ca 51mg, Fe 1.8mg, Mg 81mg, P 46mg, K 379mg, Na 213mg, Zn 0.4mg, Cu 0.2mg, Mn 0.4mg, Se 0.9µg, vitamin A 306µg RE (14692µg carotenoids), E 1.9mg, K 830mg, B_1 0.04mg, B_2 0.09mg, niacin 0.4mg, B_6 0.1mg, folate 14µg, pantothenate 0.2mg, C 30mg. A 50g serving (1 leaf) is a source of Mg, vitamin A, a good source of vitamin C.

Also used as name for blanched summer shoots of globe ARTI-CHOKE and inner leaves of CARDOON, *Cynara cardunculus*.

swordfish Oily FISH, *Xiphias gladius*.

Composition/100g: water 76g, 507kJ (121kcal), protein 19.8g, fat 4g (of which 31% saturated, 43% mono-unsaturated, 26% polyunsaturated), cholesterol 39mg, carbohydrate 0g, ash 1.5g, Ca 4mg, Fe 0.8mg, Mg 27mg, P 263mg, K 288mg, Na 90mg, Zn 1.1mg, Cu 0.1mg, Se 48.1µg, vitamin A 36µg RE

(36 µg retinal), E 0.5 mg, K 0.1 mg, B_1 0.04 mg, B_2 0.09 mg, niacin 9.7 mg, B_6 0.33 mg, folate 2 µg, B_{12} 1.8 µg, pantothenate 0.4 mg, C 1 mg. A 100 g serving is a source of vitamin B_6, a rich source of P, Se, niacin, vitamin B_{12}.

syllabub (sillabub) Elizabethan dish made from cream curdled with white wine or cider; thickened version as a dessert and a thinner version as a drink.

symbiotic Organisms (commonly micro-organisms) that have a close and obligatory relationship of mutual benefit with another organism.

See also COMMENSAL; PATHOGEN.

symptom Indication of a disease or condition noticed by the patient.

See also SIGN.

synbiotic A food or ingredient that contains both a PREBIOTIC and a PROBIOTIC.

syndrome Combination of signs and/or symptoms that form a distinct clinical picture.

syndrome X *See* METABOLIC SYNDROME.

syneresis Oozing of liquid from gel when cut and allowed to stand (e.g. jelly, baked custard or clotted blood).

Synergistic zinc^{TM} ZINC supplement that also contains COPPER and VITAMIN A, which are claimed to aid its absorption.

Synergy1^{TM} Short-chain fructose oligosaccharide used as a PREBIOTIC food additive.

synsepalum *See* MIRACLE BERRY.

synthetic rice *See* TAPIOCA-MACARONI.

syrup A solution of sugar which may be from a variety of sources, such as maple or sorghum, or stages in refining cane and beet sugar such as top syrup, refiner's syrup, sugar syrup, golden syrup or by hydrolysis of STARCH (*see* SYRUP, GLUCOSE).

syrup, glucose The concentrated solution of sugars from the acid or enzymic hydrolysis of STARCH (usually maize or potato starch); a mixture of varying amounts of glucose, maltose and glucose complexes. The CODEX ALIMENTARIUS definition is: purified, concentrated, aqueous solutions of nutritive saccharides from starch. Usually 70% total solids by weight, containing glucose, maltose and oligomers of glucose of three, four or more units. May be in dried form. Used as a sweetening agent in sugar confectionery; also termed corn syrup, corn starch hydrolysate, starch syrup, confectioners' glucose and uncrystallisable syrup.

See also DEXTROSE EQUIVALENT VALUE; SYRUP, HIGH FRUCTOSE.

syrup, high fructose Glucose SYRUP made by hydrolysis of starch and then half the glucose converted into fructose, similar to invert syrup produced from sucrose but cheaper. Also known as iso-syrups, high-fructose syrups (HFS), high-fructose corn syrups (HFCS).

See also GLUCOSE ISOMERASE.

syrup, hydrogenated Syrups produced by partial hydrolysis of starch followed by hydrogenation to yield a mixture of SORBITOL, MALTITOL and other POLYOLS. Also known as hydrogenated starch hydrolysates. Used as bulk sweeteners (*see* SWEETENERS, BULK), viscosity or bodying agents, humectants, crystallisation modifiers (*see* RETROGRADATION) and rehydration aids.

syrup, maltose Made from starch by hydrolysis with acid or bacterial maltase and a maltogenic enzyme, containing up to 75% maltose with little glucose.

T

T3, T4 Tri-iodothyronine and thyroxine (tetra-iodothyronine), the THYROID HORMONES.

Tab^{TM} Sugar-free COLA drink sweetened with CYCLAMATE, introduced 1963.

tabasco A thin piquant sauce prepared by fermentation of powdered dried fruits of chilli pepper (*see* PEPPER, CHILLI), mixed with spirit vinegar and salt.

tachycardia Rapid heartbeat, as occurs after exercise; may also occur, without undue exertion, as a result of anxiety and in ANAEMIA and VITAMIN B_1 deficiency.

tachyphagia Rapid eating.

taeniasis Infection with TAPEWORMS of the genus *Taenia*.

taette *See* MILK, FERMENTED.

tagatose D-Lyxo-2-hexulose an isomer of FRUCTOSE obtained by hydrolysis of plant gums and used as a bulk sweetener (*see* SWEETENERS, BULK); 14-times as sweet as sucrose. Not metabolised to any significant extent, so does not affect blood glucose, and has zero energy yield.

tagliatelle *See* PASTA.

tahini (tahina) Middle East; paste made from SESAME seeds, usually eaten as a dip; also used in preparation of HUMMUS.

takadiastase Or koji; an enzyme preparation produced by growing the fungus *Aspergillus oryzae* on bran, leaching the culture mass with water and precipitating with alcohol. Contains a mixture of enzymes, largely diastatic (i.e. AMYLASE), used for the preparation of starch hydrolysates.

Talin^{TM} Thaumatin, an extract of the berry *Thaumatococcus danielli*, about 3000 times as sweet as sucrose.

See also KATEMFE.

tallow, rendered Beef or mutton fat other than that from around the kidney (which gives rise to PREMIER JUS), prepared by heating with water in an autoclave. When pressed, separates to a liquid fraction, oleo oil, used in margarine, and a solid fraction, oleostearin, used for soap and candles.

tamal (tamales) Mexican; maize meal pancake, similar to TOR-TILLA, but made with fat. Traditionally cooked inside the soft husks of maize.

tamarillo Reddish yellow or purple fruit of *Cyphomandra betacea*, also called tree or English tomato.

tamarind Leguminous tree, *Tamarindus indica*, with pods containing seeds embedded in brown pulp, eaten fresh, and used to prepare beverages and seasonings in oriental cuisine (e.g. the Indian sauce, imli).

Composition/100 g: (edible portion 34%) water 31 g, 1000 kJ (239 kcal), protein 2.8 g, fat 0.6 g, carbohydrate 62.5 g (57.4 g sugars), fibre 5.1 g, ash 2.7 g, Ca 74 mg, Fe 2.8 mg, Mg 92 mg, P 113 mg, K 628 mg, Na 28 mg, Zn 0.1 mg, Cu 0.1 mg, Se 1.3 µg, vitamin A 2 µg RE (18 µg carotenoids), E 0.1 mg, K 2.8 mg, B_1 0.43 mg, B_2 0.15 mg, niacin 1.9 mg, B_6 0.07 mg, folate 14 µg, pantothenate 0.1 mg, C 4 mg.

tammy To squeeze a sauce through a fine woollen cloth (a tammy cloth) to strain it.

tandoori (tanduri) Indian term for food cooked in a clay oven (tandoor). The meat is marinated with aromatic herbs and spices before cooking.

tangelo A CITRUS fruit, cross between TANGERINE and POMELO.

tangerine A CITRUS fruit, *Citrus reticulata*, also called mandarin; satsuma is a variety of tangerine.

Composition/100 g: (edible portion 72%) water 85.2 g, 222 kJ (53 kcal), protein 0.8 g, fat 0.3 g, carbohydrate 13.3 g (10.6 g sugars), fibre 1.8 g, ash 0.4 g, Ca 37 mg, Fe 0.2 mg, Mg 12 mg, P 20 mg, K 166 mg, Na 2 mg, Zn 0.1 mg, Se 0.1 µg, vitamin A 34 µg RE (801 µg carotenoids), E 0.2 mg, B_1 0.06 mg, B_2 0.04 mg, niacin 0.4 mg, B_6 0.08 mg, folate 16 µg, pantothenate 0.2 mg, C 27 mg. A 95 g serving (1 medium) is a rich source of vitamin C.

tangleberry Wild BILBERRY, *Gaylusacia frondosa*.

tangors *See* CITRUS.

tanier *See* TANNIA.

tankage Residue from slaughterhouse excluding all the useful tissues; used as fertiliser or (formerly) animal feed.

Tanner standards Tables of height and weight for age used as reference values for the assessment of growth and nutritional status in children, based on data collected in Britain in the 1960s. Now largely replaced by the NCHS (US National Center for Health Statistics) standards.

See also ANTHROPOMETRY; HARVARD STANDARDS; NCHS STANDARDS.

tannia (tanier) The corm of *Xanthosoma sagittifolium*; known as new cocoyam or yautia in W. Africa; same family as TARO.

Composition/100 g: (edible portion 86%) water 73 g, 410 kJ (98 kcal), protein 1.5 g, fat 0.4 g, carbohydrate 23.6 g, fibre 1.5 g, ash 1.5 g, Ca 9 mg, Fe 1 mg, Mg 24 mg, P 51 mg, K 598 mg, Na 21 mg, Zn 0.5 mg, Cu 0.3 mg, Mn 0.2 mg, Se 0.7 µg, 5 µg carotenoids, vitamin B_1 0.1 mg, B_2 0.04 mg, niacin 0.7 mg, B_6 0.24 mg, folate 17 µg, pantothenate 0.2 mg, C 5 mg. A 100 g serving is a source of vitamin B_6, a good source of Cu.

tannic acid *See* TANNINS.

tannins Also called tannic acid and gallotannin. Water-soluble polyphenolic compounds (from a variety of plants, including sorghum, carob bean, unripe fruits, tea), so-called because they were originally used in leather tanning. They have an astringent effect in the mouth, precipitate proteins and are used to clarify beer and wines. Two main types: proanthocyanidins (condensed tannins) and glucose polyesters of gallic or hexahydroxydiphenic acids (hydrolysable tannins). They are potentially protective ANTIOXIDANTS, but also have potential antinutritional effects, reducing protein digestibility and impairing absorption of some minerals.

tanrogan Manx name for SCALLOPS.

tansy A herb, *Tanacetum vulgare*. Leaves and young shoots used for flavouring puddings and omelettes. Tansy cakes made with eggs and young leaves used to be eaten at Easter. Tansy tea (an infusion) was formerly used as tonic and to treat intestinal worms. Root, preserved in honey or sugar, was used to treat gout.

tapas Spanish; small savoury dishes served with wine in bars.

tapé Indonesian; sweet-sour alcoholic paste made from fermented cassava, millet or maize, using a RAGI starter. Either sun-dried and used in soups and stews or deep fried as a snack.

tapeworm Parasitic intestinal worms; infection is acquired by eating raw or undercooked infected pork (*Taenia solium*), beef (*T. saginata*) or fish (*Diphyllobothrium latum*). Eggs are shed in the faeces and infect the animal host. Cysticercosis is infection of human beings with the larval stage by ingestion of eggs from faecal contamination of food and water.

tapioca Starch prepared from the root of the CASSAVA plant (*Manihot utilissima*). The starch paste is heated to burst the granules, then dried either in globules resembling SAGO or in flakes.

The name is also used of starch in general, as in manioc tapioca and potato flour tapioca.

Composition/100 g: water 11 g, 1499 kJ (358 kcal), protein 0.2 g, fat 0 g, carbohydrate 88.7 g (3.3 g sugars), fibre 0.9 g, ash 0.1 g, Ca 20 mg, Fe 1.6 mg, Mg 1 mg, P 7 mg, K 11 mg, Na 1 mg, Zn 0.1 mg, Mn 0.1 mg, Se 0.8 µg, vitamin B_6 0.01 mg, folate 4 µg, pantothenate 0.1 mg.

tapioca-macaroni A mixture of either 80–90 parts TAPIOCA flour, with 10–20 parts of peanut flour, or tapioca, peanut and semolina, 60:15:25, baked into shapes resembling rice grains or macaroni shapes; developed in India. Also referred to as synthetic rice.

tarako Japanese; salted ROE of Alaskan pollack (*Pollachius virens*), also known as momojiko.

taramasalata Greek; fish roe (commonly smoked cod ROE), whipped with oil, garlic and lemon juice, then thickened with bread, to make a dip.

tares Traditional English name for the vetches (*Lathyrus* and *Vicia* spp.), which are PULSES.

taro Corm of *Colocasia esculenta* and *C. antiquorum*; called eddo or dasheen in Caribbean, old cocoyam in W. Africa.

Composition/100 g: (edible portion 86%) water 71 g, 469 kJ (112 kcal), protein 1.5 g, fat 0.2 g, carbohydrate 26.5 g (0.4 g sugars), fibre 4.1 g, ash 1.2 g, Ca 43 mg, Fe 0.6 mg, Mg 33 mg, P 84 mg, K 591 mg, Na 11 mg, Zn 0.2 mg, Cu 0.2 mg, Mn 0.4 mg, Se 0.7 µg, vitamin A 4 µg RE (55 µg carotenoids), E 2.4 mg, K 1 mg, B_1 0.09 mg, B_2 0.03 mg, niacin 0.6 mg, B_6 0.28 mg, folate 22 µg, pantothenate 0.3 mg, C 5 mg.

tarragon Leaves and flowering tops of the bushy perennial plant *Artemisia dracunculus*.

tartar Hard gritty deposit of PLAQUE and minerals that accumulates on and between teeth, also known as calculus. Originally the name given by alchemists to animal and vegetable concretions, such as wine lees, stone, gravel and deposits on teeth, since they were all attributed to the same cause.

tartar emetic Potassium antimonyl tartrate; produces inflammation of the gastrointestinal MUCOSA; formerly used as an emetic.

tartaric acid Dihydroxysuccinic acid, a dibasic acid. Occurs in fruits, the chief source is grapes; used in preparing lemonade, added to jams when the fruit is not sufficiently acidic (citric acid is also used) and in baking powder (E-334). Wine lees is a mixture of tartrates. Rochelle salt is potassium sodium tartrate (E-337).

See also CREAM OF TARTAR; TARTAR EMETIC.

tartrazine A yellow colour (E-102), called Yellow No. 5 in the USA.

466

taste   The tongue can distinguish five separate tastes: sweet, salt, sour (or acid), bitter and savoury (sometimes called UMAMI, from the Japanese word for a savoury flavour), owing to stimulation of the TASTE BUDS. The overall taste or flavour of foods is due to these tastes, together with astringency in the mouth, texture and aroma.

The tongue can also detect polyunsaturated fatty acids released from dietary triacylglycerol by lipase secreted by the tongue.

taste buds   Situated mostly on the tongue; about 9000 elongated cells ending in minute hair-like processes, the gustatory hairs.

Taste buds for salt have a sodium ion channel in the cell membrane, for sourness a proton channel and for umami a glutamate channel; taste buds for sweetness and bitterness have cell surface receptors that lead to production of intracellular second messengers.

tatare (steak tatare)   Dish prepared from minced beef or other meat, eaten uncooked.

taurine   Aminoethane sulphonic acid, derived from CYSTEINE by oxidation of the sulphydryl group and decarboxylation. Known to be a dietary essential for cats (deficient kittens are blind) and possibly essential for human beings, since the capacity for synthesis is limited, although deficiency has never been observed. Its main functions are in conjugation of BILE acids, and maintenance of osmotic integrity in tissues, especially the retina.

taurochenodeoxycholic acid   The TAURINE conjugate of CHENO-DEOXYCHOLIC ACID, *see* BILE.

taurocholic acid   The TAURINE conjugate of CHOLIC ACID, *see* BILE.

TBARS (thiobarbituric acid reactive substances)   Colorimetric method of determination of dialdehydes formed by breakdown of lipid peroxides, by reaction with thiobarbituric acid; used as an index of RADICAL attack on unsaturated fatty acids, and hence as an inverse index of antioxidant status.

TBA value   A measure of oxidative rancidity in fats. Thiobarbituric acid reacts with malondialdehyde formed by oxidation of polyunsaturated fatty acids to form a coloured product.

TDT   THERMAL DEATH TIME.

tea   A beverage prepared by infusion of the young leaves, leaf buds and internodes of varieties of *Camellia sinensis* and *C. assamica*, originating from China. Green tea is dried without further treatment. Black tea is fermented (actually an oxidation) before drying; Oolong tea is lightly fermented. Among the black teas, flowering Pekoe is made from the top leaf buds, orange Pekoe from first opened leaf, Pekoe from third leaves, and Souchong from next leaves. Earl Grey is flavoured with

BERGAMOT; lapsang souchong was originally produced by burning tarry ropes near the tea during processing. Up to 30% of the dry weight may be various polyphenols that have been associated with protection against cardiovascular disease.

See also CAFFEINE; TISANE; XANTHINES.

tea, Brazilian (Paraguayan) *See* MATÉ.

tea, Mexican *See* EPAZOTE.

teaseed oil Oil from the seed of *Thea sasangua*, cultivated in China; used as salad oil and for frying.

teetotal Total abstinence from alcohol, advocated by Richard Turner in a speech in Preston (Lancs) in 1833; he stammered over the word 'total'.

TEF Thermic effect of food, *see* DIET-INDUCED THERMOGENESIS.

teff A tropical MILLET, *Eragrostis abyssinica*, the dietary staple in Ethiopia; little grown elsewhere.

Teflon^{TM} *See* PTFE.

teg Two-year-old sheep, s*ee* LAMB.

tempeh SOYA bean cake fermented by *Rhizopus* spp. mould.
Composition/100 g: water 60 g, 808 kJ (193 kcal), protein 18.5 g, fat 10.8 g (of which 24% saturated, 33% mono-unsaturated, 42% polyunsaturated), carbohydrate 9.4 g, ash 1.6 g, Ca 111 mg, Fe 2.7 mg, Mg 81 mg, P 266 mg, K 412 mg, Na 9 mg, Zn 1.1 mg, Cu 0.6 mg, Mn 1.3 mg, vitamin B$_1$ 0.08 mg, B$_2$ 0.36 mg, niacin 2.6 mg, B$_6$ 0.22 mg, folate 24 µg, B$_{12}$ 0.1 µg, pantothenate 0.3 mg.

temperature, absolute A temperature scale starting from absolute zero. In the kelvin scale (K) this is –273 °C; in the Rankine scale (°R) it is –460 °F.

tempering (1) Cooling food to a temperature close to its freezing point.
(2) In chocolate manufacture, the process of re-heating, stirring and cooling to convert unstable forms of fats (polymorphs) into the stable β-forms (mp 34.5 °C). If not properly carried out, crystals of fat can separate out on the surface of the chocolate causing the harmless but unsightly effect of 'fat bloom'.

Templein^{TM} Textured vegetable protein.

tenderiser PROTEINASES (endopeptidases) used to hydrolyse COLLAGEN and ELASTIN in the SARCOLEMMA, and so tenderise meat. Enzymes used include: actinidain (EC 3.4.22.14) from KIWI fruit, bromelain (EC 3.4.22.33) from PINEAPPLE, ficin (EC 3.4.22.3) from FIGS, PAPAIN (EC 3.4.22.2) from PAWPAW, and proteases from *Aspergillus oryzae* and *Bacillus subtilis*.

tenderometer Instrument to measure the stage of maturity of peas to determine whether they are ready for cropping, or the tenderness of meat. Measures the force required to effect a shearing action.

tender stretch process   Process involving keeping the beef carcase stretched to prevent COLD-SHORTENING.

tenesmus   Persistent ineffective spasms of bladder or rectum; intestinal tenesmus commonly occurs in IRRITABLE BOWEL SYNDROME.

tensile elongation   A measure of the ability of a material to stretch.

tensile strength   The force needed to stretch a material.

tensiometer   Instrument for measuring the surface tension of a liquid.

tenuate   Anorectic (appetite suppressing, *see* APPETITE CONTROL) drug, formerly used in the treatment of OBESITY.

tepary bean   *See* FRIJOLE BEAN.

tequila   Mexican; SPIRIT (40–50% alcohol by volume) prepared by double distillation of fermented sap of the cultivated agave or maguey, *Agave tequilana*. Mescal and pulque are similar, made from various species of wild agave, and have a stronger flavour.

teratogen   A compound that is capable of causing developmental defects in the fetus *in utero*, and hence non-genetic congenital defects.

terpeneless oil   *See* TERPENES.

terpenes   Chemically consist of multiple isoprenoid (five-carbon) units. Monoterpenes consist of two isoprenoids; sesquiterpenes of three, diterpenes of four, triterpenes of six, and tetraterpenes of eight. Phytol and RETINOL are diterpenes; CAROTENES are tetraterpenes.

   Major components of the ESSENTIAL OILS of citrus fruits, but not responsible for the characteristic flavour, and since they readily oxidise and polymerise to produce unpleasant flavours, removed from citrus oils by distillation or solvent extraction, leaving the so-called terpeneless oils for flavouring foods and drinks.

terramycin   ANTIBIOTIC, also known as oxytetracycline, *see* TETRACYCLINES.

testa   The fibrous layer between the pericarp and the inner aleurone layer of a cereal grain.

test meal   *See* FRACTIONAL TEST MEAL.

tetany   Spasm of twitching of muscles, caused by over-sensitivity of motor nerves to stimuli; particularly affects face, hands and feet. Caused by low plasma ionised CALCIUM and may occur in RICKETS.

tetracyclines   A group of closely related ANTIBIOTICS including tetracycline, oxytetracycline (terramycin) and aureomycin. The last two are used in some countries for preserving food and as growth improvers, added to animal feed at the rate of a few milligrams per tonne (prohibited in the EU).

tetraenoic acid FATTY ACID with four double bonds, e.g. ARACHI-DONIC ACID.

tetramine poisoning Paralysis similar to that caused by curare, caused by a toxin in the salivary glands of the red whelk, *Neptunea antiqua* (distinct from the edible whelk *Buccinum undatum*).

tetrodontin poisoning Caused by a toxin, tetrodotoxin, in fish of the Tetrodontidae family (puffer fish) and amphibia of the Salamandridae family. Occurs in Japan from Japanese puffer fish or fugu (*Fuga rubripes*), eaten for its gustatory and tactile pleasure since traces of the poison cause a tingling sensation in the extremities (larger doses cause respiratory failure). The toxin is acquired via the food chain from bacteria in the coral reef, rather than synthesised by the fish. Lethal dose $10\,\mu g/kg$ body weight.

tetrodotoxin *See* TETRODONTIN POISONING.

tewfikose Name given to a sugar isolated from a sample of buffalo milk obtained from Egypt in 1892, later found to be an artefact; named after Tewfik Bey Pasha, Governor of Egypt.

Texatrein™**, Texgran**™ Textured vegetable proteins.

texture Combination of physical properties perceived by senses of kinaesthesis (muscle–nerve endings), touch (including mouth-feel), sight and hearing. Physical properties may include shape, size, number and conformation of constituent structural elements.

The texture profile is an ORGANOLEPTIC analysis of the complex of food in terms of mechanical and geometrical characteristics, fat and moisture content, including the order in which they appear from the first bite to complete mastication.

textured vegetable protein Spun or extruded vegetable protein, usually made to simulate meat.

***T*g** *See* GLASS TRANSITION TEMPERATURE.

TGS Trichlorogalactosucrose, *see* SUCRALOSE.

thaumatin The intensely sweet protein of the African fruit, *Thaumatococus danielli*, 1600 times as sweet as sucrose. Called katemfe in Sierra Leone and miracle fruit in the Sudan (not the same as MIRACLE BERRY).

theaflavins Reddish-orange pigments formed in TEA during fermentation; responsible for the colour of tea extracts and part of the astringent flavour.

theanine γ-*N*-Ethylglutamine, the major free amino acid in tea, 1–2% dry weight of leaf.

thearubigen Poorly characterised red-brown complex of catechin derivatives in black TEA.

theine Alternative name for CAFFEINE, when found in tea.

theobromine 3,7-Dimethylxanthine, an ALKALOID found in cocoa, chemically related to CAFFEINE, and with similar effects.

theophylline 1,3-Dimethylxanthine, an ALKALOID found in tea, chemically related to CAFFEINE, and with similar effects.

therapeutic diets Those formulated to treat disease or metabolic disorders.

therapeutic index Ratio of the dose of a drug that causes tissue or cell damage to that required to have a therapeutic effect.

therm Obsolete unit of heat $= 1.055 \times 10^8$ J.

thermal centre The point in a food that heats or cools most slowly.

thermal conductivity The rate at which heat moves through a substance.

thermal death time (TDT) Measure of heat resistance of an organism, enzyme or chemical component at a particular temperature, usually 121 °C. Also known as F-value.

thermal diffusivity The ratio of THERMAL CONDUCTIVITY of a material to its (specific HEAT CAPACITY × density).

thermal efficiency In drying of foods, the ratio of heat used in evaporation to total heat supplied in the process.

Thermamyl^{TM} Heat-stable α-AMYLASE from *Bacillus licheniformis*, active up to 100 °C; used in manufacture of glucose SYRUP from STARCH.

thermic effect of food *See* DIET-INDUCED THERMOGENESIS.

thermisation Heat treatment to reduce the number of microorganisms; less severe than PASTEURISATION; used e.g. in cheese-making.

thermoduric Bacteria that are heat resistant but not thermophilic (*see* THERMOPHILES), i.e. they survive, but do not develop, at PASTEURISATION temperatures. Usually not pathogens but indicative of unsanitary conditions.

thermogenesis Increased heat production by the body, either to maintain body temperature (by either shivering or non-shivering thermogenesis) or in response to food intake (DIET-INDUCED THERMOGENESIS).

See also ADIPOSE TISSUE, BROWN; UNCOUPLING PROTEINS.

thermogenic drugs Compounds that stimulate body heat output, and thus of potential interest in 'slimming'.

thermogenin *See* UNCOUPLING PROTEINS.

thermography Technique for measuring and recording heat output by regions of the body, using a film or detector sensitive to infrared radiation.

thermopeeling A method of peeling tough-skinned fruits in which the fruit is rapidly passed through an electric furnace at about 900 °C, then sprayed with water.

thermophiles   Bacteria that prefer temperatures above 55 °C and can tolerate temperatures up to 75–80 °C. Extreme thermophiles can live in boiling water, and have been isolated from hot springs.

thiamin   *See* VITAMIN B₁.

thiaminases   Enzymes that cleave thiamin (VITAMIN B₁). Thiaminase I (EC 2.5.1.2) is found in freshwater fish, ferns and some bacteria; it catalyses an exchange reaction between the thiazole ring and a variety of bases. Thiaminase II (EC 3.5.99.2) occurs in a small number of micro-organisms; it catalyses hydrolysis of the methylene–thiazole bond, releasing TOXOPYRIMIDINE.

thiazoles   Derivatives of five-membered heterocyclic compounds containing both N and S in the ring (C_3H_3NS) that impart green, roasted or nutty flavours to foods. May be naturally present in foods or formed by the MAILLARD REACTION.

thiazolindinediones   Group of oral hypoglycaemic agents used in treatment of type II DIABETES mellitus; they increase insulin sensitivity of tissues, and activate the PPARγ receptor and repress the synthesis of 11β-hydroxysteroid dehydrogenase in adipocytes, so reducing the formation of cortisol in ADIPOSE TISSUE.

thiobarbituric acid reactive substances   *See* TBARS.

thiobarbituric acid (TBA) value   *See* TBA VALUE.

thiobendazole   Drug used to treat intestinal infestation with *STRONGYLOIDES* spp., and, as an antifungal agent, for surface treatment of bananas.

thiochrome   Fluorescent product of the oxidation of thiamin (VITAMIN B₁) in alkaline solution; the basis of an assay of the vitamin.

thioctic acid   *See* LIPOIC ACID.

thiophenes   Derivatives of five-membered heterocyclic compounds (C_4H_4S), sulphur analogues of FURANS that impart pungent or sweet flavours to foods.

thirst   *See* WATER BALANCE.

thixotropic   A fluid whose structure breaks down with continued SHEAR STRESS, so that VISCOSITY decreases, as is the case with most creams.

    See also DILATANT; PSEUDOPLASTIC; RHEOPECTIC.

thoracic duct   One of two main trunks of the lymphatic system; receives lymph from the legs and lower abdomen, and drains into the left innominate vein. The main point of entry of CHYLOMICRONS into the bloodstream.

threonine   An essential amino acid, abbr Thr (T), M_r 119.1, pK_a 2.09, 9.10, CODONS ACNu.

thrombin   Plasma protein involved in the COAGULATION of blood, formed in the circulation by partial proteolysis of PROTHROMBIN. *See also* VITAMIN K.

thromboembolism   Condition in which a blood clot formed in the circulation becomes detached and lodges elsewhere.

thrombokinase (thromboplastin)   An enzyme (clotting factor Xa, EC 3.4.21.6) liberated from damaged tissue and blood platelets; converts PROTHROMBIN to THROMBIN in the coagulation of blood.

thrombolysis   Dissolution of blood clots.

thromboplastin   *See* THROMBOKINASE.

thrombosis   Inappropriate formation of blood clots in blood vessels. Antagonists of VITAMIN K, including WARFARIN, are commonly used to reduce clotting in people at risk of thrombosis.

thrombus   Blood clot that remains stationary in a blood vessel. *See also* EMBOLISM.

thuricide   A microbial insecticide; a living culture of *Bacillus thuringiensis* which is harmless to human beings but kills insect pests. Used to treat certain foods and fodder crops to destroy pests such as corn earworm, flour moth, tomato fruit worm, cabbage looper, etc.

thyme   The aromatic leaves and flowering tops of *Thymus vulgaris* used as flavouring.

thymidine, thymine   A PYRIMIDINE; *see* NUCLEIC ACIDS.

thymonucleic acid   Obsolete name for DNA.

thymus   Chest (neck) sweetbread; a ductless gland in the chest, as distinct from gut sweetbread or PANCREAS.

Composition/100 g: water 74 g, 636 kJ (152 kcal), protein 14.8 g, fat 9.8 g (of which 52% saturated, 42% mono-unsaturated, 6% polyunsaturated), cholesterol 260 mg, carbohydrate 0 g, ash 1.4 g, Ca 8 mg, Fe 2.3 mg, Mg 21 mg, P 400 mg, K 420 mg, Na 75 mg, Zn 1.9 mg, Cu 0.1 mg, Se 34.3 µg, vitamin B_1 0.03 mg, B_2 0.25 mg, niacin 3.7 mg, B_6 0.07 mg, folate 13 µg, B_{12} 6 µg, pantothenate 1 mg, C 18 mg. A 100 g serving is a source of Fe, Zn, vitamin B_2, pantothenate, a good source of niacin, a rich source of P, Se, vitamin B_{12}, C.

thyrocalcitonin   *See* CALCITONIN.

thyroglobulin   The protein in the thyroid gland which is the precursor for the synthesis of the THYROID HORMONES as a result of iodination of tyrosine residues. The thyroid-stimulating hormone (THYROTROPIN) stimulates hydrolysis of thyroglobulin and secretion of the hormones into the bloodstream.

thyroid hormones   The thyroid is an endocrine gland situated in the neck, which takes up IODINE from the bloodstream and synthesises two HORMONES, tri-iodothyronine (T3) and thyroxine (T4, tetra-iodothyronine). The active hormone is T3; thyroxine is converted to T3 in tissues by the action of a SELENIUM-dependent de-iodinase (EC 3.8.1.4). T3 controls the BASAL METABOLIC RATE.

Enlargement of the thyroid gland is GOITRE; it may be associated with under- or overproduction of the thyroid hormones. Severe iodine deficiency in children leads to goitrous CRETINISM.

See also HYPOTHYROIDISM; IODINE, PROTEIN-BOUND; THYROTOXICOSIS; TRANSTHYRETIN.

thyroid-releasing hormone (TRH)   *See* THYROTROPIN.

thyrotoxicosis   Overactivity of the thyroid gland, leading to excessive secretion of THYROID HORMONES and resulting in increased BASAL METABOLIC RATE. Hyperthyroid subjects are lean and have tense nervous activity. May be due to overstimulation of the thyroid gland. Iodine-induced thyrotoxicosis affects mostly elderly people who have lived for a long time in iodine-deficient areas, have a long-standing goitre, and have then been given extra iodine. Also known as Jodbasedow, Basedow's disease and Graves' disease.

thyrotropin   Thyroid-stimulating hormone secreted by the anterior pituitary; stimulates hydrolysis of THYROGLOBULIN and secretion of the THYROID HORMONES.

thyroxine   One of the THYROID HORMONES.

thyroxine binding pre-albumin   *See* TRANSTHYRETIN.

TIA   *See* TRANSIENT ISCHAEMIC ATTACK.

TIBC   Total iron binding capacity, *see* TRANSFERRIN.

tierce   Obsolete measure of wine cask; one-third of a PIPE, i.e. about 160 L (35 Imperial gallons).

tiffin   Anglo-Indian name for a light midday meal.

tiger nut   Tuber of grass-like sedge, *Cyperus esculentus*; also earth or ground almond, chufa nut, rush nut, nut sedge, 5–20 mm long, usually sold partly dried.

tikka   Indian; marinated chicken (or other meat) threaded on skewers and grilled.

til   *See* SESAME.

tilsit   Originally Dutch/German, firm textured cheese.

timbale   Round fireproof china or tinned copper mould, used for moulding meat or fish mixtures; also the dishes cooked in the mould. For hot timbales the mould is lined with potato, pastry or pasta; for cold the lining is aspic.

time–temperature indicator   Chemical, enzymic or microbiological system that undergoes an irreversible change (e.g. a change in colour) that is temperature dependent, used in food packaging to indicate cumulative exposure to high temperatures. It gives a continuous, temperature-dependent response throughout the product's history, and can be used to indicate an 'average' tem-

474

perature during storage, which may be correlated with continuous, temperature-dependent loss of quality. Critical temperature indicators (CTI) show only exposure above (or below) a reference temperature, without the time-dependence.

See also PACKAGING, INTELLIGENT.

tin   A metal; a dietary essential for experimental animals, but so widely distributed in foods that human deficiency has not been reported, and its function, is not known. In the absence of oxygen, metallic tin is resistant to corrosion, and is widely used in tinned cans for food.

tipsy cake   Sponge cake soaked in wine and fruit juice, made into a trifle and reassembled into the original tall shape. The wine and fruit juice may cause the cake to topple sideways in drunken (tipsy) fashion.

tiramisu   Italian; dessert made from coffee-flavoured sponge or biscuit filled with sweetened cream cheese (MASCARPONE) and cream, doused with syrup.

tisane   French term for an infusion made from herbs, fruits or flowers (camomile, lime blossoms, fennel seeds, etc.), believed to have medicinal properties. Also known as herb or herbal tea. Medicinal or health claims are sometimes made, largely on traditional rather than scientific grounds.

titre   A measure of the amount of antibody in an antiserum, the extent to which the antiserum can be diluted and still retain the ability to cause agglutination of the antigen.

TK$_{ac}$ Transketolase activation coefficient, the result of the TRANSKETOLASE test for VITAMIN B$_1$ nutritional status, an ENZYME ACTIVATION ASSAY.

TMA   *See* TRIMETHYLAMINE.

TNF   *See* TUMOUR NECROSIS FACTOR.

toad skin   *See* PHRYNODERMA.

TOBEC   *See* TOTAL BODY ELECTRICAL CONDUCTIVITY.

tocol   *See* VITAMIN E.

tocopherol   *See* VITAMIN E.

tocopheronic acid   Water-soluble metabolite isolated from the urine of animals fed tocopherol; has VITAMIN E activity.

tocotrienol   *See* VITAMIN E.

toddy palm (kitul)   *Caryota urens*, the source of palm sugar and sago; the sap is fermented to yield an alcoholic beverage. Young leaves are edible.

toenail analysis   Measurement of various minerals (including ZINC) in toenails has been proposed as an index of status. Adsorption of minerals from sweat confounds the results.

toffee   A sweet made from butter or other fat, milk and sugar boiled at a higher temperature than caramels. Called candy or taffy USA (originally the UK name). Variants include butter-scotch and glessie (Scots). Toffee apples are apples coated with hardened syrup (called caramel apples in USA).

tofu Originally Japanese; soybean curd precipitated from the aqueous extract of the SOYA bean.

Composition/100 g: water 85 g, 293 kJ (70 kcal), protein 8.2 g, fat 4.2 g (of which 23% saturated, 31% mono-unsaturated, 46% polyunsaturated), carbohydrate 1.7 g (0.6 g sugars), fibre 0.9 g, ash 1 g, Ca 201 mg, Fe 1.6 mg, Mg 37 mg, P 121 mg, K 148 mg, Na 12 mg, Zn 0.8 mg, Cu 0.2 mg, Mn 0.6 mg, Se 9.9 µg, vitamin B_1 0.06 mg, B_2 0.06 mg, niacin 0.1 mg, B_6 0.07 mg, folate 19 µg, pantothenate 0.1 mg. An 80 g serving is a source of Cu, P, a good source of Ca, Mn.

tolazamide, tolbutamide *See* HYPOGLYCAEMIC AGENTS.

tomatillo Or ground tomato; husk-covered fruit of *Physalis ixocarpa*; resembles a small, green tomato.

Composition/100 g: water 92 g, 134 kJ (32 kcal), protein 1 g, fat 1 g, carbohydrate 5.8 g (3.9 g sugars), fibre 1.9 g, ash 0.6 g, Ca 7 mg, Fe 0.6 mg, Mg 20 mg, P 39 mg, K 268 mg, Na 1 mg, Zn 0.2 mg, Cu 0.1 mg, Mn 0.2 mg, Se 0.5 µg, vitamin A 6 µg RE (568 µg carotenoids), E 0.4 mg, K 9.8 mg, B_1 0.04 mg, B_2 0.04 mg, niacin 1.9 mg, B_6 0.06 mg, folate 7 µg, pantothenate 0.2 mg, C 12 mg.

tomato The fruit of *Lycopersicon esculentum*.

Composition/100 g: (edible portion 91%) water 94.5 g, 75 kJ (18 kcal), protein 0.9 g, fat 0.2 g, carbohydrate 3.9 g (2.6 g sugars), fibre 1.2 g, ash 0.5 g, Ca 10 mg, Fe 0.3 mg, Mg 11 mg, P 24 mg, K 237 mg, Na 5 mg, Zn 0.2 mg, Cu 0.1 mg, Mn 0.1 mg, vitamin A 42 µg RE (3246 µg carotenoids), E 0.5 mg, K 7.9 mg, B_1 0.04 mg, B_2 0.02 mg, niacin 0.6 mg, B_6 0.08 mg, folate 15 µg, pantothenate 0.1 mg, C 13 mg. An 85 g serving (1 medium) is a source of vitamin C.

tomato, English or tree *See* KIWANO; TAMARILLO.

tomme au raisin French soft cheese covered with grape pulp, skin and pips.

tomography Technique for visualisation of organs and generation of a three-dimensional image, by analysis of successive images produced using X-rays or ultrasound sharply focused at a given depth within the body.

See also CAT SCANNING; PET SCANNING.

tonic water (Indian tonic water) A sweetened carbonated beverage flavoured with quinine, commonly used as a mixer with GIN or VODKA. Originally invented by the British in India as a pleasant way of taking a daily dose of quinine to prevent malaria.

tonka bean Seed of the S. American tree *Dipteryx odorata* with a sweet pungent smell, used like VANILLA for flavouring.

ton refrigeration   A measure of refrigeration plant performance; the rate of cooling produced when a (US) ton (2000 lb) of ice melts during a 24 h period. 1 ton refrigeration is 3.54 kW.

toothfriendly sweets   Name given to sugar confectionery made with SUGAR ALCOHOLS and/or BULK SWEETENERS which are not fermented in the mouth and so do not damage teeth.

topepo   Hybrid between tomato and sweet pepper.

tophus (plural tophi)   Hard deposit of URIC ACID under skin, in cartilage or joints, as occurs in GOUT.

toppings   *See* WHEATFEED.

topside   Boneless joint of BEEF from the top of the hind leg.

Torrymeter   *See* FISH TESTER.

torte   Open tart or rich cake mixture baked in a pastry case, filled with fruit, nuts, chocolate, cream, etc.

tortilla   (1) Mexican; thin maize pancake. Traditionally prepared by soaking the grain in alkali and pressing it to form a dough, which is then baked on a griddle. Tortillas filled with meat, beans and spicy sauce are TACOS. TAMALES are similar, but made with fat.

   (2) In Spain, an omelette made by frying potatoes and onions with eggs; may be served hot or cold; also used for a variety of filled omelettes.

torulitine   *See* VITAMIN T.

Torulopsis   Genus of yeasts that cause spoilage in various foods.

total body electrical conductivity (TOBEC)   A method of measuring the proportion of fat in the body by the difference in the electrical conductivity between fat and lean tissue. Depends on the induction of a magnetic field by a high-frequency (5 MHz) alternating current in a solenoid above the body, and detection of the evoked field by a secondary coil.

   See also BIOELECTRICAL IMPEDANCE.

total iron binding capacity   *See* TRANSFERRIN.

total parenteral nutrition (TPN)   *See* PARENTERAL NUTRITION.

total polar materials   An index of degradation of oil used in frying by measuring free fatty acids due to lipolysis.

tourte (trete, treet)   Medieval English; whole wheat bread containing both flour and husk. Often used to form the TRENCHER.

toxic oil syndrome   *See* SPANISH TOXIC OIL SYNDROME.

Toxocara   Genus of intestinal parasitic nematode worms, especially in domestic cats and dogs; human beings can become infected by larvae from eggs in the faeces of pets (toxocariasis).

toxocariasis   *See* TOXOCARA.

toxoid   Chemically inactivated derivative of the toxin produced by a pathogenic organism; harmless, but stimulates the synthesis of antibodies; used in vaccines.

toxopyrimidine   Antimetabolite of vitamin B$_6$ released by the action of THIAMINASE II on thiamin.

TPM   *See* TOTAL POLAR MATERIALS.

TPN   Total PARENTERAL NUTRITION.

TQM   Total quality management.

trabecular bone   Thin bars of bony tissue in spongy BONE.

traceability   Of foods, the ability to relate each batch of product both back to the individual ingredients, their suppliers and the delivery dates, and forward to the packages supplied and their distribution to shops and final consumers.

trace elements   *See* MINERALS, TRACE; MINERALS, ULTRATRACE.

tracers   *See* ISOTOPES.

traife   Foods that do not conform to Jewish dietary laws; the opposite of KOSHER.

Trailblazer^{TM} FAT REPLACER made from protein.

trans-   *See* ISOMERS (3).

transaminase   Enzymes (EC 2.6.1.x, also known as aminotransferases) that catalyse the reaction of transamination; the transfer of the amino group from an amino acid donor onto a keto-acid (oxo-acid) acceptor, yielding the keto-acid (oxo-acid) carbon skeleton of the donor and the amino acid corresponding to the acceptor. The enzymes are pyridoxal phosphate (VITAMIN B$_6$)-dependent, and the activation of either alanine (EC 2.6.1.2) or aspartate (EC 2.6.1.1) aminotransferase apo-enzyme in red blood cells by pyridoxal phosphate added *in vitro* provides an index of vitamin B$_6$ status. An activation coefficient above 1.25 (alanine aminotransferase) or 1.8 (aspartate aminotransferase) is indicative of deficiency.

transcription   The process whereby one strand of the region of DNA containing the information for one or more proteins is copied to yield RNA, catalysed by RNA polymerase (EC 2.7.7.6).

transcription factors   The various proteins in addition to RNA polymerase that are required for TRANSCRIPTION of DNA to form mRNA.

   See also TRANSCRIPTOMICS; TRANSLATION.

transcriptomics   The GENOME of an organism is, subject to mutation, constant, and analysis of a genome does not tell us which genes are expressed in which tissue, at what stage in development, or in response to environmental, nutritional and hormonal stimuli. This is the science of transcriptomics – identification of which genes are active (i.e. being transcribed) in the organism, tissue or cell at different times and under different conditions.

   See also GENOMICS; METABOLOMICS; PROTEOMICS; TRANSCRIPTION.

transferrin   The main IRON transport protein in plasma. Fractional saturation of transferrin with iron provides a sensitive index of iron status, but transferrin synthesis is impaired in some chronic diseases, so fractional saturation may be inappropriately high. This also limits the usefulness of transferrin measurement as an index of protein–energy nutrition. Total iron binding capacity of plasma is the sum of free plus iron-containing transferrin.

transferrin receptor   A transmembrane protein for uptake of TRANSFERRIN (and hence IRON) into cells. The extracellular region is cleaved and enters the circulation, where it can be measured by immunoassay. In early iron deficiency there is induction of the transferrin receptor, and an elevated plasma concentration of the extracellular fragment provides a sensitive index of iron status.

transgenic   A micro-organism, plant or animal genetically engineered to contain a gene from another species. *See also* AGROBAC-TERIUM TUMEFACIENS; BIOLISTICS; GENETIC MODIFICATION; ELECTROPORATION.

transient ischaemic attack (TIA)   Temporary disruption of the blood supply to part of the brain, due to EMBOLISM, THROMBOSIS or a spasm of the arterial wall.

transit time   The time taken between ingestion of a food and its elimination in faeces, commonly measured by including radio-opaque plastic markers in the test food, followed by X-ray examination of faeces.

transketolase   Enzyme (EC 2.2.1.1) in the pentose phosphate pathway of GLUCOSE METABOLISM; requires thiamin diphosphate as cofactor, so activation of apo-transketolase in red blood cells by thiamin diphosphate added *in vitro* provides an index of vitamin B_1 status. An activation coefficient above 1.25 indicates deficiency.

translation   The process of synthesising protein on the RIBOSOME, by translating the information in mRNA into the amino acid sequence.
    See also TRANSCRIPTION.

transthyretin   THYROID HORMONE binding protein in plasma, formerly known as pre-albumin. Also forms a complex with the small plasma RETINOL BINDING PROTEIN to prevent loss of bound VITAMIN A by renal filtration. It has a HALF-LIFE of 2–3 days, and may provide an index of nutritional status because synthesis decreases rapidly in protein–energy malnutrition; however, synthesis is also affected by trauma and sepsis.

trassi (trassi udang)   Sumatran; cured salted SHRIMP paste; may contain potato peelings or rice bran. Cooked with chilli peppers to make the condiment sambal goring.

treacle First product of refining of MOLASSES from beet or sugar cane extract is black treacle, slightly less bitter; will not crystallise.

trehalose Mushroom sugar, or mycose, a DISACCHARIDE of glucose. Found in some fungi (*Amanita* spp.), MANNA and some insects.

trematode *See* FLUKE.

tremorgens A group of neurotoxins produced by various moulds (*Penicillium* spp., *Aspergillus* spp., *Claviceps* spp.) which cause sustained whole body tremors leading to convulsive seizures which may be fatal. Possible cause of endemic afflictions in human beings in Nigeria and India (alfatrem from *A. flavus*, penitrem from *Penicillium* spp.).

trencher Medieval English; thick slices of (normally stale) bread, party hollowed out and used as a plate, commonly given to the poor after the meal. Later replaced by a wooden trencher.

trepang *See* BÊCHE-DE-MER.

tretinoin Synthetic RETINOID used in treatment of acne.

TRH Thyroid-releasing hormone, *see* THYROTROPIN.

triacetin Glyceryl triacetate.

triacylglycerols Sometimes called triglycerides, simple fats or LIPIDS consisting of glycerol esterified to three FATTY ACIDS (chemically acyl groups). The major component of dietary and tissue fat. Also known as saponifiable fats, since on reaction with sodium hydroxide they yield glycerol and the sodium salts (or soaps) of the fatty acids.

trichinosis (trichinellosis, trichiniasis) Disease that can arise from eating undercooked pork or pork sausage meat; due to *Trichinella spiralis*, a worm that is a parasite in pork muscle; destroyed by heat and by freezing. Adult worms live in the small intestine; larvae bore through the intestinal wall and migrate around the body, causing fever, delirium and limb pain.

trichlorogalactosucrose *See* SUCRALOSE.

trichobezoar Or hairball. A mass of swallowed hair in the stomach.
    See also BEZOAR.

trichology Study of hair; *see* HAIR ANALYSIS.

Trichomonas Genus of parasitic flagellate protozoans. *T. hominis* infests the large intestine, *T. tenax* the mouth.

trichuriasis Infestation of the large intestine by the whipworm, *Trichuris trichiura*.

tricothecenes MYCOTOXINS produced by *Fusarium sporotrichioides* and *F. graminearum* growing on cereals.

trientine Chelating agent used to enhance the excretion of COPPER in WILSON'S DISEASE.

trifluoracetyl chloride   Used to prepare volatile trifluoracetyl derivatives of AMINO ACIDS for gas–liquid CHROMATOGRAPHY.

Trifyba^TM   Processed wheat bran from husk of *Testa triticum tricum* containing 80 g dietary fibre/100 g with reduced content of PHYTIC ACID.

triglycerides   *See* TRIACYLGLYCEROLS.

trigonelline   *N*-Methyl nicotinic acid, a urinary metabolite of NICOTINIC ACID. There is a relatively large amount in green COFFEE beans, much of which is demethylated during roasting, so coffee is a significant source of NIACIN.

tri-iodothyronine   One of the THYROID HORMONES.

trimethylamine $(CH_3)_3N$ Formed by bacterial reduction of trimethylamine oxide in marine FISH as they become stale; measured as an index of freshness. People with a genetic deficiency of trimethylamine oxidase (EC 1.14.13.8) excrete trimethylamine in sweat – the so-called fish odour syndrome.

tripe   Lining of the first three stomachs of RUMINANTS, usually calf or ox. Sold 'dressed', i.e. cleaned and treated with lime. According to the part of the stomach there are various kinds such as blanket, honeycomb, book, monk's hood and reed tripe. Contains a large amount of CONNECTIVE TISSUE which forms GELATINE on boiling.

Composition/100 g: water 84 g, 356 kJ (85 kcal), protein 12.1 g, fat 3.7 g (of which 43% saturated, 50% mono-unsaturated, 7% polyunsaturated), cholesterol 122 mg, carbohydrate 0 g, ash 0.6 g, Ca 69 mg, Fe 0.6 mg, Mg 13 mg, P 64 mg, K 67 mg, Na 97 mg, Zn 1.4 mg, Cu 0.1 mg, Mn 0.1 mg, Se 12.5 µg, vitamin E 0.1 mg, B_2 0.06 mg, niacin 0.9 mg, B_6 0.01 mg, folate 5 µg, B_{12} 1.4 µg, pantothenate 0.2 mg.

triticale   Polyploid hybrid of WHEAT (*Triticum* spp.) and RYE (*Secale* spp.) which combines the winter hardiness of the rye with the special baking properties of wheat.

Composition/100 g: water 10.5 g, 1406 kJ (336 kcal), protein 13.1 g, fat 2.1 g (of which 27% saturated, 13% mono-unsaturated, 60% polyunsaturated), carbohydrate 72.1 g, ash 2.2 g, Ca 37 mg, Fe 2.6 mg, Mg 130 mg, P 358 mg, K 332 mg, Na 5 mg, Zn 3.5 mg, Cu 0.5 mg, Mn 3.2 mg, vitamin E 0.9 mg, B_1 0.42 mg, B_2 0.13 mg, niacin 1.4 mg, B_6 0.14 mg, folate 73 µg, pantothenate 1.3 mg.

tRNA (transfer RNA)   The family of small RNA species that have both an anticodon region which binds to the CODON on mRNA on the RIBOSOME and also a specific amino acid binding site, so that the appropriate amino acid is brought to the ribosome for protein synthesis (*see* TRANSLATION).

Trolox^TM   A water-soluble VITAMIN E analogue, 6-hydroxy-2,5,7,8-tetramethyl-chroman-2-carboxylic acid.

tropical oils Suggested term (USA) for vegetable oils that contain saturated, but little polyunsaturated, fatty acids, such as COCONUT and PALM oils.

trout Freshwater oily FISH, brown trout is *Salmo trutta*, rainbow trout is *S. gairdneri*.

Composition/100 g: water 71 g, 620 kJ (148 kcal), protein 20.8 g, fat 6.6 g (of which 19% saturated, 56% mono-unsaturated, 25% polyunsaturated), cholesterol 58 mg, carbohydrate 0 g, ash 1.2 g, Ca 43 mg, Fe 1.5 mg, Mg 22 mg, P 245 mg, K 361 mg, Na 52 mg, Zn 0.7 mg, Cu 0.2 mg, Mn 0.9 mg, Se 12.6 µg, I 13 µg, vitamin A 17 µg retinol, E 0.2 mg, K 0.1 mg, B_1 0.35 mg, B_2 0.33 mg, niacin 4.5 mg, B_6 0.2 mg, folate 13 µg, B_{12} 7.8 µg, pantothenate 1.9 mg, C 1 mg. A 100 g serving is a source of Cu, Se, a good source of vitamin B_1, B_2, niacin, a rich source of Mn, P, vitamin B_{12}, pantothenate.

trub *See* HOT BREAK.

truffles (1) Edible fungi (*see* MUSHROOMS) growing underground, associated with roots of oak trees; very highly prized for their aroma and flavour. Most highly prized is French, black or Perigord truffle, *Tuber melanosporum*, added to pâté de foie gras. Others include: white Piedmontese truffle, *T. magnatum*; summer truffle, *T. aestivum*; and violet truffle, *T. brumale*.

(2) Chocolate truffles; mixture of chocolate, sugar, cream and often rum, covered with chocolate strands or cocoa powder.

Trusoy^{TM} Heat-treated full-fat SOYA FLOUR.

trypsin A proteolytic enzyme (EC 3.4.21.4) in pancreatic juice, an ENDOPEPTIDASE. Active at pH 8–11. Secreted as the inactive precursor, trypsinogen, which is activated by ENTEROPEPTIDASE.

trypsin inhibitors Low molecular weight proteins in raw SOYA beans and other LEGUMES that inhibit TRYPSIN and thus impair the digestion of proteins. Inactivated by heat, but the nutritional quality of some animal feeds containing trypsin inhibitors is not improved by heating.

trypsinogen *See* TRYPSIN.

tryptophan An essential amino acid, abbr Trp (W), M_r 204.2, pK_a 2.43, 9.44, codon UGG. In addition to its role in protein synthesis, it is the precursor of the neurotransmitter 5-HYDROXYTRYPTAMINE (serotonin) and of NIACIN. Average intakes of tryptophan are more than adequate to meet niacin requirements without the need for any preformed niacin in the diet.

Destroyed by acid, and therefore not measured when proteins are hydrolysed by acid before analysis; determination of tryptophan requires alkaline or enzymic hydrolysis of the protein.

tryptophan load test For assessment of VITAMIN B_6 status; measurement of urinary excretion of xanthurenic and kynurenic acids after a test dose of 2 or 5 g of tryptophan. The enzyme kynureninase (EC 3.7.1.3) is pyridoxal phosphate-dependent, and especially sensitive to deficiency.

Tshugaeff reaction   Colorimetric reaction for CHOLESTEROL; the development of a cherry red colour on reaction with zinc chloride and acetyl chloride.

TSP   Textured SOYA protein, prepared by extrusion through fine pores to give a fibrous, meat-like, texture to the final product.

TTI   *See* TIME–TEMPERATURE INDICATOR.

TTT   Time–temperature tolerance.

tubby mouse   Genetically OBESE mouse that develops INSULIN resistance; it is also deaf and blind owing to APOPTOSIS in sensory neurons in the retina and hair cells in the cochlear organ of Corti. The role of the *tub* gene product in the development of obesity is not known.

tube feeding   *See* ENTERAL NUTRITION.

tuber   Botanical term for underground storage organ of some plants, e.g. potato, Jerusalem artichoke, sweet potato, yam.

tuberin   The major protein of POTATO, a globulin.

tumour necrosis factor   Two CYTOKINES produced by monocytes and macrophages (cachectin, TNF-α), and lymphocytes (lymphotoxin, TNF-β); cytotoxic to a variety of cancer cells, but also act on other cells. TNF action is responsible for much of the hypermetabolism seen in CACHEXIA. TNF-α, secreted by macrophages in ADIPOSE TISSUE stimulates pre-ADIPOCYTES and endothelial cells to secrete macrophage attractants, and impairs INSULIN receptor signalling.

tun   Obsolete measure; large cask holding 216 Imperial gallons (972 L) of ale; 252 gallons (1134 L) of wine.

tuna (tunny)   Species of *Thunnus* and *Neothunnus*, oily FISH. (Tuna is also an alternative name for PRICKLY PEAR.)

Composition/100 g: water 68 g, 603 kJ (144 kcal), protein 23.3 g, fat 4.9 g (of which 30% saturated, 37% mono-unsaturated, 33% polyunsaturated), cholesterol 38 mg, carbohydrate 0 g, ash 1.2 g, Ca 8 mg, Fe 1 mg, Mg 50 mg, P 254 mg, K 252 mg, Na 39 mg, Zn 0.6 mg, Cu 0.1 mg, Se 36.5 µg, I 30 µg, vitamin A 655 µg retinol, E 1 mg, B_1 0.24 mg, B_2 0.25 mg, niacin 8.7 mg, B_6 0.46 mg, folate 2 µg, B_{12} 9.4 µg, pantothenate 1.1 mg. A 100 g serving is a source of Mg, vitamin B_1, B_2, pantothenate, a good source of I, vitamin B_6, a rich source of P, Se, vitamin A, niacin, B_{12}.

tuo zaafi   African; sorghum or millet gruel left overnight to undergo a lactic acid fermentation.

Tupperware^{TM} Plastic bowls and canisters with seal that permits them to be stored on the side or upside down, introduced by American chemist Earl Tupper in 1945.

turanose   A DISACCHARIDE, α-1,3-glucosyl-fructose.

turbidimetry Measurement of the turbidity (or optical density) of a culture as an index of growth in microbiological assays.

turbidity *See* TYNDALL EFFECT.

turbot A FLATFISH, *Psetta maxima*.

Composition/100g: water 77g, 398kJ (95kcal), protein 16g, fat 3g (of which 35% saturated, 26% mono-unsaturated, 39% polyunsaturated), cholesterol 48mg, carbohydrate 0g, ash 2.1g, Ca 18mg, Fe 0.4mg, Mg 51mg, P 129mg, K 238mg, Na 150mg, Zn 0.2mg, Se 36.5µg, vitamin A 11µg retinol, B_1 0.07mg, B_2 0.08mg, niacin 2.2mg, B_6 0.21mg, folate 8µg, B_{12} 2.2µg, pantothenate 0.6mg, C 2mg. A 100g serving is a source of Mg, P, niacin, a rich source of Se, vitamin B_{12}.

turkey A poultry bird, *Meleagris gallopavo*.

Dark meat, composition/100g: (edible portion 64%) water 75g, 523kJ (125kcal), protein 20.1g, fat 4.4g (of which 39% saturated, 26% mono-unsaturated, 34% polyunsaturated), cholesterol 69mg, carbohydrate 0g, ash 0.9g, Ca 17mg, Fe 1.8mg, Mg 22mg, P 184mg, K 286mg, Na 77mg, Zn 3.2mg, Cu 0.1mg, Se 28.6µg, I 8µg, vitamin B_1 0.08mg, B_2 0.22mg, niacin 3.1mg, B_6 0.36mg, folate 11µg, B_{12} 0.4µg, pantothenate 1.2mg. A 100g serving is a source of Fe, vitamin B_2, niacin, B_6, a good source of P, Zn, pantothenate, a rich source of Se, vitamin B_{12}.

Light meat, composition/100g: (edible portion 71%) water 74g, 481kJ (115kcal), protein 23.6g, fat 1.6g (of which 42% saturated, 25% mono-unsaturated, 33% polyunsaturated), cholesterol 60mg, carbohydrate 0g, ash 1g, Ca 12mg, Fe 1.2mg, Mg 27mg, P 204mg, K 305mg, Na 63mg, Zn 1.6mg, Cu 0.1mg, Se 24.4µg, I 8µg, vitamin B_1 0.06mg, B_2 0.12mg, niacin 5.8mg, B_6 0.56mg, folate 8µg, B_{12} 0.4µg, pantothenate 0.7mg. A 100g serving is a source of pantothenate, a good source of P, vitamin B_6, a rich source of Se, niacin, vitamin B_{12}.

turkey X disease *See* AFLATOXINS.

Turkish delight Confectionery made from gelatine and concentrated grape juice (PEKMEZ), flavoured with rose water. Also sometimes made with marshmallow (Turkish *rahat lokum*).

Turkish taffy American name for TURKISH DELIGHT.

turmeric Dried rhizome of *Curcuma longa* (ginger family), grown in India and S Asia. Deep yellow and used both as condiment and food colour; used in curry powder and in prepared mustard. Its pigment is used as a dye under the name curcumin or Indian saffron (E-100).

turnip Root of *Brassica campestris* eaten as a cooked vegetable.

Composition/100g: (edible portion 81%) water 92g, 117kJ (28kcal), protein 0.9g, fat 0.1g, carbohydrate 6.4g (3.8g sugars), fibre 1.8g, ash 0.7g, Ca 30mg, Fe 0.3mg, Mg 11mg, P 27mg, K

191 mg, Na 67 mg, Zn 0.3 mg, Cu 0.1 mg, Mn 0.1 mg, Se 0.7 µg, vitamin K 0.1 mg, B_1 0.04 mg, B_2 0.03 mg, niacin 0.4 mg, B_6 0.09 mg, folate 15 µg, pantothenate 0.2 mg, C 21 mg. A 60 g serving is a good source of vitamin C.

Turnip leaves (greens) are also eaten; composition/100 g: (edible portion 70%) water 90 g, 134 kJ (32 kcal), protein 1.5 g, fat 0.3 g, carbohydrate 7.1 g (0.8 g sugars), fibre 3.2 g, ash 1.4 g, Ca 190 mg, Fe 1.1 mg, Mg 31 mg, P 42 mg, K 296 mg, Na 40 mg, Zn 0.2 mg, Cu 0.3 mg, Mn 0.5 mg, Se 1.2 µg, vitamin E 2.9 mg, K 251 mg, B_1 0.07 mg, B_2 0.1 mg, niacin 0.6 mg, B_6 0.26 mg, folate 194 µg, pantothenate 0.4 mg, C 60 mg. A 95 g serving is a source of vitamin B_6, a good source of Ca, Cu, Mn, vitamin E, a rich source of folate, vitamin C.

See also PARSLEY, HAMBURG; SWEDE.

turtle   Marine reptile; the main species for food is the green turtle, *Chelonia mydas*, so-called because of the greenish tinge of its fat. Farmed to a small extent, but mainly caught in the wild.

Composition/100 g: water 79 g, 373 kJ (89 kcal), protein 19.8 g, fat 0.5 g, cholesterol 50 mg, carbohydrate 0 g, ash 1.2 g, Ca 118 mg, Fe 1.4 mg, Mg 20 mg, P 180 mg, K 230 mg, Na 68 mg, Zn 1 mg, Cu 0.3 mg, Se 16.8 µg, vitamin A 30 µg retinol, E 0.5 mg, K 0.1 mg, B_1 0.12 mg, B_2 0.15 mg, niacin 1.1 mg, B_6 0.12 mg, folate 15 µg, B_{12} 1 µg.

Tuscorora rice   *See* RICE, WILD.

Tuxford's index   Formula for assessing height relative to weight in children. The index is >1 for heavier than average children and <1 for lighter than average. For boys, TI = [weight (lb)/height (in)] – [336 × age (months)/270]; for girls, TI = [weight (lb)/height (in)] – (308 × age (months)/235].

TVB   Total volatile bases, measured as an index of freshness of FISH.

See also TRIMETHYLAMINE.

TVP   Textured vegetable protein.

Twaddell   Scale for measurement of density of solutions; density = 1 + (°Twaddell/200). 1% salt = 1.4° Twaddell, density = 1.007; 2% salt = 2.8° Twaddell, density = 1.014; 4% salt = 5.6° Twaddell, density = 1.028; 10% salt = 14.6° Twaddell, density = 1.073; 20% salt = 30.2° Twaddell, density = 1.151.

Tweens™   Non-ionic surface active agents derived from SPANS by adding polyoxyethylene chains to the non-esterified hydroxyl groups, so making them water-soluble. Polysorbate 40 is a mixture of polyoxyethylene esters of oleic esters of sorbitol anhydrides used in medicinal products as an emulsifying agent.

TX numbers   Systematic classification of toxins produced by food poisoning bacteria according to: type of infection: 1 = intoxication, 2 = toxin produced in host without adherence, 3 = toxin produced in host with adherence to cells, 4 = toxin produced by invasive bacteria, 5 = toxin produced by bacteria causing systemic infection; type of toxin: 1 = enterotoxin, 2 = neurotoxin, 3 = nonprotein toxin; target or mechanism of action; individual toxin number. Shown as TX x.x.x.x.

Tyndall effect Dispersion of light by a colloidal suspension (*see* COLLOID), commonly determined as turbidity by measuring the light emitted at 90° to the direction of incident light.

typhoid Gastrointestinal infection caused by *Salmonella typhi*, transmitted by food or water contaminated by faeces of patients or asymptomatic carriers. Paratyphoid is due to *S. paratyphi*.

tyramine The AMINE formed by decarboxylation of the AMINO ACID TYROSINE; chemically *p*-hydroxyphenylethylamine.

tyrosinase *See* PHENOL OXIDASES.

tyrosine A non-essential AMINO ACID, abbr Tyr (Y), M_r 181.2, pK_a 2.43, 9.11, 10.13 (—OH), CODONS UAPy. Can be formed from the essential amino acid PHENYLALANINE, hence it has some sparing action on phenylalanine. In addition to its role in proteins, tyrosine is the precursor for the synthesis of melanin (the black and brown pigment of skin and hair), and for ADRENALINE and NORADRENALINE.

tyrosinosis GENETIC DISEASE due to lack of *p*-hydroxyphenylpyruvate oxidase (EC 1.13.11.27), affecting the metabolism of TYROSINE and leading to excretion of *p*-hydroxyphenylpyruvate in the urine. Treatment is by restriction of dietary intake of PHENYLALANINE and tyrosine.

tzatziki Greek; grated cucumber in yogurt, flavoured with garlic, olive oil and vinegar.

U

ubichromenol Cyclised derivatives of UBIQUINONES.

ubiquinones Coenzymes in the respiratory (electron transport) chain in mitochondria, also known as coenzyme Q or mitoquinones; widely distributed in nature. Chemically, derivatives of benzoquinone with isoprene side chains. There is no evidence that they are dietary essentials; they may have ANTIOXIDANT activity.

ucuhuba butter A yellow solid fat obtained from ucuhuba nuts, the fruit of *Myristica surinamensis*. 90% saturated, 7% mono-unsaturated, 3% polyunsaturated, vitamin E 0.6 mg/100 mL.

udon Japanese; fine transparent noodles made from wheat.

UFA Unesterified fatty acids, *see* FATTY ACIDS, NON-ESTERIFIED.

ugli   CITRUS fruit; cross between grapefruit and tangerine, also called tangelo (USA); first produced in Jamaica in 1930.

UHT   *See* ULTRA-HIGH-TEMPERATURE STERILISATION.

UL   Tolerable upper intake level of a nutrient; maximum intake (from supplements and enriched foods) that is unlikely to pose a risk of adverse effects on health.

ulcer   A crater-like lesion of the skin or a mucous membrane resulting from tissue death associated with inflammatory disease, infection or cancer. Peptic ulcers affect regions of the GASTROINTESTINAL TRACT exposed to gastric juices containing acid and PEPSIN: gastric ulcer in the stomach and duodenal ulcer in the duodenum.

Treatment was formerly conservative, with a bland diet, followed if necessary by surgery. Now treated by inhibition of gastric acid secretion using HISTAMINE RECEPTOR ANTAGONISTS or inhibitors of the PROTON PUMP. May be caused or exacerbated by infection with *Helicobacter pylori*.

ulcerative colitis   *See* COLITIS.

ullage   Air space left in cask or bottle after some liquid has been removed.

ultracentrifuge   *See* CENTRIFUGE.

ultrafiltration   Procedure for removal of low molecular weight compounds from plasma, protein solutions, etc., using a SEMIPERMEABLE MEMBRANE and either hydrostatic pressure or centrifugation.

ultra-high-temperature sterilisation (UHT)   Sterilisation at higher temperatures and for shorter times, than HIGH-TEMPERATURE SHORT-TIME sterilisation.

ultrasound   Sound above the normal range of human hearing, commonly above 20 kHz.

ultraviolet (UV) irradiation   Light of wavelength below the visible range. Wavelength for maximal germicidal action is 260 nm; poor penetrating power and of value only for surface sterilisation or sterilising air and water. Also used for tenderising and ageing of meat, curing cheese, and prevention of mould growth on the surface of bakery products. Ultraviolet from sunlight is responsible for skin tanning, and the formation of VITAMIN D from 7-dehydrocholesterol in the skin.

umami   Name given to the special taste of MONOSODIUM GLUTAMATE, some other amino acids, protein and the RIBONUCLEOTIDES (inosinate and guanylate). The Japanese name for a savoury flavour, now considered one of the five basic senses of TASTE.

umbles   Edible entrails of any animal (especially deer) which used to be made into pie, umble pie or humble pie.

uncoupling proteins   Proteins in MITOCHONDRIA that act to uncouple the processes of electron transport and oxidative phosphorylation, so permitting more or less uncontrolled oxidation of metabolic fuels, with production of heat. An important part of maintenance of body temperature by non-shivering thermogenesis, and maintenance of ENERGY BALANCE; they are stimulated by LEPTIN.

UCP-1 (thermogenin) is the best studied. It occurs in brown adipose tissue (*see* ADIPOSE TISSUE, BROWN), and is activated by free fatty acids produced in response to β-adrenergic stimulation. UCP-2 occurs in a variety of tissues, including skeletal muscle and lung; UCP-3 occurs only in skeletal muscle.

uncrystallisable syrup *See* SYRUP.

unesterified fatty acids (UFA) *See* FATTY ACIDS, NON-ESTERIFIED.

UNICEF United Nations Children's fund; web site http://www.unicef.org/.

universal product codes (UPC) Standard multidigit numbers that represent product, size, manufacturer and nature of contents, on food and other labels as machine-readable bar codes.

unsaponifiable *See* NON-SAPONIFIED.

unsaturated fatty acids *See* FATTY ACIDS.

UNU United Nations University; web site http://www.unu.edu/.

UPC *See* UNIVERSAL PRODUCT CODES.

uperisation A method of sterilising milk by injecting steam under pressure to raise the temperature to 150 °C. The added water is evaporated off.

uracil A PYRIMIDINE; *see* NUCLEIC ACIDS.

urataemia High blood concentration of URIC ACID and its salts, as in GOUT.

uraturia Urinary excretion of high concentrations of URIC ACID and its salts.

urd bean *See* GRAMS, INDIAN.

urea $CO(NH_2)_2$, the end-product of nitrogen metabolism in most mammals, excreted in the urine. Synthesised in the liver from ammonia (arising from the deamination of amino acids) and the AMINO ACID ASPARTIC ACID. It is the major nitrogenous compound in urine, and the major component of the non-protein nitrogen in blood plasma.

urease Intestinal bacterial enzyme (EC 3.5.1.5) that hydrolyses UREA to ammonia and carbon dioxide. Important in the entero-hepatic cycling of urea. Also found in some beans.

urethane Ethyl carbamate, used as intermediate in organic syntheses, as a solubiliser and as the precursor for polyurethane foam. Found in small amounts in liqueurs made from stone fruits, wines and some distilled spirits where it is formed by reaction between alcohol and nitrogenous compounds; cause for concern since it is genotoxic, and hence a potential CARCINOGEN.

uric acid   The end-product of PURINE metabolism in human beings and other apes; most other mammals have the enzyme uricase (EC 1.7.3.3), which oxidises uric acid to allantoin, which is more soluble in water. GOUT is the result of excessive formation of uric acid, and/or impaired excretion; it is only slightly soluble in water, and in excess it crystallises in joints, as gouty nodules (tophi) under the skin and sometimes in the kidney.

urobilinogen   Pigment in urine derived from the bile pigments, which, in turn, are formed from haemoglobin. When urine is left to stand, the urobilinogen is oxidised in air to urobilin.

urogastrone   Name given to a peptide found in urine that inhibits gastric secretion, (nearly) identical to epidermal growth factor.

urwaga   *See* ORUBISI.

USDA   US Department of Agriculture, created as an independent department in 1862; web site http://www.usda.gov/.

USRDA   REFERENCE INTAKES used for nutritional labelling of foods in the USA before the introduction of DAILY VALUES.

uszka   Polish; type of ravioli, egg-flour dough stuffed with mushrooms.

UV   *See* ULTRAVIOLET.

V

vacherin   (1) Circular cakes of meringue and cream.

(2) French mild cheeses made from cow's milk; traditionally moulded in flat circles and wrapped in a border of bark.

vac-ice process   Alternative name for FREEZE DRYING.

vacreation   DEODORISATION of cream by steam distillation under reduced pressure; developed in New Zealand.

vacuum contact drying   Or vacuum contact plate process, a method of drying food in a vacuum oven in which the material is heated by hot plates both above and below. As the material shrinks due to water loss, continuous contact is maintained by closing the plates; heats the food more effectively than a simple vacuum oven.

vada   Indian; spiced, deep fried balls of legume flour that has been left overnight to undergo a lactic acid bacterial fermentation, together with *Leuconostoc mesenteroides*, which produces carbon dioxide as a leavening agent.

vagotomy   Surgical cutting of part of the vagus (10th cranial) nerve, usually to reduce secretion of acid and PEPSIN by the gastric mucosa.

valerian   Extracts and the essential oil of the herbaceous perennial *Valeriana officinalis* are used as flavouring in many foods.

The root has traditionally been used as a sedative and tranquilliser, with evidence of efficacy.

valgus Any deformity that displaces the hand or foot away from the mid-line of the body; e.g. genu valgus is knock knees, as seen in RICKETS.

See also VARUS.

validity Of an assay, the extent to which a method measures what it purports to measure.

See also ACCURACY; PRECISION; SENSITIVITY; SPECIFICITY.

valine An essential amino acid, abbr Val (V), M_r 117.1, pK_a 2.29, 9.74, CODONS GUNu; rarely, if ever, limiting in foods.

valzin, valzol *See* DULCIN.

vanadium A MINERAL known to be essential to experimental animals, although sufficiently widespread for human dietary deficiency to be unknown. Its precise function is unknown, although it acts as an activator of a number of enzymes.

vanaspati Indian; purified hydrogenated vegetable oil; similar to MARGARINE and usually fortified with vitamins A and D. Also used to prepare GHEE (vanaspati ghee).

vanilla Extract of the vanilla bean, fruit of the tropical orchid *Aracus* (or *Vanilla*) *aromaticus* and related species. Discovered in Mexico in 1571 and could not be grown elsewhere, because pollination could be effected only by a small Mexican bee, until artificial pollination was introduced in 1820. Main growing regions now Madagascar and Tahiti.

The major flavouring principle is vanillin (chemically methyl protocatechuic aldehyde), but other substances present aid the flavour. Ethyl vanillin is a synthetic substance which does not occur in the vanilla bean; 3.5 times as strong in flavour, and more stable to store than vanillin, but does not have the true flavour.

vanillin *See* VANILLA.

VaporPrint™ **imaging** A graphical representation of the flavour profile obtained using a ZNOSE™ 'electronic nose'.

variety meat American name for OFFAL.

varus Any deformity that displaces the hand or foot towards the mid-line of the body; e.g. genu varus is bow legs, as seen in RICKETS.

See also VALGUS.

vasoactive intestinal peptide (VIP) Protein secreted by the PANCREAS; over-secretion can cause severe DIARRHOEA.

vasoconstriction Constriction of the blood vessels; the reverse of VASODILATATION.

vasodilatation (vasodilation) Dilation of the blood vessels; the reverse of VASOCONSTRICTION. Caused by a rise in body temperature; serves to lose heat from the body.

vasopressin   Antidiuretic hormone secreted by the pituitary; acts to increase resorption of water in the kidneys and to constrict blood vessels.

VCD   *See* VACUUM CONTACT DRYING.

VDP   Volatile decomposition products.

veal   Meat of young calf (*Bos taurus*) 2½–3 months old.

Composition/100 g: water 76 g, 456 kJ (109 kcal), protein 20.3 g, fat 2.5 g (of which 42% saturated, 42% mono-unsaturated, 16% polyunsaturated), cholesterol 84 mg, carbohydrate 0 g, ash 1.1 g, Ca 17 mg, Fe 0.9 mg, Mg 25 mg, P 213 mg, K 331 mg, Na 83 mg, Zn 3.5 mg, Cu 0.1 mg, Se 8.8 µg, vitamin E 0.3 mg, B_1 0.09 mg, B_2 0.29 mg, niacin 7.4 mg, B_6 0.45 mg, folate 13 µg, B_{12} 1.5 µg, pantothenate 1.3 mg. A 100 g serving is a source of Se, vitamin B_2, a good source of P, Zn, vitamin B_6, pantothenate, a rich source of niacin, vitamin B_{12}.

vegans   Those who consume no foods of animal origin. *See* VEGETARIANS.

Vegemite™   Australian; YEAST EXTRACT.

vegetable   *See* FRUIT.

vegetable butters   *See* COCOA BUTTER EQUIVALENTS; COCOA BUTTER SUBSTITUTES.

vegetable oyster   *See* SALSIFY.

vegetable pepsin   *See* PAPAIN.

vegetable protein products   General term to include textured SOYA and other bean products, often made to simulate meat (*see* TEXTURED VEGETABLE PROTEIN). The basic material is termed flour when the protein content is not less than 50%; concentrate, not less than 65%; isolate, not less than 90% protein.

vegetable spaghetti   *See* SPAGHETTI SQUASH.

vegetarians   Those who do not eat meat or fish, either for ethical/religious reasons or because they believe that a meat-free diet confers health benefits. Apart from a risk of VITAMIN B_{12} deficiency, there are no adverse effects of a wholly meat-free diet, although vegetarian women are more at risk of IRON deficiency than those who eat meat. Vitamin B_{12} is found only in meat and meat products, but supplements prepared by bacterial fermentation (and hence ethically acceptable to the strictest of vegetarians) are available.

The strictest vegetarians are vegans, who consume no products of animal origin at all. Those who consume milk and milk products are termed lacto-vegetarians; those who also eat eggs, ovolacto-vegetarians. Some vegetarians (pescetarians) will eat fish, but not meat; demi-vegetarians eat little or no meat, or eat poultry but not red meat.

veitchberry   Variety of LOGANBERRY.

veltol   *See* MALTOL.

venison   Meat of deer (*Odocoileus* spp.); traditionally GAME, but now mainly farmed.

Composition/100g: water 74g, 502kJ (120kcal), protein 23g, fat 2.4g (of which 43% saturated, 33% mono-unsaturated, 24% polyunsaturated), cholesterol 85mg, carbohydrate 0g, ash 1.2g, Ca 5mg, Fe 3.4mg, Mg 23mg, P 202mg, K 318mg, Na 51mg, Zn 2.1mg, Cu 0.3mg, Se 9.7µg, vitamin E 0.2mg, K 1.1mg, B_1 0.22mg, B_2 0.48mg, niacin 6.4mg, B_6 0.37mg, folate 4µg, B_{12} 6.3µg, A 100g serving is a source of Se, Zn, vitamin B_1, B_6, a good source of Cu, Fe, P, a rich source of vitamin B_2, niacin, B_{12}.

venting   Removal of air from a RETORT or RETORT POUCH before heating.

verbascose   A non-digestible tetrasaccharide, galactosyl-galactosyl-glucosyl-fructose, found in LEGUMES; fermented by intestinal bacteria and causes flatulence.

verbena   A lemon flavoured HERB, the leaves of *Lippia citroidora*.

verdoflavin   Name given to a substance isolated from grass, later shown to be riboflavin (VITAMIN B_2).

verjuice   Literally green juice; sour juice of crab apples (and sometimes unripe grapes) formerly used in cooking meat, fish and game dishes. Now normally replaced by lemon juice.

vermicelli   *See* PASTA.

vermicide   Any drug used to kill or expel intestinal parasitic worms.

vermouth   Fortified wine (about 16% alcohol by volume) flavoured with herbs and QUININE. French vermouth is dry and colourless; Italian may be red or white and is sweet. Drunk as an apéritif, either with soda or with gin or vodka (when called a martini). Name originally derived from German *Wermut* for wormwood, a toxic ingredient that was included in early vermouths (as in ABSINTHE).

Sweet or Italian vermouth, 15–17% alcohol (by volume), 12–20% sugar (by weight). Dry or French type 18–20% alcohol, 3–5% sugar.

Versene™   Ethylenediamine tetra-acetic acid, *see* EDTA.

Verv™   Calcium stearyl-2-lactate, used to reduce baking variations in flour. It produces a more extensible dough, more easily machined, and gives a loaf with better keeping properties and more uniform structure.

vervain   Herb (*Verbena officianilis*) used to make herb tea.

very low-density lipoproteins (VLDL)   *See* LIPOPROTEINS, PLASMA.

vetch   Old term applied generally to LEGUMES; originally *Vicia* spp., also called tares.

ve-tsin   *See* MONOSODIUM GLUTAMATE.

Vibrio cholerae   The causative agent of cholera, bacterium transmitted especially through water; forms an ENTEROTOXIN after adhering to epithelial cells in gut. Infective dose 10^8 organisms, onset 2–5 days, duration 4–6 days, TX 3.1.2.2.

vichyssoise   Leek and potato cream soup, served cold.

vicilin   Globulin protein in pea and lentil.

vicine   One of the toxins in broad beans, responsible for acute haemolytic anaemia or FAVISM.

victory bread   American; recipe for bread containing SOYA flour to spare wheat, in a circular published by the US Secretary of Agriculture in 1918.

Vienna flour   Specially fine flour used to make strudel PASTRY, Vienna bread and cakes.

Viennese coffee   Ground coffee containing dried figs.

viili   Finnish; YOGURT made using *Streptococcus cremoris* as the main organism.

villi, intestinal   Small, finger-like processes covering the surface of the small intestine in large numbers (20–40/mm^2), projecting some 0.5–1 mm into the lumen. They provide a surface area of about 300 m^2 for the absorption of nutrients from the small intestine.

See also GASTROINTESTINAL TRACT.

vinasses   The residual liquors from sugar beet MOLASSES; contain appreciable quantities of BETAINE.

vinegar   A solution of acetic acid (not less than 4%); the product of two fermentations, first with yeast to convert sugars into alcohol; this liquor, called gyle (6–9% alcohol), is then fermented with *Acetobacter* spp. to form acetic acid. In most countries vinegar is made from grape juice (wine vinegar, may be from red, white or rosé wine).

vinegar, balsamic   Made from grape juice that has been concentrated over a low flame and fermented slowly in a series of wooden barrels; traditionally made only around Modena, Italy.

vinegar, cider   Made from apple juice, and known simply as vinegar in the USA.

vinegar, malt   Made from malted barley and may be distilled to a colourless liquid with the same acetic acid content but a more mellow flavour.

vinegar, non-brewed (or non-brewed condiment)   A solution of acetic acid, 4–8%, coloured with caramel.

vinegar, rice   Made from SAKÉ.

vine leaves   Leaves of the GRAPE vine, *Vitis vinifera*, used in Mediterranean cuisine.

Composition/100 g: (edible portion 95%) water 73 g, 389 kJ (93 kcal), protein 5.6 g, fat 2.1 g (of which 20% saturated, 7% mono-unsaturated, 73% polyunsaturated), carbohydrate 17.3 g

(6.3 g sugars), fibre 11 g, ash 1.6 g, Ca 363 mg, Fe 2.6 mg, Mg 95 mg, P 91 mg, K 272 mg, Na 9 mg, Zn 0.7 mg, Cu 0.4 mg, Mn 2.9 mg, Se 0.9 μg, vitamin A 1376 μg RE (18 579 μg carotenoids), E 2 mg, K 108.6 mg, B_1 0.04 mg, B_2 0.35 mg, niacin 2.4 mg, B_6 0.4 mg, folate 83 μg, pantothenate 0.2 mg, C 11 mg.

vinification The process of fermentation of sugars in grape juice to make WINE.

viosterol Irradiated ergosterol; VITAMIN D_2.

VIP *See* VASOACTIVE INTESTINAL PEPTIDE.

Virginia date *See* PERSIMMON.

Virol^{TM} A vitamin preparation based on malt extract.

virpa *See* SOWANS.

viscera The organs within a body cavity, used especially for the abdominal viscera, LIVER, SPLEEN, GASTROINTESTINAL TRACT, kidneys, etc.

viscoelastic Material such as cheese, dough or gelled food, that has both viscous and elastic properties (*see* VISCOSITY); when a SHEAR STRESS is removed it does not return to its original shape, but is deformed.

viscogen Thickening agent for whipping CREAM. Two parts of lime (calcium oxide) in six parts of water, added to five parts of sugar in ten parts of water; used at the rate of 3–6 g/L of cream.

viscometer Instrument for measuring the VISCOSITY of liquids.

viscosity Of a liquid or gas, its resistance to flow. Decreases with increasing temperature for liquids, but increases for gases. Dynamic viscosity is the ratio of SHEAR STRESS : SHEAR RATE. Kinematic viscosity is dynamic viscosity/DENSITY.

   See also DILATANT; PLASTIC FLUIDS; PSEUDOPLASTIC; REYNOLDS NUMBER; RHEOPECTIC; THIXOTROPIC; VISCOELASTIC.

viscosity, dynamic (or absolute) The ratio of SHEAR STRESS : SHEAR RATE for fluids that exhibit a linear relationship between shear stress and shear rate (Newtonian flow).

vision The process of vision is mediated by photosensitive pigments formed by reaction between retinaldehyde (VITAMIN A aldehyde) and the protein opsin. The pigments are known variously as visual purple (because of its colour), rhodopsin (in the rod cells of the retina) and iodopsin (in the cone cells, with sensitivity to different wavelengths of light in different cells). Exposure to light results in bleaching of the pigment, with loss of the retinaldehyde and a conformational change in the protein, which leads to closure of a sodium channel in the retinal cell, and initiation of a nerve impulse.

visual pigments, visual purple *See* VISION.

vitafoods Foods designed to meet the needs of health-conscious consumers that enhance physical or mental quality of life and may increase health status.

vitamers Chemical compounds structurally related to a VITAMIN, and converted to the same active metabolites in the body. They thus possess the same kind of biological activity, although sometimes with lower potency.

When there are several vitamers, the group of compounds exhibiting the biological activity of the vitamin is given a GENERIC DESCRIPTOR (e.g. VITAMIN A is the generic descriptor for retinol and its derivatives as well as several CAROTENOIDS).

vitamin There are 13 organic compounds (thus excluding trace minerals) essential to human life in very small amounts. Eleven of these must be supplied in the diet (vitamins A, B_1, B_2, B_6, B_{12}, C, E, K, FOLIC ACID, BIOTIN and PANTOTHENIC ACID); two (NIACIN and VITAMIN D) can be made in the body if there is sufficient of the AMINO ACID, TRYPTOPHAN, and sunlight, respectively. The word may be pronounced either *veitamin* or *vittamin*.

Vitamins A, D, E and K are grouped together as fat-soluble vitamins, because they are soluble in lipids, but not in water. Vitamin C and the B vitamins (including pantothenic acid, biotin and folic acid) are grouped together as the water-soluble vitamins since they are all soluble in water, but not lipids.

vitamin A (*see* p. 495) Fat-soluble vitamin, occurring either as the preformed vitamin (retinol) found in animal foods or as a precursor (CAROTENES) found in plant foods. Required for control of growth, cell turnover and fetal development, maintenance of fertility and maintenance of the normal moist condition of epithelial tissues lining the mouth and respiratory and urinary tracts; essential in VISION. The main active metabolites in the body are retinaldehyde, all-*trans*- and 9-*cis*-retinoic acids.

Deficiency leads to slow adaptation to see in dim light (poor DARK ADAPTATION), later to night blindness; then drying of the tear ducts (xerophthalmia) and ulceration of the cornea (keratomalacia) resulting in blindness.

The vitamin A content of foods is expressed as retinol equivalents, i.e. retinol plus carotene; 1 μg retinol = 6 μg β-carotene = 12 μg other active carotenoids = 3.33 INTERNATIONAL UNITS.

See also CONJUNCTIVAL IMPRESSION CYTOLOGY; RELATIVE DOSE RESPONSE TEST; RETINOL BINDING PROTEIN; VISION.

vitamin A toxicity Retinol in excess of requirements is stored in the liver, bound to proteins, and is a cumulative poison. When the storage capacity is exceeded, free retinol causes damage to cell membranes. CAROTENE is not toxic in excess, since there is only a limited capacity to form retinol from carotene.

VITAMIN A

The recommended upper limits of habitual daily intake of retinol are about 12.5 × REFERENCE INTAKE for adults, but only 2.5 × reference intake for infants. Retinol is also TERATOGENIC in excess, and for pregnant women the recommended upper limit of daily intake is 3000–3300 μg.

vitamin A₂ Old name for dehydroretinol, the form found in livers of freshwater fish; has 40% of the biological activity of retinol.

vitamin B complex Old-fashioned term for the various B vitamins: VITAMIN B₁ (thiamin), VITAMIN B₂ (riboflavin), NIACIN, VITAMIN B₆, VITAMIN B₁₂, FOLIC ACID, BIOTIN and PANTOTHENIC ACID. These vitamins occur together in cereal germ, liver and yeast; function as coenzymes; and historically were discovered by separation from what was known originally as 'vitamin B'; hence, they are grouped together as the B complex.

vitamin B₁ Thiamin. Thiamin diphosphate is a coenzyme in metabolism of glucose, and in the citric acid cycle. Thiamin triphosphate has a role in nerve conduction, by activating a chloride channel. Deficiency, especially when associated with a carbohydrate-rich diet, results in the disease BERIBERI, degeneration of the sensory nerves in the hands and feet, spreading through the limbs, with fluid retention and heart failure. Relatively acute deficiency, especially associated with alcohol abuse, results in central nervous system damage, the WERNICKE–KORSAKOFF SYNDROME.

See also THIOCHROME; TRANSKETOLASE.

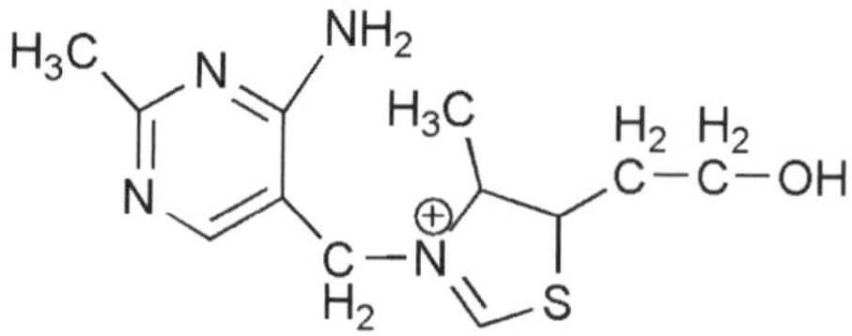

VITAMIN B$_1$

vitamin B$_1$ dependency syndromes A very small number of children have been reported with a variant form of MAPLE SYRUP URINE DISEASE in which the defect is in the binding of thiamin diphosphate to the branched chain keto acid dehydrogenase (EC 1.2.4.4). These children respond well to supplements of large amounts of vitamin B$_1$, without the need for strict control of their intake of the amino acids.

vitamin B$_2$ Riboflavin. Coenzyme in a wide range of oxidation reactions of fats, carbohydrates and amino acids, as riboflavin phosphate (flavin mononucleotide), flavin adenine dinucleotide or covalently bound riboflavin at the active site of the enzyme. Riboflavin-dependent enzymes are collectively known as flavoproteins.

Deficiency impairs energy-yielding metabolism and results in a group of symptoms known as ariboflavinosis, including cracking of the skin at the corners of the mouth (angular stomatitis), fissuring of the lips (cheilosis) and tongue changes (glossitis); seborrhoeic accumulations appear around the nose and eyes. Not fatal because there is very efficient recycling of riboflavin in deficiency.

See also GLUTATHIONE REDUCTASE; LUMICHROME; LUMIFLAVIN.

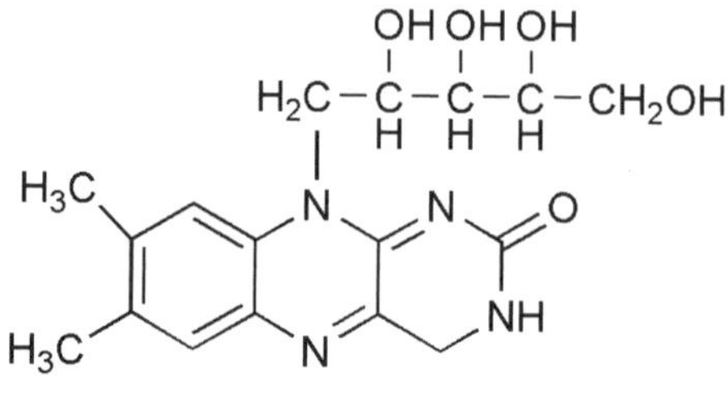

VITAMIN B$_2$

vitamin B₃ Term once used for PANTOTHENIC ACID and sometimes, incorrectly, used for NIACIN.

vitamin B₄ Name given to what was later identified as a mixture of the amino acids ARGININE, GLYCINE and CYSTINE.

vitamin B₅ Name given to a substance later presumed to be identical with vitamin B₆ or possibly nicotinic acid: also sometimes used for PANTOTHENIC ACID.

vitamin B₆ Generic descriptor for three compounds (chemically derivatives of 2-methylpyridine): the hydroxyl (alcohol) compound, pyridoxine (previously known as adermin and pyridoxol); the aldehyde, pyridoxal; and the amine, pyridoxamine; and their phosphates. All are equally active biologically. The active metabolite is pyridoxal 5′-phosphate, which acts as a coenzyme in decarboxylation and transamination of amino acids, and in glycogen phosphorylase (EC 2.4.1.1), it also has a role in terminating the actions of STEROID hormones.

Deficiency causes abnormalities in the metabolism of the amino acids TRYPTOPHAN and METHIONINE; in rats convulsions and skin lesions (acrodynia) and in dairy cows and dogs, anaemia with abnormal red blood cells. Dietary deficiency leading to clinical signs is not known in human beings, apart from a single outbreak in babies fed a severely overheated preparation of formula milk in the 1950s; they showed abnormalities of amino acid metabolism and convulsions resembling epileptic seizures, which responded to supplements of the vitamin.

See also METHIONINE LOAD TEST; TRANSAMINASE; TRYPTOPHAN LOAD TEST.

VITAMIN B₆

vitamin B₆ dependency syndromes A very small number of children suffer from GENETIC DISEASES affecting the binding of pyridoxal phosphate to just one of the pyridoxal phosphate-dependent enzymes. The abnormality is corrected by the administration of large supplements of vitamin B_6.

vitamin B_6 toxicity   High intakes of supplements of vitamin B_6, in excess of 200–1000 mg/day (far in excess of what could be obtained from foods) cause peripheral sensory neuropathy.

vitamin B_7, B_8 and B_9   In the early days of nutrition research, when a new factor was discovered that was claimed to be essential for chick growth and feathering, the claimant stated that since nine factors were known the new factors should be called vitamins B_{10} and B_{11}. In fact, the B vitamins had been numbered only up to B_6, hence B_7, B_8 and B_9 have never existed. B_9 is sometimes (incorrectly) used for FOLIC ACID.

vitamin B_{10} and B_{11}   The names given to two factors claimed to be essential for chick growth and feathering; they were later shown to be a mixture of vitamin B_1 and folic acid.

vitamin B_{12}   (*see* p. 499) Cobalamin; coenzyme for methionine synthetase (EC 2.1.1.13, important in metabolism of FOLIC ACID), methylmalonyl CoA mutase (EC 5.4.99.2) and leucine aminomutase (EC 5.4.3.7).

Deficiency leads to pernicious ANAEMIA when immature red blood cells are released into the bloodstream, and there is degeneration of the spinal cord. The anaemia is the same as seen in folate deficiency, and is due to impairment of folate metabolism. There is also urinary excretion of METHYLMALONIC ACID.

Absorption of vitamin B_{12} requires INTRINSIC FACTOR, a protein secreted in the gastric juice. Failure of absorption, rather than dietary deficiency, is the main cause of pernicious anaemia. However, B_{12} is found only in animal foods so strict VEGETARIANS are at risk.

See also dUMP SUPPRESSION TEST; METHYL FOLATE TRAP; SCHILLING TEST.

vitamin B_{13}   Orotic acid, an intermediate in PYRIMIDINE synthesis; no evidence that it is a dietary essential; not a vitamin.

vitamin B_{14}   Not an established vitamin; name originally given to a compound found in human urine that increases the rate of cell proliferation in bone marrow culture.

vitamin B_{15}   PANGAMIC ACID; no evidence that it has any physiological function in the body; not a vitamin.

vitamin B_{16}   This term has never been used.

vitamin B_{17}   AMYGDALIN (laetrile); no evidence that it has any physiological function in the body; not a vitamin.

vitamin B_C   Obsolete name for FOLIC ACID.

vitamin B_D   Called the antiperosis factor for chicks, but can be replaced by MANGANESE and CHOLINE (not a dietary essential for human beings).

VITAMIN B$_{12}$

vitamin B$_T$ CARNITINE; an essential dietary factor for the meal-worm *Tenebrio molitor*, and certain related species, but not a dietary essential for human beings.

vitamin B$_W$ Or factor W; probably identical to BIOTIN.

vitamin B$_X$ Non-existent; has been used in the past for both PANTOTHENIC ACID and *PARA*-AMINO BENZOIC ACID.

vitamin C ASCORBIC ACID. For formula, *see* p. 39. It functions as a cofactor for a group of hydroxylases that also catalyse the decarboxylation of 2-oxoglutarate (including the hydroxylation of LYSINE and PROLINE in the synthesis of COLLAGEN, and two hydroxylases in the synthesis of CARNITINE); in these reactions it is consumed, but not stoichiometrically with substrates. It is also the coenzyme for dopamine β-hydroxylase (EC 1.14.17.1) in the synthesis of NORADRENALINE, and peptidyl glycine hydroxylase (EC 1.14.17.3) in the post-synthetic modification of a number of peptide hormones. It is a general (non-enzymic) antioxidant, including the reduction of oxidised VITAMIN E in cell membranes.

Deficiency results in SCURVY: seepage of blood from capillaries, subcutaneous bleeding, weakness of muscles, soft, spongy gums and loss of dental cement, leading to loss of teeth and in advanced cases deep bone pain. A lesser degree of deficiency results in impaired healing of wounds.

The requirement to prevent scurvy is less than 10 mg/day; REFERENCE INTAKES range between 30 and 85 mg/day, depending on the criteria of adequacy adopted and the assumptions made in the interpretation of experimental data. At intakes above 100 mg/day the vitamin is excreted in the urine; there is no evidence of any adverse effects at intakes up to 4000 mg/day.

Fruits and vegetables are rich sources; also used in curing ham, and as an antioxidant and bread improver.

See also DICHLOROPHENOL INDOPHENOL; ERYTHORBIC ACID; IRON; *O*-PHENYLENE DIAMINE; OXALIC ACID.

vitamin D   (*see* p. 501) Vitamin D_3 is calciol or cholecalciferol; formed in the skin by the action of ultraviolet light on 7-DEHYDROCHOLESTEROL, hence not strictly a vitamin. However, in northern latitudes sunlight exposure may not be adequate to meet requirements, and a dietary source becomes essential.

Vitamin D_2 (ercalciol or ergocalciferol) is a synthetic VITAMER produced by irradiation of ergosterol. The name vitamin D_1 was given originally to an impure mixture and is not used now.

The main storage form of the vitamin is the 25-hydroxy derivative, calcidiol, in plasma; the active metabolite is the 1,25-dihydroxy derivative, calcitriol. Formation of calcitriol is regulated by the state of CALCIUM balance.

The function of calcitriol is mainly in regulation of calcium metabolism; it acts via nuclear receptors, like a STEROID hormone, and also via cell-surface receptors. Stimulates absorption of dietary calcium from the small intestine and calcium turnover in bone, by activating osteoblasts to mobilise calcium, then later recruiting and stimulating differentiation of osteoblast precursors for bone formation. Acting to regulate intracellular calcium concentrations, it is important in control of the secretion of insulin and other hormones. It also has a role (together with VITAMIN A) in regulation of cell differentiation and replication, and control of the cell cycle.

Deficiency causes RICKETS in young children, OSTEOMALACIA in adults.

Not widely distributed in foods; egg yolk, butter, oily fish and enriched margarine are the only significant sources. Reference

VITAMIN D

intakes are 10–15 µg/day for adults, amounts that are unlikely to be obtained from unsupplemented diets.

The obsolete international unit of vitamin D = 25 ng calciol; 1 mg calciol = 40 IU.

vitamin D resistant rickets *See* RICKETS.

vitamin D toxicity Excessive intake of vitamin D results in disturbance of calcium metabolism, resulting in hypercalcaemia, dangerously raised blood calcium concentrations, leading to raised blood pressure, and calcinosis, inappropriate deposition of calcium in soft tissues, leading to brain and kidney damage. Excessive exposure to sunlight does not lead to excessive formation of vitamin D because previtamin D undergoes further light-catalysed reactions to inactive compounds, and there is only limited availability of 7-DEHYDROCHOLESTEROL in the skin.

vitamin E (*see* p. 502) Two main groups of compounds have vitamin E activity: the tocopherols and the tocotrienols; there are four isomers of each: α-, β-, γ- and δ-tocopherols and α-, β-, γ- and δ-tocotrienols, with differing potencies.

Deficiency symptoms vary considerably in different animal species; sterility in mouse, rat, rabbit, sheep and turkey; muscular dystrophy in several species; capillary permeability in chick and turkey; anaemia in monkey. Human dietary deficiency is unknown, but hereditary lack of β-lipoprotein leads to functional deficiency, with severe neurological damage. Premature infants may show haemolytic ANAEMIA as a result of vitamin E deficiency.

Functions as an ANTIOXIDANT in cell membranes, protecting unsaturated FATTY ACIDS from oxidative damage. It also has membrane-specific functions, and a role in cell signalling and modulation of gene expression.

The vitamin E content of foods is expressed as milligrams α-tocopherol equivalent (based on the different potency of the different vitamers). The obsolete INTERNATIONAL UNIT of vitamin E

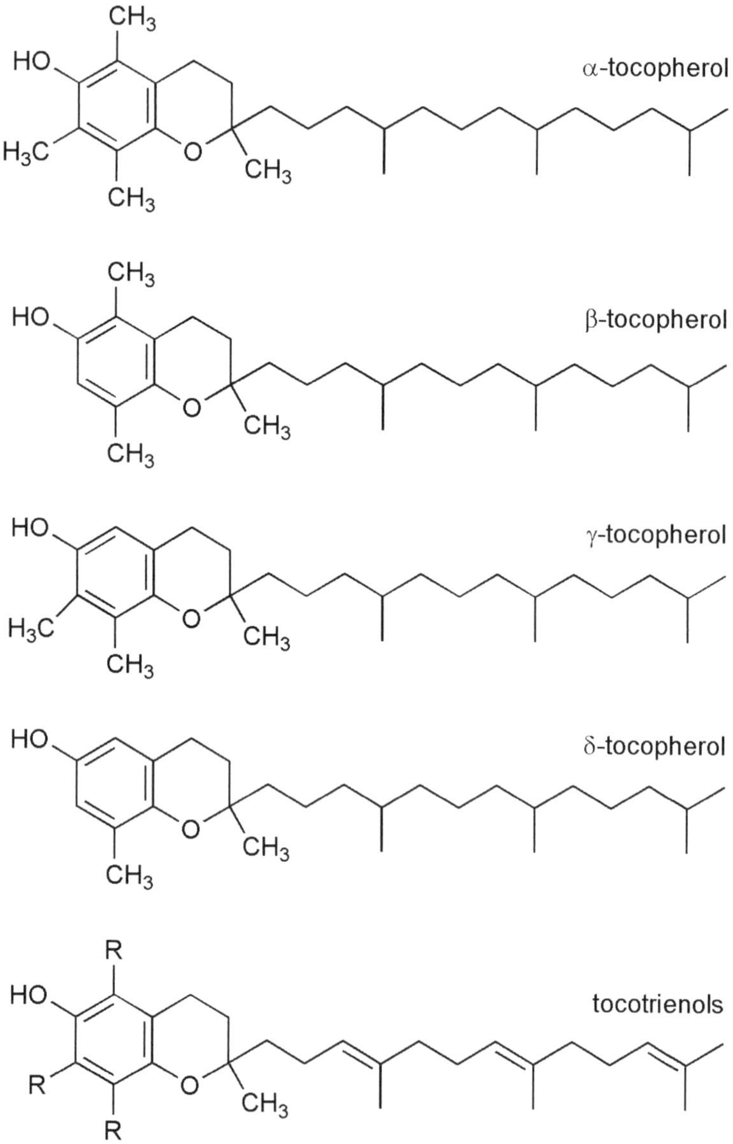

502

α-tocopherol

β-tocopherol

γ-tocopherol

δ-tocopherol

tocotrienols

activity was equal to 1 mg of synthetic α-tocopherol; on this basis natural source α-tocopherol is 1.49 IU/mg.

vitamin F   Sometimes used for the essential FATTY ACIDS.

vitamin G   Obsolete name for VITAMIN B$_2$.

vitamin H *See* BIOTIN.

vitamin K Two groups of compounds have vitamin K activity: phylloquinones (vitamin K_1), found in all green plants, and a variety of menaquinone (vitamin K_2) synthesised by intestinal bacteria. Vitamin K_3 is a synthetic analogue, MENADIONE.

Functions as coenzyme in carboxylation of glutamate to γ-CARBOXYGLUTAMATE in a number of calcium binding proteins, including PROTHROMBIN and other proteins involved in the BLOOD CLOTTING system, the bone protein OSTEOCALCIN, and the product of the growth arrest-specific gene (*Gas-6*), which is important in regulation of growth and development.

Dietary deficiency is unknown, except associated with general malabsorption diseases. However, some newborn infants are at risk of developing haemorrhagic disease as a result of low vitamin K status, and it is general practice to give a single relatively large dose of the vitamin by injection.

See also ANTICOAGULANTS; DICOUMAROL; WARFARIN.

VITAMIN K

vitamin L Factors extracted from yeast and thought at the time to be essential for lactation; they have not become established vitamins.

vitamin M Obsolete name for FOLIC ACID.

vitaminoids Name given to compounds with 'vitamin-like' activity; considered by some to be vitamins or partially to replace vitamins. Include FLAVONOIDS (VITAMIN P), INOSITOL, CARNITINE, CHOLINE, LIPOIC ACID and the essential fatty acids (*see* FATTY ACIDS,

ESSENTIAL). With the exception of the essential fatty acids, there is no evidence that any of them is a dietary essential.

vitamin P   Name given to a group of plant FLAVONOIDS (sometimes called bioflavonoids) that affect the strength of blood capillaries: rutin (in buckwheat), hesperidin, eriodictin and citrin (a mixture of hesperidin and eriodictin in the pith of citrus fruits). Now considered that the effect is pharmacological and that they are not dietary essentials, although they have ANTIOXIDANT activity. Called vitamin P from the German *permeabilitäts vitamin*, because of the effect on capillary permeability and fragility.

vitamin PP   The PELLAGRA-preventing vitamin, an old name for NIACIN before it was identified.

vitamin Q   *See* UBIQUINONE.

vitamin T   Factor found in insect cuticle, mould mycelia and yeast fermentation liquor, claimed to accelerate maturation and promote protein synthesis. Also known as torulitine. Said to be a mixture of folic acid, vitamin B_{12} and deoxyribosides (DNA); hence not a particular vitamin.

vitellin   The major protein of egg yolk; approximately 80% of the total; a phosphoprotein accounting for 30% of the phosphorus of egg yolk.

VLDL   Very low-density lipoprotein, *see* LIPOPROTEINS, PLASMA.

VOC   Volatile organic compounds

vodka   Made from neutral spirit, i.e. alcohol distillate mainly from potatoes, with little or no acid, so that there is no ester formation and hence no flavour. Polish vodka is flavoured with a variety of herbs and fruits.

voidage   The fraction of the total volume occupied by air (the degree of openness) of a bed of material in fluidised-bed drying.

Vol^{TM} Commercial ammonium carbonate, a mixture of ammonium bicarbonate and carbamate. Used as aerating agent in baking, as it breaks down to carbon dioxide, ammonia and steam on heating, without leaving any residue.

volvulus   Twisting of part of the GASTROINTESTINAL TRACT, leading to partial or complete obstruction.

votator   Machine used for the continuous manufacture of margarine; the fat and water are emulsified, and the subsequent conditioning process carried out in the same machine.

VP   Vacuum packaging.

VSP   Vacuum skin packaging.

W

wähe   Swiss; tarts made from yeast-leavened dough filled with fruit, vegetables or cheese.

waist:hip circumference ratio   Simple method for describing the distribution of subcutaneous and intra-abdominal ADIPOSE TISSUE.

wakame   Japanese; lobe leaf seaweed, normally dried.

Composition/100 g: water 80 g, 188 kJ (45 kcal), protein 3 g, fat 0.6 g, carbohydrate 9.1 g (0.6 g sugars), fibre 0.5 g, ash 7.2 g, Ca 150 mg, Fe 2.2 mg, Mg 107 mg, P 80 mg, K 50 mg, Na 872 mg, Zn 0.4 mg, Cu 0.3 mg, Mn 1.4 mg, Se 0.7 µg, vitamin A 18 µg RE (216 µg carotenoids), E 1 mg, K 71.7 mg, B_1 0.06 mg, B_2 0.23 mg, niacin 1.6 mg, folate 196 µg, pantothenate 0.7 mg, C 3 mg.

walnuts   The rough shelled English walnut, black walnut, HICKORY NUT and BUTTERNUT are all botanically walnuts. Common English walnut (so-called because carried round the world for centuries in English ships) is *Juglans regia*.

Black walnuts, composition/100 g: (edible portion 24%) water 4.6 g, 2587 kJ (618 kcal), protein 24.1 g, fat 59 g (of which 6% saturated, 28% mono-unsaturated, 66% polyunsaturated), carbohydrate 9.9 g (1.1 g sugars), fibre 6.8 g, ash 2.5 g, Ca 61 mg, Fe 3.1 mg, Mg 201 mg, P 513 mg, K 523 mg, Na 2 mg, Zn 3.4 mg, Cu 1.4 mg, Mn 3.9 mg, Se 17 µg, vitamin A 2 µg RE (33 µg carotenoids), E 1.8 mg, K 2.7 mg, B_1 0.06 mg, B_2 0.13 mg, niacin 0.5 mg, B_6 0.58 mg, folate 31 µg, pantothenate 1.7 mg, C 2 mg. A 20 g serving (3 nuts) is a source of Mg, P, a good source of Cu, a rich source of Mn.

English walnuts, composition/100 g: (edible portion 45%) water 4.1 g, 2738 kJ (654 kcal), protein 15.2 g, fat 65.2 g (of which 10% saturated, 14% mono-unsaturated, 76% polyunsaturated), carbohydrate 13.7 g (2.6 g sugars), fibre 6.7 g, ash 1.8 g, Ca 98 mg, Fe 2.9 mg, Mg 158 mg, P 346 mg, K 441 mg, Na 2 mg, Zn 3.1 mg, Cu 1.6 mg, Mn 3.4 mg, Se 4.9 µg, vitamin A 1 µg RE (21 µg carotenoids), E 0.7 mg, K 2.7 mg, B_1 0.34 mg, B_2 0.15 mg, niacin 1.1 mg, B_6 0.54 mg, folate 98 µg, pantothenate 0.6 mg, C 1 mg. A 20 g serving (3 nuts) is a good source of Cu, Mn.

Walnut oil is 10% saturated, 24% mono-unsaturated, 66% polyunsaturated, contains 0.4 mg vitamin E, 15 mg vitamin K/100 g.

wappato   *See* ARROWHEAD.

Warfarin   Synthetic compound that acts as a VITAMIN K antagonist, by inhibiting vitamin K epoxide reductase (EC 1.1.4.1). Used clinically to impair blood clotting in patients at risk of THROMBOSIS, and as a rodenticide. Named for the Wisconsin Alumnus Research Fund, which sponsored the research that led to its discovery (1951).

Use of Warfarin in pregnancy can lead to fetal abnormalities (the fetal Warfarin syndrome) as a result of inhibition of the vitamin K-dependent carboxylation of the product of the growth arrest-specific (*Gas-6*) gene, which is important in regulation of growth and development.

wari   Indian, Pakistani; dried balls of legume and cereal flour that has undergone a yeast fermentation; can be stored for some months, then deep fried.

wasabe   Japanese; pungent condiment prepared from dried HORSERADISH and MUSTARD.

wash, spent   *See* SPENT WASH.

wassail   (1) Spiced ale.

(2) Salutation or toast drunk to a person's health.

wastel   Medieval English; fine white bread made from sifted flour.

water activity (a_w)   Ratio between vapour pressure of water in the food and that of pure water at the same temperature. Most bacteria cannot grow at a_w below 0.9, yeasts below 0.85 and moulds below 0.7. So-called dehydrated foods have a_w lower than 0.6.

water balance   The balance between intake and excretion of fluids. Average daily intakes are: as drinks 1–1.5 L; as aqueous part of food, 0.5 L; and formed in the body by oxidation of foodstuffs (METABOLIC WATER), 300–500 mL; total 2–3 L. Losses from the lungs, 400–500 mL; through the skin 400–500 mL; in faeces 80–100 mL; in urine 1–1.8 L.

Total body water is 500 (female)–600 (male) mL/kg body weight. Of this, 57% is intracellular and 43% extracellular; 7% of the total is in blood plasma.

The kidney controls the volume of extracellular water by excreting water. Ingestion of sodium chloride (SALT) raises the OSMOTIC PRESSURE of the extracellular water, causing thirst.

water binding capacity   *See* MEAT, WATER BINDING CAPACITY.

water biscuit   *See* CRACKERS.

water, bound   Water that is physically or chemically bound to the food matrix, so that it has a lower vapour pressure than would be expected.

waterbrash   Sudden filling of the mouth with dilute SALIVA.

water chestnut   Seeds of *Trapa natans* and *T. bicornis*; *see* CHESTNUT.

watercress   Leaves of *Nasturtium officinale* (green watercress, remains green in autumn and is susceptible to frost) and *N. microphyllum × officinale* (brown or winter watercress); eaten raw in salads.

Composition/100 g: (edible portion 92%) water 95 g, 46 kJ (11 kcal), protein 2.3 g, fat 0.1 g, carbohydrate 1.3 g (0.2 g sugars), fibre 0.5 g, ash 1.2 g, Ca 120 mg, Fe 0.2 mg, Mg 21 mg, P 60 mg, K 330 mg, Na 41 mg, Zn 0.1 mg, Cu 0.1 mg, Mn 0.2 mg, Se 0.9 µg, vitamin A 235 µg RE (8587 µg carotenoids), E 1 mg, K 250 mg, B_1 0.09 mg, B_2 0.12 mg, niacin 0.2 mg, B_6 0.13 mg, folate 9 µg, pantothenate 0.3 mg, C 43 mg. A 20 g serving (quarter bunch) is a source of vitamin C.

water, demineralised Water that has been purified by passage through a bed of ION-EXCHANGE RESIN or treatment by reverse osmosis (*see* OSMOSIS, REVERSE), which removes mineral salts. Demineralised or deionised water is at least as pure as distilled water.

See also WATER, REMINERALISED.

water, extracellular, intracellular *See* WATER BALANCE.

water-glass Sodium silicate; used at one time to preserve eggs, by forming a layer of insoluble calcium silicate around the shell, so sealing the pores.

water hardness Soap-precipitating power of water due to the formation of insoluble calcium and magnesium salts of the soap. Temporary hardness (carbonates) is removed by boiling, permanent hardness (sulphates) is not. May be measured in degrees Clarke; one degree = 10 ppm calcium carbonate.

water holding capacity *See* MEAT, WATER HOLDING CAPACITY.

water ice *See* SORBET.

water lemon *See* PASSION FRUIT.

waterless cooking Cooking in a heavy pan with tightly fitting lid, with a steam vent; only a minimal amount of cooking liquid is needed, but the food is not cooked under pressure.

Waterlow classification A system for classifying PROTEIN–ENERGY MALNUTRITION in children based on wasting (the percentage of expected weight for height) and the degree of stunting (the percentage of expected height for age).

See also GOMEZ CLASSIFICATION; WELLCOME CLASSIFICATION.

watermelon Fruit of *Citrullus vulgaris*.

Composition/100 g: (edible portion 52%) water 91 g, 126 kJ (30 kcal), protein 0.6 g, fat 0.2 g, carbohydrate 7.6 g (6.2 g sugars), fibre 0.4 g, ash 0.3 g, Ca 7 mg, Fe 0.2 mg, Mg 10 mg, P 11 mg, K 112 mg, Na 1 mg, Zn 0.1 mg, Se 0.4 µg, vitamin A 28 µg RE (4921 µg carotenoids), E 0.1 mg, K 0.1 mg, B_1 0.03 mg, B_2 0.02 mg, niacin 0.2 mg, B_6 0.05 mg, folate 3 µg, pantothenate 0.2 mg, C 8 mg. A 120 g serving is a source of vitamin C.

water, metabolic Produced in the body by the oxidation of foods. 100 g of fat produces 107.1 g, 100 g of starch produces 55.1 g and 100 g of protein produces 41.3 g of water.

See also WATER BALANCE.

water, mineral Natural, untreated, spring waters, some of which are naturally carbonated, may be slightly alkaline or salty. Numerous health claims have been made for the benefits arising from the traces of a large number of minerals found in solution. They are normally named after the town nearest the source. Examples are Evian, Malvern, Apollinaris, Vichy, Vittel, Perrier. Sparkling mineral water may either contain the gases naturally present at the source or may be artificially carbonated (SODA

WATER, Seltzer water or club soda). Carbonated beverages are sometimes called minerals.

water, remineralised Bottled water that has been demineralised (*see* WATER, DEMINERALISED) by reverse osmosis (*see* OSMOSIS, REVERSE), then had specific minerals added.

waxes ESTERS of FATTY ACIDS with long-chain monohydric alcohols (fats are esters of fatty acids with the trihydric alcohol glycerol). For example, beeswax, myricyl palmitate; spermaceti, cetyl palmitate. Animal waxes are often esters of the steroid alcohol CHOLESTEROL.

waxing Coating fruits and vegetables with a thin layer of edible wax. In the case of apples and oranges this replaces the natural wax that is removed when the crop is washed; in the case of vegetables it is an addition; in both instances the waxing prevents loss of moisture, prolongs storage life and improves the appearance.

waxy flour Flour prepared from varieties of rice and maize that have starch with waxy adhesive properties, and acts as a stabiliser in sauces.

See also CORNFLOUR.

WBC *See* MEAT, WATER BINDING CAPACITY.

WCRF World Cancer Research Fund, an international alliance of organisations dedicated to the prevention and control of cancer through healthy diets and lifestyles. Web site http://www.wcrf.org/.

weaning foods Foods specially formulated for infants aged between 3 and 9 months for the transition between breast or bottle feeding and normal intake of solid foods.

Weende analysis *See* PROXIMATE ANALYSIS.

weenie American name for small sausages, abbreviation of wienerwurst.

weight, desirable (ideal) Standardised tables of desirable (or ideal) weight for height for adults are based on life expectancy; both undernutrition and obesity are associated with increased risk of premature death.

See also BODY MASS INDEX.

weight-for-age An index of the adequacy of the child's nutrition to support growth. Standard weight-for-age is the 50th centile of the weight-for-age curves of well-fed children.

See also ANTHROPOMETRY; NCHS STANDARDS.

weight-for-height For children, can be used as an alternative to WEIGHT-FOR-AGE as an index of nutritional adequacy; for adults it is the only acceptable way of expressing weight relative to ideal or desirable weight.

See also ANTHROPOMETRY; BODY MASS INDEX; NCHS STANDARDS; WEIGHT, DESIRABLE.

weighting oils *See* BROMINATED OILS.

weisse *See* BEER.

Wellcome classification A system for classifying PROTEIN–ENERGY MALNUTRITION in children based on percentage of expected weight for age and the presence or absence of OEDEMA. Between 60 and 80% of expected weight is underweight in the absence of oedema, and is kwashiorkor if oedema is present; under 60% of expected weight is marasmus in the absence of oedema, and is marasmic kwashiorkor if oedema is present.

See also GOMEZ CLASSIFICATION; WATERLOW CLASSIFICATION.

Welsh rarebit (Originally rabbit); melted cheese, mixed with mustard powder, pepper and brown ale, served on toast. Buck rarebit is Welsh rarebit topped with a poached egg.

Wensleydale English hard CHEESE, originally made from sheep or goat milk, now cow milk; may be blue veined.

Wernicke–Korsakoff syndrome The result of brain damage due to VITAMIN B₁ deficiency, commonly associated with alcohol abuse. Affected subjects show clear signs of neurological damage, including NYSTAGMUS with psychiatric changes (KORSAKOFF'S PSYCHOSIS) characterised by loss of recent memory and CONFABULATION, the invention of fabulous stories.

See also ALCOHOLISM; BERIBERI.

Wesson oil Cottonseed oil deodorised by a high temperature vacuum process developed by David Wesson in 1899.

western blot *See* BLOTTING.

wet bulb temperature Temperature measured by a wet thermometer in an air–water vapour mixture, as a means of determining HUMIDITY.

wettability The ability of a powder to absorb water and start the process of reconstituting a dried material.

Wetzel Grid Children are grouped by physique into five groups, ranging from tall and thin to short and thick-set. A healthy child will grow, as measured by height and weight, along one of these channels at a standard rate, if s/he deviates from the channel, malnutrition is suspected.

See also ANTHROPOMETRY; WEIGHT-FOR-AGE; WEIGHT-FOR-HEIGHT.

wey Obsolete measure; 48 bushels of oats or 40 bushels of salt or corn.

WHC *See* MEAT, WATER HOLDING CAPACITY.

wheat The most important of the cereals and one of the most widely grown crops. Many thousand varieties are known but there are three main types: *Triticum vulgare,* used mainly for BREAD; *T. durum* (durum wheat), largely used for PASTA; and *T. compactum* (club wheat), too soft for ordinary bread. The berry is composed of the outer branny husk, 13% of the grain, the germ or embryo (rich in nutrients) 2%, and the central endosperm (mainly starch) 85%.

Composition/100 g (varying between red and white varieties, and spring or winter sown): water 9–13 g, 1370–1430 kJ (330–340 kcal), protein 10–15 g, fat 1.5–2 g (of which 27% saturated, 18% mono-unsaturated, 55% polyunsaturated), carbohydrate 68–75 g (0.4 g sugars), fibre 12–13 g, ash 1.5–1.9 g, Ca 25–32 mg, Fe 3–5 mg, Mg 90–130 mg, P 290–490 mg, K 360–430 mg, Na 2 mg, Zn 2.7–3.5 mg, Cu 0.4 mg, Mn 4 mg, Se 30–70 µg, 225 µg carotenoids), vitamin E 1 mg, K 1.9 mg, B_1 0.4–0.5 mg, B_2 0.1 mg, niacin 4–5 mg, B_6 0.3–0.4 mg, folate 40 µg, pantothenate 1 mg. European wheats are lower in Se than those grown in N America.

Wheat germ oil is 20% saturated, 16% mono-unsaturated, 65% polyunsaturated, vitamin E 149.4 mg, K 24.7 mg/100 g.

See also FLOUR, EXTRACTION RATE; GERM, WHEAT.

wheatfeed   Also called millers' offal and wheat offals; by-product from milling of WHEAT, other than the GERM; bran of various particle sizes and varying amounts of attached endosperm.

wheatmeal, national   *See* FLOUR, WHEATMEAL.

whelks   SHELLFISH; several types of spiral-shelled marine MOLLUSCS, especially *Buccinum undatum, Fusus antiquus*.

Composition/100 g: water 66 g, 573 kJ (137 kcal), protein 23.8 g, fat 0.4 g, cholesterol 65 mg, carbohydrate 7.8 g, ash 2 g, Ca 57 mg, Fe 5 mg, Mg 86 mg, P 141 mg, K 347 mg, Na 206 mg, Zn 1.6 mg, Cu 1 mg, Mn 0.4 mg, Se 44.8 µg, vitamin A 26 µg RE (26 µg retinal), E 0.1 mg, K 0.1 mg, B_1 0.03 mg, B_2 0.11 mg, niacin 1 mg, B_6 0.34 mg, folate 6 µg, B_{12} 9.1 µg, pantothenate 0.2 mg, C 4 mg. An 85 g serving is a source of Mn, P, vitamin B_6, a good source of Mg, a rich source of Cu, Fe, Se, vitamin B_{12}.

whey   The residue from milk after removal of the casein and most of the fat (as in cheese-making); also known as lactoserum. Contains about 1% protein (lactalbumin and lactoglobulin) together with all the lactose, water-soluble vitamins and minerals, and therefore has some food value, although it is 92% water.

Whey cheese (e.g. RICOTTA) is made by heat coagulation of the protein and whey butter from the small amount of fat (0.25%). Dried whey is added to processed cheese; much whey is fed in liquid form to pigs, and it is also used to produce nutritional supplements and beverages..

Whipple's disease   Rare GENETIC DISEASE occurring only in males, in which intestinal absorption is impaired, accompanied by skin pigmentation and arthritis.

whipworm   Whip-like nematode worm (*Trichuris trichiura* or *Trichocephalus dispar*) parasitic in the large intestine.

whiskey, whisky   A grain SPIRIT distilled from BARLEY, RYE, MAIZE or other cereal that has first been malted (*see* MALT) and then fermented. Most brands of whisky are a blend of malt whisky with spirit distilled from grain. The distilled spirit is diluted to about 62% alcohol and matured in wooden casks; Irish and Scotch whisky, made from malted barley, are matured for at least three years. Bourbon, made from malted maize, for at least one year. Sour mash bourbon is made from mash that has yeast left in it from a previous fermentation. Other American and Canadian whiskies are made from rye.

Diluted after maturation and generally around 40% ALCOHOL by volume, 920 kJ (220 kcal)/100 mL.

Both spellings permitted but generally whisky is the Scotch variety and whiskey the Irish and American varieties. Name derived from the Gaelic *uisge beatha*, water of life.

whitebait   A mixture of young HERRINGS and SPRATS (fresh or frozen); they are caught together and are impossible to separate on a commercial scale.

white blood cells   *See* LEUCOCYTES.

whitefish   Oily freshwater FISH, *Coregonus* spp.

white foots   Fine white precipitate of calcium and other salts deposited in jars of meat cured with rock salt.

white pudding   Sausage made from white meat (chicken, rabbit, pork), cereal and spices. The French version, *boudin blanc*, includes eggs and onions. Irish white pudding is made from flake or leaf lard and oatmeal, spiced; served sliced and fried.

white spirits   Distilled SPIRITS from fermented fruit; *eau de vie* or *alcool blanc* in French, *schnapps* in German.

whiting   White FISH, *Merlangius merlangus*.

WHO   World Health Organization, headquarters in Geneva; web site http://www.who.int/en/.

wholefoods   Foods that have been minimally refined or processed, and are eaten in their natural state. In general nothing is removed from, or added to, the foodstuffs in preparation. Wholegrain cereal products are made by milling the complete grain.

wholesome   Description applied to food that is fit for human consumption.

wholewheat meal   Flour or meal prepared by milling the whole wheat grain, i.e. 100% extraction rate. *See* FLOUR, EXTRACTION RATE.

whortleberry   *See* BILBERRY.

Wilson's disease   GENETIC DISEASE due to deficiency of ceruloplasmin, affecting COPPER metabolism, leading to accumulation of copper in liver and brain. Also known as hepatolenticular degeneration.

WIN Weight-control Information Network of the National Institute of Diabetes and Digestive and Kidney Diseases; web site http://www.niddk.nih.gov/health/nutrit/nutrit.htm/.

windberry *See* BILBERRY.

wine Fermented juice from grapes (varieties of *Vitis vinifera*), also made with other fruits and even vegetables with the addition of sugar. Red wines are made by fermenting the juice together with the skins at 21–29 °C; white wines normally from white grapes by fermenting the juice alone at 15–17 °C; rosé by removing the skins after 12–36 h, or by mixing red and white wines.

Beverages made by fermenting other fruit juices and sugar in the presence of vegetables or leaves or roots are also called wines (elderberry, elder flower, parsnip, peapod, rhubarb, etc.), although the legal definition may be restricted to the fermented grape. *See* ALCOHOLIC BEVERAGES.

Wines generally contain 9–14% alcohol, dry wines 290 kJ (70 kcal), sweet wines 500 kJ (120 kcal), and about 1 mg iron/ 100 mL; only traces of vitamins.

wine, apéritif Slightly bitter-tasting fortified wines drunk before meals, VERMOUTH, including (trade names) Amer Picon, Bonal, Byrrh, Campari, Dubonnet, Fernet-Branca, Martini, Saint Raphaël. Made from red or white wine fortified with spirit and flavoured with herbs and quinine. 15–25% alcohol by volume, 5–10% sugars, 75–130 kcal (320–550 kJ) per 100 mL.

wineberry Orange coloured fruit of the Japanese and Chinese wild raspberry, *Rubus phoenicolasius*, and now also hybrids with European cultivated raspberries.

wine, British Made in Great Britain from imported grape juice or concentrated grape juice, as distinct from English wine, which is made from grapes grown in England.

wine classification Many of the major wine-producing countries have legally enforced systems of classification of wines based on grape varieties used and regions of production. Other countries have a system of denomination of origin for wines grown in defined regions which may or may not reflect quality. The national classifications are as follows (in increasing order of quality for each country).

wine classification, Austria As for Germany (*see* WINE CLASSIFICATION, GERMANY), with an additional classification of QmP wines, ausbruch, intermediate in sweetness between beerenauslese and trockenbeerenauslese.

wine classification, Bulgaria Three grades: wines of declared variety of brand; wine of declared geographical origin (DGO); controliran, which are specific varieties grown in specific areas.

The best of DGO and controliran wines can be offered as reserve, and in exceptional years as special reserve.

wine classification, Canada Wines from specified areas (three designated areas in Ontario and four in British Columbia) are labelled VQA (Vintners' Quality Alliance, Canada). Wines must be made from classic grape varieties or preferred hybrids, and the wine must contain at least 85% of the variety named on the label. Wines described as estate-bottled must be made only from grapes owned or controlled by the winery; if a particular vineyard designation is used, the site must be within a recognised viticultural area and all the grapes must come from the designated vineyard. Ice wine (*see* EISWEIN) made from grapes that have frozen on the vine, very sweet.

wine classification, France Vin de table (or vin ordinaire); vin de pays (subdivided into vin de pays de zone for wines from a single area; départementaux for wines from one département; régionaux for wines from more than one département); vin délimité de qualité supérieure (VDQS); appellation contrôlée (AC) or appellation d'origine contrôlée (AOC) for wines from a specified area, from specified grape varieties grown under controlled conditions.

wine classification, Germany Tafelwein (Deutscher Tafelwein is of German origin; wine labelled simply as Tafelwein may be of mixed origin); Landwein (dry or half-dry wines from one of 15 designated areas); Qualitätswein bestimmer Anbaugebeite, QbA (from 11 designated areas and approved grape varieties, sugar may be added to increase sweetness, each bottle carries a batch number (*Amtliche Prüfungsnummer*, AP), as proof that it complies with QbA status); Qualitätswein mit Prädikat, QmP (with six quality gradings based on the level of natural sugar at harvest and extra sugar may not be added: kabinett, light, fruity and delicate, usually dry; spätlese, late picked grapes, dry to sweet; auslese, selected late picked grapes, rich and sweet; beerenauslese, late picked grapes affected by 'NOBLE ROT' (*Botrytis cinerea*), always sweet; trockenbeerenauslese, late picked grapes that have dried to raisins on the vine, strong and sweet; EISWEIN, rare, made from grapes that have frozen on the vine, very sweet.

wine classification, Italy Vini de tavola (Vdt); vini di tavola con indicazione geografica (from a particular area); vini tipici (equivalent to French vin de pays); denominazione di origine controllata (DOC, from specified areas and grape varieties); denominazione di origine controllata e garantita (DOCG, as DOC but with more stringent regulations and control).

wine classification, Luxembourg Appellation contrôlée wines must carry a vintage; bottles carry a neck label awarded by the state controlled Marque Nationale after tasting, according to the strength of the wine; in order of increasing alcohol content the grades are: non admis, marque nationale, vin classé, premier cru, grand premier cru.

wine classification, Portugal Indicação de proveniencia regulamentada (IPR); região demarcada (RD, the same as appellation contrôlée). Table wines are vinho de mesa, wines aged more than 1 year are vinho maduro.

wine classification, South Africa Classification by variety of grape and area of production; coloured seals used as: blue band indicates that origin is certified; red band guarantees vintage year; green band certifies grape varieties; 'estate' certifies that it is from one estate; 'superior' on gold seal indicates superior quality. Wines also carry identification numbers to testify that controls have been adhered to during production.

wine classification, Spain Vinos de la tierra (two-thirds of the grapes must come from the region named on the label); denominacion de origen (DO).

wine classification, USA Each state has its own appellation of origin; in addition *American wine* or *vin de table* is blended wine from one or more areas; multistate appellation is wine from two or three neighbouring states (the percentage from each must be shown on the label); for State and County appellation at least 75% must come from the designated area. *Approved viticultural areas* must have defined boundaries, specific characteristics and a proven reputation for quality; 85% of the grapes used must come from the defined area; when an individual vineyard is named, 95% of the grapes must have been grown there. A vintage year may be declared if at least 95% of the wine has been fermented in the calendar year claimed. For tax purposes a table wine must be between 10 and 14% alcohol, stronger wines are classified as dessert wines, even if dry; dessert wines between 17 and 21% alcohol are classified by alcoholic strength, not sweetness. US Wines may be sold by a generic classification (e.g. Chablis or Loire); such names are prohibited from export to the EU.

wine, fortified Made by adding BRANDY or SPIRITS to increase the ALCOHOL content of the wine to 15–18% and so prevent further fermentation (to acids) in warm climates, e.g. MADEIRA, marsala, PORT, SHERRY.

wine, sparkling Wine containing bubbles of carbon dioxide, bottled under pressure. Three methods of production:

(1) The méthode champenoise in which the wine undergoes a second fermentation in the bottle. Wine produced outside

the Champagne region of France may not be called champagne, even if made by this method.

(2) The tank or bulk method, in which the wine is bottled while still fermenting slightly.

(3) The addition of carbon dioxide gas while bottling.

Lightly sparkling wines are known as pétillante or frizzante; they are often young wines, bottled while still fermenting.

wine, sweetness The UK Wine Promotion Board classifies white and rosé wines from 1 for very dry wines (0.6% sugars) to 9 (very sweet, 6% sugars).

For red wines the classification is from A (light and dry) to E (full-bodied heavy wines).

German and Austrian labelling is: trocken (dry), halbtrocken (half dry), halbsüss or lieben (medium sweet) and süss (very sweet).

winkle (periwinkle) Small, snail-like, marine MOLLUSCS, *Littorina littorea.*

winter berry Fruit of the American evergreen shrub *Gaultheria procumbens*, red, with a spicy flavour; used mainly for pies and sauces.

winterization Process involving slow cooling of oils and removal of the precipitated fats with a relatively high melting point, so that the final product remains clear when refrigerated.

wisdom teeth Third molar tooth on each side of both jaws; usually erupt in late adolescence.

witches' milk Secretion of the mammary gland of the newborn of both sexes, because of the presence of the hormone prolactin which travels from the blood of the mother into the fetus. Also known as sorcerers' milk.

witchetty grubs Australian edible grubs, species of longicorn beetle (*Xylentes* spp.).

witloof *See* CHICORY.

WOF Warmed over flavour.

wok Chinese vessel for STIR FRYING; a shallow bowl-shaped pan in which food can be fried rapidly in a small amount of oil over a high heat.

wood alcohol *See* METHANOL.

wood sugar *See* XYLOSE.

wool green S A green COLOUR, Green S (E-142).

worcester berry American species of GOOSEBERRY, *Ribes divaricatum.*

Worcestershire sauce Thin spicy sauce; recipes are usually 'secret' but basically soya, tamarinds, anchovies, garlic and spices, plus sugar, salt and vinegar, traditionally matured in oak casks.

work *See* ENERGY.

wormseed *See* EPAZOTE.

wort Aqueous extract of MALT in brewing. *See* BEER.

WPC WHEY protein concentrate.

wraplings *See* WUNTUN.

WTO World Trade Organization, web site http://www.wto.org/.

wuntun (wonton) Chinese; small dough parcels containing meat, boiled or deep fried. Also known as chiao-tzu or wraplings.

X

Xangold^{TM} Natural source esters of the carotenoids XANTHOPHYLL and LUTEIN.

xanthaemia *See* CAROTINAEMIA.

xanthan gum Complex polymer made by bacterial fermentation; stable to wide range of pH and temperatures; used as thickening agent to form gels, increase viscosity in foods.

xanthelasma Yellow fatty plaques on the eyelids, due to HYPERCHOLESTEROLAEMIA.

xanthine A PURINE, intermediate in the metabolism of adenine and guanine to URIC ACID. CAFFEINE (in coffee and tea) is 1,3,7-trimethylxanthine; THEOPHYLLINE (in tea) is 1,3-dimethylxanthine; THEOBROMINE (in cocoa) is 3,7-dimethylxanthine.

xanthoma Yellow skin lesion associated with disorders of lipid metabolism, and especially HYPERCHOLESTEROLAEMIA.

xanthophylls Hydroxylated CAROTENOIDS. Occur in all green leaves together with CHLOROPHYLL and CAROTENE, also present in egg yolk, CAPE GOOSEBERRY, etc. Most have no VITAMIN A activity. Include flavoxanthin (E-161a), lutein (161b), cryptoxanthin (E-161c, is vitamin A precursor), rubixanthin (161e), rhodoxanthin (161f), canthaxanthin (161g).

xanthoproteic reaction Test for proteins (actually for the aromatic rings of PHENYLALANINE, TYROSINE and TRYPTOPHAN). Yellow colour on boiling with nitric acid, turns orange on adding ammonia.

xanthosis Yellowing of the skin associated with high blood concentrations of CAROTENE.

Xenical^{TM} *See* ORLISTAT.

xenobiotic Substances foreign to the body, including drugs and some food additives.

xerophilic *See* OSMOPHILES.

xerophthalmia Advanced VITAMIN A deficiency in which the epithelium of the cornea and conjunctiva of the eye deteriorates because of impairment of the tear glands, resulting in dryness then ulceration, leading to blindness.

xerosis Abnormal dryness of conjunctiva, skin or mucous membranes.

xerostomia Dry mouth, a common side effect of a variety of drugs.

See also PTYALISM.

X-ray diffraction Technique for determination of crystal structures (e.g. of proteins) by analysis of the diffraction pattern of a beam of X-rays shone through the crystal.

xylanase Mixture of enzymes of fungal or bacterial origin that hydrolyse XYLANS: β-1,4-endoxylanase (EC 3.2.1.8) and β-D-xylosidase (EC 3.2.1.32). Sometimes added to poultry and pig feed to increase the digestibility of cereal NON-STARCH POLYSACCHARIDES.

xylans Polysaccharides of XYLOSE, not digested, part of NON-STARCH POLYSACCHARIDE; a major component of HEMICELLULOSE.

xylitol A five-carbon SUGAR ALCOHOL found in raspberries, endive, lettuce; 80–100% of the sweetness of sucrose; used in sugar-free hard sweets and gelatine gums. Apart from being of low cariogenicity, xylitol is said to have an effect in suppressing the growth of some of the bacteria associated with dental CARIES (*see* TOOTH-FRIENDLY SWEETS).

xyloascorbic acid Term used for ASCORBIC ACID (VITAMIN C) to distinguish from isoascorbic acid (*see* ERYTHORBIC ACID), which is araboascorbic acid and has only slight vitamin C activity.

xyloglucan One of the hemicelluloses in plant cell walls, linking CELLULOSE fibres. A component of NON-STARCH POLYSACCHARIDE.

xylose Pentose (five-carbon) sugar found in plant tissues mainly as polysaccharides (XYLANS); 40% as sweet as sucrose. Also known as wood sugar. Mainly excreted unmetabolised, and used to test carbohydrate absorption.

xylulose Pentose (five-carbon) sugar occurring as a metabolic intermediate in the PENTOSE PHOSPHATE PATHWAY.

Y

YAC Yeast artificial chromosome, a specialised cloning vector that can carry large DNA inserts.

Yakult™ YOGURT containing live *Lactobacillus* spp. which are PROBIOTICS. Originally Japanese name for yoghurt fermented with *L. casei*.

yam Tubers of perennial climbing plants of a number of species of *Dioscorea*, *D. rotundala* white yam, and *D. cayenensis*, yellow or Guinea yam, water, trifoliate or Chinese yam. A major food in parts of Africa and also the Far East. In USA sweet potatoes (*see* POTATO, SWEET) are sometimes called yam.

518

Composition/100 g: (edible portion 86%) water 70 g, 494 kJ (118 kcal), protein 1.5 g, fat 0.2 g, carbohydrate 27.9 g (0.5 g sugars), fibre 4.1 g, ash 0.8 g, Ca 17 mg, Fe 0.5 mg, Mg 21 mg, P 55 mg, K 816 mg, Na 9 mg, Zn 0.2 mg, Cu 0.2 mg, Mn 0.4 mg, Se 0.7 μg, vitamin A 7 μg RE (83 μg carotenoids), E 0.4 mg, K 2.6 mg, B_1 0.11 mg, B_2 0.03 mg, niacin 0.6 mg, B_6 0.29 mg, folate 23 μg, pantothenate 0.3 mg, C 17 mg. A 130 g serving is a source of vitamin B_6, folate, a good source of Cu, Mn, a rich source of vitamin C.

yang *See* MACROBIOTIC DIET.

Yarmouth bloater *See* RED HERRINGS.

yautia *See* TANNIA.

yeast Unicellular organisms, sometimes grouped with the fungi; eukaryotic organisms with more complex subcellular organisation than BACTERIA. Some types are of major importance in the food industry. *Saccharomyces cerevisiae* and *S. carlsbergensis* are used in brewing, wine-making and baking.

Yeasts such as *Candida utilis* (formerly *Torula utilis*) are grown on carbohydrate or hydrocarbon media as animal feed and potential human food, since they contain about 50% protein (dry weight) and are very rich in B vitamins.

Some yeasts are pathogenic (especially *Candida* spp., which cause thrush); many are used in biotechnology for production of hormones (*see* HORMONES, HUMAN) and other proteins.

yeast extract A preparation of the water-soluble fraction of autolysed brewers' YEAST, valuable both as a source of B vitamins and for its strong savoury flavour; used as a drink or a breadspread.

Composition/100 g: water 37 g, 661 kJ (158 kcal), protein 27.8 g, fat 0 g, carbohydrate 11.8 g, fibre 3 g, ash 23.4 g, Ca 86 mg, Fe 3.7 mg, Mg 180 mg, P 104 mg, K 2600 mg, Na 3600 mg, Zn 2.1 mg, Cu 0.3 mg, Se 18 μg, vitamin B_1 9.7 mg, B_2 14.3 mg, niacin 97 mg, B_6 1.3 mg, folate 1010 μg, B_{12} 0.5 μg. A 6 g serving is rich source of vitamin B_1, B_2, niacin, folate.

yeast fermentation, bottom Or deep fermentation; fermentation during the manufacture of BEER with a yeast that sinks to the bottom of the tank. Most beers are produced this way; ale, porter and stout being the principal beers produced by top fermentation.

Yeastrel^{TM}, **Yeatex**^{TM} *See* YEAST EXTRACT.

yeheb A nut, fruit of *Cordeauxia edulis*, originally from the Horn of Africa.

yellow fats *See* SPREAD, FAT.

yerba dulce The leaves of the Paraguayan shrub, *Stevia rebaudiana*, the source of STEVIOSIDE and REBAUDIOSIDE.

yerba maté *See* MATÉ.

Yersinia enterocolitica Food poisoning organism that invades intestinal epithelial cells. Infective dose 10^6–10^7 organisms; onset 3–5 days; duration weeks; TX 4.1.3.1.

Yestamin™ A variety of preparations of dried debittered brewers' YEAST (*Saccharomyces* spp.) used to enrich foods.

yield Weight of food after processing as a percentage of unprocessed material.

yin *See* MACROBIOTIC DIET.

ylang-ylang oil Aromatic oil from flowers of Philippine tree *Cananga odorata* used as a flavouring in soft drinks, confectionery and baked goods.

YN A synthetic PHOSPHOLIPID (ammonium phosphatide) developed by Cadbury to replace LECITHIN as an emulsifying agent in CHOCOLATE manufacture.

yogurt Milk (from a variety of animals but usually cows) coagulated and fermented with two types of bacteria, *Streptococcus thermophilus* and *Lactobacillus bulgaricus*. The two organisms are symbiotic; each produces compounds that promote the growth of the other. Both act to precipitate and gel proteins; main flavour development is from the slower formation of D-lactic acid by *L. bulgaricus*, although *S. thermophilus* has a greater capacity to metabolise LACTOSE to L-lactate. Stirred yogurt is prepared in bulk; set yogurt is fermented in the plastic containers in which it will be sold. Strained (Greek style) yogurt is prepared by removing some of the whey by straining through a cloth or by centrifugation. Drinking yogurt is a low-viscosity drink made by blending yogurt with fruit juice and sugar.

May be pasteurised, when most of the bacteria are destroyed, otherwise termed live yogurt. Bioyogurts also contain *Lactobacillus acidophilus* (*see* MILK, ACIDOPHILUS) and *Bifidobacterium bifidum*, which are claimed to enhance the growth of beneficial bacteria in the intestine.

See also MILK, FERMENTED.

yolk index Index of freshness of an egg; ratio between height and diameter of yolk under defined conditions. As the egg deteriorates, the yolk index decreases.

youngberry Cross between BLACKBERRY and DEWBERRY.

yukwa Korean; snack food made by deep frying dried dough prepared by steeping waxy rice for 1–2 weeks.

yusho disease Caused by leakage of polychlorinated biphenyls which contaminated edible oil on the Japanese island of Kyushu in 1968.

Z

zabaglione (zabaione) Italian; frothy dessert made from egg yolks, sugar and wine (usually marsala) whisked over gentle heat until thick. French sabayon is similar.

ZAG Zinc α2 glycoprotein, secreted by various tumours; activates lipolysis and contributes to loss of ADIPOSE TISSUE in CACHEXIA.

zampone Italian; pork SAUSAGE in which meat is stuffed into a boned pig's trotter instead of casing.

zearalenone Trichothecene MYCOTOXIN produced when cereals are infected with *Fusarium* spp.

zeaxanthin One of the CAROTENOID pigments in maize, egg yolk and *Physalis* (CAPE GOOSEBERRY); has no vitamin A activity; used as a colouring.

See also LUTEIN.

zébrine Variety of AUBERGINE with purple and white stripes.

zedoary root Root of the Indian plant *Curcuma zedoaria*, a member of the ginger family. Used in the manufacture of flavours and BITTERS.

zeer Sudanese; earthenware vessel used for preparation of KAWAL.

zein A PROLAMIN, the major protein of MAIZE (*Zea mays*), very poor in lysine and tryptophan.

Z-enzyme Enzyme (β-1,3-glucosidase, EC 3.2.1.58) found associated with AMYLASES, that hydrolyses the few β-1,3-links present in AMYLOSE. Pure, crystalline β-amylase will convert only 70% of amylose to maltose; it requires the presence of the Z-enzyme for complete conversion.

Zeocarb™ An ION-EXCHANGE RESIN.

zest Outer skin of citrus fruits. *See* FLAVEDO.

zinc An essential mineral which forms the PROSTHETIC GROUP of a large number of enzymes, and the nuclear receptor proteins for STEROID and THYROID HORMONES and VITAMINS A and D. Deficiency results in hypogonadism and delayed puberty, small stature and mild anaemia; it occurs mainly in subtropical regions where a great deal of zinc is lost in sweat, and the diet is largely based on unleavened wholemeal bread, in which much of the zinc is unavailable because of the high content of PHYTIC ACID. Intestinal absorption of zinc requires an (as yet unidentified) organic zinc binding ligand secreted in pancreatic juice. Deficiency may also lead to functional vitamin A deficiency because of impaired synthesis of RETINOL BINDING PROTEIN.

zitoni *See* PASTA.

zizanie *See* RICE, WILD.

zNose™ A surface acoustic wave-based sensor that permits extremely rapid gas chromatography with very high sensitivity – an 'electronic nose'.

See also ENOSE.

Zollinger–Ellison syndrome Excessive secretion of gastric acid due to high levels of circulating GASTRIN secreted by a pancreatic tumour.

zomotherapy Treatment of convalescents with raw meat or meat juice, long since discontinued.

zoopherin Obsolete name for VITAMIN B₁₂.

zooplankton *See* PLANKTON.

zucchini Italian variety of MARROW developed to be harvested when small. American and Australian name for COURGETTE.

Zucker rat A genetically obese strain of rat used in research.

z value *See* DECIMAL REDUCTION TIME.

zwieback German; twice-baked bread or rusk.

zwitterions An ionised molecule with both positive and negative charges, e.g. the AMINO ACIDS.

Zygosaccharomyces Yeasts that grow in high concentrations of sugar (osmophilic) that cause spoilage of honey, jams, and syrups.

zymase Obsolete name for the mixture of enzymes in YEAST which is responsible for FERMENTATION.

zymogens The inactive form in which some enzymes, especially the protein digestive enzymes, are secreted, being activated after secretion. Also called proenzymes, or enzyme precursors.

zymotachygraph An instrument that measures the gas produced in a fermenting dough and the amount escaping from the dough, as an index of bread-making properties.

Appendix

Table 1 Units of physical quantities and multiples and submultiples of units

Physical quantity	Unit	Symbol	Definition
Amount of substance	mole	mol	SI base unit
Electric charge	coulomb	C	$s\,A$
Electric conductance	siemens	S	$A\,V^{-1}$
Electric current	ampere	A	SI base unit
Electric potential difference	volt	V	$J\,A^{-1}s^{-1}$
Electric resistance	ohm	Ω	$V\,A^{-1}$
Electrical capacitance	farad	F	$A\,s\,V^{-1}$
Energy	joule	J	$m^2\,kg\,s^{-2}$
	calorie	cal	$4.186\,J$
Force	newton	N	$J\,m^{-1}$
Frequency	hertz	Hz	s^{-1}
Illuminance	lux	lx	$cd\,sr\,m^{-2}$
Length	metre	m	SI base unit
	ångstrom	Å	$10^{-10}\,m$
Luminous flux	lumen	lm	$cd\,sr$
Luminous intensity	candela	cd	SI base unit
Magnetic flux	weber	Wb	$V\,s$
Magnetic flux density	tesla	T	$V\,s\,m^{-2}$
Mass	kilogram	kg	SI base unit
Plane angle	radian	rad	SI base unit
Power	watt	W	$J\,s^{-1}$
Pressure	pascal	Pa	$N\,m^{-2}$
	bar	bar	$10^5\,Pa$
Radiation dose absorbed	gray	Gy	$J\,kg^{-1}$
Radioactivity	becquerel	Bq	s^{-1}
Solid angle	steradian	sr	SI base unit
Temperature	degree Celsius	°C	thermodynamic temperature $-273.15\,K$
Temperature (thermodynamic)	kelvin	K	SI base unit
Time	second	s	SI base unit
Volume	litre (cubic decimeter)	L or (dm^3)	$10^{-3}\,m^3$

multiple	prefix	symbol	submultiple	prefix	symbol
10^1	deca	da	10^{-1}	deci	d
10^2	hecta	h	10^{-2}	centi	c
10^3	kilo	k	10^{-3}	milli	m
10^6	mega	M	10^{-6}	micro	μ
10^9	giga	G	10^{-9}	nano	n
10^{12}	tera	T	10^{-12}	pico	p
10^{15}	peta	P	10^{-15}	femto	f
10^{18}	exa	E	10^{-18}	atto	a
10^{21}	zetta	Z	10^{-21}	zepto	z

Table 2 Labelling reference values for foods

	USA: reference daily intake	European Union: proposed by Scientific Committee for Food, 1993	European Union: required by EU Directive
Vitamin A, µg	1500	500	800
Vitamin D, µg	10	5	5
Vitamin E, mg	30	–	10
Vitamin C, mg	60	30	60
Thiamin, mg	1.5	0.8	1.4
Riboflavin, mg	1.7	1.3	1.6
Niacin, mg	20	15	18
Vitamin B$_6$, mg	2.0	1.3	2.0
Folate, µg	400	140	200
Vitamin B$_{12}$, µg	6.0	1.0	1.0
Biotin, µg	300	–	150
Pantothenic acid, mg	10	–	6
Calcium, mg	1000	550	800
Copper, mg	2.0	0.8	–
Iodine, µg	150	100	150
Iron, mg[a]	18	7, 14	14
Magnesium, mg	400	–	300
Phosphorus, mg	1000	–	800
Selenium, µg	–	40	–
Zinc, mg	15	7.5	15

[a] The Scientific Committee for Food proposed separate figures for iron for women (14 mg) and men (7 mg).

Table 3 US/Canadian recommended dietary allowances and acceptable intakes, 1997–2001

Age	Vit A µg	Vit D µg	Vit E mg	Vit K µg	Vit B₁ mg	Vit B₂ mg	niacin mg	Vit B₆ mg	folate µg	Vit B₁₂ µg	Vit C mg	Ca mg	P mg	Mg mg	Fe mg	Zn mg	Cu µg	Se µg	I µg	Cr µg	Mn mg	Mo µg
0–6 months	400	5	4	2.0	0.2	0.3	2	0.1	65	0.4	40	210	100	30	–	2	200	15	110	0.2	–	2
7–12 months	500	5	5	2.5	0.3	0.4	4	0.3	80	0.5	50	270	275	75	11	3	220	20	130	5.5	0.6	3
1–3 years	300	5	6	30	0.5	0.5	6	0.5	150	0.9	15	500	460	80	7	3	340	20	90	11	1.2	17
4–8 years	400	5	7	55	0.5	0.6	8	0.6	200	1.2	25	800	500	130	10	5	440	30	90	15	1.5	22
Males																						
9–13 years	600	5	11	60	0.9	0.9	12	1.0	300	1.8	45	1300	1250	240	8	8	700	40	120	25	1.9	34
14–18 years	900	5	15	75	1.2	1.3	16	1.3	400	2.4	75	1300	1250	410	11	11	890	55	150	35	2.2	43
19–30 years	900	5	15	120	1.2	1.3	16	1.3	400	2.4	90	1000	700	400	8	11	900	55	150	35	2.3	45
31–50 years	900	5	15	120	1.2	1.3	16	1.3	400	2.4	90	1000	700	420	8	11	900	55	150	35	2.3	45
51–70 years	900	10	15	120	1.2	1.3	16	1.7	400	2.4	90	1200	700	420	8	11	900	55	150	30	2.3	45
>70 years	900	15	15	120	1.2	1.3	16	1.7	400	2.4	90	1200	700	420	8	11	900	55	150	30	2.3	45
Females																						
9–13 years	600	5	11	60	0.9	0.9	12	1.0	300	1.8	45	1300	1250	240	8	8	700	40	120	21	1.6	34
14–18 years	700	5	15	75	1.0	1.0	14	1.2	400	2.4	65	1300	1250	360	15	9	890	55	150	24	1.6	43
19–30 years	700	5	15	90	1.1	1.1	14	1.3	400	2.4	75	1000	700	310	18	8	900	55	150	25	1.8	45
31–50 years	700	5	15	90	1.1	1.1	14	1.3	400	2.4	75	1000	700	320	18	8	900	55	150	25	1.8	45
51–70 years	700	10	15	90	1.1	1.1	14	1.5	400	2.4	75	1200	700	320	8	8	900	55	150	20	1.8	45
>70 years	700	15	15	90	1.1	1.1	14	1.5	400	2.4	75	1200	700	320	8	8	900	55	150	20	1.8	45
Pregnant	770	5	15	90	1.4	1.4	18	1.9	600	2.6	85	1000	700	350	27	11	1000	60	220	30	2.0	50
Lactating	900	5	16	90	1.4	1.6	17	2.0	500	2.8	120	1000	700	310	9	12	1300	70	290	45	2.6	50

Figures for infants under 12 months are Adequate Intakes (AI), based on the observed mean intake of infants fed principally on breast milk; for nutrients other than vitamin K figures are RDA, based on estimated average requirement + 2 SD; figures for vitamin K are AI, based on observed average intakes. Figures for calcium, chromium, manganese are AI.

Table 4 EU population reference intakes of nutrients, 1993

Age	Protein g	vit A µg	vit B₁ mg	vit B₂ mg	niacin mg	vit B₆ mg	folate µg	vit B₁₂ µg	vit C mg	Ca mg	P mg	Fe mg	Zn mg	Cu mg	Se µg	I µg
6–12 months	15	350	0.3	0.4	5	0.4	50	0.5	20	400	300	6	4	0.3	8	50
1–3 years	15	400	0.5	0.8	9	0.7	100	0.7	25	400	300	4	4	0.4	10	70
4–6 years	20	400	0.7	1.0	11	0.9	130	0.9	25	450	350	4	6	0.6	15	90
7–10 years	29	500	0.8	1.2	13	1.1	150	1.0	30	550	450	6	7	0.7	25	100
Males																
11–14 years	44	600	1.0	1.4	15	1.3	180	1.3	35	1000	775	10	9	0.8	35	120
15–17 years	55	700	1.2	1.6	18	1.5	200	1.4	40	1000	775	13	9	1.0	45	130
18+ years	56	700	1.1	1.6	18	1.5	200	1.4	45	700	550	9	9.5	1.1	55	130
Females																
11–14 years	42	600	0.9	1.2	14	1.1	180	1.3	35	800	625	18	9	0.8	35	120
15–17 years	46	600	0.9	1.3	14	1.1	200	1.4	40	800	625	17	7	1.0	45	130
18+ years	47	600	0.9	1.3	14	1.1	200	1.4	45	700	550	16*	7	1.1	55	130
Pregnant	57	700	1.0	1.6	14	1.3	400	1.6	55	700	550	*	7	1.1	55	130
Lactating	63	950	1.1	1.7	16	1.4	350	1.9	70	1200	950	16	12	1.4	70	160

*8 mg iron post-menopausally; supplements required in latter half of pregnancy.

Table 5 UK reference nutrient intakes, 1991

Age	vit B₁ mg	vit B₂ mg	niacin mg	Vit B₆ mg	Vit B₁₂ μg	folate μg	vit C mg	vit A μg	vit D μg	Ca mg	P mg	Mg mg	Na mg	Fe mg	Zn mg	Cu mg	Se μg	I μg
0–3 months	0.2	0.4	3	0.2	0.3	50	25	350	8.5	525	400	55	210	1.7	4.0	0.2	10	50
4–6 months	0.2	0.4	3	0.2	0.3	50	25	350	8.5	525	400	60	280	4.3	4.0	0.3	13	60
7–9 months	0.2	0.4	4	0.3	0.4	50	25	350	7	525	400	75	320	7.8	5.0	0.3	10	60
10–12 months	0.3	0.4	5	0.4	0.4	50	25	350	7	525	400	80	350	7.8	5.0	0.3	10	60
1–3 years	0.5	0.6	8	0.7	0.5	70	30	400	7	350	270	85	500	6.9	5.0	0.4	15	70
4–6 years	0.7	0.8	11	0.9	0.8	100	30	500		450	350	120	700	6.1	6.5	0.6	20	100
7–10 years	0.7	1.0	12	1.0	1.0	150	30	500		550	450	200	1200	8.7	7.0	0.7	30	110
Males																		
11–14 years	0.9	1.2	15	1.2	1.2	200	35	600		1000	775	280	1600	11.3	9.0	0.8	45	130
15–18 years	1.1	1.3	18	1.5	1.5	200	40	700		1000	775	300	1600	11.3	9.5	1.0	70	140
19–50 years	1.0	1.3	17	1.4	1.5	200	40	700		700	550	300	1600	8.7	9.5	1.2	75	140
50+ years	0.9	1.3	16	1.4	1.5	200	40	700	10	700	550	300	1600	8.7	9.5	1.2	75	140
Females																		
11–14 years	0.7	1.1	12	1.0	1.2	200	35	600		800	625	280	1600	14.8	9.0	0.8	45	130
15–18 years	0.8	1.1	14	1.2	1.5	200	40	600		800	6254	300	1600	14.8	7.0	1.0	60	140
19–50 years	0.8	1.1	13	1.2	1.5	200	40	600		700	550	270	1600	14.8	7.0	1.2	60	140
50+ years	0.8	1.1	12	1.2	1.5	200	40	600	10	700	550	270	1600	8.7	7.0	1.2	60	140
Pregnant	+0.1	+0.3				+100	+10	+100	10									
Lactating	+0.1	+0.5	+2		+0.5	+60	+30	+350	10	+550	+440	+50			+6.0	+0.3	+15	

529

Table 6 Recommended nutrient intakes for vitamins, FAO 2001

Age	Vit A µg	Vit D µg	Vit K µg	Vit B_1 mg	Vit B_2 mg	niacin mg	Vit B_6 mg	folate µg	Vit B_{12} µg	Vit C mg	panto mg	biotin µg
0–6 months	375	5	5	0.2	0.3	2	0.1	80	0.4	25	1.7	5
7–12 months	400	5	10	0.3	0.4	4	0.3	80	0.5	30	1.8	6
1–3 years	400	5	15	0.5	0.5	6	0.5	160	0.9	30	2.0	8
4–6 years	450	5	20	0.6	0.6	8	0.6	200	1.2	30	3.0	12
7–9 years	500	5	25	0.9	0.9	12	1.0	300	1.8	35	4.0	20
Males												
10–18 years	600	5	35–55	1.2	1.3	16	1.3	400	2.4	40	5.0	30
19–50 years	600	5	65	1.2	1.3	16	1.3	400	2.4	45	5.0	30
50–65 years	600	10	65	1.2	1.3	16	1.7	400	2.4	45	5.0	30
>65 years	600	15	65	1.2	1.3	16	1.7	400	2.4	45	5.0	30
Female												
10–18 years	600	5	35–55	1.1	1.0	16	1.2	400	2.4	40	5.0	25
19–50 years	600	5	55	1.1	1.1	14	1.3	400	2.4	45	5.0	30
50–65 years	600	10	55	1.1	1.1	14	1.5	400	2.4	45	5.0	30
>65 years	600	15	55	1.1	1.1	14	1.5	400	2.4	45	5.0	30
Pregnant	800	5	55	1.4	1.4	18	1.9	600	2.6	55	6.0	30
Lactating	850	5	55	1.5	1.6	17	2.0	500	2.8	70	7.0	35

Table 7 Food additives permitted in the EU

Colours

Yellow and orange colours
E100	Curcumin
E101	(i) Riboflavin, (ii) Riboflavin-5′-phosphate (vitamin B_2)
E102	Tartrazine (= FD&C Yellow no. 5)
E104	Quinoline yellow
E110	Sunset Yellow FCF; Orange Yellow S (= FD&C Yellow no. 6)

Red colours
E120	Cochineal; Carminic acid; Carmines
E122	Azorubine; Carmoisine
E123	Amaranth
E124	Ponceau 4R; Cochineal Red A
E127	Erythrosine (= FD&C Red no. 3)
E128	Red 2G
E129	Allura Red AC (= FD&C Red no. 40)

Blue colours
E131	Patent Blue V
E132	Indigotine; Indigo Carmine (= FD&C Blue no. 2)
E133	Brilliant Blue FCF (= FD&C Blue no. 1)

Green colours
E140	Chlorophylls and chlorophyllins (the natural green colour of leaves)
E141	Copper complexes of chlorophyll and chlorophyllins
E142	Green S

Brown and black colours
E150a	Plain caramel
E150b	Caustic sulphite caramel
E150c	Ammonia caramel
E150d	Sulphite ammonia caramel
E151	Brilliant Black BN; Black PN
E153	Vegetable carbon
E154	Brown FK
E155	Brown HT

Derivatives of carotene
E160a	Carotenes
E160b	Annatto; Bixin; Norbixin
E160c	Paprika extract; Capsanthian; Capsorubin
E160d	Lycopene
E160e	Beta-apo-8′-carotenal (C30)
E160f	Ethyl ester of beta-apo-8′-carotenoic acid (C30)

Other plant colours
E161b	Lutein
E161g	Canthaxanthin
E162	Beetroot Red; Betanin
E163	Anthocyanins

Other compounds used as colours
E170	Calcium carbonate
E171	Titanium dioxide
E172	Iron oxides and hydroxides
E173	Aluminium

532

Table 7 (*continued*)

E174	Silver
E175	Gold
E180	Litholrubine BK

Preservatives

Sorbic acid and its salts

E200	Sorbic acid
E202	Potassium sorbate
E203	Calcium sorbate

Benzoic acid and its salts

E210	Benzoic acid
E211	Sodium benzoate
E212	Potassium benzoate
E213	Calcium benzoate
E214	Ethyl *p*-hydroxybenzoate
E215	Sodium ethyl *p*-hydroxybenzoate
E216	Propyl *p*-hydroxybenzoate
E217	Sodium propyl *p*-hydroxybenzoate
E218	Methyl *p*-hydroxybenzoate
E219	Sodium methyl *p*-hydroxybenzoate

Sulphur dioxide and its salts

E220	Sulphur dioxide
E221	Sodium sulphite
E222	Sodium hydrogen sulphite
E223	Sodium metabisulphite
E224	Potassium metabisulphite
E226	Calcium sulphite
E227	Calcium hydrogen sulphite
E228	Potassium hydrogen sulphite

Biphenyl and its derivatives

E230	Biphenyl; diphenyl (for surface treatment of citrus fruits)
E231	Orthophenyl phenol (for surface treatment of citrus fruits)
E232	Sodium orthophenyl phenol (sodium biphenyl-2-yl oxide)

Other preservatives

E234	Nisin
E235	Natamycin (NATA, for surface treatment of cheeses and dried cured sausages)
E239	Hexamethylene tetramine (hexamine)
E242	Dimethyl dicarbonate
E1105	Lysozyme (an antibacterial enzyme found in tears)

Pickling salts

E249	Potassium nitrite
E250	Sodium nitrite
E251	Sodium nitrate
E252	Potassium nitrate (saltpetre)

Acids and their salts

E280	Propionic acid
E281	Sodium propionate
E282	Calcium propionate

533

Table 7 (*continued*)

E283	Potassium propionate
E284	Boric acid
E285	Sodium tetraborate; borax

Antioxidants
Vitamin C
E300	Ascorbic acid
E301	Sodium ascorbate
E302	Calcium ascorbate
E304	Fatty acid esters of ascorbic acid (a lipid-soluble derivative of the vitamin)

Vitamin E
E306	Tocopherols (natural source, mixed isomers)
E307	Alpha-tocopherol
E308	Gamma-tocopherol
E309	Delta-tocopherol

Other antioxidants
E310	Propyl gallate
E311	Octyl gallate
E312	Dodecyl gallate
E315	Erythorbic acid (the D-isomer of vitamin C, little vitamin activity)
E316	Sodium erythorbate
E320	Butylated hydroxyanisole (BHA)
E321	Butylated hydroxytoluene (BHT)

Sweeteners
Sugar alcohols used as bulk sweeteners
E420	(i) Sorbitol, (ii) Sorbitol syrup
E421	Mannitol
E953	Isomalt
E965	(i) Maltitol, (ii) Maltitol syrup
E966	Lactitol
E967	Xylitol

Intense (synthetic) sweeteners
E950	Acesulfame K
E951	Aspartame
E952	Cyclamic acid and its Na and Ca salts
E954	Saccharin and its Na, K and Ca salts
E957	Thaumatin
E959	Neohesperidine DC

Emulsifiers, stabilisers, thickeners and gelling agents
E322	Lecithins (found especially in egg yolk and soya bean)

Alginates
E400	Alginic acid
E401	Sodium alginate
E402	Potassium alginate
E403	Ammonium alginate
E404	Calcium alginate
E405	Propane-1,2-diol alginate

Table 7 (*continued*)

Plant gums (soluble fibre)
E406	Agar
E407	Carrageenan
E407a	Processed eucheuma seaweed
E410	Locust bean gum; carob gum
E412	Guar gum
E413	Tragacanth
E414	Acacia gum; gum arabic
E415	Xanthan gum
E416	Karaya gum
E417	Tara gum
E418	Gellan gum
E425	Konjac

Polysorbates
E432	Polyoxyethylene sorbitan monolaurate; Polysorbate 20
E433	Polyoxyethylene sorbitan mono-oleate; Polysorbate 80
E434	Polyoxyethylene sorbitan monopalmitate; Polysorbate 40
E435	Polyoxyethylene sorbitan monostearate; Polysorbate 60
E436	Polyoxyethylene sorbitan tristearate; Polysorbate 65

Cellulose derivatives
E460	Cellulose
E461	Methyl cellulose
E463	Hydroxypropyl cellulose
E464	Hydroxypropyl methyl cellulose
E465	Ethyl methyl cellulose
E466	Carboxy methyl cellulose, Sodium carboxy methyl cellulose
E468	Cross-linked sodium carboxy methyl cellulose
E469	Enzymatically hydrolysed carboxy methyl cellulose

Fatty acid derivatives and modified fats
E470a	Sodium, potassium and calcium salts of fatty acids
E470b	Magnesium salts of fatty acids
E471	Mono- and diglycerides of fatty acids
E472a	Acetic acid esters of mono- and diglycerides of fatty acids
E472b	Lactic acid esters of mono- and diglycerides of fatty acids
E472c	Citric acid esters of mono- and diglycerides of fatty acids
E472d	Tartaric acid esters of mono- and diglycerides of fatty acids
E472e	Mono- and diacetyltartaric acid esters of mono- and diglycerides of fatty acids
E472f	Mixed acetic and tartaric acid esters of mono- and diglycerides of fatty acids
E473	Sucrose esters of fatty acids
E474	Sucroglycerides
E475	Polyglycerol esters of fatty acids
E476	Polyglycerol polyricinoleate
E477	Propane-1,2-diol esters of fatty acids
E479b	Thermally oxidised soya bean oil interacted with mono and diglycerides of fatty acids
E481	Sodium stearoyl-2-lactylate
E482	Calcium stearoyl-2-lactylate
E483	Stearyl tartrate

Table 7 (*continued*)

E491	Sorbitan monostearate
E492	Sorbitan tristearate
E493	Sorbitan monolaurate
E494	Sorbitan monooleate
E495	Sorbitan monopalmitate

Other compounds

E440	Pectins (found naturally in fruit, especially apples)
E442	Ammonium phosphatides
E444	Sucrose acetate isobutyrate
E445	Glycerol esters of wood rosins
E1103	Invertase

Other additives
Acid, acidity regulators, anti-caking agents, anti-foaming agents, bulking agents, carriers and carrier solvents, emulsifying salts, firming agents, flavour enhancers, flour treatment agents, foaming agents, glazing agents, humectants, modified starches, packaging gases, propellants, raising agents and sequestrants

Acidity regulators
Carbon dioxide and carbonates

E170	Calcium carbonates
E290	Carbon dioxide
E500	Sodium carbonates
E501	Potassium carbonates
E503	Ammonium carbonates
E504	Magnesium carbonates

Acetic acid and its salts

E260	Acetic acid (vinegar is dilute acetic acid)
E261	Potassium acetate
E262	Sodium acetate
E263	Calcium acetate

Lactic acid and its salts

E270	Lactic acid (the acid of sour milk)
E325	Sodium lactate
E326	Potassium lactate
E327	Calcium lactate

Citric acid and its salts

E330	Citric acid
E331	Sodium citrates
E332	Potassium citrates
E333	Calcium citrates
E380	Triammonium citrate

Tartaric acid and its salts

E334	Tartaric acid (L-(+))
E335	Sodium tartrates
E336	Potassium tartrates (cream of tartar)
E337	Sodium potassium tartrate
E353	Metatartaric acid
E354	Calcium tartrate

536

Table 7 (*continued*)

Phosphoric acid and its salts
E338   Phosphoric acid
E339   Sodium phosphates
E340   Potassium phosphates
E341   Calcium phosphates
E343   Magnesium phosphates
E450   Diphosphates
E451   Triphosphates
E452   Polyphosphates
E541   Sodium aluminium phosphate

Malic acid and its salts
E296   Malic acid
E350   Sodium malates
E351   Potassium malate
E352   Calcium malates

Adipic acid and its salts
E355   Adipic acid
E356   Sodium adipate
E357   Potassium adipate

Hydrochloric acid and its salts
E507   Hydrochloric acid
E508   Potassium chloride
E509   Calcium chloride
E511   Magnesium chloride
E512   Stannous chloride

Sulphuric acid and its salts
E513   Sulphuric acid
E514   Sodium sulphates
E515   Potassium sulphates
E516   Calcium sulphate
E517   Ammonium sulphate
E520   Aluminium sulphate
E521   Aluminium sodium sulphate
E522   Aluminium potassium sulphate
E523   Aluminium ammonium sulphate

Other acids and their salts
E297   Fumaric acid
E363   Succinic acid
E385   Calcium disodium ethylene diamine tetra-acetate; calcium disodium
            EDTA

Alkalis
E524   Sodium hydroxide
E525   Potassium hydroxide
E526   Calcium hydroxide
E527   Ammonium hydroxide
E528   Magnesium hydroxide
E529   Calcium oxide
E530   Magnesium oxide

Table 7 (*continued*)

Other salts
E535   Sodium ferrocyanide
E536   Potassium ferrocyanide
E538   Calcium ferrocyanide

Compounds used as anticaking agents and other uses
E422   Glycerol (used as a humectant, also for its sweetness)
E431   Polyoxyethylene (40) stearate
E459   Beta-cyclodextrin

Silicon salts
E551   Silicon dioxide
E 552   Calcium silicate
E553a   (i) Magnesium silicate, (ii) Magnesium trisilicate
E553b   Talc
E554   Sodium aluminium silicate
E555   Potassium aluminium silicate
E556   Aluminium calcium silicate

Other compounds
E558   Bentonite
E559   Aluminium silicate; kaolin
E570   Fatty acids
E574   Gluconic acid
E575   Glucono delta-lactone
E576   Sodium gluconate
E577   Potassium gluconate
E578   Calcium gluconate
E579   Ferrous gluconate
E585   Ferrous lactate

Compounds used as flavour enhancers
Amino acids
E620   Glutamic acid
E621   Monosodium glutamate
E622   Monopotassium glutamate
E623   Calcium diglutamate
E624   Monoammonium glutamate
E625   Magnesium diglutamate
E640   Glycine and its sodium salt

Nucleotides
E626   Guanylic acid
E627   Disodium guanylate
E628   Dipotassium guanylate
E629   Calcium guanylate
E630   Inosinic acid
E631   Disodium inosinate
E632   Dipotassium inosinate
E633   Calcium inosinate
E634   Calcium 5'-ribonucleotides
E635   Disodium 5'-ribonucleotides

538

Table 7 (*continued*)

Other compounds
E650   Zinc acetate

Compounds used as glazing agents
E900   Dimethylpolysiloxane
E901   Beeswax, white and yellow
E902   Candelilla wax
E903   Carnauba wax
E904   Shellac
E905   Microcrystalline wax
E912   Montan acid esters (for surface treatment of citrus fruits)
E914   Oxidised polyethylene wax

Compounds used to treat flour
E920   L-Cysteine (an amino acid)
E927b   Carbamide

Propellant gases
E938   Argon
E939   Helium
E941   Nitrogen
E942   Nitrous oxide
E943a   Butane
E943b   Iso-butane
E944   Propane
E948   Oxygen
E949   Hydrogen

Modified starches (used as thickening and gelling agents)
E1404   Oxidised starch
E1410   Monostarch phosphate
E1412   Distarch phosphate
E1413   Phosphated distarch phosphate
E1414   Acetylated distarch phosphate
E1420   Acetylated starch
E1422   Acetylated distarch adipate
E1440   Hydroxyl propyl starch
E1442   Hydroxy propyl distarch phosphate
E1450   Starch sodium octanoyl succinate
E1451   Acetylated oxidised starch

Miscellaneous compounds
E999   Quillaia extract
E1200   Polydextrose
E1201   Polyvinylpyrrolidone
E1202   Polyvinylpolypyrrolidone
E1505   Triethyl citrate
E1518   Glyceryl triacetate; triacetin
E1520   Propan-1,2-diol; propylene glycol

Table 8 Fatty acid nomenclature

Trivial name	Systematic name	Shorthand code
Acetic	ethanoic	C2:0
Propionic	propanoic	C3:0
Butyric	butanoic	C4:0
Caproic	hexanoic	C6:0
Caprylic	octanoic	C8:0
Capric	decanoic	C10:0
Lauric	dodecanoic	C12:0
Myristic	tetradecanoic	C14:0
Palmitic	hexadecanoic	C16:0
Stearic	octadecanoic	C18:0
Arachidic	eicosanoic	C20:0
Behenic	docosanoic	C22:0
Lignoceric	tetracosanoic	C24:0
Palmitoleic	9-hexadecenoic	C16:1 ω7
Oleic	9-octadecenoic	C18:1 ω9
Elaidic	*trans*-9-octadecenoic	*trans*-C18:1 ω9
Vaccenic	11-octadecenoic	C18:1 ω7
Petroselinic	6-octadecenoic	C18:1 ω6
Gadoleic	9-eicosaenoic	C20:1 ω9
Erucic	13-docosenoic	C22:1 ω9
Brassidic	*trans*-13-docosenoic	*trans*-C22:1 ω9
Cetoleic	11-docosenoic	C22:1 ω11
Nervonic	15-tetracosenoic	C24:1 ω9
α-Linolenic	9,12,15-octadecatrienoic	C18:3 ω3
Parinaric	9,11,13,15-octadecatetraenoic	C18:4 ω3
Eicosapentaenoic (timnodonic)	5,8,11,14,17-eicosapentaenoic	C20:5 ω3
Docosapentaenoic (clupanodonic)	7,10,13,16,19-docosapentaenoic	C22:5 ω3
Docosahexaenoic (cervonic)	4,7,10,13,16,19-docosahexaenoic	C22:6 ω3
Linoleic	9,12-octadecadienoic	C18:2 ω6
γ-Linolenic	6,9,12-octadecatrienoic	C18:3 ω6
α-Eleostearic	9,11 *trans*, 13, *trans*-octadecatrienoic	*trans*-C18:3 ω6
Dihomo-γ-linolenic	8,11,14-eicosatrienoic	C20:3 ω6
Arachidonic	5,8,11,14-eicosatetraenoic	C20:4 ω6
Docosatetraenoic (adrenic)	7,10,13,16-docosatetraenoic	C22:4 ω6
Docosapentaenoic	4,7,10,13,16-docosapentaenoic	C22:5 ω6
Mead	5,8,11-eicosatrienoic	C20:3 ω9

24 Hour
Check-out